PRAISE FOR
EXPECTING 411

"*Expecting 411* was my go to book when I found out I was knocked up. It's funny, easy to read, and alleviated all my baby anxiety. It's a must have on your nightstand if you have a little one on the way."

—Kristen Bell

"This book was by my bedside the whole time I was pregnant . . . it's as if your very best girlfriend was a brilliant OB and wrote a book for you."

—Kerry Washington

"*Expecting 411* answered all of my questions in the most comforting and personal way, even though it was co-written by one of the most brilliant, and not to mention, glamorous OB-GYNs, Dr. Michele Milovina. No woman should go through pregnancy without reading it—even my husband loved it!"

—Rachel Zoe

"Dr. Brown's knowledgeable and straightforward counsel makes her an invaluable resource for all things parenting. *Expecting 411* is a must-read for the mom-to-be looking for clear, concise answers to her many questions and wanting honest advice on the healthiest, safest ways to approach pregnancy."

—Lacey Major, editor-in-chief, *Pregnancy & Newborn*

"Unlike other pregnancy books, *Expecting 411* gives moms-to-be the latest medical advice with a lighthearted girlfriend-to-girlfriend tone and accessible format. Dr. Milovina and Dr. Brown—young moms themselves who offer both an obstetrician's and a pediatrician's perspective—answer all the questions that couples might be too embarrassed to ask, and empowers them with comprehensive information in a non-alarmist way."

—Diane Debrovner, former deputy editor-in-chief, *Parents* magazine

"This is an impressive wealth of knowledge in a very readable, up-to-date style. This book answers all your questions clearly and precisely. It probably answers questions you haven't even thought about yet! I see myself using this as a reference in my role as an advice nurse."

—Nancy Edelman, RN, OB phone triage nurse

"Finally, a book for pregnant women and their families that's accurate and informative without being stuffy or alarmist: hard to believe it's written by doctors, but it is—and they've done a great job. It's on target and will even make you laugh out loud at times (appropriately, though . . .)!"

—Lawrence Platt, MD, FACOG, professor of maternal and fetal medicine, UCLA, obstetrician/gynecologist

"*Expecting 411* is today's guide to pregnancy and childbirth for all women! This book provides all women the great opportunity I have—to constantly ask one of LA's hottest OB-GYNs a 'million' questions (including some we may not feel comfortable to ask). I am one of Michele Milovina's patients and think she is both brilliant and practical. She is one of us, including her love for shoes (which I bought her when she delivered one of my girls). If I had this book when I was pregnant, it would have cut down on a lot of phone time!"

—Jodi Weingarten, mother of three

"*Expecting 411* is straightforward, funny, and informative. It's the perfect pregnancy guide for women in the twenty-first century."

—Rebecca Waldman, attorney, mother of three

EXPECTING 411

Also by Ari Brown, MD

Baby 411

Toddler 411

— 5th Edition —

EXPECTING 411

The Insider's Guide to Pregnancy and Childbirth

Michele Milovina, MD
Ari Brown, MD

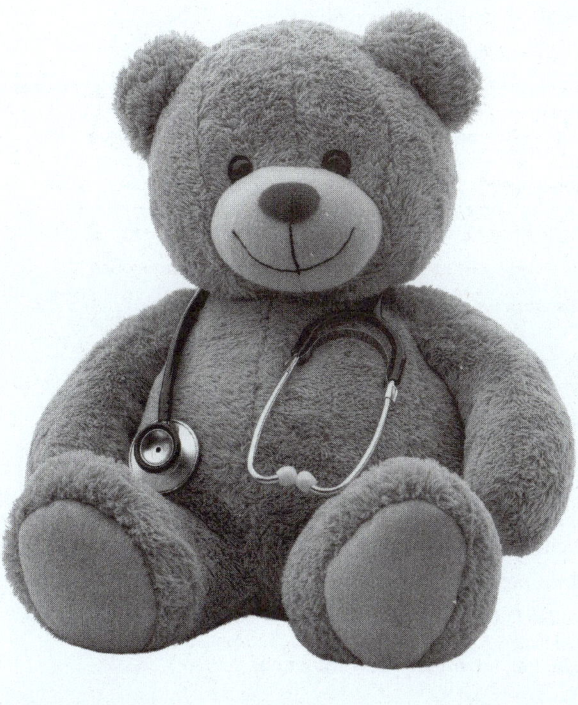

RODALE
NEW YORK

Rodale Books
An imprint of Random House
A division of Penguin Random House LLC
1745 Broadway, New York, NY 10019
rodalebooks.com | randomhousebooks.com

A Rodale Trade Paperback Original

Earlier editions of this work were published in the United States by Windsor Peak Press, Boulder, CO from 2010 through 2017.

ISBN 9780593980927
Ebook ISBN 9780593980934

Printed in the United States of America

1st Printing

Book Team: Production editor: Cassie Gitkin • Managing editor: Allison Fox • Production manager: Kevin Garcia • Copy editor: Rebecca Maines • Proofreaders: Caryl Schwartz, Kyndle Fuller, Ella Maoz, Rachel Twersky, Pam Feinstein • Indexer: Gina Guilinger

Book design by Ralph Fowler

The authorized representative in the EU for product safety and compliance is Penguin Random House Ireland, Morrison Chambers, 32 Nassau Street, Dublin D02 YH68, Ireland. https://eu-contact.penguin.ie

To all moms, moms-to-be, and dads, this is no easy feat.
We are honored to help and be a part of your village.

CONTENTS

PART TWO

Life Goes On

PART THREE

Getting Ready for the Big Event

PART FOUR

The Big Event

PART FIVE

Special Concerns and Problems

INTRODUCTION

Why Read This Book?

Congratulations! You have a precious little being growing within you for whom you are now responsible. And they haven't even peed on you yet . . . or asked for the car keys.

Everyone tells you that becoming a parent will change your life—and they're right. But what you may not realize is that the change happens *now*. We're not talking about nine months down the road—we're talking about this very moment. Your health during pregnancy affects your baby. So your first job as a parent is to take good care of yourself.

If you are the person carrying the bundle of joy, welcome to *Invasion of the Body Snatchers*. You will look in the mirror sometimes and wonder who is staring back at you.

If you are the partner supporting that pregnant person, you too may wonder who is staring back at you (and occasionally yelling and crying . . . while simultaneously demanding a foot massage).

After forty weeks of aches, pains, and emotional outbursts, you will be rewarded with the most amazing experience of your life. And if that wasn't enough, you'll next embark on life's most challenging, frustrating, uplifting, delightful journey—parenthood!

As the mothers of four children (young when we first wrote this book and all in their late teens and twenties now), we know what you are going through. If you are anything like us, you quickly realize pregnancy is equal parts exciting . . . and terrifying.

Most of all, we realize you have questions. Lots of questions. And that's why we are here.

You need solid advice on what's best for you and your baby. And you want the *latest* information and research about pregnancy, not outdated advice from ten years ago or, worse, from your own parents' generation!

Of course, there's no shortage of advice for pregnancy—you hear it from your friends, co-workers, or strangers at the grocery store. Then there's the web . . . and the zillions of other pregnancy books out there.

So why write another book on pregnancy? What can we possibly say here that hasn't already been said in those other thick pregnancy tomes? And can't you just get advice online for free?

Funny you should ask! Let's discuss.

Does the World Need Another Pregnancy Book?

Yes, it does.

Sure, there are dozens of other pregnancy books out there. You could scroll through the pregnancy section at your favorite online bookseller and go into labor before you're done.

But take a closer look at the other pregnancy books. As experts on pregnancy and babies, we found many pregnancy books to be . . . well, *lacking*.

Some are out of date, leaving you to base important decisions on ancient medical history (that is, anything more than a few years old).

Other books are written by well-meaning authors who don't deliver babies for a living. It is one thing to *research* pregnancy, labor, and delivery and another to actually dedicate your career to caring for pregnant women and their babies! Trust us, there's a big difference.

And then there is the original sin of too many pregnancy books: the freak-out factor. Their aim to catalog every possible terrible thing that can go wrong with pregnancy ends up scaring the heck out of every reader. But what's often missing is *perspective*: How common are these complications? Is a risk real . . . or merely hypothetical?

That's why we decided to write *Expecting 411*. Our goal: give you the most up-to-date advice on pregnancy and childbirth—while taming the freak-out factor. Best of all, this advice is from two women who spend their days and nights caring for pregnant women and their babies.

Meet the Authors

Healthy pregnancies produce healthy babies. So it's key to get the facts straight. You need a reliable source you can trust.

Who better to write a book about giving birth than an obstetrician and a pediatrician? While that sounds obvious, *Expecting 411* is the first pregnancy book to be authored by both a baby doc and a doc who delivers babies. The combined expertise gives you a 360-degree view of this crazy process we call having a baby.

Let's take a second to introduce you to Dr. Michele Milovina, OB-GYN, and Dr. Ari Brown, pediatrician.

Meet Dr. M, OB-GYN and mom: I'm an obstetrician-gynecologist who has been practicing in Beverly Hills, California, for more than twenty years. I received my training at UCLA Cedars-Sinai Medical Center in Los Angeles. In addition to authoring several articles on pregnancy, I also appeared in *Little Man*, an award-winning documentary on preterm labor and premature birth and was honored by the March of Dimes in 2015 as a Prematurity Champion.

I decided to become an obstetrician because I love the bond that develops between a woman and her OB-GYN as they work together to navigate the ups and downs of puberty, pregnancy, and childbirth, even menopause (but who wants to think about that right now!). And it's an absolute honor to be present to help women through pregnancy, labor, and delivery.

After having two kids of my own, I bring a real-world perspective to pregnancy and delivery that they don't teach you in medical school. Morning sickness, heartburn, varicose veins, labor pains—yes, I've been there, done that!

And I am passionate about educating pregnant couples. It has been a labor of love to share my knowledge and expertise with you.

Meet Dr. B, pediatrician and mom: I am a pediatrician in practice for thirty years after training at Harvard Medical School and Boston Children's Hospital. I practice in Austin, Texas, and started writing books in 2003.

Besides authoring the bestsellers *Baby 411* and *Toddler 411*, I am also a spokesperson for the American Academy of Pediatrics. I have two grown children, but believe me, I remember my pregnancies just like they were yesterday!

I love my job because I get to participate in a family's birth experience and help babies grow up healthy and thrive.

Why do we have *both* an OB and pediatrician authoring this book? We share the same patient: your baby. Dr. M (the OB) handles moms-to-be and the baby-in-the-womb, and Dr. B (the pediatrician) handles care once the baby is born. Both of us combine our expertise on the best things you can do during pregnancy to ensure a healthy baby. And we can prepare you for newborn issues and decisions that arise before or shortly after delivery. Having two expert perspectives makes this book unique.

We've also recruited additional experts for special must-read sections. For breastfeeding, we turn to a certified lactation consultant. For home births, a certified nurse midwife will walk you through this experience.

Seven Reasons to Buy This Book

Now that you've met the authors, let's talk about what makes this book different.

1. **Easy-to-find answers.** You've got questions—and you want to find the answers quickly. We've organized the basics of your pregnancy into three chapters, each covering a trimester. But many questions don't fit so easily into a week-by-week or month-by-month format.

   That's why the rest of the book is organized by topics so you can actually find the information you need. If you are wondering if a symptom is normal, check out Chapter 5, "Is This Normal?" Curious about a test your doctor has ordered? Yep, that's in a chapter cleverly titled "Tests" (Chapter 6). And you'll easily be able to find info on exercise in Chapter 9, "Lifestyles."

2. **Better than scrolling on the internet.** Yes, there's a lot of free pregnancy advice online. But that free advice is often worth the price you've paid.

   Why? It is exceedingly difficult to find a trusted messenger that offers detailed, science-based guidance. This book gives you the depth and facts you need to make wise decisions.

   Many pregnancy websites are supported by advertising. And many influencers create content based on their corporate sponsorships. We don't, so we promise to tell you like it is.

3. **Frequent updates.** Medicine moves at light speed these days—upending what was common practice just a few years ago.

We update *Expecting 411* periodically. When you buy the most recent edition of the book, you can be assured you are not reading advice that is dated.

We also have a website (Expecting411.com) with updates *between* editions. And follow us on our socials for the latest breaking news.

4. **Paranoia, tamed.** Nothing is more terrifying than reading about the myriad of things that can go wrong with pregnancy. Even if these complications are rare, you can lose endless hours of sleep worrying about your baby (as if you didn't have enough issues with getting some shut-eye).

   To solve this problem, we put all the scary stuff into one section at the end of this book. That way, you don't have to read about these problems unless it is absolutely necessary.

   And to help lower the fear level, we also mark other potentially unsettling content with a special warning icon. (You'll learn more about the icon system in the next section.) Feel free to skip this material, which is included for readers who want the whole story.

   When it comes to risks to your pregnancy, we separate the hypothetical from reality. We'll tell you if science backs up a warning or not.

5. **Questions you are too embarrassed to ask.** Let's be honest—when you are face-to-face with your OB, it can be embarrassing to discuss what's really on your mind.

   As two mamas who've been there, we know you wonder about items that seem silly to discuss with your doc. Like . . . can you wax down there? How about oral sex? No, it won't kill you (contrary to what other books might say). We've got answers to more embarrassing questions than anyone else!

6. **Your partner wants to read, too!** We know that partners are much more involved in pregnancy and childbirth than in past generations. And you want useful tips that go beyond "be supportive" and "hold partner's hand during labor."

   That's why we've scattered partner tips throughout this book—we assume both of you are reading it. And we promise to treat you with the intelligence and respect you deserve.

7. **Parenthood prep.** Yep, your job as parents starts when you conceive. While you may spend eight months picking out that perfect paint hue for your baby's nursery, what happens when you actually hold that newborn in your arms for the first time?

   Many of us are clueless when it comes to preparing to be a parent. (We sure were when we were first parents.) Newborn screening. Cord blood banking. Childcare. Breastfeeding. Circumcision. Vaccinations. These are just a few decisions that lie ahead. Don't worry—we will walk you through all of these topics, since you often have to make these decisions while you're still pregnant. As always, the secret sauce of the 411 series is reader feedback. Many of the questions you see in this book are real-life queries from Dr. M's and Dr. B's patients and from readers who have reached out to us.

How to Use This Book

Before we get rolling, let's go over a few details on how to get the most out of *Expecting 411*.

First, this book contains some big, ugly Latin words and medical terminology. You can't discuss medical issues and pregnancy without whipping out a few complex medical terms, which conveniently are often in Latin. What? You didn't study Latin in college?

Okay, to keep the jargon from overwhelming you, we have a handy glossary at the end of this book. When you see a ***word*** in bold italics, turn to the back to get a quick definition.

Second, if you flip through the chapters, you'll find different tip boxes and sidebars to highlight key information, takeaways, and tips, for both you and your partner. There are also note boxes with opinions from Dr. M or Dr. B. As it sounds, these are the authors' opinions on several hot-button issues. Feel free to disagree with these thoughts, but they are based on years of seeing real-world patients and delivering thousands of babies. Unlike some other pregnancy books, we think readers deserve to know where the line is drawn between fact and opinion. You can then decide what works for you and your partner. We've created an icon system to help you find this info in a hurry:

Helpful Hint

Reality Check

Red Flags

Feedback from the Real World

Fact Check

Insider Secret

New Parent-to-Be 411

Partner Tip

Warning: Disturbing Material Ahead

Dr. B's Opinion

Dr. M.'s Opinion

We also have a quick note on language. While we use the terms "women" or "partner" throughout the text, you may use other terms to describe yourself. We use these terms to streamline the editorial process, but we see and welcome everyone who is about to enter parenthood.

Dr. M and Dr. B share their respective expertise in obstetrics-gynecology and in pediatric medicine. You'll see some content that is written in first person, reflecting and sharing knowledge in our particular specialty. You can assume that the "I" refers to Dr. M when we discuss pregnancy and adult medicine, and the "I" refers to Dr. B when we talk about newborns and pediatric medicine.

Finally, let's talk about citations—we are transparent about the sources used throughout this book. Our mantra is "show us the science!" We want our readers to feel confident that the guidance throughout this book is based on reputable, peer-reviewed, large-scale studies that reflect solid evidence and best practices. The complete citation list is located in the back of this book in case you want to read more about a particular study or source.

What's New in This Edition

Because we are committed to giving our readers the most up-to-date guidance, we have plenty of new and revised content for you! For this edition of *Expecting 411*, we have major updates on prenatal tests. We'll go over the gold standard tests as well as the latest optional tests that are better at detecting chromosomal issues. We have significantly expanded the section on environmental exposures and ways to reduce risk. And we have also added content to reflect the questions today's parents have about vaccines given during pregnancy and to their newborn.

Major Legal Disclaimer

No medical book is complete without that ubiquitous legal disclaimer, so here's ours:

The information we provide in this book is intended to help you understand the medical issues around pregnancy and childbirth. It is not intended to replace the advice of your doctor, midwife, or OB provider taking care of you during your pregnancy. Before you start any medical treatment, always check in with your OB provider who can counsel you on the specific needs for your pregnancy and baby.

We have made a tremendous effort to give you the most up-to-date medical info available. However, medical research is constantly providing new insights into healthcare.

Okay, enough of the introductions. First up: Chapter 1, "It's Positive . . . Now What Do I Do?"

PART ONE

I'm Pregnant! Now What?

From the moment you discover that positive result on the home pregnancy test, your mind is filled with questions. This section explores what to do first, including meeting your OB provider, prenatal care, and all of the decisions you have to make (Birthing classes? Where to have the birth? Hiring a doula?). We'll take a week-by-week look as you go through your first, second, and third trimesters. And we'll prepare you for what lies ahead. Finally, let's look at what's normal (and what's not) for your changing body, plus all of those tests you'll take over the next nine months.

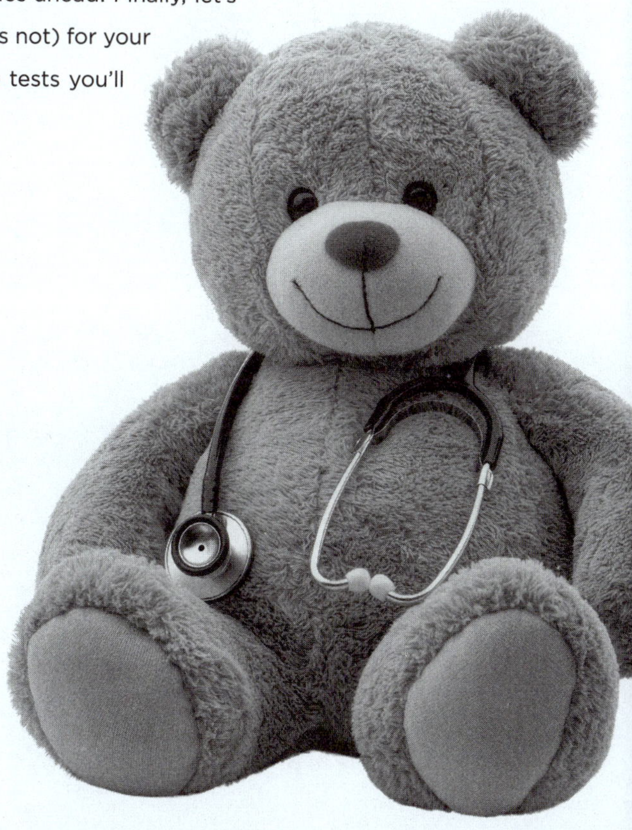

CHAPTER 1

It's Positive . . . Now What Do I Do?

"It sometimes happens, even in the best of families, that a baby is born. This is not necessarily cause for alarm. The important thing is to keep your wits about you and borrow some money."

—Elinor Goulding Smith

What's in This Chapter

- **Are you really pregnant?**
- **Calculating your due date**
- **The birds and the bees**

There's probably one big question running through your mind right now: "I think I'm pregnant. Now what?"

For many of you (and trust us, we felt this way, too) seeing those two lines on the pregnancy test is quite a shock. So let's take a deep breath and then read on.

Some pregnancies are strategically planned, others just . . . happen.

In an ideal world, you and your partner have a pre-conception visit (a visit that occurs prior to pregnancy) with your OB provider. The OB provider reviews your medical conditions, information about any previous pregnancy or gynecological issues, immunization history, list of medications you are taking, lifestyle issues that may be risky for an unborn baby and mom-to-be (such as drug use, alcohol use, smoking, environmental/work exposures), nutrition, exercise habits, and both partners' family medical histories to assess for potential genetic disease risks.

Then the OB provider recommends that you start taking prenatal vitamins and change any poor lifestyle habits.

Wouldn't it be nice if we all did this? Let's get real. For many of us, pregnancy is a pleasant surprise, which happens without starting those prenatal vitamins or changing bad habits. Don't panic. That's why we are here—we will bring you up to speed.

This introductory chapter is a crash course in pregnancy before we discuss your life for the next forty weeks. Yes, some of this is pretty boring stuff (especially if you never liked science or health class). But it is helpful for you to understand what is going on with your body and your baby right from the start. Let's get rolling.

Am I Really Pregnant?

This question will hit you when you either: a) miss your period; b) feel like you ate some bad takeout; or c) yell at your loved ones for no apparent reason. Then, like all of us, you will run out and buy one (or three) home pregnancy tests to confirm your suspicions.

If your test is clearly positive, congratulations! You can pass go and skip to the next section. But sometimes it's not that clear-cut. Let's talk about how those home pregnancy tests work.

Q. What does the pregnancy test actually test for?

The test looks for ***human chorionic gonadotropin (beta-hCG)*** in the urine. Beta-hCG is a hormone the body makes during pregnancy. It circulates through the body and then gets eliminated in the urine. In most normal pregnancies, the levels of beta-hCG increase by at least 50 percent every forty-eight hours until about ten weeks of pregnancy. So, by the time a woman misses her period, there is plenty of beta-hCG in her urine to make a test turn positive.

Your OB provider can also order a blood test that measures beta-hCG (obviously not something one does in your own bathroom).

Q. When is the most accurate time to do a home pregnancy test?

Anytime after a missed period. We know it's hard to wait, especially if you have been trying and are eager to see if those two lines are there. Truthfully, many home pregnancy tests can detect beta-hCG a few days *before* a missed period, but doing the test too early could give you inaccurate results. In English: You're pregnant, but the test doesn't detect it yet. Besides being unnecessarily disappointed and wasting a few bucks, testing too early may lead you to resume habits that could be dangerous for a new pregnancy (like drinking alcohol).

BOTTOM LINE: Be patient. Wait until you miss your period to do the test.

Q. What if the first home pregnancy test is negative but I really feel pregnant?

Early in pregnancy, some women feel the way they do just before they get their period. You may have tender breasts, cramps, moodiness, and cravings.

If you have these symptoms, miss your period, and your first pregnancy test is negative, you've got two options.

- Option 1: Wait a few days and take another urine pregnancy test at home.
- Option 2: See your OB provider and get a blood pregnancy test. Because the blood test looks at actual blood levels of beta-hCG, it detects this pregnancy hormone a few days sooner and confirms pregnancy earlier than a urine pregnancy test.

Q. What if there is only a faint line?

A faint line means that there is some beta-hCG in your urine.

You may get one of those "faintly positive" tests (where you have to squint your eyes and put the stick up to the sunlight to see the line) if you do a home pregnancy test a few days before a missed period or very close to the date of the missed period. Or you could have ovulated later than you thought, so you are not as far along as you anticipated. This is common in women who have menstrual cycles that are longer than twenty-eight days.

It's common for the first few home pregnancy tests to be light (where the test result line is lighter than the control line) because the hormone levels are lower in the early stages of pregnancy. I say the "first few tests" because if you are like most women (and Dr. M includes herself here, as she took eight with her first pregnancy!), you will not take just one test. You will take *ten* before you even get to your first doctor's visit! Some women test multiple brands to make sure that they all are positive. I've even had a patient make her husband pee on one to act as the control!

Regardless of which test kit(s) you use, it is important to follow the instructions correctly.

Reality Check

Read the test results within five to ten minutes. If you let the pregnancy test sit for an hour and then go back to read it (or pull it out of the trash can to check just one more time—it's okay, I [Dr. M] did that, too), you may see a faint line that is actually a false positive. The faint line does not mean anything if the test has been sitting for an hour.

Q. What if the first one is faintly positive and the next one is negative?

The most likely reason is that you *were* pregnant, but you had an abnormal pregnancy. Many women have what doctors informally call a ***chemical pregnancy.*** A chemical pregnancy means your body made enough beta-hCG to produce a positive test but not a viable baby. You actually were pregnant, but there was a very early miscarriage that occurred before anything could even be detected by ultrasound. This is common. The good news: It doesn't usually happen repeatedly. You don't have to see your OB provider if this happens, but you should call the office and let them know.

What's My Due Date?

Q. How do I figure out my due date?

A full-term pregnancy is about forty weeks or 280 days long. Docs start counting from the first day of your last menstrual period. Back in the good old days before ultrasounds and pregnancy tests, a birth date or due date was calculated by this equation:

1. Take the first day of your ***last menstrual period (LMP)***.
2. Subtract three months.
3. Add seven days.

That date is your estimated due date or ***estimated date of delivery (EDD)***. This is also sometimes referred to as the ***estimated date of confinement (EDC)***, which is an old Victorian term used when women really were confined for birth.

While this is an easy way to do it, it's not perfect. It assumes that a woman has a twenty-eight-day menstrual cycle (which many of us don't) and doesn't consider leap years or months with fewer than thirty-one days.

If you and math haven't gotten along since eighth grade algebra, you can use a due date calculator such as one found at uptodate.com/contents/calculator-estimated-date-of-delivery-edd-patient-education.

Your OB provider has something called a "pregnancy wheel" that is kind of a cheat sheet for us. We routinely whip one of these plastic wheels out of our white coats many times during the course of your pregnancy and intensely spin it around to calculate how far along you are. In fact, we are pretty incapacitated without one!

Nowadays, we calculate a patient's due date using a combination of the first day of the last known menstrual period (LMP) and an ultrasound.

Don't be alarmed if you can't remember when your last period was or if you have irregular periods. Your OB provider can make a pretty good approximation after doing an exam and ultrasound. It may sound odd, but your OB provider will have a better idea about dates the *earlier* an ultrasound is performed.

Women who have conceived with assisted reproductive technology (like in vitro fertilization) have their due date calculated by their fertility specialist. That date is based on the date of the procedure, the stage of the embryo being implanted (for IVF), and early ultrasounds.

BOTTOM LINE: It's crucial to have accurate dates for a pregnancy because most tests must be done during a specified window of time during pregnancy.

Helpful Hint

To figure out when you need to make your first prenatal appointment, call your OB provider's office and give them your LMP (the first day of your last menstrual period) and the date of your first positive pregnancy test. They will then know when to schedule the appointment.

Reality Check

If you are in Vegas, do not bet on your due date being your baby's birthday. You have a 5 percent chance of actually delivering on that day. You read that right; that wasn't a typo. In fact, I know a local obstetrician who won't even give his patients a due date. Instead, he gives them a two-week window when the probability is highest that they will deliver. But this nebulous date should at least give you a ballpark idea of when to have your nursery ready.

NEW PARENT-TO-BE 411:

Pregnancy Lingo

Yes, there is a whole glossary in the back of this book for you to refer to at your leisure or to use as a sleeping aid. But here are a few terms that are routinely tossed around so you can follow along in this chapter.

Conception: This is when the sperm and egg meet. It's also sometimes called fertilization.

C-section (cesarean section): This is a surgical procedure used to deliver a baby. The obstetrician makes a small cut or incision in a woman's lower abdomen and uterus to remove the baby.

Ectopic pregnancy: An embryo implants in the wrong place. Instead of the embryo setting up shop and growing in the uterus (womb), it settles elsewhere—most commonly in the fallopian tube. Except in extremely rare cases, ectopic pregnancies cannot go to completion and are medical emergencies.

Embryo: This is what your unborn baby is called from the time of conception through the first eight weeks of development.

Fetus: This is what your unborn baby is called from nine weeks of development until birth.

Gestation: The period of time that the embryo/fetus develops in the womb. Gestational age refers to the number of weeks or days the embryo/fetus has been in the womb.

Placenta: Organ that forms after fertilization occurs. It is your baby's life support system. It brings in nourishment and oxygen, while removing waste from the unborn baby (fetus). The umbilical cord, which contains blood vessels, is the conduit between the placenta and the fetus.

Postpartum: The six- to eight-week window after a woman gives birth.

OB provider: To simplify things, we will refer to your healthcare provider as "your OB provider." This refers to your obstetrician ("OB"), family OB provider, nurse OB provider, nurse midwife, or lay midwife who serves as your main healthcare provider during the course of your pregnancy and immediately afterward.

Preconception: Before you are pregnant.

Prenatal: The time from conception until birth.

Trimesters: Your pregnancy lasts about forty weeks. That time is divided into three stages or trimesters, and each is about thirteen weeks. The first trimester is zero to thirteen weeks; the second is fourteen to twenty-seven weeks; and the third is twenty-eight to forty weeks.

Uterus: The female organ commonly known as the womb. It is where the developing baby grows until they are born.

Vaginal delivery: A baby is delivered after traveling through the birth canal (the vagina). The vagina is basically a muscular tube that goes from the uterus and cervix to the outside.

Q. How long am I actually going to be pregnant?

For 280 days. That is divided up into three trimesters, ten lunar months, or forty weeks. Any way you slice or dice it, it's a long time. By the end, you will be wishing you were a seahorse, one of the few species where the males carry the babies!

Q. Why do you refer to everything in weeks instead of months?

Counting by month can be very confusing. Pregnancy is not exactly nine months, and the number of days in each month varies, so it's more accurate to follow your pregnancy by the week and not the month. A pregnancy that goes to term (also called ***full term***) is thirty-seven to forty weeks.

BOTTOM LINE: Just tell your friends how many weeks along you are and let them figure out when to plan your baby shower.

The Birds and the Bees

Q. How does a baby become, well, a baby?

In most cases a woman releases an egg from one of her two ovaries. Her female hormones elegantly control this monthly event. After the egg is released, it leaves the ***ovary*** and travels through the ***fallopian tube***. That's called ***ovulation***.

Once that egg starts its journey, it has to find a nice sperm to pair up with while it is in the fallopian tube. Sperm can live in a woman's body for as long as five days. Eggs are on a tighter time schedule, however. Once an egg heads out of the ovary, it has to be fertilized by a sperm within twenty-four hours.[1] If the sperm does not reach and penetrate the egg, the egg dies, and a woman menstruates (that is, gets her ***menstrual period***) about fourteen days later.

If a sperm finds the egg, which seems easy enough because there are usually anywhere from 20 million to 200 million per batch, voilà! Fertilization can occur.

This is, however, a difficult feat for sperm . . . they have to navigate through the top of the ***vagina*** into the ***cervix*** (a few good men are lost there). Then they swim up into the body of the ***uterus***, and some choose the wrong fallopian tube, while others choose the right one.

This is as tough as it sounds. There are no road signs or GPS systems to rely on.

Of the millions of sperm that are released during sexual intercourse, fewer than 200 get anywhere near that little egg.[2] Of the remaining sperm that make it into the correct fallopian tube, only one (and in rare cases two) actually break down the hard outer shell of the egg (the *zona pellucida*) and fertilize it. That's called ***conception***.

The fertilized egg (***embryo***) then enters the uterus and attaches (called ***implantation***) to the uterine lining about seven days later. That little fertilized egg is now your baby.

Of course, that's the old-fashioned way. Today, there are more options to accomplish this goal! There is a whole chapter devoted to multiples (twins or more) in Chapter 21, "Multiples." We'll explain how Mother Nature makes that happen (and how your friendly fertility specialist can do the same thing).

Fertilization and Implantation

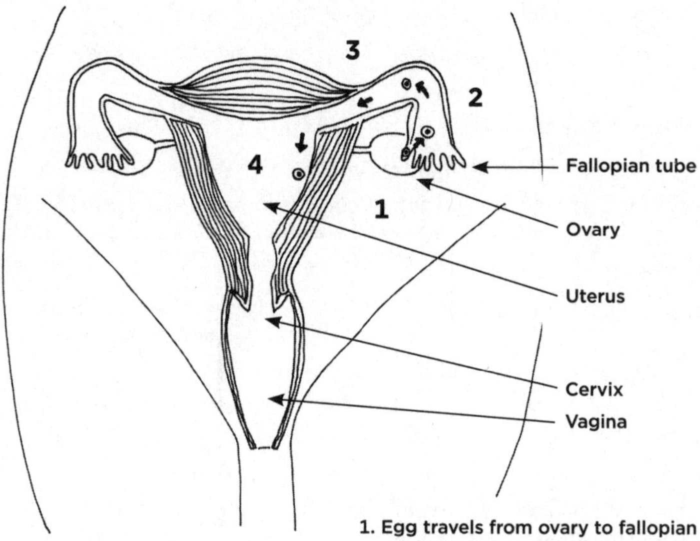

1. Egg travels from ovary to fallopian tube (ovulation).
2. Egg meets sperm in fallopian tube (fertilization).
3. Fertilized egg (embryo) moves through fallopian tube.
4. Embryo attaches to uterine lining.

Reality Check

The time between when a woman ovulates (releases a mature egg for fertilization) and when she menstruates (gets her period) is remarkably consistent for all of us. It is usually fourteen days. It's the time between when you get your period and when you ovulate that varies a bit—which explains why one woman may have a twenty-eight-day cycle and another might have a thirty-four-day cycle. We mention this just in case you want (or don't want) to get pregnant again! Subtract fourteen days from the first day of your last period and you will know how many days into your cycle you are ovulating.

Fact Check

You'll have better odds of conceiving if your partner is on top (missionary position).

The truth: You'll have better odds of conceiving if you have vaginal intercourse while you are ovulating, no matter which position you are in.

NEW PARENT-TO-BE 411:

The Nitty Gritty Details of How It All Works

So how does a human become a human? Let's do a brief review in case you were sleeping through your high school biology class.

- Chromosomes are our body's blueprints. They carry genetic material (our genes) made from DNA (deoxyribonucleic acid).
- Human cells have twenty-three pairs (or forty-six total) of chromosomes.
- The two chromosomes that make up pairs one to twenty-two are identical.
- The two chromosomes that make up the twenty-third pair are the sex chromosomes. Girls have two identical X sex chromosomes. Boys have one X and one Y sex chromosome.
- The egg (ovum) and the sperm are special human cells because they are the only cells in the body that have half the number of chromosomes that all other cells do: Eggs have twenty-three chromosomes (twenty-two plus an X sex chromosome), and sperm have twenty-three chromosomes (twenty-two plus either an X or a Y sex chromosome).
- When an egg and a sperm meet, their single chromosomes pair up with each other. Pairs one to twenty-two find each other as does pair twenty-three. The twenty-third pair is either XX or XY. Each baby gets half of their genetic blueprints from the egg and half from the sperm. However, the X- or Y-carrying sperm is what ultimately determines the sex of the baby.
- Once the egg and sperm unite, the fertilized egg (embryo) starts dividing and growing about twenty-four hours later to become a ball of cells.
- This little ball follows its highly complex blueprint to become a human and enters the world about thirty-seven weeks later.

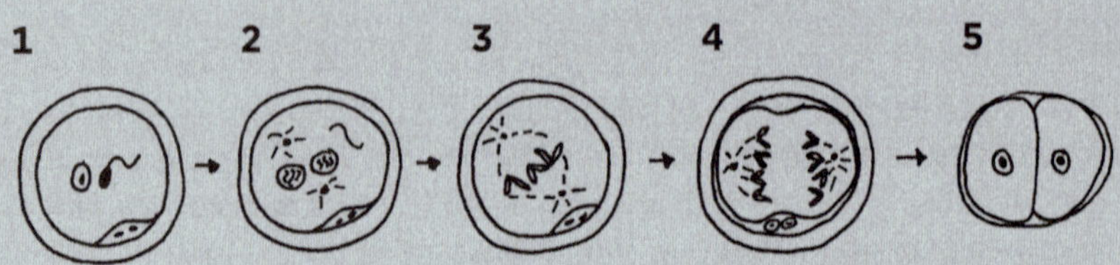

1. Egg and sperm meet.

2. They begin sharing their genetic material.

3. The chromosomes pair up.

4. A new cell is made.

5. The cell begins to divide.

There will be a quiz on this next Monday.

Q. How does my OB provider know how far along I am?

There are two ways to follow your growing baby's development.

- **Fertilization age:** Day 1 starts when the egg and sperm meet (that is, fertilization or conception). It takes 266 days or thirty-eight weeks for a fetus to complete its development.
- **Gestational age:** Day 1 starts on the first day of your last menstrual period (LMP). For the sake of simplicity, this is what we use because we don't usually know the exact day that fertilization/conception happened. It takes 280 days or forty weeks to complete development if you look at it this way. This is how your OB provider follows your baby's progress, so that's what we will do in this book. Confusing, we know. It's true, you are not carrying a fertilized egg for the first two weeks of this time period—but any time you get two free weeks without nausea or the urge to pee, consider it a blessing!

Tales from the Womb: Your Growing Baby[3]

EMBRYO

Gestational Age	Size	Weight	Milestone
Day 1	N/A	N/A	First day of last menstrual period
1 week	N/A	N/A	Egg not yet released from ovary
2 weeks	N/A	N/A	Egg and sperm meet (fertilization)
3 weeks	N/A	N/A	Embryo implants
4 weeks	0.06* inch	N/A	Brain/spine/nerves develop
5 weeks	0.1* inch	N/A	Heart/eyes/ears/budding arms develop
6 weeks	0.2* inch	N/A	Face/arms/organs form, heart beats
7 weeks	0.3* inch	N/A	Lower legs, intestines, bladder form
8 weeks	0.6* inch	0.04 ounce	Heart has four chambers, throat forms, teeth buds
9 weeks	0.8* inch	0.07 ounce	Inner ear, nose, fingers form
10 weeks	1.3* inches	0.14 ounce	Doppler detects heartbeat

FETUS

Gestational Age	Size	Weight	Milestone
11 weeks	1.9* inches	0.3 ounce	Eyelids fused together
12 weeks	2.4* inches	0.5 ounce	Some organs working, mouth forms
14 weeks	3.4* inches	1.5 ounces	External genitals visible
16 weeks	4.7* inches	3.8 ounces	Sucks thumb, swallows, breathes, pees
18 weeks	5.5* inches	7 ounces	Bones harden, ovaries make eggs
22 weeks	10.9 inches	1 pound	Head/body hair and body fur appears, fetal kicking begins
24 weeks	11.8 inches	1.4 pounds	Hearing develops, rapid eye movements occur
26 weeks	14.2 inches	1.8 pounds	Lungs begin maturing, fingernails form

Gestational Age	Size	Weight	Milestone
28 weeks	14.8 inches	2.2 pounds	Eyes open and close
30 weeks	15.7 inches	2.9 pounds	Bone marrow works
32 weeks	16.7 inches	3.7 pounds	Pupils respond to light
34 weeks	17.7 inches	4.6 pounds	Eyes close with sleep
36 weeks	18.6 inches	5 pounds	Lungs mature, testes descend
38 weeks	19.6 inches	6.4 pounds	Fat accumulates, breasts protrude
40 weeks	20.2 inches	7.5 pounds	Ready to go!

*Your OB provider measures your baby's length from their head to their heinie—called crown rump length, or CRL—on ultrasounds until about fourteen weeks. Starting at twenty weeks, it's possible to estimate your baby's length from head to toe. (All measurements are averages. Don't obsess about them.)

Tales from the Womb: Your Growing Baby

We have a handy table (see previous page and above) of your growing baby. Below is a table of *your* growing body for the next forty weeks, just to give you the big picture of it all. Here is a rough timeline of the changes to come:

FIRST TRIMESTER (0–13 WEEKS)

Week (Gestational Age)	How Your Body Changes
4 weeks	Home pregnancy test positive
6 weeks	Sore breasts, frequent urination, food aversions
8 weeks	Nauseated, grumpy, severe fatigue, constipated
10 weeks	Enlarging breasts, enlarging waistline (pants that buttoned in the morning will not close by late afternoon)
12 weeks	Uterus can be felt above the pelvis, increased vaginal discharge
13 weeks	Risk of miscarriage diminishes, baby bump may appear

SECOND TRIMESTER (14–27 WEEKS)

Week (Gestational Age)	How Your Body Changes
14 weeks	Nausea and mood changes usually end, more energy
16 weeks	Growing and feeling good, increased appetite, onset of heartburn, aches and pains
20 weeks	Center of gravity changes, clumsiness, start to feel fetal movement
24 weeks	Skin changes, swollen feet at the end of a long day

THIRD TRIMESTER (28–40 WEEKS)

Week (Gestational Age)	How Your Body Changes
28 weeks	Back pain, leg cramps
30 weeks	Heartburn worsens, constipation returns, swollen veins around the anus (***hemorrhoids***) bless us with their presence
32 weeks	Leaking early breast milk is possible, practice contractions may begin (called ***Braxton-Hicks contractions***)

Week (Gestational Age)	How Your Body Changes
34 weeks	Fatigue returns, shoes don't fit, stretch marks may appear
36 weeks	Vaginal discharge increases again, may start to leak urine
37 weeks	Practice contractions begin or continue, mucus blocking cervix may come out, hard to find a comfortable position
38 weeks	Peeing every one to two hours, hemorrhoids enlarge, can't sleep
39 weeks	Everything we've already said taken to another level!
40 weeks	You'll be praying to every holy being in every religion to please make you go into labor!

CHAPTER 2

The First Trimester

"No one told me I would be coming home in diapers, too."

—Chrissy Teigen

What's in This Chapter

- **Week by week**
- **Food and beverages to avoid**
- **Your first prenatal visit**
- **When to tell friends and family**

Welcome to your first trimester of pregnancy!

Here's our goal for this chapter (and the two that follow). By trimester, we'll look at body changes, common questions, your health-care needs (called prenatal care), decisions you will need to make, and what is going on with your growing baby. And we will guide you to where you will find info on specific topics covered in later chapters.

Week by Week: The First Trimester

Let's start with an overview of what's to come over the next several weeks.

Zero to Two Weeks

Technically, you haven't even conceived yet. But the forty-week countdown begins on the first day of your menstrual period. You get two free weeks right at the start!

Three Weeks

This is the week the fertilized egg implants into your womb (uterus). Some women experience light spotting (a few drops of blood that stain a panty liner or undies) when this happens. This is called ***implantation bleeding***. You probably don't even realize that you are pregnant at this point because you have not missed your period yet. If you have been trying to become pregnant, you should already be avoiding unhealthy habits and taking prenatal vitamins.

Four to Five Weeks

Congratulations! You've missed your period and discover you have a positive pregnancy test. Enjoy the elation.

Signs of pregnancy are heading your way soon. If you aren't already taking daily prenatal vitamins, put this book down right now and go buy some (later in this chapter we offer tips on which ones to buy). Stop any habits that are bad for you and even worse for your unborn baby. See Chapter 8, "Environmental Health," for details.

Call your OB provider to set up your first prenatal visit. For most of you, your first appointment will be when you are between seven to ten weeks pregnant. If you have a chronic medical condition or are considered a high-risk pregnancy, your first appointment may be sooner than that.

If you have any vaginal bleeding or severe abdominal pain, don't wait for your first prenatal appointment. Call your OB provider now. (See Chapter 22, "When It Doesn't Work," and Chapter 16, "Pregnancy 911," for symptoms of ***miscarriage***.)

If you have conceived with the help of a fertility specialist, that doctor will probably care for you until eight to twelve weeks. Once released from your fertility specialist's care, you will start seeing your OB provider.

Contemplating sushi or continuing with your lattes during pregnancy? Check out Chapter 8, "Environmental Health." Wondering if you need to cancel your hair highlights or manicure/pedicure appointments? See Chapter 10, "Self-Care."

Curious to know if you can still take that Caribbean cruise while pregnant? See Chapter 9, "Lifestyles." Want to know how to eat a healthy diet and gain the right amount of weight during pregnancy? It's all there in Chapter 7, "Nutrition."

Six to Seven Weeks

One of the first clues you are pregnant is that your breasts will be sore and tender. See Chapter 5, "Is This Normal?" for ways to relieve your discomfort. You will also need to pee more than usual. You may need to get up a few times a night to urinate. Again, see Chapter 5 for what is normal and what warrants a visit to your OB provider. You may also start having quite a bit of vaginal discharge. Sorry, but this will continue throughout your pregnancy.

Eight to Nine Weeks

Pregnancy should be in full swing now. Many women experience severe fatigue, all-day nausea (who are we kidding by calling it morning sickness?), and general grumpiness. Some women also experience mild pelvic cramps. See Chapter 5 to sort out what to do about these typical symptoms. You'll have to live with some of these unpleasant issues for the next four weeks or so.

If you have excessive vomiting, you should call your OB provider now. See Chapters 16, "Pregnancy 911," and Chapter 17, "The Complicated Pregnancy," for details on morning sickness gone south (***hyperemesis gravidarum***).

You'll have your first prenatal visit this week or soon after. Be sure to bring your partner with you to this visit, and block out your morning or afternoon (it's usually a long appointment). Check out details in this chapter for a list of questions to ask your OB provider.

Yes, lab tests are a fact of life for all pregnant moms. See Chapter 6, "Tests," for details on all the routine tests as well as optional ones you may want to request.

Plan on routine appointments with your OB provider about once a month until you are twenty-eight weeks, when they become more frequent.

Ten to Eleven Weeks

This is the week of the enlarging breasts and waistline. You may enjoy the look of your new shapely breasts, but they may feel pretty sore and tender to the touch. See Chapter 5, "Is This Normal?" for some reassurance and tips to relieve discomfort.

You will notice that you can button your pants in the morning, but not in the afternoon. If you haven't spilled the beans to family, friends, or your boss yet, you won't be able to hide your body changes much longer. Read later in this chapter for concerns about telling family and friends. See Chapter 9, "Lifestyles," about telling your boss and to learn more about employee medical leave rights.

If you are thirty-five years of age or older (aka "***advanced maternal age***," ugh!), you may want to learn about optional tests that screen for chromosomal abnormalities like the first trimester screening test, ***chorionic villus sampling (CVS)***, non-invasive prenatal screening (NIPS), or ***amniocentesis.*** See Chapter 6, "Tests," for all you need to know about these specialized tests. Even if you are under thirty-five, you may want to read this section.

The first trimester screening test is done between ten and thirteen weeks, and CVS is done at about the same time, so get reading.

Twelve to Thirteen Weeks

You are almost done with your first trimester! Hooray! If you have made it this far, it's much less likely you will miscarry. Your little baby bump may start to appear . . . Yes, you are really going to have a baby.

Your OB provider will begin listening to your baby's heartbeat with a Doppler device at each visit. This is really fun (and very reassuring) to hear. You'll start showing between thirteen and twenty weeks, depending on your body stature, whether this is your first baby or not, and how many babies you are carrying. Normal complaints in the first trimester include headaches, lightheadedness, forgetfulness, all-day nausea, constipation, excessive gas and burping, lots of vaginal discharge, lots of peeing, acne, and, of course, moodiness and fatigue. You'll be happy to head into your second trimester. Pregnant life does get better!

Aches, Pains, and Changes in the First Trimester (Zero to Thirteen Weeks):

- Moody, emotional
- Headaches
- Difficulty sleeping
- Frequent urination, urinating at night
- Nausea, vomiting (morning sickness)
- Vaginal discharge starts and continues for the duration
- Acne, splotchy marks on the face
- Tired
- Gas, burping, constipation
- Tender, growing breasts

Common Questions About the First Trimester

We know you've got a million questions right now! And you won't be seeing your healthcare provider for a little while, so this section should ease your mind until that first appointment.

Q. My home pregnancy test was positive. When should I schedule an appointment with my OB provider?

Most OB providers see newly pregnant patients anywhere between seven to ten weeks of pregnancy. You can calculate this from the first day of your last menstrual period (see "What's My Due Date?" in Chapter 1, "It's Positive . . .").

If you conceived by assisted-reproductive technologies, like in vitro fertilization (IVF), your fertility specialist will see you at frequent intervals during the early part of your pregnancy. You will then be released into the care of your OB provider anywhere between eight and twelve weeks of ***gestation***.

If you have a ***high-risk pregnancy***, you may need to see your OB provider sooner rather than later. Not sure if you fit into that category? Check out our handy box below or call your OB provider. She can tell you when to come in for that first appointment.

NEW PARENT-TO-BE 411:

Do I Have a High-Risk Pregnancy?

The answer is yes if you:

- Are having twins, triplets, or even more multiples.
- Have a history of repeated miscarriages.
- Conceived by assisted-reproductive technology/with the help of a fertility specialist.

(continued)

- Are having vaginal bleeding.
- Have chronic medical issues like lupus, preexisting diabetes, or high blood pressure.
- Have a complication arise during your current pregnancy (like placenta previa).
- Are thirty-five years old or older (I know, that seems extreme), although some docs consider only women over age forty to be high risk.
- Have a history of an ectopic pregnancy.

Q. Are there any foods or beverages I need to avoid now that I am pregnant?

Short answer: Yes.

The long answer to what you should and shouldn't eat gets an entire chapter later in this book (Chapter 8, "Environmental Health"). But below is a list to review before you see your OB provider for the first time so you don't have any early anxiety attacks.

Here's a prime example: I received an emergency page from a patient's husband on a Friday night. Why? His wife ate some soybeans that had been sitting in the same take-out box as his sushi. Did this put the pregnancy at risk? (Answer: No!)

Given the high anxiety level about this topic, here's the brief thirty-second version of what to avoid eating when pregnant:

- **Avoid eating fish with high mercury levels—and limit the amount of fish with moderate and low mercury levels.** That list is featured in Chapter 8, "Environmental Health".
- **Avoid raw or undercooked meat and fish.** Sorry, that means sushi is a no-no. Seared fish and rare meat are also off-limits. And avoid anything made with raw eggs. That includes freshly made Caesar salad dressing, hollandaise sauce, and homemade eggnog.
- **Avoid unpasteurized dairy products and juices.** Some fancy cheeses fit into this category. These can include Brie, Camembert, feta, Gorgonzola, queso blanco, and Roquefort.
- **Wash all fruits and vegetables thoroughly before eating.** Unwashed or poorly washed fruit and veggies can expose you to toxoplasma, listeria, salmonella, and norovirus, all of which can lead to serious infections for you and your baby.
- **Thoroughly cook pre-sliced deli meat and hot dogs before eating.** Microwave these until they're steaming before eating for the same reason as above.
- **Avoid alcoholic beverages.** Even small amounts of alcohol during pregnancy have been associated with fetal alcohol spectrum disorders (FASD), including autism and learning differences.
- **Avoid caffeine if possible.** If that sounds daunting (we're doctors, we understand caffeine), limit your consumption to one or at most two caffeinated beverages a day, especially in the first trimester.

- **Stop smoking.** If that has been tough, talk with your OB provider about other options to help quit. (This one we won't budge on.)

Your OB provider will discuss and/or give you a list of all the banned food and beverages during pregnancy at your first visit. But you can get started with your new pregnancy diet with this information in hand. We will explain why you have to avoid all these foods in detail when you get to Chapter 8, "Environmental Health".

Reality Check

If you smoke, drink alcohol, or use drugs, now is the time to stop.

Q. Are there any medications I need to stop using now that I am pregnant?

The short answer is yes.

There is an expansive list in Appendix A, "Medications," that covers both over-the-counter and prescription medications with safety ratings for pregnancy and breast-feeding.

Certain medications are absolute no-nos, especially in the first trimester (thirteen weeks), because they can cause birth defects.

For other medications, the risk to the unborn baby must be weighed against the benefit of the mother-to-be's health. The OB provider handling your pregnancy can discuss possible alternative medications with your other healthcare providers if there is a significant risk with what you are currently taking.

If you have health or mental health issues that require you to take daily medication, call the physician prescribing it and notify them of your pregnancy right now—just in case you need to stop that medicine. And you or your physician can always call your obstetrician to double-check on medications that are safe to take during pregnancy.

Q. How about herbal medication? Can I continue or start taking those meds?

Check with your OB provider if you are currently taking or want to start taking any herbal, homeopathic, or alternative medicine. Seemingly innocuous supplements such as ginseng and St. John's wort have the potential to cause bleeding and should not be used during pregnancy. Check out the list of alternative remedies and their safety/risks during pregnancy in Appendix B, "Complementary Medicines and Therapies."

Until you have your first prenatal appointment, I suggest holding off on these products.

Q. Are there any vitamins or nutritional supplements I need now?

Yes! Until you visit your OB provider and get their advice, I recommend taking a daily dose of any over-the-counter prenatal vitamin containing 300 mg of ***DHA*** (fish oil or omega-3 fatty acid), at least 400 mcg of methylated folate or folic acid, and *less than*

5,000 IU a day of vitamin A (unless in the form of beta-carotene, which is very safe). I also recommend picking up a vitamin D supplement: 800 IU to 1,000 IU of vitamin D is a good addition to your prenatal vitamin and your diet.

If you planned this pregnancy, you should already be taking prenatal vitamins. The latest research shows that taking prenatal vitamins containing at least 400 mcg of methylated folate for three months before conception lowers the risk of certain birth defects, like ***neural tube defect***, and some pregnancy-associated health issues, such as preterm births. If your pregnancy was a pleasant surprise, put down this book and go buy some prenatal vitamins.

Don't get overwhelmed when you go to the pharmacy. There are several choices when it comes to prenatal vitamins, and most pills are similar. Some contain a stool softener (which is usually a welcome treat in the first trimester, as constipation is a frequent side effect of pregnancy). Some contain DHA, which has health benefits for both mom and baby. What's most important is to check for the amount of folic acid (make sure it's methylated) and vitamin A.

We cover prenatal vitamins and other supplements in greater depth in Chapter 7, "Nutrition." Pop over there for some very helpful tips!

After you go to your first prenatal visit, you may also need to take an iron supplement if you are anemic. Your OB provider will let you know based on a blood test taken at your first or second visit.

Helpful Hint

Do not take your prenatal vitamin and iron supplement (if needed) simultaneously. Take them at least two hours apart so the iron is more effectively absorbed.

INSIDER SECRET:

Take Your Vitamins with Food

Do prenatal vitamins make you feel queasy? The label on your prenatal vitamin probably tells you to take the pill on an empty stomach so the vitamins will be better absorbed. This will, ten times out of ten, make you vomit. Believe us, we've tried it! We suggest taking your prenatal vitamin on a full stomach, with your biggest meal of the day. Or at the very least, have some pudding or crackers to coat your stomach first.

Q. When am I going to start gaining weight, and how much should I gain?

Read about this topic in depth in Chapter 7, "Nutrition." But here is the quick answer: The amount you should gain depends on your pre-pregnancy weight. And yes, you will start to gain weight in your first trimester.

If you were a healthy weight, you should gain about three to five pounds in the first trimester.

Q. Will I start feeling bad before I get in to see my doctor?

Probably. Most women see their OB providers between seven and ten weeks of pregnancy. And some women begin having pregnancy symptoms right away. Here are some things you might suffer from . . . uh, we mean experience, before you get to see your OB provider:

1. **Fatigue.** And we mean severe fatigue . . . like the life has been sucked out of you. Don't be surprised if you are ready to go to bed at 6:30 p.m. Try to catch a nap if you can. Your body needs it.
2. **Cramping in your lower belly.** You may feel like you're having menstrual cramps. Most of the time, you feel this because your uterine muscles are stretching and growing. Occasionally it can be a sign of a problem—especially if you are having vaginal bleeding with those cramps or pain only on one side. See the "Red Flags" section on page 23 for details and to determine whether you need to call your OB provider.
3. **Lots of pee.** Pregnant women pee a lot. And yes, that happens even in the early stages of your pregnancy. You may need to get up two or three times a night to use the bathroom. If it hurts or burns when you urinate, call your OB provider. You need to be tested for a ***bladder infection***.
4. **Big, tender breasts.** You may be used to getting some breast tenderness before your period. But you ain't seen nothing like this. Some women's breasts and nipples are so tender that water running over them in the shower or a sheet sitting on them in bed is excruciating. You may want to warn your partner that they are a touch-free zone. You may also notice that the veins on the skin of your breasts and surrounding chest area become very prominent and often resemble a road map. No need to worry—that's to accommodate the increased blood flow to your naturally enhanced breasts.
5. **Sensitivity to odors.** You and your dog can now compete for who smells food first. Pregnant women have bionic powers of smell and can pick up a scent a mile away. That sounds cool, except that most of those smells (which never bothered you before) may send you running for the nearest place to vomit. When I was pregnant, I was bothered by the metal smell of my keys. I had to hold my nose until I placed my key into the front door of my house. I'm sure my neighbors thought I was odd, but that was better than throwing up on my lawn every day.
6. **"Morning" sickness.** If only it happened just in the morning, ha! Many pregnant women feel nauseated or have queasy stomachs all day long. In fact, it is often worse at the end of the day. Some women just *think* they are going to puke, and others are unlucky enough to actually do it. This feeling starts around the sixth or seventh week of pregnancy and usually lasts until the first trimester ends. I'll see some women in my office for their first prenatal visit who claim to feel great—but it's a different story when I see them for their next visit a few weeks later. Look for tips on combating morning sickness in Chapter 5, "Is This Normal?"
7. **Emotional roller coaster.** Pregnant women should have a sign posted on them that says, "Pregnant woman—stay back 200 feet." Take those PMS symptoms

you are used to and multiply them by 1,000. You could go through periods of feeling weepy, bitchy, elated, and detached all in a span of thirty minutes. And yes, your partner is often the recipient of this hormonal behavior—so you might want to issue a warning! We hurt the ones we love the most. All of these feelings are normal. Since those hormones start surging right at the beginning of pregnancy, so will these emotional ups and downs. You (and your partner) should know that things start to smooth out by week fourteen.

BOTTOM LINE: Yes, you may "feel" pregnant before you see your OB provider for the first visit. However, here is a key fact: 30 percent of women don't have any symptoms of pregnancy other than a missed period. Don't panic. Lacking symptoms isn't a sign that something is wrong.

Q. People say I am eating for two. But with this morning sickness, I can't even eat for one right now! What do I do?

We won't lie: You can feel pretty queasy during the first trimester. Around ten weeks, you will feel like you want to crawl into a hole and wake up next spring.

Many women are extremely nauseated and eat only what makes them feel better. Whether that is Taco Bell (Dr. M's first pregnancy) or Coke and Cheetos (Dr. M's second pregnancy), you do what you've gotta do to get through it. We don't recommend the Coke and Cheetos diet, however, once you have gotten over morning sickness.

Focus on diet and nutrition in the *second* trimester when your gut feels better and life returns to something closer to normal. We'll cover all of your nutrition questions and concerns in Chapter 7, "Nutrition."

For your first trimester, remember that when people say you are "eating for two," you are actually eating for one and a few millimeters . . . so you do need to eat more but within reason.

Q. I am having food aversions. Anything that has a strong smell makes me sick to my stomach. Is this normal? Why does this happen?

It is very common, particularly in the first trimester, to have very strong aversions to smells.

Your stomach might turn with the faintest whiff of cigarette smoke, meat, fish, or anything overwhelming in the kitchen pantry. Think of it as nature's way of preventing pregnant women from ingesting something potentially dangerous.

Here's the theory: Hundreds of years ago (before refrigeration and the FDA), our ancestors relied on their sniffers to determine if something was rotten or poisonous—in other words, something you shouldn't eat. Since a pregnant woman is at greater risk of harm (to herself and the unborn baby) from ingesting something bad, her sense of smell is now in overdrive.

Of course, our food supply today is quite a bit safer, and we can read labels to avoid potentially dangerous foods. Yet our instincts often take over despite modern food safety.

FEEDBACK FROM THE REAL WORLD:
Food Aversions

One of Dr. M's patients (who is also a great friend) couldn't come within a mile of chicken during her first pregnancy. Seeing, touching, smelling, or eating chicken was impossible. To this day, she steers clear of chicken, which is comical, since her family is in the meatpacking business!

Red Flags: The First Few Weeks

Contact your OB provider immediately if you experience:

- **Vaginal bleeding.** Most of the time, a little spotting does not mean something serious is going on. But call your OB provider if you have *any* bleeding from your vagina and let your OB provider decide what to do. Heavy bleeding, like the volume you see when you get your period, can be a sign of pregnancy loss (***miscarriage***), the implantation of the embryo in the wrong place (***ectopic pregnancy***), or a separation of the placenta from the wall of the uterus (***subchorionic hematoma***). Your OB provider will need to see you, do an exam, check your blood type, and, most of the time, perform an ultrasound. Miscarriage and ectopic pregnancies are discussed in detail in Chapter 22, "When It Doesn't Work."

  If all is well upon exam and testing, the heavy bleeding is presumed to be from a placental separation, and you might be placed on bed rest or asked to limit your activity (modified bed rest).
- **Severe cramps.** Most pregnant women have occasional cramps in their pelvic area, most noticeably in the first trimester. These feel like menstrual cramps and are usually normal.

  Severe pain isn't normal. Pain located on one side more than the other also isn't normal. Call your OB provider. This can be a sign of miscarriage or ectopic pregnancy—especially if severe, painful cramps arrive along with heavy vaginal bleeding.
- **Persistent vomiting.** Pregnant women are nauseated. And some pregnant women vomit. But a few can't stop vomiting (***hyperemesis gravidarum,*** see Complication #1 in Chapter 17, "The Complicated Pregnancy"). Those women are dehydrated and malnourished because nothing will stay down. Sometimes hospitalization is required to break the vomiting cycle and help rehydrate a woman with nutrition and fluid given through a vein (***intravenous fluid***). Call your OB provider if you can't keep anything down for twenty-four hours or more.

Red Flags: Ectopic Pregnancy

An ectopic pregnancy occurs when a fertilized egg implants in the wrong place, outside of the uterus. This is a dangerous medical complication. Symptoms include severe abdominal pain, particularly on just one side, or even painless vaginal bleeding with a missed period and positive pregnancy test. See Chapter 16, "Pregnancy 911," and Chapter 22, "When It Doesn't Work," for details.

Prenatal Care

As we discussed earlier, the first visit is about seven to ten weeks from the first day of your last menstrual period. Once your home pregnancy test(s) is positive, go ahead and schedule your first prenatal appointment. (Prenatal care is the official term for all those healthcare appointments prior to labor and childbirth.) Yes, those few weeks before you see your OB provider feel like forever!

Wondering which OB provider you should see for your prenatal care? We cover that in the "Decisions" section later in this chapter.

Q. Are there any reasons why I might need to see my OB provider before the standard first visit?

Yes. See if you fit into any of the categories below, and if so, call your OB provider as soon as you know you are pregnant.

1. You have a chronic medical condition, such as lupus, diabetes, heart disease, or high blood pressure.
2. You are having vaginal bleeding.
3. You have severe abdominal (belly or lower belly) pain.
4. You cannot stop vomiting.
5. You conceived by assisted reproductive technologies—IUI (intrauterine insemination) or IVF (in vitro fertilization).
6. You know you are carrying multiples (twins, triplets, etc.).
7. You have a history of an ectopic pregnancy.

Those of you in categories #5 and likely #6 have a fertility specialist who will probably continue to care for you until you are eight to twelve weeks pregnant, at which time you will be released into the care of your obstetrician for your prenatal care.

Helpful Hint

If you have preexisting medical conditions, call your OB provider as soon as you know you are pregnant. Pregnancy can make some medical conditions worse, and it can make some conditions better. Your OB provider can advise you right at the start once she knows you are pregnant. She may want to see you earlier than seven to ten weeks. This is especially important if you are having a flare-up of your disease or need to take medication on a daily basis.

Q. What happens at the first visit?

I'll walk you through what I do for a typical first visit. While this may vary a little from OB provider to OB provider, this should give you the basic idea of what an obstetrician will do. Let's pretend you are my patient.

I start by visiting with you (and hopefully your partner) in my office before going into an exam room. I find it easier to have a conversation with you when you aren't naked, sitting under a wispy paper gown in a freezing exam room!

I thoroughly review your personal medical history, your partner's medical history, both of your family medical histories, and discuss any potential issues, such as never having had certain childhood illnesses or having cats at home. This helps me determine if this is a high-risk pregnancy and allows me to advise you of any special concerns.

Then we move into an exam room to do a breast exam if one is needed, pelvic (internal) exam, and then an ultrasound. (FYI: That breast exam at the first visit is pretty uncomfortable because most women have extremely tender breasts in the first trimester.)

During the pelvic exam, I may take a few swabs from the ***cervix*** (opening of the womb/uterus) to test for infections like gonorrhea and chlamydia. I'll also do a Pap smear if one has not been done recently.

Next, a ***transvaginal ultrasound*** is done (see Chapter 6, "Tests," for a more complete explanation) if this is your first visit early in your pregnancy. The ultrasound probe is inserted into your vagina (as opposed to placing the probe on top of your belly) because at this point the fetus is too small to see any other way.

This ultrasound tells me several things: I can see that the growing fetus is in the uterus where it should be and is not implanted in the wrong place (see ***ectopic pregnancy***). I can figure out if the size of the fetus is appropriate based on the date of your ***last menstrual period (LMP).*** I can document whether the fetus has a detectable heartbeat. (This depends on how many weeks along you are when you have your first visit.) And I can see if the other internal female organs (fallopian tubes and ovaries) are normal.

Occasionally, twins or other multiples can be seen during this ultrasound, too. The excitement over seeing your baby for the first time will probably make you forget that you have a probe in your vagina!

Next, you get your blood drawn for several screening tests (details in Chapter 6, "Tests"). Some of my patients dread this more than the transvaginal ultrasound! When the lab results are completed several days later, you should get a phone call.

Assuming all is well, we go back into my office (with paper gown in the trash and clothes back on!), and I give out my standard pregnancy dos and don'ts advice sheets (good news: they are included in this book!), information on the hospital where I perform deliveries, the reason for and dates of upcoming screening tests, and resources for childbirth/breastfeeding/first aid classes. You'll schedule your next appointment for two to four weeks later.

Reality Check

Be sure to take off a morning or afternoon from work for your first appointment—you will be there for a while. I also suggest that you eat a good breakfast, drink a lot of water, and turn your head the other way when you get your blood drawn!

NEW PARENT-TO-BE 411:

How to Prepare for Your First Visit

- Bring a list of medications you are taking.
- Compile a family health history for both you and your partner to give your OB provider.
- Compile your own health history to share with your OB provider.
- Bring your partner!

Q. What are the standard tests done in the first trimester?

The American College of Obstetricians and Gynecologists (ACOG) recommends several screening tests during pregnancy. These tests will be explained in full detail in Chapter 6, "Tests." But here is the basic rundown:

TEST	WHEN IT'S DONE
Blood pressure, weight, urinalysis	Every visit
Prenatal blood panel*	First or second prenatal visit
Pap smear	First prenatal visit
Cervical cultures	First prenatal visit

*Includes a complete blood count, blood typing, an infectious disease panel (HIV, syphilis, Hepatitis B, hepatitis C, rubella), a urinalysis, and a urine culture.

Q. Are there any optional tests that can be done?

Yes. There are other tests that may be useful, depending on your personal medical history, age, or ethnicity. These may raise (or lower) the risk of certain disorders. Chapter 6, "Tests," provides a full explanation of your choices. But these are the tests to consider:

1. **First trimester screening test.** A blood test and an ultrasound to help calculate the odds of having a baby with ***Down syndrome*** (trisomy 21), Edwards syndrome (trisomy 18), trisomy 13, certain sex chromosome abnormalities and microdeletions. This test is usually done between ten and thirteen weeks.
2. **Chorionic villus sampling (CVS).** A physician performs a minor procedure to obtain tissue from the placenta. The test diagnoses 99 percent of all chromosome abnormalities, as well as some other disorders. Test occurs at ten to thirteen weeks.
3. **Additional infection panel.** These specific tests identify exposure and/or immunity for other infections. Example: Cat owners may get tested for toxoplasmosis. Tests occur at first visit or whenever necessary.
4. **Other screening tests.** Tests for sickle cell anemia carriers, cystic fibrosis carriers, and other screens may be recommended, depending on your health history and ancestry. Tests are done either prior to pregnancy or at the first prenatal visit.

Q. Will I have a pelvic (internal exam) every time?

No. That's the good news!

It's standard protocol to have a pelvic exam during the first appointment. Then, as long as there are no particular concerns, there won't be another pelvic exam until the home stretch of your pregnancy.

Q. Will I get an ultrasound each time?

Usually not.

Although you might want to sneak a peek at your baby every time you visit your OB provider, this isn't necessary for routine pregnancies.

Most docs do an ultrasound at the first visit, and sometimes one at the next visit.

There are a couple of screening tests that also utilize ultrasounds—one is called the first trimester screening test (done at ten to thirteen weeks), and the other evaluates all the fetus's body parts at twenty to twenty-two weeks. Those studies are discussed in Chapter 6, "Tests."

However, there are special situations that call for an ultrasound as part of each visit. Example: women with twins or triplets.

Q. How often will I see my OB provider after the first visit?

Although all OB providers do things a little differently, here is the American College of Obstetricians and Gynecologists recommended schedule of routine visits for a typical pregnancy:

- Office visit every four weeks from seven to ten weeks up to twenty-eight weeks
- Office visit every two weeks from twenty-eight weeks to thirty-six weeks
- Office visit once a week from thirty-six weeks until delivery

If you have a high-risk pregnancy, such as if you're carrying twins or have high blood pressure, you get to visit your OB provider more often. And if any problems arise (fever, pain with urination, etc.) between those routine visits, you may have a few more appointments.

Q. After the first visit, what usually happens at prenatal appointments?

You will get used to the routine when you walk into your OB provider's office. Yes, this varies depending on your OB provider, but this is what will happen in most cases if you see a physician or nurse OB provider.

First, you will get handed a plastic cup for a urine sample. Believe it or not, we can learn a lot from your pee. We can make sure you don't have a bladder infection (UTI), which can be relatively symptom-free in pregnancy. And we can tell if you are dehydrated or in need of some extra calories.

Next, you get to weigh in. I'm not going to lie—this isn't fun. You will start to see weights on the scale you have never seen before. At one point during my second pregnancy, I weighed more than my brother-in-law and made the mistake of telling him that. To this day, I have never lived it down! The important thing here is to know that you are supposed to gain weight in pregnancy, and your OB provider will make sure you are gaining the right amount.

You'll also get your blood pressure measured at every visit.

Next, your OB provider will visit with you, feel your belly, and listen for the baby's heartbeat. Finally, there is an opportunity to ask any burning questions that are keeping you up at night. So write down your list and remember to bring it in to your appointment (or jot it in your smartphone).

Q. When can I hear the baby's heartbeat?

It depends. Hearing your baby's heartbeat is different than seeing it. If your first appointment is at seven weeks of pregnancy and you have an ultrasound, you should be able to see the baby's heartbeat. Some ultrasound machines have an audio component that allows you to hear the heartbeat at this point as well.

Most OB providers use a handheld Doppler ultrasound after ten weeks that is placed on mom-to-be's belly. Your baby's heartbeat is much faster than yours. It's ticking at about 120–160 beats per minute and sounds like a galloping horse. The Doppler may also pick up your own, much slower, heart rate of 60–90 beats per minute. After having several of these, you will learn the difference in the rates and noises.

Q. Can I buy my own Doppler?

Yes, but we don't recommend it.

First of all, they are very expensive. Second, using the Doppler requires the experienced hands of someone who has used one about a thousand times. And even in those experienced hands, it can be hard to find the baby's heartbeat, especially early in pregnancy.

What ends up happening is that the pregnant couple can't detect the baby's heartbeat at home and they frantically rush into their OB provider's office. Other times, couples listen cheerfully to mom's pulse instead of baby's heartbeat!

So skip the panic (you'll have your share of that as new parents) and save your money—you'll need it for the college fund.

Q. Should I bring my spouse/partner with me to every visit? Are there some that are more important than others?

It's nice to have both members of the pregnant couple present at every visit, but let's face it, that isn't always possible. It's often hard enough just to fit all those prenatal visits into one person's crazy schedule—coordinating two schedules can be impossible sometimes. (By the way, this will prepare you for juggling your child's future baseball games, dance lessons, and band practice into your own busy lives and getting everyone where they need to be on time and fed . . . but we digress.)

You may have to pick and choose which visits are the most important ones for both partners to attend. Here are the visits I think are the critical ones for the first trimester:

1. **First prenatal appointment.** This is key, especially if this is your first child. The information dispensed is both important and sometimes overwhelming. Four

ears hear more than two. This way, everyone's questions get answered (yes, spouses and partners have questions, too), and both of you can together see your baby for the first time. Yes, your baby may look like a "blob," "speck of dust," "blueberry," or "peanut"—but it's your peanut!

2. **First trimester screening test**. FYI: This is not a routine test, so it doesn't apply to everyone. And there are several different strategies to approaching these tests—here's a brief overview.

   There are two parts to this. The first is a blood test, called a non-invasive prenatal screening test (NIPT or NIPS). It is typically done between ten and thirteen weeks (but can be done anytime after ten weeks and, in some cases, even a little earlier). Blood is drawn and sent to one of many different companies (different OB providers use different companies). This test is a screening test that looks at cell-free fetal DNA found in mom's circulation. It looks at your baby's chromosomes and helps to rule out things like Down syndrome (trisomy 21), Edwards syndrome (trisomy 18), a few sex chromosome abnormalities, as well as some microdeletions. And yes, this is the test that can let you know whether you are carrying a little boy (46XY) or a little girl (46XX).

   The second part of the first trimester screening involves having a perinatologist perform an ultrasound between eleven and thirteen and a half weeks. They check the overall size of the fetus, the thickness of the back of the fetus's neck (***nuchal lucency***) and looks to see whether or not the nasal bone is present. These assessments help the perinatologist determine if a fetus is at higher risk for certain genetic syndromes, birth defects, or miscarriage. More on this in Chapter 6, "Tests." Then, be prepared for more blood to be drawn.

   It's really important for the couple to be present so that a thorough medical history can be obtained from both of you. If you have an egg donor or a sperm donor, bring all the medical information about the donor. And together, you can be advised of any high-risk pregnancy issues. Occasionally, an abnormality is found and additional testing is recommended on the spot. It's nice to have your partner there (or your mom, sister, or best friend) to help make decisions if need be.

Helpful Hint

It's also helpful for your partner to be present at the twenty- to twenty-two-week ultrasound and the thirty-four- to thirty-six-week prenatal visit. We'll explain why in the chapters covering the second and third trimesters.

Partner Tip

Find out what the person carrying the baby *really* wants you to do. She might say she doesn't mind if you can't make it to an appointment (but she really does . . . you know how that goes!). Then try your best to be there!

DR. M'S OPINION:
Partners and Prenatal Visits

Most of the other prenatal visits are pretty routine. If your partner, a trusted family member, or a close friend is able to be there for all the visits, that's great! You may or may not want your partner there for your weigh-ins, blood draws, and urine tests—which, by the end of your pregnancy should be considered an Olympic sport. Crouching over the toilet trying to aim your pee into a teeny, tiny cup gets harder and harder as you get bigger and bigger!

Decisions

As parents-to-be, you will have many decisions to make. Being major planners ourselves, we think it's a good idea to be prepared so you and your partner don't have any surprises. We will put these items on your radar screen for each trimester (and head over to Chapter 11, "Parenthood Prep," for even more decisions to make)! Our advice: Make decisions as a couple. Believe us, unilateral decision-making is not great for maintaining good relations with your beloved. Here are some good conversation starters.

Q. Should we tell all our family and friends we are pregnant, or is it better to wait until I am further along in the pregnancy?

This is a question that comes up often—pretty much with every newly pregnant couple. And it's not an easy answer. We'll give you the facts, and then you can decide for yourself.

Most ***miscarriages*** (loss of pregnancy) occur before the eighth week of pregnancy. Here are the stats: There is a 15 to 33 percent chance of having a miscarriage when someone first finds out they are pregnant.

There are even more miscarriages that happen before someone knows they are pregnant or has taken a pregnancy test. When you add those undiscovered pregnancies into the mix, some experts estimate that up to 50 percent of all pregnancies don't make it.

Obviously, the risk of miscarriage is higher in women who have had previous miscarriages, medical problems, or have ongoing drug or alcohol use. The risk of miscarriage is also higher for women in their thirties and forties. Women who are pregnant with multiples (twins, triplets, or more) also have a higher rate of miscarriage.

> DR. M'S OPINION
>
> *I suggest waiting at least until your first prenatal visit when a heartbeat is detected on a pelvic ultrasound before you announce the pregnancy.*

Now, you may be so excited to discover you are pregnant that you've already told your parents, siblings, the mailman, and everyone in line at your local grocery store. But if you haven't blabbed yet, here is what those stats mean for you. Your OB provider will likely do an ultrasound at your first prenatal visit (seven to ten weeks of pregnancy). The ultrasound determines if the baby's size matches the date of your last menstrual period (LMP). If a heartbeat is detected and the baby's size is equivalent to how many weeks along you are supposed to be, the risk of miscarriage is much lower. That may be all you need to hear before you tell the world the good news.

For other women who fit into the "advanced maternal age" (that is, the over age thirty-five club—don't take it personally) or fertility specialist–assisted pregnancy categories, you may want to wait a few more weeks until more tests are done (first trimester screening test, explained in Chapter 6, "Tests") before everyone finds out your little secret.

Once you've made it to thirteen weeks, the odds are very low that you will miscarry and very high that you won't be able to hide that growing bulge for much longer. So if you really want to wait until the last minute to divulge, you'll have to endure some lengthy stares while people wonder if are you pregnant or just getting thick around the middle.

Obviously, this is your call—just remember that if you decided to announce your pregnancy and then have a miscarriage, you will have to deal with the inevitable questions. While some couples feel it is therapeutic to share their grief with family and close friends, others find talking about a miscarriage to be a painful reminder of their loss. Consider how both of you might handle this situation.

DR. B'S OPINION:

Sharing the News with a Young Child

If you already have a young child/children at home, I suggest waiting to share the news with them until you are actually showing. Pregnancy itself is a fairly abstract concept to a young child. Having a visual aid to follow is helpful. Waiting until after thirteen weeks also increases your odds that the pregnancy is successful. (It's very sad and confusing for the older sibling-to-be if you have to tell them that the baby is "no longer in mommy's tummy.")

I always remind parents that young children have no concept of time—hence the famous "Are we there yet?" line you will hear incessantly from the back seat of your car. Once you tell your older child that a new baby is coming, the sibling-to-be will be rather impatient for that day to come. The later in pregnancy this is announced, the less you will have to deal with the daily explanation!

Reality Check

Here are the stats on spilling the beans to co-workers and employers, from a BabyCenter.com survey:

- 23 percent tell immediately.
- 23 percent wait a few weeks until reality sets in.
- 36 percent wait until after the first trimester (thirteen weeks).
- 14 percent wait until they are starting to show.

Q. Which OB provider should I use for my pregnancy and delivery?

There are many different types of healthcare providers who care for pregnant women. Some provide prenatal care and deliver babies, while others provide prenatal care or support, but don't actually do deliveries. Let's review the different types of providers, and explain their training and background.

- **Obstetricians** ("OB" or "OB-GYN" for short) are medical doctors (MD) or doctors of osteopathic medicine (DO) who have at least eight years of medical training after completing a bachelor's degree in college. They complete four years of medical school, four years in a specialty residency in obstetrics and gynecology, and then complete licensing and board certification. Obstetricians provide prenatal care, perform deliveries (both vaginal and cesarean) and postpartum care. Most OBs take care of both low-risk and high-risk pregnancies, but this varies in different parts of the country. OBs deliver babies in hospitals and carry malpractice insurance.
- **Family OB providers** are also medical doctors (MD) or doctors of osteopathy (DO). After graduating from college, they complete four years of medical school, three years of family practice residency, then licensing and board certification. Some, but not all, programs offer training in obstetrics. Simply put, not all family practice docs take care of pregnant women and deliver babies. Family OB providers who practice obstetric medicine typically only care for routine pregnancies (not high-risk ones). Family practice docs also deliver their babies in hospitals and carry malpractice insurance.

NEW PARENT-TO-BE 411:

Who Is ACOG Anyway?

ACOG stands for the American College of Obstetricians and Gynecologists, a nonprofit organization that represents more than 50,000 obstetricians (doctors who treat pregnant women) and gynecologists (doctors who treat women's health issues). ACOG makes recommendations for the highest standards of medical care for women, including during pregnancy.

To become a member, or fellow, of ACOG, doctors must graduate from an accredited medical school, complete a residency in obstetrics and gynecology, have an active license to practice medicine, and successfully pass the national board examination in obstetrics and gynecology. And most importantly, these docs should be doing annual recertification with ACOG. If your doc was certified thirty years ago and hasn't done anything since, you may want to find someone who has kept up with their credentialing. Look for the letters FACOG after a doctor's name as proof of their credentials.

Being a fellow of ACOG myself, I will refer to ACOG guidelines for pregnancy throughout the book. If you are in the market to find a doctor certified by ACOG, you can ask your primary care doctor or other healthcare professional for a recommendation.

- **Nurse OB providers (NPs)** are registered nurses who have completed additional advanced nursing education (generally a master's degree). In the United States, NPs have state licensing and board certifications. They see patients on their own, under the supervision of a physician. Most nurse OB providers do not deliver babies, although they do provide prenatal and postnatal care. If you use an obstetrician for your prenatal care, your doc may have an NP who sees you for one or more of your visits (especially if the doc has to run out to deliver someone else's baby during office hours!).
- **Midwives.** There are many different types of midwives. We'll go over each type below.
- **Certified nurse midwives (CNMs)** graduate from college, then complete nursing and midwifery training. Some CNMs have a master's or doctoral degree in nurse-midwifery. They attend births in hospitals (although not all hospitals allow midwives to deliver), birthing centers, and at home. CNMs either practice under the supervision of a physician or independently. They offer prenatal and postnatal care. CNMs do not perform ***cesarean sections***. Almost all CNM-assisted deliveries occur in a hospital setting. All fifty states require CNMs to be licensed. Some accept health insurance, and all of them must carry malpractice insurance.
- **Certified professional midwives (CPMs)** either train at an accredited midwifery school or through an apprenticeship, meeting standards of the North American Registry of Midwives (NARM) and the Midwives Alliance of North America (MANA). Individual states regulate credentialing, so there is some variability in the way CPMs practice in each state. CPMs practice independently. They offer prenatal care, home deliveries, and postpartum care. CPMs typically do not take insurance, nor do they carry malpractice insurance.
- **Certified midwives (CM)** have no requirement for previous nursing training or experience. They do have formal midwifery training. Not all states certify or license CMs. Licensed midwives and registered midwives are titles used in some states for the same thing.
- **Traditional midwives (lay midwives)** learn their trade from other midwives or on their own. They rely mainly on the wisdom of thousands of years of midwives before them. Traditional midwives may not have a college degree or any certification. They may perform deliveries in the home or at a birthing center. Let's be clear: There's no requirement to have any formal medical training to call yourself a midwife.
- Lastly, there are **doulas**. Doulas do not provide prenatal care or deliver babies. They are women who offer prenatal and postpartum support, education, breastfeeding counseling, and "labor support." Simply put, a doula will help coach you through your labor. Doulas are great additions to the labor team, especially if a woman wants to attempt labor and delivery without pain medication.

Reality Check

Since a doula will be with you and your partner through the entire labor and delivery, make sure you both like this person and agree with their philosophies.

DR. M'S OPINION:

Who Should Deliver Your Baby?

What type of OB provider should deliver your baby? This is strictly my opinion, and I admit that I am biased based on the method in which I was trained. Here's my take: Most deliveries should occur in a hospital with a physician or a certified nurse midwife.

Why do I feel this way? I trained at Cedars-Sinai Medical Center where approximately 7,000 deliveries take place each year. After four years of work, I saw it all—the good, the bad, and the ugly.

Most of the time, deliveries go great. Mom feels fine . . . baby is perfect . . . bonding occurs . . . everyone goes home elated.

But when something does go wrong in obstetrics, there isn't much time to act. Oftentimes a seemingly normal, low-risk delivery has a completely unforeseen complication at the last minute that takes everyone by surprise. When this happens, it is my opinion that the safest place to be is at a hospital.

Yes, the list of possible complications is long (and we'll discuss these in more detail later in this book). But just consider one possibility: bleeding so severe after delivery (***postpartum hemorrhage***) that the mother needs a blood transfusion and requires a surgical procedure in an operating room. You can't do that at home.

Again, the point is not to scare you. The truth is 95 percent of the time, none of the scary stuff happens. However, you should make an educated decision about who assists you during birth and where your baby is born.

DR. B'S OPINION:

Ditto That

As a pediatrician, I agree with Dr. M and also admit to being biased as a doctor who has seen it all.

While most deliveries are fairly textbook, the occasional emergency is a real emergency. Bad things can happen within the first five minutes of a baby's life that have potential lifelong consequences (like brain damage from lack of oxygen) or can even be fatal. From a pediatrician's perspective: Do you really want to deliver anywhere that is more than five minutes away from a neonatologist (a medical doctor who cares for premature and high-risk newborns) or a neonatal intensive care unit (NICU)?

I delivered both my kids at a hospital that had a NICU right down the hall from the newborn nursery. I never needed their services, but I was glad they were there. This is particularly important if you have a high-risk pregnancy (like having twins). You are more likely to need a NICU, and you won't want to be at one hospital and have your baby/babies transferred to another.

Top Questions to Ask Yourself When Deciding on an OB Provider

1. **Where do you want to deliver?** Do you have a preference for delivering in a hospital, birthing center, or at home? That may influence your provider choice. For instance, if you want to deliver in a hospital, having a midwife may not be an option (it depends on the hospital's policies). If you want to have your baby at home, know that most, if not all, OBs carry malpractice insurance that will not cover home deliveries. And if you have your heart set on one particular hospital, make sure your OB provider does deliveries there. One more thing to consider: Some community hospitals do not have in-house anesthesiologists, neonatologists, or neonatal intensive care units (NICUs). Larger city hospitals and academic institutions routinely have these features available 24/7. Find out what your prospective delivery site offers.
2. **Who did your friends use?** If all roads point to the same OB provider in your circle of friends, you will probably like this person, too. However, if you are the first among your friends to have a baby, call the hospital where you plan to deliver and ask to speak to a friendly labor and delivery nurse. L&D nurses know better than almost anyone which OB providers are competent and nice (even at three a.m.).
3. **Do you have a high-risk pregnancy?** Take a look at the high-risk pregnancy box earlier in this chapter. If the answer is yes, you need an obstetrician, and you should deliver at a hospital.

   Of course, it's possible to start out as a routine, low-risk pregnancy and become high risk if you develop a condition along the way (see Chapter 17, "The Complicated Pregnancy"). If you want to deliver with a midwife or your family OB provider, you'll need to have a backup plan for an obstetrician and a delivery hospital if this happens.
4. **What type of obstetric practice are you looking for?** Obstetric practices come in several flavors. There are solo OB providers, small group practices, and large group practices.

   Some doctors do their own patients' deliveries on weekdays and let the on-call OB handle deliveries on weekends. Others have a delivery-doc-of-the-day every day. And a few doctors, like me, deliver (almost) all their own babies.

   Spoiler alert for the movie *Knocked Up*: Even if your doctor does all their own deliveries, they may still take an occasional vacation or attend a bar mitzvah in San Francisco when you go into labor.

   In any obstetric practice, it's possible to have one doctor do all your prenatal care visits and end up with the doc du jour doing your delivery. Yes, you may be meeting that person for the first time when you are in labor. When you are in the midst of pushing, you probably won't care who the heck is there, as long as that person gets you and your baby through it!

   Some practices utilize nurse OB providers to keep your appointment from being canceled when your doc gets called to a delivery ten minutes before your appointment time. These same nurse OB providers sometimes handle postpartum care (hospital visits after birth). This might be fine . . . or you may prefer a practice where only your doc sees you for all your appointments, knowing that there is a good chance you will have at least one or two appointments rescheduled because someone else's baby is coming.

BOTTOM LINE: Find out with whom your doctor shares on-call responsibilities so you know who may be there for your delivery. Ask to be introduced to the other doc(s).

---

5. **How am I going to pay for this?** Some OB providers accept health insurance; others don't. Even if you have health insurance, you could have to pay a deductible or a portion of the costs for your prenatal visits and delivery. So be sure to check your insurance benefits carefully. When people say having a baby is expensive, they aren't just talking about the cost of diapers!

   All-cash practices (that is, those docs who don't accept insurance) may offer longer office visits and other added services (such as a pledge by your doc to be there at delivery, barring a natural disaster).
6. **Do you prefer a male or female OB provider?** If you have a major preference here, remember to find out with whom your prospective OB provider shares on-call responsibilities. You may or may not be able to control the gender of the OB provider who does your delivery.
7. **If you choose a physician, are they board-certified? If you choose a midwife, are they certified?** While there are no absolute guarantees in life, having an OB provider who is certified should mean they have a certain level of competency and know their stuff. Again, it is important not only to check your OB provider's initial certification but also make sure whomever you choose continues their annual certification. Medicine changes rapidly, and what we learned fifteen or twenty years ago is not usually how we take care of people today.
8. **How much experience does the OB provider have?** Has this OB provider done ten deliveries or 1,000? Being the delivery attendant during medical training counts in these numbers. So even if your obstetrician has entered private practice recently, they've probably logged in at least a couple hundred deliveries during their training. Obstetricians definitely have more hands-on experience (particularly in high-risk pregnancies and deliveries) than family OB providers just by the nature of the medical training they receive.
9. **Does the OB provider have children?** This is certainly not a requirement, but it helps! One doesn't need to have undergone quadruple-bypass surgery to be a great cardiac surgeon. But I can tell you that I learned an enormous amount from going through two pregnancies myself.

   This doesn't just pertain to female OB providers. My ex-husband is also an OB-GYN (you can only imagine what our dinner table conversations used to be—on second thought, don't), and he has told me that he absolutely approaches his pregnant patients differently, with more empathy and with more helpful advice, since we've had children.

   Being pregnant or living with a pregnant person is on-the-job training. There is so much that isn't taught in school or in textbooks. Bottom line: Going through a pregnancy changes your perspective!

10. **Do you feel comfortable with the OB provider?** By far, this is *the* most important question we've asked. After your first appointment, ask yourself—is this OB provider a good fit?

    Having a child is one of the most amazing experiences you will ever have. You want someone you trust, you like, and who will take good care of you.

Top Questions to Ask Your OB provider

You and your selected OB provider need to have the same vision for your birth experience. This is an opportunity to see if this is a good fit. A patient should have the opportunity to discuss their vision for birth at the first visit, but I'm afraid that's not actually the case for some. It may be due to time restraints on the side of the OB provider, or a patient is too scared, nervous, or forgetful to ask. Either way, there should be time for this. If the provider answer is not your cup of tea, one option is wait for a second visit to see if kinks can be ironed out or, yes, schedule another meet-and-greet with a different provider.

We'll put it all together in forty questions to consider asking:

For Doctors

1. Will I see you for all my prenatal visits?
2. Do you have nurse midwives or nurse OB providers on staff?
3. Are there other doctors in your practice?
4. Are there other doctors outside your practice with whom you share on-call responsibilities?
5. What gender are the doctors in your on-call group? (If this is important to you.)
6. If you may not be delivering me, will I have a chance to meet all of the doctors in your practice or on-call group?
7. Where will I deliver?
8. If you perform deliveries in a hospital, is it a teaching hospital or academic center?
9. Will there be residents and medical students present and participating in my labor or delivery?
10. How long have you been in practice?
11. How many deliveries have you done?
12. How do I reach you in case of an emergency?
13. What are your recommendations on pregnancy nutrition, vitamins, and how much weight I should gain?
14. When do you recommend I stop traveling?
15. I work as a ________ (fill in the blank). Are there any risks for my pregnancy due to my occupation?
16. I smoke, drink alcohol, or ________. (Be honest here!) What risks do I face? Do you have any suggestions to help me stop?
17. I take ________ medications regularly. Are these safe to take during pregnancy?

FIRST TRIMESTER

18. I have ________ disease/disorder. Are my symptoms going to worsen during my pregnancy? Will it affect my pregnancy?
19. I had _________ with a previous pregnancy. Is this something I need to worry about with this pregnancy?
20. I have a family medical history of _____________. Do I need to have any special tests done during my pregnancy?
21. My spouse/spouse's family has ____________ medical problem. Do I need to have any special tests done during my pregnancy?
22. How do you feel about inducing my labor?
23. How do you feel about doing an "elective" or scheduled ***cesarean section*** (surgical procedure to remove the baby) without a medical reason for it? (If this interests you.)
24. How do you feel about using ***epidural anesthesia*** (pain medication that numbs the lower part of the body)?
25. Do you work with doulas? Do you have any you recommend?
26. Do you work with acupuncturists? Chiropractors?
27. Do you accept my health insurance plan?
28. If you don't accept my health insurance plan, how much is your fee? Will your office help me get reimbursed by my insurance plan?
29. What are the general costs for a vaginal delivery and for a cesarean section?
30. Are there any other costs for prenatal care, labor, and delivery I should anticipate? (These include blood tests, cultures, imaging studies like ultrasounds, hospital charges, anesthesiologist, etc.)

For Midwives and Home Births

1. How much experience do you have?
2. What was your training like?
3. Are you licensed or certified?
4. Do you work with other midwives?
5. Do you cover for one another?
6. Will you have someone with you at the time of my delivery, or will you be alone?
7. Which prenatal tests do you perform or recommend for your patients?
8. What happens if there is an unexpected complication/emergency during delivery?
9. Do you have an obstetrician you work with in case a problem arises with my pregnancy or delivery?
10. Where is the nearest hospital, and what type of emergency transportation do you have lined up should my baby or I need immediate medical attention?

What's Going on Down There?

For each trimester, we'll give you the 411 on your growing baby. There are some pretty amazing things going on inside your body right now. Let's take a look.

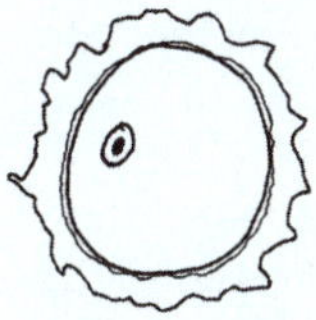

One Week: The egg.

The forty-week countdown for ***gestational age*** has already started, even though the egg and sperm haven't met yet.

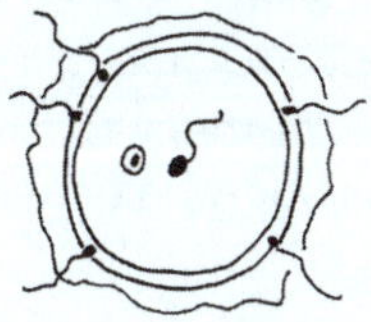

Two Weeks: The egg and sperm meet (fertilization).

Fertilization occurs in the fallopian tube. The fertilized egg begins rapidly dividing, making new cells while it travels toward the uterus.

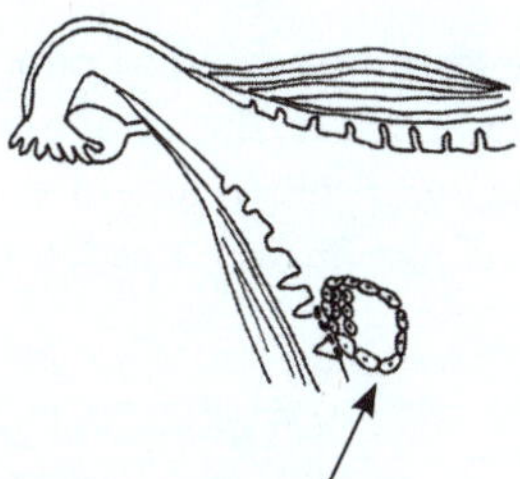

Fertilized egg (morula)

Three Weeks: Implantation.

The ball of rapidly dividing cells (your future baby) is called a morula at this stage. Later, it's called the embryo . . . then the fetus . . . then Jack or Ava. The cellular ball attaches to the lining of the uterus and gets cozy. Three membranes start to form to protect and feed the embryo (their technical terms: yolk sac, ***amnion***, and ***chorion***). Specialized cells invade the wall of your uterus to begin forming the placenta.

Neural tube

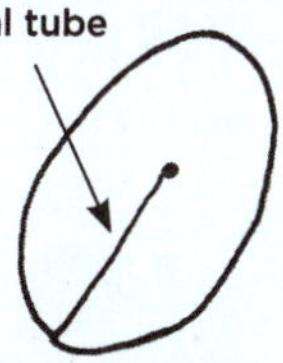

Four Weeks: The embryo.

You can call the ball of cells an embryo now. The embryo already has the crude beginnings of a brain, spinal cord, and nerves (called the ***neural tube***).

Neuropore

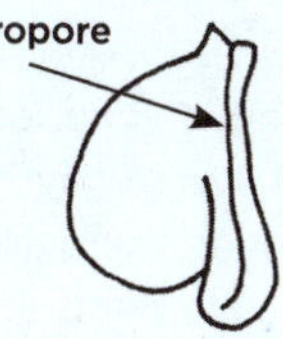

Five Weeks: The embryo.

The embryo has a top end (cranial neuropore) and a bottom end (caudal neuropore). The heart, eyes, ears, and budding arms begin to develop.

Head

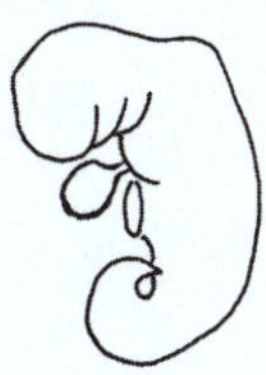

Tail

Six Weeks: The embryo.

The face, arms (including elbows and fingers), and legs start to develop. The crudely formed heart beats (it doesn't have four chambers yet nor a circulatory system to transport blood).

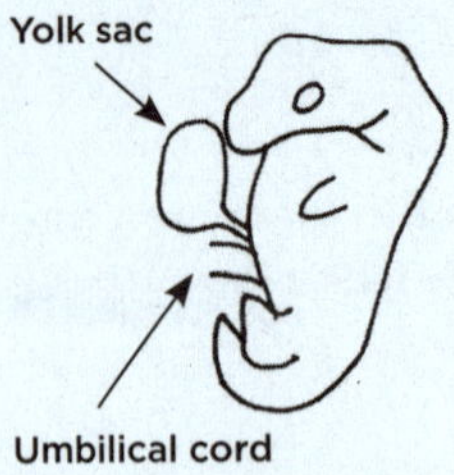

Seven Weeks: The embryo.

Your embryo (baby) now has the beginnings of a nose, mouth, throat, intestines, pancreas, liver, bladder, fingers, and toes. Your embryo also has a little tail (don't worry, that will go away). And their intestines bulge into the umbilical cord. In case you are wondering, the umbilical cord is about fifty centimeters long (just under two feet).

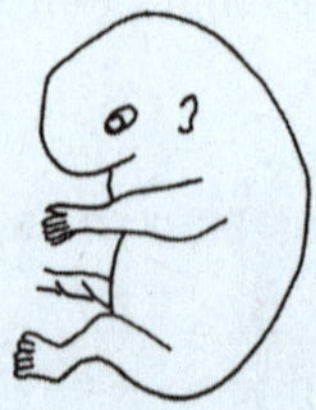

Eight Weeks: The embryo.

The genitals finally start to grow, even though the sex of the embryo was determined way back at fertilization. The heart has four chambers now. The throat forms. The teeth begin developing, although you won't see them until several months after birth.

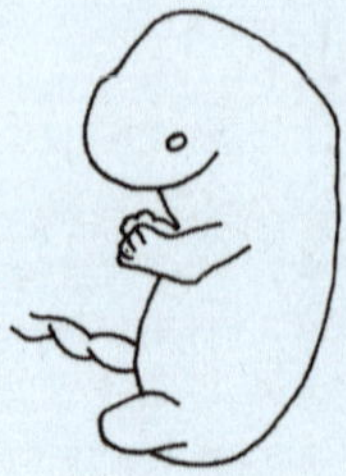

Nine Weeks: The embryo.

All body organs and systems are present. At this point, they develop more and begin functioning. The inner ear develops. Your baby has a nose with nostrils, and an anus that is open. Your little one has fingers, but their toes are still webbed.

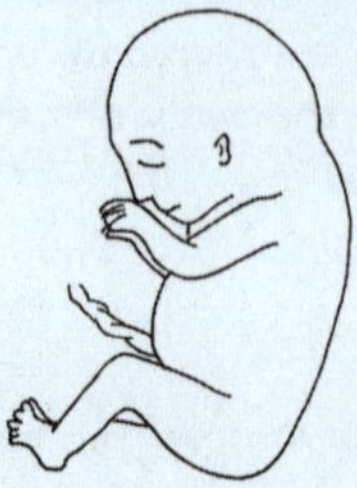

Ten Weeks: The fetus.

Your baby is now a fetus. You can hear their heart beating by Doppler. Their tail is gone, and their taste buds are forming.

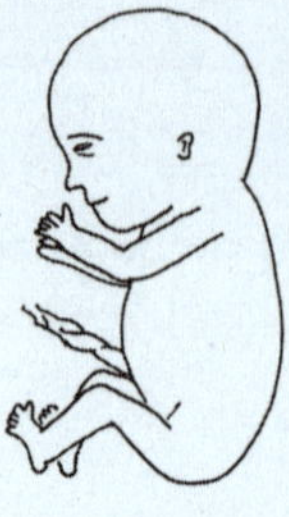

Twelve Weeks: The fetus.

Your baby's mouth is forming. They have vocal cords (although you won't hear what they have to say for a while). Some body organs, like the liver, gallbladder, and pancreas are working. Arms and legs bend at the elbows and the knees.

Q. What's the difference between an embryo and a fetus?

An ***embryo*** is your baby for the first eight weeks after fertilization. Lots of cells divide and organize into future body organs and systems, and believe it or not, most of this organization is complete after just eight short weeks.

After ten weeks gestation, your baby is now called a ***fetus***. In many ways, the die has already been cast. The brain and nervous system, however, are still sensitive to injury throughout pregnancy.

The main job of the fetus is to grow and mature. The fetus will have the most growth in length from three to five months. And they will gain the most weight at eight to nine months. Their head will be half of the body size at eight weeks. At birth, it will be about a quarter of their entire body size.

Reality Check

Unfortunately, you may not even realize that you are pregnant while your baby is in this critical window. So, naturally, you might start to freak out.

Here's our message: relax. Odds are your baby will still be born with ten fingers and ten toes . . . even if you had a martini last week or an X-ray at the dentist.

There's something called the "all or nothing effect" when it comes to potential ***teratogens*** (something that has a negative effect during embryo/fetal development) early in the first trimester. That is, pregnancies where embryos have a significant amount of damage often end up miscarrying rather than going to term and resulting in a newborn with a major abnormality.

Of course, if you find out you're pregnant around four to five weeks, it's time to make some healthy lifestyle changes.

Your baby is most susceptible to exposures that can lead to improper development or malformations (birth defects) during weeks five to ten of gestation—that's the critical period of development. By exposures, we are talking about infections, medications, drug use, vitamin/nutritional deficiencies, environmental toxins, X-rays/radiation, etc.

Critical Periods in Your Baby's Development[1]

The table on the following pages deserves a warning icon since it is discussing birth defects! These are all the things that can go wrong during your growing baby's development. The table demonstrates when certain body parts and systems are developing in the embryo and fetus. The white bar is the most sensitive window of time where body parts or systems are at risk of having an adverse event occur during development. If the birth defect is severe, the embryo will not survive. The gray bar is a less sensitive window of time, but malformations or anomalies can still occur to these body parts or systems.

Critical Periods in Your Baby's Development

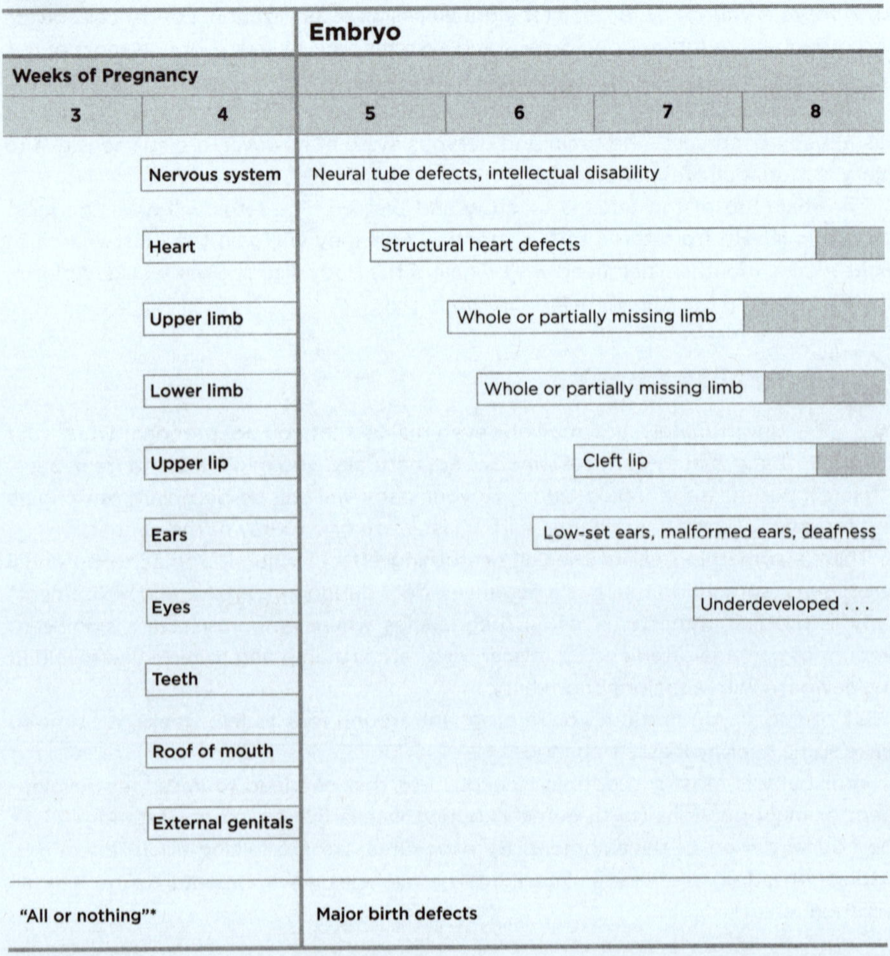

*Either the damage is so great that the embryo dies, or it has little effect and the baby develops without defects.

Q. How does the baby get nutrition while they are growing in the womb?

The ***placenta*** is the middleman between mom and baby. It grows from cells that are originally part of the embryo. The placenta becomes a full-fledged body organ (as you will see at delivery, if you dare!). A blood vessel network is formed between the placenta and the uterus.

The ***umbilical cord*** is the tissue that connects the placenta to the baby with three blood vessels. One blood vessel (the umbilical vein) delivers the food, oxygen, and your antibodies (cells that help fight infection) to the baby. Two blood vessels (the umbilical arteries) send the baby's waste products (including carbon dioxide) back to the placenta. The placenta processes the waste and dumps it into mom's bloodstream again for removal.

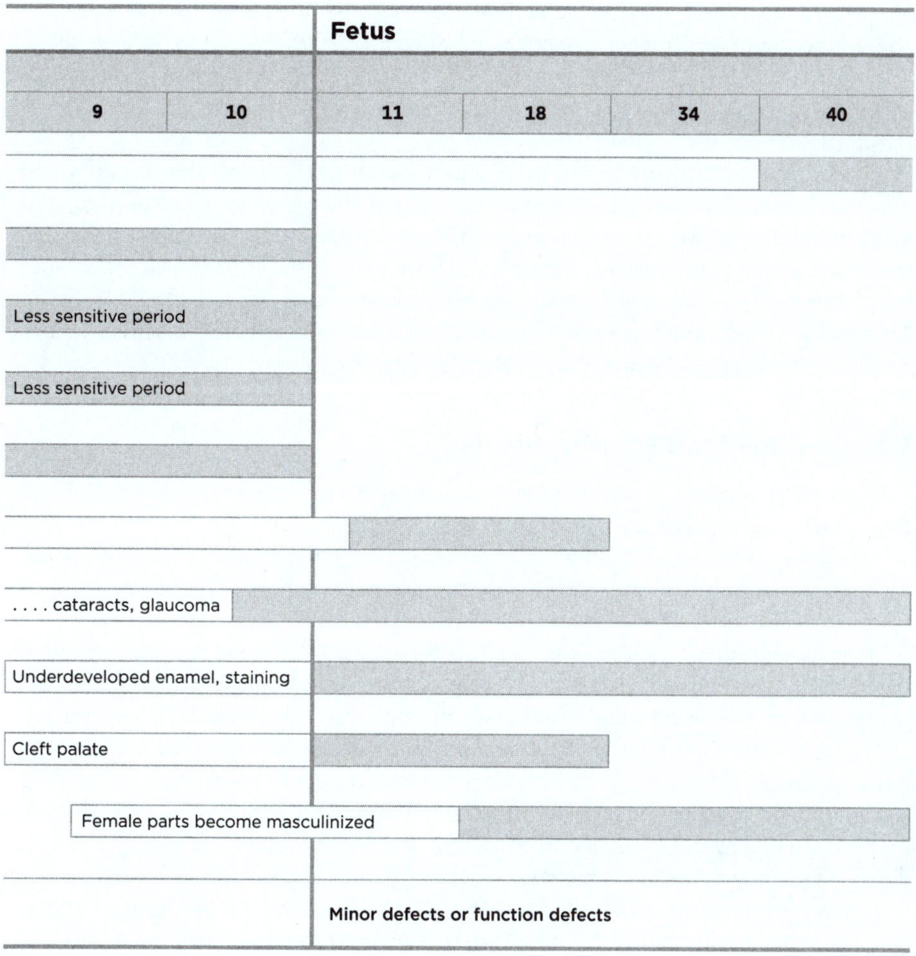

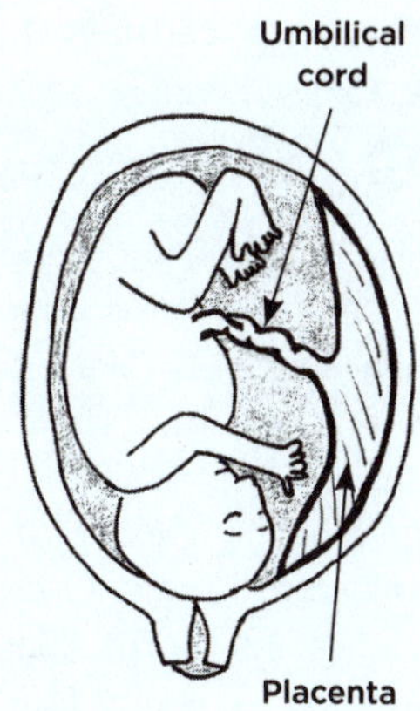

This elaborate system allows mom's body to feed and supply oxygen to the baby and allows baby to eliminate waste, usually without a direct mingling of mother and baby's blood. (There are certain situations where direct mingling occurs, and that's covered in Chapter 17, "The Complicated Pregnancy.") The placenta also makes hormones that nurture pregnancy and initiate labor and delivery.

When your baby is born, they stay attached to the placenta by the umbilical cord. Someone (your healthcare provider or maybe your support person) will cut the cord after placing two clamps on it so the baby will not lose any blood from the blood vessels that remain temporarily intact. And FYI, after you deliver your baby, you will then have to deliver the placenta about three to fifteen minutes later. While it's not nearly as large as the baby (it's about a pound or so), it does have to come out, too.

Reality Check

The good news is that your antibodies travel through the placenta and protect your baby. The bad news is that the placenta is not perfect, and some infections, as well as certain drugs and medications, use that same transit system. Most infections (like the common cold) have no significant health effect on your baby. The ones that can cause problems for your baby are discussed in Chapter 18, "Infections." There are also certain medications that can cross the placenta—these should be avoided. See Appendix A, "Medications," for details.

Q. Does the fetus actually breathe?

This is a trick question. Yes, your fetus practices breathing while in the womb. But, no, they won't breathe in air and get oxygen the way you do.

Your fetus gets oxygen from your blood when they are hanging out in your uterus. You breathe oxygen into your lungs, and that oxygen enters your bloodstream. Your red blood cells carry it through the arteries of your body to all of your organs.

If you are pregnant, the oxygen-rich red blood cells also travel to your placenta. It's here (through an amazing system) that oxygen leaves your red blood cells, attaches to fetal red blood cells, then travels through the umbilical vein to your fetus.

You may catch your fetus breathing on an ultrasound—where their chest wall moves in and out. They are actually taking ***amniotic fluid*** into their lungs, not air. This is very reassuring to see on ultrasound. In fact, it is one of the things we look for if we are concerned about the well-being of a baby. "Practice breathing" is one part of fetal life that tells us your baby is healthy.

When your baby takes their first breath at birth, they begin to get rid of all of that fluid from their lungs. Your little one will also cough and sneeze to help get it out, too, and that's kind of cute to watch! That first breath also triggers a major change in blood flow (circulation) to the lungs to let your baby breathe in air and exchange oxygen for carbon dioxide.

Q. Does the fetus eat, sleep, pee, or poop?

Yes, yes, yes, and hopefully, no.

Yes, your fetus eats, but not through their mouth. There's an all-you-can-eat buffet available 24/7 (like a cruise, minus the food poisoning) through mom's bloodstream. Everything that you take into your body is processed, absorbed into your bloodstream, filtered by the placenta, and taken via the umbilical vein straight to baby. This continues up until birth, when the umbilical cord is cut. That's the first time your baby will actually have to exert some energy and work to eat—breast milk or formula.

Yes, your fetus sleeps. In fact, some researchers think fetuses may start dreaming as early as twenty-four weeks gestation, because they begin to have rapid eye movements around this time.[2] Fetuses have sleep cycles that can last up to ninety minutes,

NEW PARENT-TO-BE 411:

Amniotic Fluid—Your Baby's Private Swimming Pool

Your unborn baby is swimming around in a watery substance called amniotic fluid. After about ten weeks, it is composed of a liquid containing proteins and other vital minerals and nutrients.

Early on, the placenta makes amniotic fluid—although some of it comes from fetal urine (more on that later). By the end of pregnancy, most of the amniotic fluid is composed of fetal urine.

The amniotic fluid levels are maintained by mom's fluid intake and by the fetus's intact digestive tract (esophagus/stomach/intestines/anus) and urinary system (kidneys/ureter/bladder/urethra). The fetus drinks the amniotic fluid, and it then goes through its digestive tract, helping the fetus to form ***meconium*** (the baby's first poop).

The fetus makes urine in their kidneys the same way that we do, and after it's eliminated via the bladder and urethra, it adds to the pool of amniotic fluid. The fetus also breathes amniotic fluid in and out of their lungs. In fact, this is essential for normal lung development.

but unfortunately, they don't always correspond to your sleep patterns. So you might have a sleeping fetus at two p.m. and an active one at two a.m.!

Yes, your fetus urinates. That urine dumps right into the amniotic sac (also known as "the water bag") and helps make up some of the amniotic fluid. The fetus also drinks almost half a quart a day of amniotic fluid. It's kind of gross to think about drinking recycled urine, but it's clean stuff. What we mean by "clean" is that there are no waste products (remember, you and your placenta filter out all the waste) and no bacteria. That same sterile fluid goes in and out of the lungs.

While your fetus does have the ability to poop while inside the womb, they usually don't, and no one wants them to! See information in Chapter 17, "The Complicated Pregnancy."

CHAPTER 3

The Second Trimester

"Women who miscalculate are called mothers."

—Abigail Van Buren

What's in This Chapter

- **Expected weight gain**
- **Six helpful pregnancy purchases**
- **Fundal height**
- **Key decisions: Three good classes**

Welcome to your second trimester (fourteen to twenty-seven weeks)! You're probably feeling a bit more confident and used to being pregnant at this point. But we know you still have a ton of questions. What's going on with your body? When will you start to show (if you haven't already)? How much weight will you gain? Here we go.

Week by Week: The Second Trimester

Fourteen to Fifteen Weeks

Ahh. This is the beginning of the trimester where you will feel your best. Morning sickness should end, and you will feel more energetic than you have for the past several weeks. If you had a healthy ***body mass index (BMI)*** before pregnancy, you should gain about one pound a week from here on out—sometimes a little more, sometimes less. See Chapter 7, "Nutrition," for the scoop on that.

Enjoy being intimate with your partner while it is still fun. See Chapter 9, "Lifestyles," for some take-home tips. Many women develop vaginal infections during pregnancy, so if you have itching or burning down there, check out Chapter 18, "Infections," for some troubleshooting on yeast infections and other causes of unpleasant vaginal discharge.

You will be offered the option of specialized testing (Second Trimester Screen, Amniocentesis) to screen for and/or diagnose chromosome abnormalities. These tests are done between fifteen and twenty weeks. For details, see Chapter 6, "Tests."

Sixteen to Seventeen Weeks

"Are you going to finish that?" You never thought liver and onions would look appealing, and now you want seconds. Your appetite will really pick up, and strange cravings may begin. Visit Chapter 7, "Nutrition," to get a handle on what it means to have a healthy pregnancy diet now that you feel like eating again.

While we are on the subject of mealtime, you also may get some heartburn (and that's not just if you overindulge on Taco Bell). See Chapter 5, "Is This Normal?" for details.

Eighteen to Twenty Weeks

Let the aches and pains begin. Some women start to have back pain, side pain, groin pain, and leg cramps. Not to mention shooting pain around the belly button. Fun, no? See Chapter 5, "Is This Normal?" to figure out if you are just pregnant, or if your symptoms need to be checked out further.

With your expanding belly, your center of gravity starts to change. You will suddenly feel clumsy. Be careful to support yourself and wear comfortable shoes (no more heels, ladies) to avoid falls.

Between eighteen and twenty-two weeks, you will start to feel your baby kicking. Women who have been pregnant before often feel it by fifteen to sixteen weeks. At first, it might feel like gas bubbles. But it will become clear as time goes on that you've got an active baby on your hands.

Your OB provider will begin measuring your baby bump at each visit with a tape measure (***fundal height***). Somewhere between now and twenty-two weeks, you'll likely have a detailed ultrasound to thoroughly assess all of the baby's body parts.

Twenty-one to Twenty-three Weeks

Some women experience mild pelvic cramping (like period cramps) in the second trimester. Sometimes it's just the uterine muscle cramping due to the baby's growth. Or it's early practice contractions (***Braxton-Hicks contractions***). Rarely, it is a sign of preterm labor. The cramps usually go away with some rest and lots of fluids. But you should always let your OB provider decide—pick up the phone. See Chapter 5, "Is This Normal?" and Chapter 16, "Pregnancy 911," for details.

The same rule goes for any time you have spotting or vaginal bleeding during your pregnancy.

This is a good time talk to your OB provider about sleeping on your side and the proper use of seat belts.

Twenty-four to Twenty-five Weeks

If you deliver today, your baby has good odds of surviving. But we do want you to keep that bun in the oven a little while longer.

Between now and twenty-eight weeks, you'll take a test to screen for gestational diabetes (see Chapter 6, "Tests").

If this is not your first pregnancy, you might start feeling practice contractions (***Braxton-Hicks contractions***) now. See Chapter 5, "Is This Normal?" and Chapter 16, "Pregnancy 911." If there is any concern that you might be having signs of preterm labor, call your OB provider.

Between twenty-four and twenty-six weeks, you should feel your baby moving around regularly. That's when it's a good idea to check ***fetal kick counts*** every day. The official recommendation says you should relax for an hour each day and feel ten movements. A more realistic goal: You should feel movement within every twelve-hour period. If you don't sense any movement, or your baby's normal pattern of movement has changed, lie down on your left side, hydrate, have a sugary snack, and see what happens over the next hour. If there is still little or no movement, call your OB provider right away. Check out Chapter 6, "Tests," for a complete discussion.

Twenty-six to Twenty-seven Weeks

You might start having some odd complaints. Here are a few of them: feelings of pins and needles (or numbness) in the legs/feet/hands, a constantly stuffy nose, or frequent nosebleeds and bleeding gums with brushing. Yep, we warned you these are weird. Check out Chapter 5, "Is This Normal?" to see if you are, indeed, normal.

You have very good odds of having a viable baby if they are born right now. If you go into preterm labor (or deliver a premature baby), you will want to read Chapter 20, "Preterm Labor and Babies," for your special concerns.

A few women start to develop high blood pressure as they enter their third trimester. Just as they have been doing the whole time, your OB provider will check your blood pressure at every visit. If you do encounter this problem, check out Chapter 17, "The Complicated Pregnancy" (see Complications #20 and #21).

Remember to do daily fetal kick counts or at least be aware of your baby's movements every twelve hours.

Aches, Pains, and Changes in the Second Trimester (Fourteen to Twenty-seven Weeks)

- Stuffy nose
- Hemorrhoids
- Swollen/bleeding gums
- Darker nipples, leaking early milk
- Feet swelling, if you are on your feet all day
- Belly pain, hip pain, groin pain, back pain, wrist pain, leg cramps
- Itching, chafing, skin tags, red palms and soles, stretch marks
- Nosebleeds
- Heartburn
- Vulvar itching (outer genitals)

Fact Check

Rubbing a pregnant woman's belly gives you good luck.

The truth: It may work for Buddha, but we can't promise the same fortune after rubbing a pregnant person's belly. This won't stop people, though. Folks from all walks of life will stroll up to you and—often without permission—reach a hand out to stroke your tummy.

Be prepared with a courteous way to say, "Hands off."

Common Questions About the Second Trimester

Q. When am I going to start showing? Right now, I just look and feel fat!

This depends on whether this is your first pregnancy, if you are carrying one baby or multiples, and your pre-pregnancy body stature. A tall woman carrying one baby with her first pregnancy may not have a baby bump until twenty weeks. A short woman carrying twins with a second pregnancy may show as early as ten weeks and will be cursing her less vertically challenged friends. *On average, women start showing between thirteen and twenty weeks.*

Unfortunately, for women of all shapes and sizes, you will look chunky—not pregnant—before that cute little baby bump appears. You will have to endure that chunky look (and feeling) through the first trimester and part of the second trimester. Buy a T-shirt that says, "Yes. I am pregnant!" if it makes you feel better.

If this is your first pregnancy, you may not fit into maternity clothes until your second trimester. That's when it will be obvious you have a baby on board. If it's not your first rodeo, pull out those maternity clothes earlier!

Q. How much weight am I supposed to gain this trimester?

Read Chapter 7, "Nutrition," for all the details. It depends on what you weighed (and what your body mass index, or BMI, was) before you were pregnant. But do not get obsessed about it, as these are general guidelines.

Women at a healthy BMI before pregnancy should gain about one pound per week.

Women who are underweight to begin with should probably gain a little more than the standard goal (about one to two pounds per week). Women who are carrying twins or multiples will also gain more. Women who were overweight or obese before pregnancy should gain less than one pound per week.

Partner Tip

Both members of the expectant couple often gain weight during pregnancy. If you want to avoid the equivalent of the proverbial "Freshman 10" for pregnancy, watch what you eat. You are not eating for two!

Q. I am definitely having food cravings! Is this normal? Why does this happen?

Yes, this is very normal. And the basis for all those pickles and ice cream pregnancy jokes.

But why do you have cravings? Your pregnant body needs more calories, and you will feel much hungrier than before.

And sometimes, you will find yourself needing to eat the strangest things . . . and we mean needing. Some women go for weeks at a time just wanting to eat citrus fruits (it was tangerines in Dr. M's case). Others only want pasta. Some can't get enough burgers or fast food. (Taco Bell is a particular favorite among pregnant women for some reason.)

Occasionally, your body will need certain vitamins or nutrients. As an example, it is not uncommon for vegetarians to start craving meat because the body says it needs more iron. Although docs don't know exactly what causes some of the stranger cravings, you can probably blame elevated hormone levels circulating in your body.

BOTTOM LINE: Aim for a well-balanced diet, plus a craving indulgence here or there.

Reality Check

If you begin craving and chewing ice, it may be a sign of iron-deficiency ***anemia***. Let your OB provider know so they can decide whether or not you need a blood test. As strange as it sounds, sometimes an anemic patient will even begin eating detergent, clay, soil, chalk, paper, salt, or soap.

Q. I've heard it's unhealthy for me to sleep on my back. Is this true?

After twenty weeks, avoid lying on your back all night. This prevents your big ol' pregnant uterus from putting pressure on your major blood vessels (the aorta and vena cava). It's best to lie on your left side for optimal blood circulation, but the right side is okay as well.

If you wake up and realize you have ended up sleeping on your back, don't panic! Just roll over, get comfy, and go back to sleep.

Q. When will I feel my baby kicking?

If this is your first pregnancy, you should feel the baby moving (called ***quickening***), between eighteen and twenty-two weeks. If you've done this pregnancy thing a time or two already, you may feel quickening as early as fifteen to sixteen weeks.

The first time you feel this sensation, you may think it's gas. It may feel like little bubbles, little thumps, or perhaps a flick against your belly. But you won't be able to see action happening on the outside of your belly—yet. That type of movement, which will begin to look like something out of the movie *Alien,* won't happen until you are about twenty-eight weeks.

If you were overweight pre-pregnancy or if your placenta lies closer to your belly and in front of the baby (anterior placenta), rather than under the baby (posterior placenta), it may take a few more weeks before you feel this sensation.

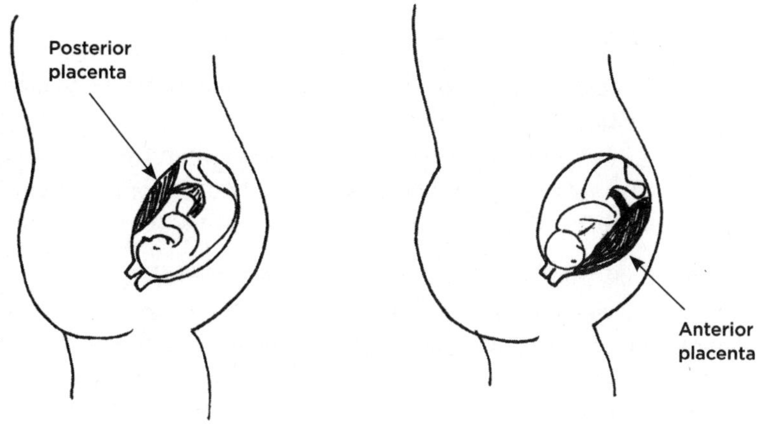

Q. When is it possible to determine the sex of the baby?

It depends on what testing you have done. If you want to know your baby's gender (and you are lucky), your doc can sometimes identify the girl or boy parts as early as twelve weeks on an ultrasound. A later ultrasound done between sixteen to seventeen weeks has better odds of showing the family jewels.

Don't get your hopes up, though. The fetus has to be willing to show off. If you have a more modest fetus, who sits with their legs crossed, you may not be able to see anything. (That was the case with both of Dr. M's kids. Dr. B wanted to be surprised.)

If you are over the age of thirty-five (and sometimes even if you are younger), you may be offered one of a few blood tests that can detect fetal DNA in your blood. Therefore, your doc can tell you (with over 99 percent certainty) not only that there aren't any major chromosomal problems but also whether you are having a boy or a girl! Amazing, no?

If you have a ***chorionic villus sampling*** (see Chapter 6, "Tests,") between ten and thirteen weeks, you can find out without question whether your baby has XX (girl) or XY (boy) chromosomes. An ***amniocentesis*** (see Chapter 6, "Tests") at fifteen to twenty weeks can determine gender from the chromosomes as well.

Today, many parents-to-be want to find out the baby's sex in advance. Dr. M rarely gets to say "It's a boy" or "It's a girl" at the delivery anymore, as did OBs of yesteryear. That said, there are no rules here on whether you should know or not. It's helpful if you want to know which color to paint the nursery or if you need to make a circumcision decision. However, this is a personal decision that you need to make as a couple. We don't recommend having one partner know, while the other partner's in the dark. The secret is bound to slip out!

Speaking of which, if you *don't* want to know the sex of your baby, tell your OB provider to write in big, bold letters across the top of the chart, "Patient does not want to know sex of baby!" And feel free to remind anyone remotely involved with ultrasounds, looking in your chart, or providing you with lab results.

Fact Check

You can tell the sex of the baby depending on how fast the baby's heart beats.

The truth: The heart rate of a fetus is usually between 120 and 160 beats per minute. Just like us, that rate increases with activity. A faster heart rate might mean you have an active baby on your hands—but it doesn't tell you the sex of your baby.

You can tell the sex of the baby based on how you are carrying.

The truth: The way you carry (the shape and distribution of your baby bump) during your pregnancy is based on a few things, but the baby's sex isn't one of them.

A woman with a deep pelvis can hide a pregnancy longer and look like she is carrying lower. A woman who is heavier than her ideal body weight pre-pregnancy may have more fatty tissue over her belly, and this can change the shape. A woman pregnant with her first doesn't show as quickly as with her third.

BOTTOM LINE: People can guess about the baby's sex, but your shape won't predict whether you are having a boy or girl.

Six Really Helpful Pregnancy Purchases

1. **Bump-friendly underwear.** When you already feel bad about how you look, it can be really demoralizing to outgrow your sexy little thong undies. You may end up biting the bullet if you find it more comfortable to wear maternity underwear. However, we've come a long way in the underwear department, baby! There are a few styles of thong underwear that are actually comfortable to wear during pregnancy. For example, Hanky Panky and Cosabella brand thongs are low enough that they sit below a blossoming belly. Some pregnancy stores even sell maternity thongs.
2. **Maternity belt.** Meet your new best friend. As your belly grows, it can start to ache—both in the front and back.

   The curvature of your spine changes, and so does your center of gravity. The bigger your belly gets, the more you will feel the aching. This usually happens earlier and earlier with each subsequent pregnancy.

   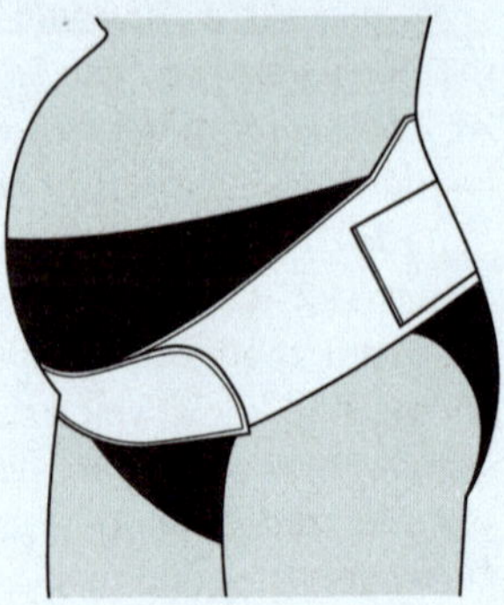

   I am a big believer in maternity belts. You can buy them at most maternity stores. They really help lift the belly up and relieve some of the pressure and discomfort. But you have to wear them correctly to get relief. You need to try on many different styles and decide what fits best before you purchase. Don't buy one online!

   Note: An extra pair of hands is invaluable when

trying to put on the belt. You will need to lift your belly up, and the extra pair of hands you are borrowing for the moment (your partner, friend, neighbor, or completely uninterested third grader) can adjust the Velcro on the belt.

It can be a real quality-of-life-saver for pregnant women who have belly, back, and leg pains.

3. **Nursing pads.** Although you won't be breastfeeding until after delivery, your breasts may start to make and leak fluid (***colostrum***) as early as the end of your second trimester. If you'd like to keep your breast incontinence (that is, wet spots on your blouse) a secret from co-workers and friends, nursing pads are a wise investment. And even if you don't use them much now, you'll definitely need them after delivery.
4. **Support hose.** This is another unattractive fashion accessory for the well-dressed pregnant gal. Compression socks or stockings help reduce swelling in your feet and improve blood flow in your legs. They come in white, beige, or black knee-highs and white only thigh-highs (there's no need for a garter belt—they have tight elastic at the top). You can buy them at most pharmacies. Some women wear them only at night; others wear them all day long. You'll thank us for recommending them around the beginning of your third trimester or anytime you take a plane trip.
5. **Pregnancy pillow.** Sleep is tough throughout your entire pregnancy. Getting comfortable and falling asleep is hard from the first trimester on, but as your body changes and your belly grows, finding a good position at night to sleep well is a mounting challenge. A pregnancy pillow or maternity pillow is a large curved pillow with support for your back, legs, belly, head, and hips. It can be paramount in helping you get into just the right position to get some good sleep. You can find one online or in one of many chains like Walmart or Target. Warning: It's a pretty big pillow and may temporarily replace your partner or dog on the bed!
6. **Large water bottle/thermos.** Water intake is a big deal in pregnancy. Not only does your blood volume double, but you are making amniotic fluid for your baby, and both of these feats require extra water. It's also common to get dizzy and fatigued without enough water intake. Carrying a large insulated water bottle with you throughout your day, in your car, and to work can help ensure you are getting enough water. A quick rule of thumb to know how much water you'll need is to divide your weight in pounds by two. That number is the number of ounces you need per day. You can see that as you continue to gain weight, your water need will increase.

Prenatal Care

You will visit your OB provider every four weeks in the second trimester. If you have an uncomplicated pregnancy, typically you'll have a total of four visits. Although it varies a bit, plan on appointments around fourteen to fifteen weeks, eighteen to nineteen weeks, twenty-two to twenty-three weeks, and twenty-six to twenty-seven weeks of pregnancy.

Q. What happens at my prenatal appointments during this trimester?

These visits are pretty routine if all is going well. You will get weighed (you don't have to look), and you will need to pee in a little cup (you do have to look) at every visit. You'll also get your blood pressure measured at every visit. Some women have high blood pressure before pregnancy. Others may develop it during pregnancy. Doing this simple test makes sure any elevation is detected.

Next, your OB provider will visit with you, feel your belly, listen for the baby's heartbeat, and, if you are beyond twenty weeks, measure the baby's size by measuring the ***fundal height*** (see box below). Then you can ask questions and discuss aches, pains, and other fun body changes you are experiencing.

Q. Are there any routine tests done in the second trimester?

Yes. There are two important tests:

- **The one-hour glucola test.** This involves drinking a sugary liquid and then getting your blood drawn to assess for pregnancy-related diabetes (***gestational diabetes***). This test occurs between twenty-four and twenty-eight weeks.
- **Fetal kick counts.** Your OB provider will instruct you to tune in to your baby's movements on a daily basis, starting at twenty-four to twenty-six weeks. This is a critical indicator that your baby is thriving, and it's kind of fun.

We will discuss both of these tests in detail in Chapter 6, "Tests."

Q. Are there any additional tests that I need to ask my OB provider about?

Yes, and you should learn more about these tests Chapter 6, "Tests."

- **Second trimester screen** (also known as ***AFP***, expanded AFP, QUAD screen, full-integrated screen). This blood test assesses the chances of a fetus having ***Down syndrome***, trisomy 18, and a few serious abnormalities. Testing occurs between fifteen and twenty weeks.
- **Ultrasound.** Also known as the anatomy scan. While it isn't routine, it is very common to perform a comprehensive ultrasound between twenty and twenty-two weeks to examine all the body parts of the fetus.
- **Amniocentesis.** Using a minor procedure, a doctor obtains amniotic fluid that can diagnose chromosome defects and some medical conditions in the fetus. Testing occurs between fifteen and twenty weeks.

Q. Are there any more ultrasounds?

Many (but not all) OB providers will perform an ultrasound at the end of the second trimester (twenty-eight weeks) or in the early third trimester (thirty-two weeks) to assess fetal growth and measure the amniotic fluid.

There are also special situations that require ultrasounds at every visit. For example, women who have had preterm labor with a previous pregnancy may need regular

NEW PARENT-TO-BE 411:

Fundal Height

Fundal height is the measurement from the pubic bone to the top of the uterus (called the uterine fundus).

Your OB provider will get out a little tape measure and push on the top of your belly to determine the fundal height. It is a very old but useful technique to estimate the size of both the baby (fetus) and the other contents of the uterus (placenta, amniotic fluid). Fundal height is measured in centimeters (cm), starting at about twenty weeks, which is when the top of the uterus is at the level of your belly button. At each visit, the number measured in centimeters should be roughly equal to your pregnancy in weeks. For example, if you are thirty-two weeks along, your fundal height should be roughly thirty to thirty-four centimeters.

There are always exceptions to the rule, but in general, it is a quick and easy way to assess the growth of a fetus and uterus. For instance, if you have been on target with all of your measurements and suddenly measure three weeks smaller in centimeters than would be appropriate for your dates, an ultrasound would be warranted to make sure your baby is growing well and that there is an appropriate amount of amniotic fluid.

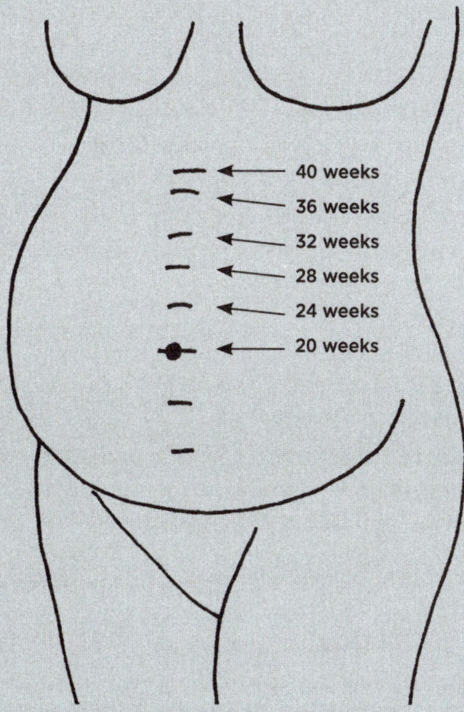

ultrasounds to assess the length of their ***cervix***. This may also apply to women who have had procedures on their cervix (LEEP, conization) or who have a history of ***cervical insufficiency***. Women carrying more than one fetus also get more ultrasounds. We'll pontificate about issues of the cervix later in this book (see Complication #34 in Chapter 17, "The Complicated Pregnancy").

Q. Which visits are the most important for my partner to attend?

We personally vote for the twenty- to twenty-two-week ultrasound. If you did not have a first trimester ultrasound, this is a great time to catch your baby looking like a baby for the first time on screen. But beware, from some angles, your baby will look . . . well, extraterrestrial (you'll know what we mean when you see the ultrasound pics).

But seriously, this ultrasound evaluates every little part and organ of your baby from the brain to the toes. It's amazing to see your baby moving around on the screen. In fact, it's priceless.

Decisions

This section covers the classes we recommend taking before going into labor. The only decision you need to make is when you and your partner can both attend!

- **Childbirth classes.** If this is your first baby, take these classes. Note: There are different ways to approach labor and the childbirth process. Do your homework by reading Chapter 13, "Home Stretch," to see which type of class is right for you. It's best to take these classes between twenty-eight and thirty-four weeks of pregnancy. Sign up now so you can graduate from childbirth class before you go into labor! You have a couple of options here.
    1. Community hospitals usually offer small-group sessions that meet several times over a period of weeks or one mega-weekend/couples retreat. If you and your partner have busy schedules, it can be a challenge to coordinate. That leads to Option #2.
    2. Hire a childbirth educator to come to your home for a private class. If you've hired a doula to help you with birth, she will most likely offer these sessions with you and your partner.
- **Breastfeeding classes.** These classes help to prepare for breastfeeding before baby arrives. They are also useful to scope out breast pumps and identify a lactation consultant. Your OB and/or pediatrician can provide recommendations, if need be.

    While your body may be naturally prepared for breastfeeding, your brain is not. Think of a breastfeeding class like driver's ed. You won't get to use your skills until you get behind the wheel for the first time.

    The best time to take a breastfeeding class is thirty-two to thirty-eight weeks. And yes, the class is for both partners. The non-breastfeeding partner will learn how to aid the breastfeeding partner and baby.

- **Infant CPR class.** All new parents should take an infant CPR class. Of course, it's easiest to carve out time to take it before your baby is born. You'll thank us for telling you to do this when your baby crawls over to the dog food bowl, digs in, and chokes on a morsel. Yes, this happened to Dr. B with her first baby!

What's Going on Down There?

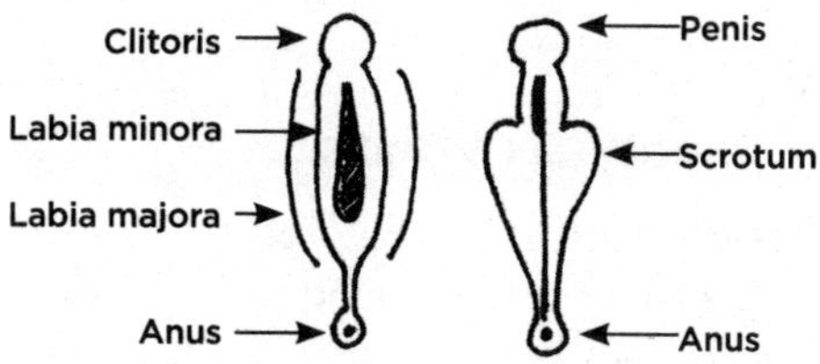

FEMALE ANATOMY **MALE ANATOMY**

Fourteen Weeks.

Big news! We can now easily see if you are carrying a boy or a girl. If you have a boy, you might catch a glimpse of his penis and scrotum on ultrasound. Don't be disappointed if your OB provider can't tell you what you are having yet, though, as it's often tough to see until about sixteen weeks. The testes sit inside the abdomen for several more weeks and then migrate down to the scrotum as your fetus nears the end of his development. For girls, the clitoris and labia form on the outside and the ovaries mature inside the abdomen.

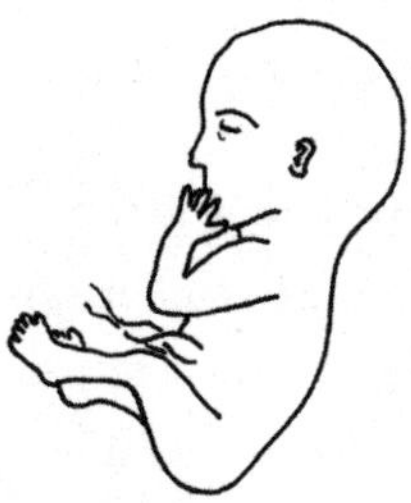

Sixteen Weeks.

The fetus can suck their thumb, swallow, "breathe," and pee. Their lungs practice inhaling and exhaling, even though amniotic fluid (not air) is going in and out. The circulatory system (that transports blood throughout the body) functions now. And your baby's kidneys start making urine.

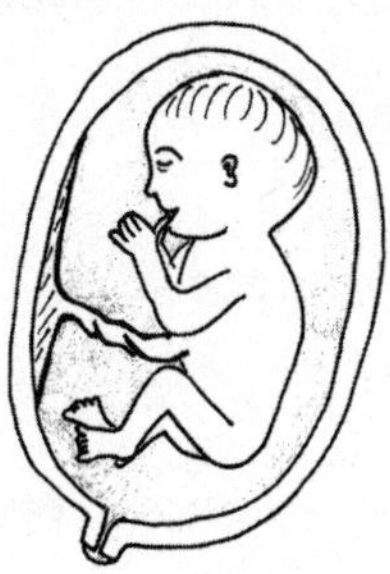

Twenty Weeks.

A cheesy covering (***vernix***) appears, protecting the skin from the watery environment of the amniotic fluid. Your baby has head and body hair, including eyebrows. They are making brown fat, which they will use for heat production as a newborn. Their bones are hardening.

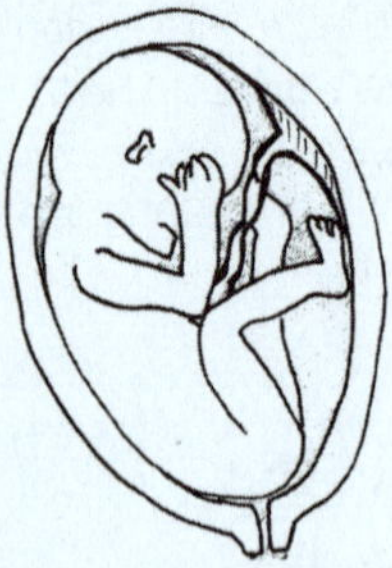

Twenty-four Weeks.

Your baby has reached viability. It's possible that they can survive life outside the womb at this point if they are delivered prematurely. The fetus can use their ears to hear and their legs to kick (you'll feel that "quickening" occasionally!). They now have rapid eye movements and blink/startle in response to noise.

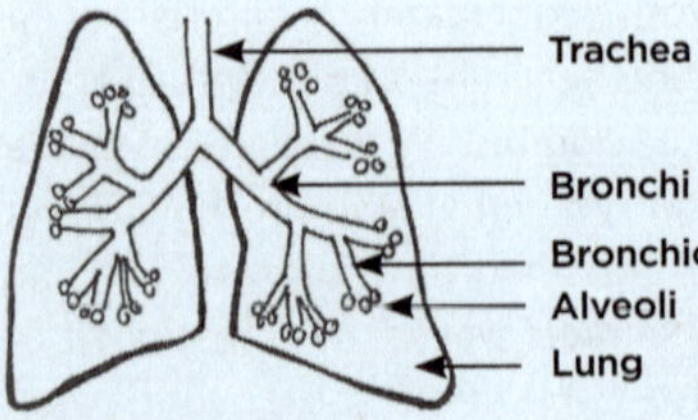

THE LUNGS

Twenty-six Weeks.

Surfactant is the big news this week. Special cells in the lungs make a soapy substance called surfactant, which keeps the tiny airways open. Surfactant is critical to helping lungs do their job outside the womb. (Remember this when we discuss prematurity later on in the book.)

Q. When can a fetus survive outside the womb?

The official term is ***viability***. It's based on both the ***gestational age*** (number of weeks in pregnancy) and fetal weight. ACOG and the Society for Maternal-Fetal Medicine carefully and thoughtfully review the data, and their most recent findings are:[1]

- Babies at twenty-three weeks gestation have a 23–27 percent survival rate.
- Babies at twenty-four weeks have a 42–59 percent survival rate.
- Babies at twenty-five weeks have a 67–76 percent survival rate.

The Eunice Kennedy Shriver National Institute of Child Health and Human Development has a useful tool to calculate survival rates based on several factors. Find it here: nichd.nih.gov/research/supported/EPBO/use.

Of note, babies who are born extremely early and survive may face significant neurodevelopmental impairment.

For details, see Chapter 20, "Preterm Labor and Babies."

Q. Is it true that my baby will recognize my voice when they are born?

Yes.

The ear is completely formed by twenty-four weeks gestation, but studies show that hearing may begin as early as sixteen weeks. And a mother's voice reaches her fetus with much more strength and intensity than music, the dog barking, or even the jackhammer down the street. Your voice will even resonate above the sound of rushing blood in your blood vessels, your heart beating, and your gurgling digestive tract. It's a wonder that a fetus can sleep with this cacophony!

So whether you are singing your unborn baby a lullaby or yelling at the car in front of you as they abruptly cut you off, your baby will hear you and recognize your voice at birth.

CHAPTER 4

The Third Trimester

"Children are a great comfort in your old age—
and they help you reach it faster, too."

—Lionel Kauffman

What's in This Chapter

- **Sleeping troubles**
- **Real versus practice contractions**
- **Why your undies are wet**
- **Key decisions timeline**

That's it for the second trimester! Let's count down the final weeks of pregnancy.

Week by Week: The Third Trimester

Twenty-eight Weeks

If you have a routine pregnancy, you will start visiting your OB provider every two weeks now until about thirty-five to thirty-six weeks, when visits become weekly.

Here is a little insight into your last trimester: Your baby may start having hiccups, which you will feel. They can last for a few minutes or even a few hours. They might feel like repetitive little flicks or spasms against your belly. No worries.

You may start to feel short of breath, even at rest, as your enlarging uterus and baby push against the muscle that sits below your lungs. Swelling of the legs, feet, or fingers is common now. Your genital area may swell as well.

It's normal to retain some fluid, but check out Chapter 5, "Is This Normal?" to learn when a little swelling has become too much. You may also start to have low back pain, as the curvature of your spine changes. If you haven't discovered a maternity belt yet, get one now.

Some women become anemic around this time, so if you are feeling more fatigued (than usual) or begin craving or chewing ice, be sure to tell your doctor. See Complication #13 in Chapter 17, "The Complicated Pregnancy."

Your blood type was tested at your first prenatal visit. If your blood type is Rh negative, you will need an injection of the medication RhoGAM at twenty-eight weeks to prevent your body from mounting a potential immune response against any future babies. See Complication #14 in Chapter 17, "The Complicated Pregnancy." You'll get another shot after delivery if your baby is Rh positive.

Start interviewing potential pediatricians. Take childbirth classes within the next six weeks. Consider taking a breastfeeding class and infant CPR class as well. While you probably have another ten to twelve weeks before you deliver, it's better to be prepared. Read Chapter 11, "Parenthood Prep," for details.

If you want to hire a doula (delivery assistant), now is the time to start doing interviews.

Be aware of fetal movements—continue checking fetal kick counts.

Twenty-nine to Thirty Weeks

You might start to become constipated again (especially if you are taking iron supplements). And constipation only makes hemorrhoids worse—yes, hemorrhoids show up around this time. Work on increasing fiber and water intake. You may even need a stool softener.

This is the time in your pregnancy when your skin might change. Your nipples may get darker, or you might get a dark line from just above your pubic hair to your belly button. You may also see some strange hair growth on your face, arms, belly, or around your nipples. Great, huh? At least the hair on your head and your fingernails get some benefits while you are pregnant—they grow like weeds. See Chapter 5, "Is This Normal?" for details.

Check fetal kick counts every day.

Thirty-one to Thirty-three Weeks

You might start leaking fluid from your breasts (***colostrum***). That's just your body's way of preparing you for the weeks ahead. If you plan on breastfeeding, be sure to read up on things you can do now to make it a success. See Chapter 12, "Feeding Your Newborn."

Your uterus may harden up intermittently—and you'll feel it. These are called ***Braxton-Hicks contractions***. While these are technically contractions, they will feel different from the real deal when you are in labor. This chapter will help you figure out the difference. And check out Chapter 5, "Is This Normal?" for more info. If you have any concern that you might be in preterm labor, pick up the phone and call your OB provider.

Your baby is still swimming around in amniotic fluid. They will start moving to their planned position for birth in the next few weeks.

Now is the time to think about circumcision—will you want to have it done? Who will perform the procedure? You will want to discuss this with your OB provider.

Decide if you want your newborn to receive optional screening tests after birth—if so, you will need to order a collection kit. The same goes for cord blood banking. See Chapter 11, "Parenthood Prep," for details.

Check fetal kick counts every day.

Thirty-four Weeks

Any energy you had during your second trimester is a distant memory now. Fatigue returns to your body (which is a bit larger than your body of yesteryear), and it's difficult to get comfy for a good night's rest.

Stretch marks start to make their appearance. Your skin, especially your belly skin, might get itchy. Some women even get chafing around rolls of skin they never had previously. Check out Chapter 5, "Is This Normal?" to see if it is okay and Chapter 10, "Self-Care," to see what you can do about it. You also may need to buy some new shoes because your pre-pregnancy ones might not fit anymore! While you are at it, pick up some support stockings to reduce wicked leg cramps, varicose veins, and swelling.

If you deliver today (up until thirty-seven weeks), you will have a ***late preterm infant***. See Chapter 20, "Preterm Labor and Babies," for what that means for you and your baby.

Read Chapter 13, "Home Stretch," and Chapter 14, "Labor Day," to prepare for the big day. If you are a real planner, read Chapter 15, "Postpartum: What's Next?" Your OB provider will probably sit down with you and discuss your labor and childbirth goals and desires around your thirty-two- to thirty-four-week office visit.

We know you know, but keep checking fetal kick counts daily.

Thirty-five Weeks

If this is your first pregnancy, your baby may start to head downward into your pelvis this week (***lightening***). Don't believe your friends when they tell you that once the baby drops, labor is right around the corner. Some babies drop five weeks in advance; others (especially when it's not your first baby) won't drop until labor begins. Once this happens, you may start to feel better. Why? Shortness of breath and heartburn may go away. But now your baby is pushing against your bladder, so you will be urinating even more often (seems absolutely impossible, doesn't it?).

Keep checking daily fetal kick counts. Time to pack your hospital bag and get that car seat installed!

Thirty-six Weeks

Feeling wet down there? It might be because your body is making even more vaginal discharge or because you are leaking urine. Concerned your water may have broken? Look for "Wet Undies 411" in the "Common Questions About the Third Trimester" section in this chapter. If you are still unsure, it's always good to talk with your provider.

You are entering the home stretch! You will see your OB provider once a week until you deliver. You'll have an internal exam at some of these visits, so you can mentally prepare for that.

Between now and 37 6/7 weeks, your OB provider will do a culture to see if you carry a bacteria called ***Group B strep***.[1] If you are a carrier, you'll need to take antibiotics, but only when you go into labor (see Chapter 6, "Tests").

The internal exam will also help assess your body's readiness for delivery. Your OB provider will be able to tell if your cervix is ripening (getting softer and opening up).

They will determine if your baby is starting to move down toward the exit and what position they plan to be in (hopefully, head first—called ***vertex***). Spotting after an exam like this is frightening, but it's normal. See Chapter 17, "The Complicated Pregnancy."

Keep up those fetal kick counts.

Thirty-seven Weeks

Your baby is considered "early term," which means your baby is likely to have mature lungs (if your dates are exact). Even so, every week counts. You may still be pregnant until your due date (or beyond). You'll be hot and sweaty from here until delivery day, even if you are fortunate enough to deliver in the winter.

You might discover a clear glob in the toilet after you've peed for the umpteenth time this week. That's your ***mucous plug,*** which seals off your cervix and protects your uterus throughout pregnancy. As your cervix ripens (softens and opens), the plug might fall out. Sorry, but it doesn't mean you are in labor. It can fall out as your body makes its final preparations for childbirth. That could be tomorrow or in three weeks. Some women never see their mucous plug come out, and sometimes it comes out at delivery.

Make sure you read Chapter 13, "Home Stretch," Chapter 14, "Labor Day," and Chapter 15, "Postpartum: What's Next?," if you have not gotten around to it yet.

Have we mentioned to check fetal kick counts every day?

Thirty-eight Weeks

You are probably peeing every couple of hours now. And thus, you are not sleeping more than a couple of hours at a time.

Even though you are more than ready to give birth, your baby is more likely to be ready to go at thirty-nine to forty weeks. Don't beg, plead, or try to bribe your OB provider into an early induction or scheduled ***C-section***. Sometimes, dates are off, and you might have a baby who is younger than billed. Those babies can potentially end up with longer hospital stays or problems not normally encountered with a full-term baby. Be patient. You are almost there.

Fetal kick counts!!

Thirty-nine Weeks

Don't plan any major events. You could go into labor any day! On the flip side, you could also be sitting around twiddling your fingers for another week or two.

If you start having regular contractions and pass blood-tinged discharge (***bloody show***), you are going into labor. Congratulations! See Chapter 14, "Labor Day," for what happens next.

It's especially important now to continue checking daily fetal kick counts.

Forty Weeks

This may be the week you meet your baby for the first time (we hope!) . . . or maybe not. Your baby cannot stay in your womb until kindergarten, so it's just a matter of time. Hang in there!

You and your OB provider may start having a conversation about inducing labor if there's no activity going on down there. You may also be hooked up to a few monitors to have a non-stress test (NST) and an ultrasound to make sure your baby can safely continue in the uterus. Read Chapter 13, "Home Stretch," to learn about the ***Bishop score,*** which can predict if you will have a successful induction.

Check fetal kick counts until you deliver.

Forty-one Weeks

Still pregnant? Check out information on post-term babies in Chapter 17, "The Complicated Pregnancy" (see Complication #48), and being induced in Chapter 13, "Home Stretch."

Aches, Pains, and Changes in the Third Trimester (Twenty-eight to Forty Weeks)

- **Moody, tired, emotional again**
- **Stuffy nose**
- **Swollen/bleeding gums**
- **Heart palpitations**
- **Spider veins, varicose veins**
- **Mild shortness of breath without chest pain**
- **Practice contractions (Braxton-Hicks)**
- **Frequent urination, urinating at night, leaking urine**
- **Itching, chafing, stretch marks, sweatiness**
- **Belly pain, hip pain, groin pain, back pain, wrist pain, leg cramps**
- **Enlarging breasts with darker nipples, prominent veins, stretch marks**
- **Constipation, gas, burping, heartburn, hemorrhoids, shooting pain in the vagina and rectum**
- **Trouble sleeping**
- **Nosebleeds**
- **Early breast-milk leaking**
- **Swollen hands, fingers, feet**
- **Pelvic cramps**

Common Questions About the Third Trimester

Q. How much weight am I going to gain?

In the final leg of this journey, you will probably gain about one pound a week if you were at a healthy weight before pregnancy. Don't be surprised, though, if your weight plateaus near the very end. And occasionally, women may even lose a pound or two right before a due date is reached.

Q. I am having trouble sleeping. Any advice?

At some point during your pregnancy, you will dread going to bed at night. Trying to fall asleep (and stay asleep) will be priceless. Here are some tried and true tricks to help you sleep through the night:

Create a nest of pillows—one under your head, one between your knees, one to hug, and one under your feet. Buying a body pillow (sold at big-box stores as well as online) may be a good investment—most are modestly priced. One reader favorite is the Leachco Snoogle Total Body Pillow.

As you build a fortress of pillows around yourself to get cozy, your bed partner will get shoved farther and farther away—perhaps onto the couch or into another bedroom if you don't have a king-size bed! Note to partners: Remember, it's not about you.

Avoid caffeine altogether. Even having an iced tea at lunch can sometimes be enough to keep you up at night.

Empty your bladder right before hopping into bed (okay, we know, it's more of a rolling motion). Yes, you will still have to get up at some point to go to the bathroom, but at least you can get a few good hours in a row at the beginning of the night.

Avoid lying on your back all night. If you awaken and you are on your back, do not freak out—just roll over.

Reality Check

No matter which side you wake up on, you will ache every morning as your pregnancy progresses. Chalk it up to the sacrifices of parenthood. Yes, it will all be worth it very soon.

Q. I feel my uterus tighten up occasionally. My OB says they are just practice contractions. How will I be able to tell the difference between these and the real thing?

Because your uterus has a large muscle layer, it contracts or tightens from time to time, whether you are pregnant or not. When you weren't pregnant, you probably only felt those contractions during your menstrual period or occasionally with an orgasm. Braxton-Hicks contractions are the special name for uterine contractions not associated with labor.

It is very normal to experience Braxton-Hicks contractions during your pregnancy. The more children you have had, the earlier in the pregnancy you may feel them and the stronger they may be. They tend to occur when you or your baby are moving around. They can also happen if you are dehydrated, have a bladder infection, or after an orgasm.

If you've noticed several Braxton-Hicks contractions in a row, kick your feet up and relax with a nice big glass of water. They eventually go away.

Real uterine contractions prepare your cervix for the birth process. Your cervix will start to thin out and open with these contractions.

Will you be able to tell the difference between these contractions and the real deal contractions? That can be tricky sometimes, but here are some key differences:

Braxton-Hicks Contractions

- These can be annoying but usually don't hurt.
- Your belly gets hard (like your chin), then relaxes and softens again.
- You can sit, breathe, and talk through them.
- They happen sporadically.
- They do not get more intense over time.
- They can last a long time—five or ten minutes, sometimes even up to thirty minutes.

Real Labor Pains

- These hurt—like really bad menstrual cramps or terrible low back pain.
- You won't want to sit, breathe, talk (or do much of anything) during one.
- They happen at more regular intervals and only last for one to one and a half minutes.
- Their intensity and frequency increase with time.
- They most often occur in the third trimester, although they are possible at any point in the pregnancy.

If you aren't sure which contractions you are having, it is always a good idea to check with your OB provider.

Q. I am leaking fluid from my breasts. Is it breast milk?

While you won't make mature breast milk until two to five days after delivery, you might produce and leak some early milk (called ***colostrum***) at the end of your second or early in your third trimester.

We'll talk more about colostrum and preparation for breastfeeding in Chapter 12, "Feeding Your Newborn." But for now, don't be alarmed if you see a thin, clear-yellow substance leaking from your nipples. You also shouldn't be alarmed if you don't see it! Some pregnant women leak while other women start after delivery when their baby begins to nurse. Leaking during pregnancy does not determine whether or not you will breastfeed successfully.

INSIDER SECRET: Nursing Pads

If you are leaking, it's time to buy some nursing pads. There are two options: disposable pads or reusable (washable) 100 percent cotton pads. There are pros and cons to each option.

Disposable pads are cheap and you can just throw them away once they are used. But they can make you look a little lumpy in a tight-fitting shirt. You can pick up a pack of sixty disposable pads online or at a big-box store.

Reusable pads are softer and a bit more form-fitting. But they are more expensive, and you have to wash them every day—you'll have to buy several unless you like doing laundry all the time. You also have to watch out that they don't migrate out of your bra, since they have no adhesive backing. It's not so attractive to have a nursing pad make its way to daylight during a business meeting or while grocery shopping!

Q. Um, my undies are a little wet. Did I just pee, or did my water break?

Wet undies are due to one of four things: 1) urine, 2) vaginal discharge, 3) amniotic fluid (this means your water has broken), or 4) sweat. Early in pregnancy, it's usually #1 or #2. To help you figure it out, we present to you:

Wet Undies 411

1. **Urine.** It's never fun to be incontinent, but this is something that can happen throughout pregnancy. As your baby gets bigger, they put more pressure on your bladder. That pressure can be more than the muscle that prevents leakage can handle. Your baby's movements can also trigger leakage. Either way, the urine just comes right on out, and you'll be darting for the nearest place to change your underwear. For the first time in your life, you'll actually be jealous that you can't wear a "Stadium Pal" (yes, it is true—a contraption billed as "a portable urinal" so guys don't have to miss an important fourth down play during a football game).
2. **Vaginal discharge.** Both the cervix and the vagina make and secrete more discharge during pregnancy. This looks yellowish-white and can be thick and mucusy on the underwear. Urine and amniotic fluid are waterier.
3. **Amniotic fluid.** If your water breaks (called ***rupture of the amniotic sac***), you'll see clear, watery fluid. It doesn't look or smell like urine. It can happen at any point during pregnancy and must be immediately diagnosed and addressed by your OB provider. Always call your OB provider if you aren't sure. There is a simple test that can be done to figure it out.
4. **Sweat.** Your baseline body temperature is higher. You are hotter than anyone around you and may threaten anyone nearby who attempts to up the thermostat a few degrees. You will sweat more than you ever have in your life thus far. There isn't a nice way to say this, but your excess sweat will pool under your

arms and between your legs. This is often mistaken for wet underwear and a broken water bag.

It's really tough to know sometimes. As an OB-GYN, I have seen many patients in the office and sent a few to the hospital (in the middle of the night) because the complaint is "wet underwear" or leaking water from the vagina. If you are unsure, the best thing to do is to call your OB provider, describe your symptoms, and let them decide with a few tests.

Here's how OB providers figure it out:

First, we look inside the vagina with a speculum to see if there is any pooling. We will ask you to cough. If your bag is broken, a lot of fluid often pools in the vagina.

We might take some of that fluid and put it on litmus-like paper, testing its pH. Amniotic fluid has a pH of 7–7.5, and our little yellow piece of paper turns dark blue. That's what we are looking for.

There are also other ways of checking that involve using individually wrapped sterile swabs impregnated with a sensitive pH indicator, such as Amnicator or AmnioTest.

Your OB may also perform an ultrasound to see how much amniotic fluid still remains inside your uterus around your baby.

Taking all this information into account, your OB provider will be able to decide if you have in fact ruptured your amniotic sac or if the less important (but more embarrassing) condition has occurred: You peed in your pants.

Q. I used to have a cute "innie" belly button. Now I have an "outie." Is this permanent?

No, it's probably not permanent. Chances are, it will look (relatively) normal again as your body returns to its pre-pregnancy shape.

As your uterus starts to grow, it pushes your belly out. With that expansion, your belly button (officially, the ***umbilicus***) may disappear and become flush with the rest of your skin or may pop out. This is one of the reasons we recommend taking out your belly button piercing, if you have one. See Chapter 10, "Self-Care," for details.

Your belly button will return to something similar to its original shape after delivery, but it might be a little bit bigger. So as much as we would love to, we can't guarantee you will look exactly the same in a bikini before and after childbirth.

Q. Are there any products I can use to prevent stretch marks?

We are all desperate when it comes to preventing stretch marks and will do just about anything to avoid getting them. I used a crazy combination of creams and oils, one on top of another, that made me smell like a slightly minted rosemary-eucalyptus tree when I went to bed at night! But remember this: There is no one "wonder cream" that will prevent stretch marks (despite all the hype out there).

Prenatal Care

You will visit your OB provider every two weeks from twenty-eight to thirty-six weeks, and then once a week until you deliver. You will be an old pro at this point. Get weighed. Pee in a cup. Roll up your sleeve and check blood pressure. Measure fundal height. Listen to baby's heartbeat. Ask questions.

But your OB provider will add a pelvic (internal) exam to this routine, starting at thirty-seven to thirty-eight weeks. Good times. You won't look forward to these exams because they are fairly uncomfortable. Your OB provider will probably say something like, "You're going to feel a little bit of pressure," to prepare you for it.

FYI: The word "pressure" in obstetrics is code for "this is going to be pretty darn uncomfortable."

But it's important to do these exams in the last stage of pregnancy so your OB provider can figure out if your body is getting ready for delivery. Your OB provider can determine if your cervix is starting to open up and soften (we call it ripening—yes, like a fruit).

The exam also helps your OB provider know what position your baby plans to be in (95 percent of the time, that is headfirst—called ***vertex***).

At one of these visits, you (and your partner, hopefully) will sit down with your OB provider to discuss your upcoming labor and delivery. This is also your chance to discuss the childbirth experience.

Q. Are there any more routine tests?

Yes. Between thirty-six and thirty-eight weeks, your OB provider will do a swab of your vagina/rectum for a ***Group B streptococcus***, or ***GBS***, culture. The details of this test are in Chapter 6, "Tests." In short, if you are a carrier of this bacteria, it will be recommended that you receive antibiotics during labor to prevent spreading it to your baby in the birth process.

In addition, you need to keep monitoring your baby's fetal kick counts, which are also covered in Chapter 6, "Tests."

Q. Any more ultrasounds?

If you have a routine pregnancy, the answer might be no. Some OBs also do one more ultrasound at thirty to thirty-four weeks to assess the baby's size and to be sure there is an appropriate amount of amniotic fluid surrounding the baby.

Q. Which visits are the most important for my partner to attend?

If you can pick only one, go for the thirty-four to thirty-six week visit. This is the big "what will happen in delivery" talk. Check with your OB provider to see when they like to have this discussion.

In my practice, this is the visit when I discuss all the nitty-gritty details about labor and delivery. That includes what going into labor feels like, when to call me, when to go to the hospital, what your pain control options are, how I monitor mother and baby during labor, what interventions are used for complicated deliveries, and why cesarean sections happen. Then I answer all the who/what/when/where/why questions you have about the big day.

You can see why both of you should be at this appointment!

Decisions

There are some pretty important health and parenting decisions that you and your partner need to tackle—ideally, before your baby arrives. For some decisions, your healthcare team needs to know what you want at or just after delivery (which is no time to make rational decisions!). For others, you need to plan ahead so you will have the most options available to you. Bottom line: You are about to become parents, and you can no longer procrastinate.

You can find detailed information on these topics in Chapter 11, "Parenthood Prep," but here is the list:

DECISION	WHEN TO DECIDE	CONSIDERATIONS
Cord blood banking	Any time before delivery	You will need to plan ahead if you want to explore the various cord blood banks and select the one that suits you.
Circumcision (for males)	Before 36 weeks	While this decision can occur at any time in your child's life, newborn circumcisions are typically performed in the first days or weeks as an outpatient procedure or a religious ritual. If this is of interest to you, you will need to determine who performs the procedure in your community (obstetrician, pediatrician, urologist) or arrange for a mohel.
Expanded newborn screening	Before delivery	Every state requires a standard newborn screening blood test for a variety of disorders. If you want additional screening, you need to obtain the filter paper from a private laboratory that collects the blood specimens. Blood is obtained at twenty-four hours of life.
Select a pediatrician	28–34 weeks	Surprise! A pediatrician will see your baby once they are born! This person will meet your baby for the first time at the hospital or in the first 2–4 days of life. It's time to line up that healthcare provider now.
Work/childcare options	Now	You can always change your mind, but considering your options now can make life a little less stressful later.
Make a will	Now	Life is uncertain. You are now responsible for a little human being. Have a plan for the unexpected.

Reality Check

Real talk from a pediatrician (Dr. B): I am constantly amazed and surprised that parents-to-be spend so much time preparing for childbirth and outfitting the baby's nursery, yet they fail to have a healthcare provider lined up for their newborn when the baby is born! My office frequently gets calls from frantic parents who have not established care, and they need an appointment for their newborn.

It's true that many newborns will have their first physical examination and care provided by the pediatric hospitalist service. (Some pediatricians still make newborn hospital visits in their communities, although it is less common these days.) But once you head home, your newborn will need to see their own pediatrician for an office visit at two to four days of life.

Planning ahead is helpful for many reasons. It gives you time to find a doctor that you like, who accepts new patients, and who accepts your insurance. Your pediatrician-to-be can also help answer questions and concerns you may have about newborn healthcare. You don't want to be hunting for a pediatrician in the midst of delivering a baby!

Q. Do I need to hire a doula? And what's a doula?

A doula is a person who is trained to provide emotional, physical, and educational support during pregnancy and delivery, and sometimes even into the postpartum period. And yes, it is time to identify someone now if you want to have a doula.

Some couples decide they want to have a doula in addition to their OB provider at one or all phases of their birth experience. Doulas are invaluable if you are planning to go through labor without pain medication, but they are also helpful even if you are planning to get an epidural. Of course, it would be wise to make sure both of you want to have a doula.

Ask your OB provider for recommendations—you'll want to make sure that if the doula has worked with your OB provider before, they have a good relationship.

You can also talk to friends who have used doulas during their pregnancies. Start interviewing doulas now if you have not done so already, and meet with as many as you need to until you both feel comfortable with one.

What's Going on Down There?

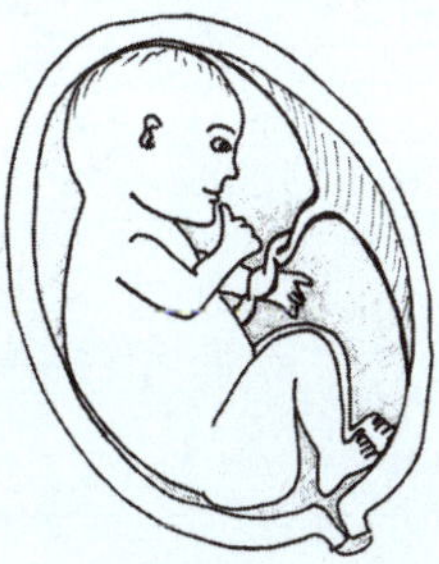

Twenty-eight Weeks.

The eyes open and close. They have eyelashes.

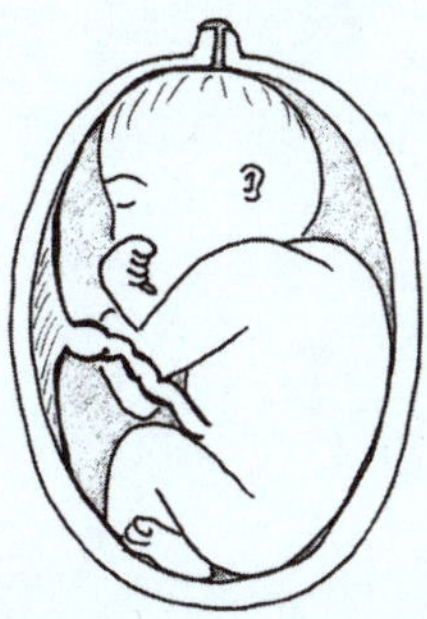

Thirty-two Weeks.

Your baby's pupils respond to light now. They are getting bigger and more cramped in their little home—so they curl into a ball called the fetal position.

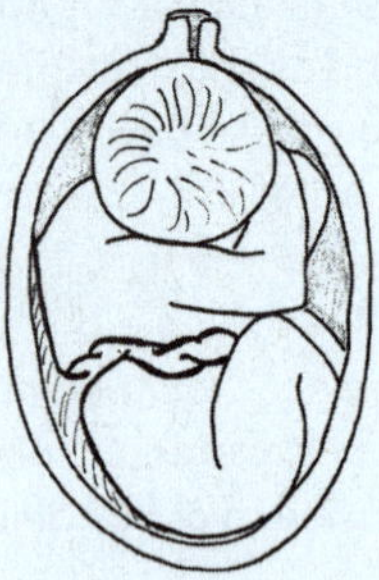

Thirty-six Weeks.

Your baby's lungs are now mature and could function outside the womb. For boys, testes have migrated into the scrotum. Your baby starts fattening up.

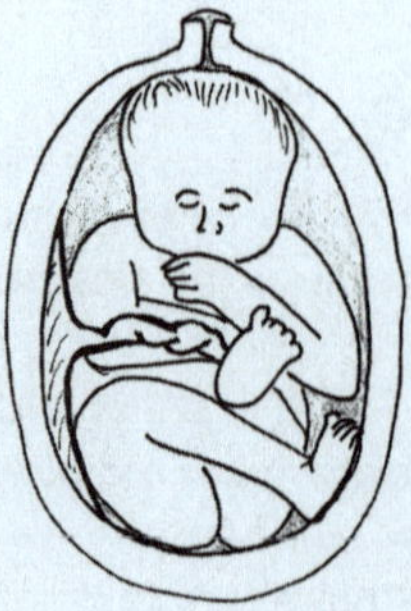

Forty Weeks.

Your baby is good to go.

CHAPTER 5

Is This Normal?

Sid: "My feet are sweaty."
Manny: "Do we have to get a newsflash every time your body does something?"
—Ice Age

What's in This Chapter

- **Why are my feet swelling?**
- **When to worry and when to call your doc**
- **Fifty more weird things you might worry about**

Your body is undergoing a major metamorphosis. Okay, that's not exactly a surprise. What you may not realize, however, is your *whole body* is changing—not just the female parts! And as long as you have a growing human being inside, you will not feel entirely normal.

For instance, your heart and blood vessels have to accommodate the increased blood flow to your growing baby. Your gut has to deal with hormones that will increase heartburn and decrease bowel movements. You'll have aches and pains in places you've never felt before. Those are just a few examples of the *many* changes to come.

This chapter will tell you what is normal and what is not, so you'll know when you need to call your OB provider . . . and when you can relax.

And since some of these symptoms aren't the most pleasant to endure, we'll also cover what to do about them (other than just living with them—which, unfortunately, is sometimes the answer).

Below is a little synopsis of your body changes for the next forty weeks, so you won't be alarmed when these weird symptoms arise. You'll also see Red Flags called out with each symptom. As you would guess, Red Flags are not normal and must be addressed immediately. You can find details on these complications in Chapter 16, "Pregnancy 911." If you have a Red Flag issue, you need to call to your OB provider.

Yes, this is a lengthy chapter. To make it easier to use, we have divided it by body system—from head to toe.

Common Body Changes and Complaints

Note: With your second pregnancy, all these body changes happen earlier.

BRAIN

SYMPTOM	WHEN IT HAPPENS, BY TRIMESTER
Moodiness	First and third trimester
Headaches	First trimester
Dizziness	First and third trimester
Fatigue	First and third trimester (fatigue during the second trimester can be a sign of anemia or a thyroid condition)
Trouble sleeping	First and third trimester
Forgetfulness	Throughout pregnancy

EYES

SYMPTOM	WHEN IT HAPPENS, BY TRIMESTER
Blurry vision	Throughout pregnancy

EAR, NOSE, THROAT

SYMPTOM	WHEN IT HAPPENS, BY TRIMESTER
Stuffy nose	Late second and third trimester
Nosebleeds	Second and third trimester
Gums swollen/bleeding	Second and third trimester

BREASTS

SYMPTOM	WHEN IT HAPPENS, BY TRIMESTER
Tenderness	First and early second trimester
Enlargement	First and third trimester
Darker nipples	Second and third trimester
Blue veins	Throughout pregnancy
Leaking early milk (colostrum)	Second and third trimester
Stretch marks	Third trimester and after breastfeeding is completed

LUNGS

SYMPTOM	WHEN IT HAPPENS, BY TRIMESTER
Shortness of breath	Late second and third trimester

HEART AND BLOOD VESSELS

SYMPTOM	WHEN IT HAPPENS, BY TRIMESTER
Swollen body parts (edema)	Second trimester if you are on your feet all day; third trimester
Heart palpitations	Any time, and always notify your OB provider

STOMACH AND INTESTINES

SYMPTOMS	WHEN IT HAPPENS, BY TRIMESTER
Morning sickness (nausea, vomiting)	First, early second, rarely through third trimester
Constipation	First and third trimester
Hemorrhoids	Second and third trimester*
Gas	First and third trimester
Burping	First and third trimester
Heartburn (acid reflux)	Rarely first, mainly second and third trimester
Umbilical pain	Second trimester
Shooting pains in vagina/rectum	Third trimester

**If you escape them during pregnancy, they will appear while pushing at delivery!*

FEMALE GENITALS

SYMPTOMS	WHEN IT HAPPENS, BY TRIMESTER
Pelvic cramps	Throughout pregnancy
Braxton-Hicks contractions	Usually third, but second trimester if it's not your first baby
Vaginal discharge	Throughout pregnancy
Varicose veins in outer genitals	Late second and third trimester
Spotting	Any time, and always notify your OB provider
Swelling/discomfort	Late second and third trimester
Shooting pains in vagina/rectum	Third trimester
Itching in outer genital area	Often second and third trimester, and always notify your OB provider

KIDNEYS AND BLADDER

SYMPTOMS	WHEN IT HAPPENS, BY TRIMESTER
Frequent urination	First and third trimester
Leaking urine (incontinence)	Late second and third trimester
Urinating at night	First and third trimester

SKIN, HAIR, NAILS

SYMPTOMS	WHEN IT HAPPENS, BY TRIMESTER
Increased hair growth	Throughout pregnancy
Nail growth	Throughout pregnancy
Glowing skin	For some women, throughout pregnancy; never for others
Acne	First trimester
Blotchy marks on face (melasma)	First, second, and third trimester
Dark line on belly (linea nigra)	Late second and third trimester
Stretch marks	Second and third trimester
Itching	Second and third trimester
Red palms and soles	Second and third trimester
Skin tags	Second and third trimester
Darker, more prominent moles	Second and third trimester, and always notify OB provider
Chafing/intertrigo	Second and third trimester
Spider veins	Second and third trimester
Varicose veins	Second and third trimester
Sweatiness	Second and third trimester

MUSCLES, BONES, AND NERVES

SYMPTOMS	WHEN IT HAPPENS, BY TRIMESTER
Hip pain (round ligament pain)	Late first and early second trimester
Groin pain	Second trimester
Pubic/leg pain	Third trimester
Low back pain/sacral pain	Late second and third trimester
Sciatic pain	Late second and third trimester
Leg cramps	Late second and third trimester
Wrist pain (carpal tunnel syndrome)	Late second and third trimester

IMMUNE SYSTEM

SYMPTOMS	WHEN IT HAPPENS, BY TRIMESTER
Illnesses last longer	Throughout pregnancy

Reality Check

Your body changes with pregnancy, and it may not return to exactly your same ol' body when the pregnancy is over. No, you won't be exactly the same as you were before, but with some work, you can get close. Our babies change us, and that's okay.

Brain

- **Moodiness**
- **Headaches**
- **Dizziness and light-headedness**
- **Fatigue**
- **Trouble sleeping**
- **Forgetfulness**
- **Baby blues**

Q. I'm eight weeks pregnant and my partner tells me I am acting like I'm getting my period—really moody and short-tempered. Is this normal?

Symptom: Moodiness. You yell at your partner for not getting dinner and rubbing your feet at the same time.

Usual time of onset: First trimester. Occasionally it can last throughout pregnancy.

Cause: Changes in your hormone levels, particularly elevations of estrogen and progesterone trigger moodiness.

Treatment:

- Have an open conversation with your partner, and be thankful this person loves you.
- Exercise.
- Get more sleep.
- Rarely, some women benefit from antidepressant medication.

Red Flags:

- Crying all the time.
- Cannot carry out activities of daily living (bathing, cooking, eating, dressing, working).
- Unable to get out of bed.
- Loss of appetite or weight loss.
- Withdrawal from friends or loved ones.
- Thoughts of harming yourself or others.

If you have any of the above Red Flag symptoms, talk to your OB provider immediately.

Partner Tip

Your partner is growing a human being inside of her and may not seem like herself anymore. The dramatic hormonal surges occurring in her body are changing her emotions faster than an Indy 500 racecar. Be patient. Be calm. Help her as much as you can. Don't take it personally. It's not about you. This will end (at some point!).

Q. I am getting really bad headaches. Is there anything I can take for them?

Symptom: Headaches.

Usual time of onset: First trimester.

Cause: Thank your elevated hormone levels again. Other causes include dehydration, increased stress, abruptly ending your caffeine intake, or a change in your sleep habits. Occasionally, pregnancy causes the shape of the lens in your eye to change, resulting in strained vision. This can give you a headache, too.

Treatment:

- Sleep more.
- Exercise.
- Stay well hydrated.
- Ask your partner for a massage (or pay for one).
- Medication options: acetaminophen (Tylenol) on occasion or consume a caffeinated beverage.
- Consider getting your vision checked.

Red Flags:

- The worst headache you have ever had.
- Headache that wakes you up from sleep.
- Headache that doesn't go away with hydration and pain meds.
- Headache that lasts more than a few hours or returns frequently.
- Abdominal pain with a headache.
- Vision changes with a headache.
- Fever with a headache.

NEW PARENT-TO-BE 411:

Migraines and Pregnancy

If you are a migraine sufferer, take note. Migraines, like many other chronic medical issues, follow the "rule of thirds" in pregnancy: one-third of pregnant migraine sufferers say that symptoms improve, one-third say they stay the same, and one-third have symptoms that worsen.

Unfortunately, ibuprofen (Motrin, Advil) is ***not*** recommended during pregnancy.

It's safe to take acetaminophen (Tylenol) on occasion, but most migraine sufferers do not get relief from Tylenol alone.

If you are one of the unlucky ones, there are some prescription migraine medications that are acceptable to take if nothing else is working. See Appendix A, "Medications," for details. Always check with your OB provider ***before*** taking any prescribed migraine medication.

Since your medication options are limited, try putting a cold towel on your head and resting in a quiet, dark room once a migraine hits.

As for prevention, avoid things that you know may trigger your migraines, such as cheese, chocolate, stress, and lack of sleep. You may also want to try meditation, yoga, acupuncture, or a regular exercise program.

Q. I have moments of feeling really lightheaded, as if I am going to faint. What can I do to prevent this feeling?

Symptom: Dizziness or lightheadedness.

Usual time of onset: First and third trimesters.

Cause: Hormones and/or dehydration. High levels of the hormone progesterone can cause the veins in your legs to dilate and blood pressure to drop. You may have less blood flow to your head and more to your feet, especially if you are standing up. If you are dehydrated, there is less volume circulating in your bloodstream, which can also make you feel lightheaded.

Treatment:

- Sit or lie down.
- Drink more water and electrolytes.
- Consider wearing support stockings if this happens regularly.
- If symptoms persist, put your head between your knees so it is lower than your heart. This will bring blood back to your head, relieving your symptoms in most cases. Memo: We realize this is easier in your first trimester than in your last one!

Red Flags:

- Dizziness and shortness of breath.
- Dizziness and chest pain.

- Dizziness and calf or leg pain.
- Dizziness and heavy vaginal bleeding.
- Actual fainting.

Q. I am tired constantly. Is anything wrong with me?

Symptom: Fatigue . . . as if the life is being sucked out of you!

Usual time of onset: First and third trimesters, with the worst of it happening in the first.

Cause: Most of your energy stores are being used to grow a human being inside of you. That doesn't leave much energy for you.

Treatment:

- Exercise. That will be the last thing you want to do, but it may help you recharge.
- Rest. If your schedule permits, take a nap when you are tired, and go to bed early to get a good night's sleep.
- No matter what you do, it gets better with time. The severe fatigue you have in the first trimester goes away as you enter the second trimester. It does return in your third, but not to the degree you experienced in the first trimester.

Red Flags:

- Severe fatigue during the second trimester.
- Severe fatigue upon awakening (especially second or third trimester).
- Fatigue and depressed mood.

Q. I just can't get a good night's sleep. What can I do about it?

Symptom: Sleep disruption. Constant waking and difficulty returning to sleep.

Usual time of onset: First and third trimesters.

Cause: There are several reasons.

- It's hard to get comfortable and then stay comfortable.
- You need to pee all the time.
- You have relentless heartburn that gets worse when you are lying down.
- You feel slightly short of breath until the baby drops down into your pelvis (***lightening***) toward the end of pregnancy.
- Many women report not being able to fall back to sleep because they have racing thoughts about what lies ahead.

All of these issues conspire to turn your evening's rest into a real nightmare.

Treatment:

- Buy a body pillow.
- Sleep with your head slightly elevated, particularly if you are suffering from heartburn.

- Take a relaxing bath before bed.
- Get a massage just before bed.
- Exercise during the day—not right before bed.
- If all else fails, talk to your OB about using a medication like diphenhydramine (Benadryl); doxylamine (Unisom); magnesium L threonate (500 mg nightly); or, in very severe cases, Ambien. See Appendix A, "Medications."

Red Flags:

- Unable to fall asleep without medication.
- Getting less than four to five hours of sleep a night on a chronic basis.
- Disrupted sleep with weepy/sad mood and lack of interest in activities.

Helpful Hint

Some pregnant women suffer from obstructive sleep apnea. If your partner complains about your snoring, tell your doctor (even if it's embarrassing). You may need help!

Q. Sometimes I feel like I am losing my mind, and I'm not a forgetful person. Does this get better after I deliver?

Symptom: Forgetfulness. You can't find your keys, remember your neighbor's last name, or recall the questions for your OB provider that you just thought of five minutes ago.

Usual time of onset: First, second, and third trimesters (and even into the postpartum period).

Cause: During pregnancy, it may be due to those elevated hormone levels. The "pregnancy brain" or "placenta brain" as one of Dr. M's patients likes to call it, persists after delivery thanks to having a newborn in the house. Anything that interferes with getting a solid night's sleep for three to four months (or more) can make anyone a bit forgetful.

Treatment: Write everything down. If you have trouble remembering what your OB provider told you after you've left the office, ask for handouts or booklets to take home, or take notes while they talk.

Red Flags: None.

Q. I've heard about women having postpartum depression, but I'm still pregnant and already feeling the blues. Shouldn't I be excited about having this baby?

Symptom: Depressed mood.

Usual time of onset: Third trimester, although it's possible at any point in the pregnancy.

Cause: Let's see, you are about to deliver a baby (which can cause anxiety, even if you have done it before), you are about to be totally responsible for a helpless little being, your sleep gets disrupted every night, and your hormone levels are off the charts. If it is your second child, sprinkle in some guilt about having to divide your love. Is that enough? Those emotions and hormones can override the excitement for what lies ahead. Also, if you have a personal history of depression, you may have changed your medication dosages or the type of medication that you take. You may not be on any medication at all at this point. This can all lead to an increase in the severity of your symptoms.

Treatment:

- Exercise (we know you're sick of us saying this by now).
- Talk about your feelings with your partner.
- Tell your OB provider how you feel. Speak to your therapist or get a referral for one. People can't help you if they don't know what is going on.

Red Flags:

- Crying all the time.
- Cannot carry out activities of daily living (bathing, dressing, working).
- Cannot get out of bed.
- Loss of appetite or weight loss.
- Withdrawing from friends.

Eyes

Q. I wear glasses/contacts. All of a sudden things seem blurry. Is that normal?

Symptom: Blurry vision. It may be associated with a mild headache.

Usual time of onset: First, second, or third trimester.

Cause: Elevated hormone levels can make the lenses in your eyes swell. This is temporary but can cause significant changes in your vision, particularly if you already wear glasses or contacts.

Treatment: Get a cheap new pair of eyeglasses from your eye doctor. Don't waste your money on a super expensive pair, because your vision will probably go back to baseline after you deliver. Always tell your OB about any vision changes so they can check for potential medical issues.

Red Flags:

- Sudden onset of blurry vision.
- Seeing flashes of light or blind spots.
- Severe headache and blurry vision/vision changes.
- Abdominal pain and vision changes.

Ear, Nose, and Mouth

- Stuffy nose
- Nosebleeds
- Swollen, bleeding gums

Q. My nose is constantly stuffy. I don't feel sick or have any other allergy symptoms, it's just my nose. What do I do?

Symptom: Stuffy nose or nasal congestion.

Usual time of onset: Second and third trimesters.

Cause: Elevated levels of estrogen and progesterone cause many body parts to swell, including your sinus and nasal passages.

Treatment:

- Use saline nose spray as often as needed to loosen nasal secretions.
- Put a humidifier in your bedroom to help loosen mucus.
- It is okay to use diphenhydramine (Benadryl) periodically, but it may not help. Check with your OB provider about using other antihistamines.

Red Flags:

- Fever and congestion.
- Severe facial pain/headache and congestion.
- Persistent sore throat and congestion.

Q. I've started having nosebleeds. Is this unusual?

Symptom: Nosebleeds.

Usual time of onset: Second and third trimesters.

Cause: Elevated estrogen and progesterone levels enlarge and soften your blood vessels. As a result, those blood vessels become more fragile. Just blowing your nose or breathing in dry, cold air can irritate the lining of your nose and cause a nosebleed.

Prevention:

- Keep the skin inside your nostrils nice and moist.
- Use saline nose drops or nasal spray liberally (several times daily).
- Use a Q-tip to apply a small amount of coconut oil or Aquaphor to the lining of your nostrils twice daily—especially at night.
- Sleep with a warm-mist humidifier in your room.

Red Flags:

- Daily nosebleeds.
- A nosebleed that you cannot control or stop after twenty to thirty minutes. This kind of nosebleed likely requires medical attention.

How to handle a nosebleed: Lean forward slightly and pinch your nose, squeezing your nostrils together for five minutes. If bleeding continues, repeat. Decongestant nose spray (like Afrin) can stop a nosebleed, but you should only use it after asking your OB provider. The decongestant shrinks the blood vessels in the nose, but if used frequently, it can have the same effect on the blood vessels in the placenta. Afrin can also become addictive.

Q. I brush and floss my teeth regularly, but my gums are swollen and bleeding. Am I doing something wrong?

Symptom: Swollen and bleeding gums.

Usual time of onset: Second and third trimesters.

Cause: Elevated hormone levels increase blood flow and cause your gums to swell. Swollen gums bleed more easily.

Treatment:

- Brush regularly (at least twice a day) with a soft-bristle toothbrush.
- Floss. Yes, every day. According to Dr. M's dad (who also happens to be a dentist), it's even more important than brushing!
- See your dentist for routine checkups and cleanings.
- Rinse your mouth periodically with a warm saltwater solution.
- Continue getting regular dental exams and cleanings.

Red Flags:

- Severe pain with brushing.
- Pain or bleeding in only one area.
- Pain or bleeding and fever.

Reality Check

Dental issues are more common in pregnancy. There's more stomach acid in the back of the throat, more vomiting, more snacking, more glucose/sugar secretion in saliva, more gum inflammation due to elevated hormone levels, and reduced saliva production. All of these things conspire to make it harder to fight oral bacteria. If a problem arises, see your dentist. Periodontal disease and abscesses may lead to preterm labor and delivery.

Breasts

- Tenderness
- Enlargement (growth)
- Dark nipples
- Blue veins
- Leaking milk (colostrum)
- Stretch marks

Q. I'm outgrowing my bras. My breasts are also really tender. When will this growth spurt end?

Symptom: Breast enlargement and tenderness. Your nipples may be especially sensitive. You'll get those boobs you've always dreamed of (temporarily) when you are pregnant.

Usual time of onset: First and third trimesters.

Cause: Elevated hormone levels (particularly estrogen) make milk ducts and breast tissue grow and enlarge.

Treatment:

- Wear a bra to bed for extra support. Bras without underwires are best, such as an exercise bra.
- Avoid hot water in the shower.
- Apply vitamin E directly to your nipples.
- Time. Most women get some relief after the first trimester is over.

Red Flags:

- Breast mass.
- Nipple discharge (although it's usually early milk, which is normal—see ***colostrum***).
- Nipple or breast tissue dimpling.
- Significant skin discoloration, other than darkening of the ***areolae*** and nipples (see below).

Reality Check

It's difficult to do breast self-exams during pregnancy because there is so much growth of your breast tissue. But do let your OB provider know if something looks or feels odd.

Q. My nipples have suddenly become discolored. Any concerns?

Symptom: Dark nipples.

Usual time of onset: Second and third trimesters.

Cause: Pregnancy increases melanin production (the pigment that gives skin its color). This excess melanin causes certain areas on the body that are already pigmented to become darker, including your nipples.

Treatment: None. It usually goes away on its own about three to six months after delivery.

Red Flags: Skin changes on the breast other than the nipple and areola (that circular area around the nipple).

Reality Check: Seeing Black

You may find several body areas get darker—underarms, ***vulva*** (outer genital area), belly button, and even the line from your belly button to your pubic hair (see ***linea nigra*** in the skin section later in this chapter.) Occasionally, women get a dark line on the back of their legs mimicking the seam of a pair of panty hose! If you have darker-toned skin to begin with, you're more likely to see these changes.

Fact Check

You can't get breast cancer while you are pregnant.

The truth: Breast cancer diagnosed during pregnancy is rare but possible. And although it is the most common type of cancer diagnosed during pregnancy, it is estimated to occur only once in every 3,000 pregnancies.[1] But any change in color or dimpling of the breast tissue itself should be checked out, as should any new lumps. If you notice any of these symptoms, you should have your OB provider take a look.

Q. I am also starting to see some big veins popping up on my chest. Is this permanent?

Symptom: Blue veins. You may begin to look like a road atlas.

Usual time of onset: First trimester.

Cause: Elevated hormone levels cause both the breast tissue and the vessels within them to expand.

Treatment: None. After you deliver and stop breastfeeding, those veins shrink back to their old size again.

Red Flags: None.

Q. I've been told that leakage coming from my breasts is a sign of breast cancer. I have a clear fluid leaking from them now. Do I need to worry?

Symptom: Colostrum production.

Usual time of onset: Occasionally second trimester but usually third.

Cause: Nope, you don't need a mammogram. You need some bra pads. Hormonal changes tell your breast tissue to make colostrum. Your body starts making it, and it may start to leak out.

Treatment: None. Just wear nursing bra pads to soak everything up so that everyone on the street doesn't know you are leaking colostrum! Sometimes if a woman is leaking a ton, she can collect it and save it for her baby in the freezer.

Red Flags:

- Bloody or blood-tinged discharge from nipples.
- Green discharge from nipples.
- Nipple discharge and pain, skin changes, or a breast mass.

Q. As my breasts grow, I am starting to develop stretch marks. Will these go away?

Symptom: Stretch marks.

Usual time of onset: First or third trimesters, as well as right after delivery.

Cause: Hormones, again. They make your breasts grow rapidly. And that rapid growth causes the dermis (the layer of skin under the top layer, or epidermis) to tear, leading to stretch marks. They usually start out looking like dark purple or red streaks on the skin. Over time, they often fade to a lighter pink, white, or silver color.

Treatment: Moisturize and support. Keep skin moistened with lotions, oils, or creams. Wear a bra that supports your enlarging breasts. See the section on stretch marks later in this chapter (in the skin section). Although they may fade, unfortunately they don't really ever go away completely.

Red Flags: None.

Lungs

Q. I'm having difficulty catching my breath, even at rest. Should I call my doctor?

Symptom: Shortness of breath.

Usual time of onset: Late second and third trimesters.

Cause: As your uterus gets bigger, it starts to push on your diaphragm (the muscle that sits below your lungs that shares the same name). Pushing the diaphragm upward reduces the volume of air you can breathe into your lungs. At the same time, your pregnant body needs more oxygen. To accommodate, your body forces you to take more frequent breaths.

Treatment:

- Rest as much as possible.
- Sit up straight with shoulders back and take a few deep breaths.
- Breathe in slowly and really expand your chest.
- Take yoga classes, which can help focus on breathing.
- Avoid situations that are physically exerting, like climbing stairs or vigorous exercising.

Red Flags:

- Rapid and labored breathing or shortness of breath that does not improve with rest or after a few minutes.
- Chest pain and shortness of breath.
- Heart racing (palpitations) or a rapid pulse (see "How to check your pulse," on page 440) and shortness of breath.
- A bluish discoloration around your lips or fingers and shortness of breath.
- A cough and shortness of breath with or without fever/chills.
- Coughing up blood and shortness of breath.
- Pain or swelling in one or both legs and shortness of breath.
- Shortness of breath in people with asthma whose flare-ups have become more severe, more often, or more difficult to control.

If you have any of the above Red Flag symptoms, notify your OB provider immediately.

Heart and Blood Vessels

- **Swelling (*edema*)**
- **Heart racing (palpitations)**

Q. I can't wear my regular shoes anymore because my feet are so swollen. Will I ever get back into my Manolos?

Symptom: Swelling of body tissues (***edema***). Layman's term: fluid retention.

Usual time of onset: Second and third trimesters.

Cause: The answer is complicated, but it boils down to two things: extra water and extra salt. A pregnant woman has a greater volume of blood in order to meet the needs of the growing fetus. We're talking between 1.5 and 2 liters of extra fluid. A pregnant woman also retains more sodium (salt) due to a process that controls blood pressure. While your body is doing what it is supposed to, you get the unwelcome side effect of fluid retention. Usually, swelling occurs in the legs and feet. Sometimes your hands, fingers, and face will swell, too.

Treatment: See the Insider Secret box on page 89.

Red Flags:

- Severe swelling that develops overnight.
- Rapid swelling in one leg or foot more than the other, with or without pain. This can signal a ***deep venous thrombosis (DVT)*** or blood clot.
- Severe swelling in the hands and face.
- Chest pain and severe swelling.
- Blurred vision or a severe headache and swelling.
- Sudden onset of swelling in your legs, feet, hands, and face. This can be a symptom of ***preeclampsia*** (high blood pressure with accompanying protein in

urine), and it may be the only symptom you notice. These are both good reasons to call your OB provider in a jiffy. See Chapter 17, "The Complicated Pregnancy," Complications #18 and #20, to learn more.

DR. M'S OPINION

As a diehard shoe-lover, I know this is depressing—but your feet will thank me.

Fact Check

Your shoe size changes after pregnancy.

The truth: During pregnancy, your feet swell so much you may only be able to wear flip-flops, UGG boots, or, like one of my patients, her husband's orange Crocs, by the end. But for most of us, foot swelling goes away a couple of weeks after delivery. You'll be back in your old shoes in no time.

A few women increase their foot size permanently. Elevated estrogen levels could lengthen the plantar ligaments in the feet.

DR. M'S OPINION

Luckily, this wasn't the case for me because as anyone who knows me will tell you, I have invested way too much money in shoes!

FEEDBACK FROM THE REAL WORLD:

Rings and Things

You may want to wear your wedding ring on a necklace if your fingers get swollen. I have seen the diamonds go a-flying in the ER when a pregnant woman waits too long to take off a beloved ring and ends up having an ER doc cut the ring off with a small saw. Don't wait.

INSIDER SECRET:

Soothing Swollen Feet

Virtually all pregnant women find that their feet swell during pregnancy (*edema*)—it is particularly noticeable at the end of a long day. Expect it to get worse if you spend all day on your feet or if you wear shoes that are too tight.

Here are a few tips that can help:

- **Get bigger shoes.** Wear comfortable, well-fitting shoes. Yes, you may have to buy a pair that is a half or whole size bigger than normal, and they probably shouldn't be Christian Louboutins. Think Birkenstocks (or a comfy pair of sneakers or clogs).
- **Cut the salt.** Cut back on excess salt in your diet. You may have to kiss chips and salsa goodbye temporarily.
- **Pick your feet up.** Elevating your legs on a pillow or two when you are sitting can help.

(continued)

- **Buy some lovely compression socks or stockings.** Purchase support stockings. Available in most pharmacies, these help reduce swelling. Some women benefit from wearing them at night, while others wear them all day long. And no, they aren't the sexiest hose on the market—but they'll help you feel better!

The only thing that permanently solves your swelling problem is giving birth. But don't panic if your legs and feet are even more swollen a few days ***after*** delivery. It's normal to have edema for seven to ten days after you deliver. All that excess fluid from pregnancy, as well as IV fluids given during labor, takes time to be eliminated (a nice way to say you will pee it out).

Q. Every once in a while, I feel my heart racing. It's pretty unsettling. Should I worry about this?

Symptom: Heart palpitations. It feels like your heart is beating out of your chest—similar to how you would feel after drinking a double shot espresso.

Usual time of onset: Any time during pregnancy, but particularly in the first and third trimesters.

Cause: Remember, you've got an extra 1.5 liters of blood that has to be moved around. Your heart works extra hard to pump that excess volume. It beats faster to accomplish this goal.

Treatment: Rest. Drink plenty of water. And yes, anything that contains caffeine can make the palpitations worse. Avoid coffee and other caffeinated beverages as well as excessive amounts of chocolate (sorry!). If happening daily, mention this to your OB provider, who may send you to a cardiologist for a checkup.

Red Flags:

- Chest pain and heart palpitations.
- Shortness of breath and heart palpitations.
- An irregular heartbeat and palpitations.
- Dizziness and heart palpitations.
- Underlying heart disorder and palpitations.

NORMAL?

Stomach and Intestines

- Morning sickness
- Constipation
- Hemorrhoids
- Gas
- Burping
- Acid reflux/heartburn
- Umbilical pain

Q. I'm in my first trimester, and I feel queasy on and off all day long. Is this "morning" sickness?

Symptom: Morning sickness (nausea and/or vomiting).

Usual time of onset: Six to fourteen weeks.

Cause: The triple shot of raging pregnancy hormones: ***beta-hCG***, estrogen, and progesterone. Progesterone in particular relaxes the smooth muscles that line your entire gastrointestinal tract. The result: belching, nausea, vomiting, heartburn, gas, and constipation. Don't be fooled by the name—many women suffer from nausea all day long. It happens more often in women who are pregnant with multiples, women who get queasy easily (particularly when taking birth control pills), and, anecdotally, in women carrying girls.

Treatment:

- Eat several small meals throughout the day.
- Eat the moment you awaken.
- Try ginger tea or candy.
- Keep saltine crackers at your nightstand.
- Add some lemon or lime juice to water or suck on a lemon drop or sour candy.
- Exercise (yes, it works for just about every malady).
- Take over the counter vitamin B6, 25 to 50 mg, three times a day.
- Try Sea-Bands (acupressure bands worn on the wrists).
- Consider acupuncture.
- Use an over-the-counter antihistamine like diphenhydramine (Benadryl) or doxylamine (Unisom). Note: Both of these can make you pretty sleepy, so only use them at night.
- If you are in agony, ask your doctor for a prescription anti-nausea medication, such as Diclegis or ondansetron (Zofran). See Appendix A, "Medications."

DR. M'S OPINION

I had a patient who was so nauseated in her first trimester that she carried a lemon with her at all times so she could scratch and sniff it to combat her urge to purge. You have to do whatever works!

Red Flags:

- Vomiting repeatedly for more than six hours.
- Urinating less than once every eight hours.

- Weight loss of more than 5 percent of your pre-pregnancy weight.
- Vomiting daily and unable to keep down food or liquids.
- Vomiting blood.
- Fever and vomiting.
- Severe abdominal pain and vomiting.
- Diarrhea and vomiting.
- Second or third trimester nausea/vomiting long after morning sickness is over. Nausea and vomiting in the second or third trimester is probably something other than morning sickness.

NEW PARENT-TO-BE 411:

Morning Sickness Intel

1. **You are more likely to have morning sickness if your mom suffered from it.** If your mom or sister had morning sickness or excessive vomiting (***hyperemesis gravidarum***, see Reality Check below), you are more likely to have it, too.
2. **It is more common to get morning sickness with multiples.** Research suggests that higher levels of a specific pregnancy hormone (beta-hCG) lead to morning sickness. The more babies you are carrying, the more beta-hCG you produce, and the more nauseated you get.
3. **If you have morning sickness, you are having a girl.** Maybe! There are studies currently underway looking at this interesting phenomenon to see if it's actually true (and if so, why).[2] Don't paint the nursery pink because you are puking, however—many women carrying boys have terrible nausea as well. But Dr. M can tell you from professional and personal experience that in general, girls make their moms sicker than boys do!
4. **If you suffer from migraines, you are more likely to have morning sickness.** Migraine-prone women have a greater chance of suffering from both morning sickness and excessive vomiting. Motion sickness–prone women also have more morning sickness.
5. **You are less likely to miscarry if you feel sick.** If there is any silver lining to all this vomit . . . you probably have a well-functioning placenta that produces higher levels of hormones. Numerous studies show that you're less likely to miscarry if you have morning sickness.

Reality Check

Up to 75 percent of pregnant women have morning sickness, but only about five in 1,000 pregnant women are unlucky enough to go above and beyond typical morning sickness (***hyperemesis gravidarum***).

These women vomit so much that they lose at least 5 percent of their pre-pregnancy weight and have nutritional and metabolic abnormalities. OB providers need to rule out other medical causes and aggressively treat this condition. See Complication #1 in Chapter 17, "The Complicated Pregnancy."

Q. I've never had a problem having regular bowel movements until now. Is this normal?

Symptom: Constipation.

Usual time of onset: Worst in first trimester. Also shows up in the third trimester.

Cause: Elevated levels of progesterone relax the smooth muscle lining the gastrointestinal tract, making it move in slow motion. An added bonus: Iron supplements (taken to treat anemia) can make things even worse.

Treatment:

- Eat more fiber. See Chapter 7, "Nutrition," for high-fiber food list. To get you started: Try blueberries, chia seeds, prunes, and high-fiber cereals.
- Drink more water.
- Try Metamucil or Benefiber natural fiber supplements.
- Take an over-the-counter stool softener like docusate (Colace).
- Ask your doctor for lactulose (Kristalose), a prescription laxative.
- If you need to take iron supplements, consider trying a less constipating type, such as Slow Fe or iron prepared in a liquid solution.

Red Flags:

- Pooping less than once every four to five days.
- Severe abdominal pain and constipation.
- Bloody poop and constipation.
- Really black (not dark brown) poop and constipation.*

Q. I think I might have a hemorrhoid. There is a little bit of blood when I wipe after a bowel movement. What can I do about it?

Symptom: Hemorrhoids (swollen veins, also called varicose veins, around the anus).

Usual time of onset: They only get worse as pregnancy progresses, and even if you aren't blessed with them during your pregnancy, they often appear when pushing during labor. They are nearly impossible to avoid!

Causes:

- Constipation and hemorrhoids go hand in hand. When you're constipated, you push harder to get the poop out. Pushing makes the veins around the anus swell up.
- Increased body weight and an enlarged uterus put pressure on these veins and interfere with blood circulation in the lower part of your body. This makes all the

*Iron supplements can make your poop (stool) color turn dark brown.

veins dilate (that's why you can get varicose veins in the feet, legs, vulva, vagina, and rectum).

- That darn progesterone dilates all your blood vessels, including those around your butt.

Treatment:

- Avoid severe constipation (see tips above in constipation section).
- Use a stool softener like docusate (Colace) to limit pushing while pooping.
- Use soothing witch hazel pads (brand name: Tucks Medicated Pads).
- Apply a numbing/anti-inflammatory cream (for example, Preparation H, Pro-cort, Analpram, Rectogel—you gotta love these names!). See Appendix A, "Medications."

Red Flags:

- Sudden, severe pain in the hemorrhoid (yes, it's a pain in the ass).
- Hemorrhoid(s) that is extremely tender to the touch.

Q. I'm burping and passing gas quite a bit. Is it from all the fiber I'm taking to avoid constipation?

Symptom: Burping and excessive gas. You could easily win a sports bar belching contest.

Usual time of onset: Burping/belching happens in the first trimester. Gas happens the whole way through.

Cause: Your GI tract is in slow motion, thanks to your progesterone surge.

Treatment: Avoid foods that will add to the problem: beans, other legumes, dried fruit, carbonated drinks, broccoli. (Yes, this is a contradiction—high-fiber foods like beans help avoid constipation . . . but then contribute to this issue!)

Red Flags: No real red flags here. But your other half may wave the white flag of surrender after being in the same room as you for a few minutes!

Q. I have an uncomfortable sensation in my chest, and I can sometimes taste food I've eaten hours ago. What is this?

Symptom: Acid reflux/heartburn/***gastroesophageal reflux disease (GERD)***. Burning pain in upper abdomen or chest. Occasionally people complain of a chronic cough or a bitter, metallic taste in the back of the throat or mouth, instead of heartburn.

Usual time of onset: Throughout pregnancy.

Cause: There are three reasons:

- There's a muscle at the junction of the esophagus and stomach called the lower esophageal sphincter (see illustration at right) that usually keeps stomach acid where it belongs. Pregnancy hormones relax that muscle, allowing the acid to move up into the esophagus (reflux).

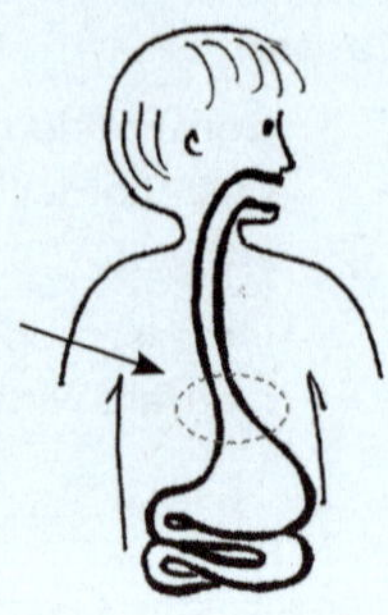

- The whole gastrointestinal tract slows down in pregnancy, giving both food and stomach acid more time to sit around and move up into the esophagus.
- The growing fetus and uterus push up on the stomach, which doesn't help matters.

Treatment:

- Avoid food and drinks that can worsen symptoms: caffeine, chocolate, citrus fruits, acidic foods, tomatoes and tomato sauce, and greasy or fried food. We know, all the good stuff!
- Sleep with your head and chest slightly elevated, on pillows or a wedge.
- Try over-the-counter antacids like Tums, Maalox, or Mylanta.
- Consider over-the-counter H2 blocker acid reducers like famotidine (Pepcid) or cimetidine (Tagamet).
- Probiotics may be helpful—these are pills, powders, or liquids.
- If you are miserable, try an over-the-counter proton pump inhibitor acid reducer, such as Prilosec, or ask your doc for a prescription medication in the same category called rabeprazole (Aciphex). Lastly, you can try a medication called metoclopramide (Reglan) that helps food move more quickly through the stomach. See Appendix A, "Medications."

Red Flags:

- Severe chest pain that isn't related to meals.
- Vomiting blood and heartburn or chest pain.
- Shortness of breath and chest pain.

Fact Check

If you have heartburn, you will have a hairy baby.

The truth: This may be true. Heartburn-afflicted pregnant women usually make more progesterone than their friends. It is the high levels of progesterone that act to relax and open the lower esophageal sphincter, allowing acid to creep up out of the stomach and cause heartburn. That same progesterone also stimulates hair growth in the fetus. So, yes, if you have really bad heartburn, you just might deliver a baby with a full head of hair!

Reality Check

It is fairly common for pregnant women to experience sharp pain or an uncomfortable sensation around their belly buttons. Some pregnant belly buttons are very sensitive to touch, similar to your nipples. This usually happens somewhere smack dab in the middle of the second trimester. If you aren't having any other symptoms (nausea, vomiting, pain elsewhere in your abdomen or back, diarrhea, fever, or pain with urination), don't worry. This will go away soon.

If you are experiencing shooting pains in your rectum, you'll find the info you need in the following gynecologic section.

Girl Parts

- Pelvic cramps
- Braxton-Hicks contractions (practice contractions)
- Vaginal discharge
- Varicose veins in the outer genital area (vulva)
- Spotting
- Swelling/discomfort
- Shooting pains in vagina/ rectum
- Itching of outer genital area

Q. I'm seven weeks and having some mild cramps, like when I get my period. Is this okay?

Symptom: Pelvic cramps.

Usual time of onset: First trimester.

Cause: Your uterus is growing to accommodate the fetus. Since most of the uterus is made up of muscle, it often "cramps" during this process.

Treatment: None, it's totally normal.

Red Flags:

- Vaginal bleeding and pelvic pain.
- Severe pelvic pain.
- Pelvic pain on one side (left or right) rather than in the middle.

Contact your OB provider if you have one of these red flag symptoms and read Chapter 16, "Pregnancy 911," for details.

Q. I'm twenty-two weeks and having some mild cramps, like when I get my period. Is this normal?

Symptom: Pelvic cramps.

Usual time of onset: Late second trimester.

Cause: There are several possibilities:

- Often, it's the same reason as before: your baby is growing, causing your uterus to expand—again, feels like mild cramps.
- Sometimes, the uterus is practicing for labor (***Braxton-Hicks contractions***).
- Occasionally, a ***bladder infection*** can cause uterine cramping as the bladder sits right on top of the uterus. This may be your only symptom.
- Sometimes, the uterus can contract after intercourse, particularly if you had an orgasm.
- Rarely, it's premature labor.

Treatment: Rest, drink lots of fluids, and notify your OB provider. Most of the time, there is nothing to worry about and you may have just overdone it during the day . . . but let your OB provider decide.

Red Flags:

- You feel your uterus getting hard with or without vaginal bleeding and pelvic cramps.
- Increased vaginal discharge and pelvic cramps.
- Vaginal bleeding with pelvic cramps.
- Watery fluid leaking from the vagina and pelvic cramps.
- Severe, constant abdominal pain.
- Painful urination and pelvic cramps.
- Vomiting and pelvic cramps.
- Fever and pelvic cramps.
- Diarrhea and pelvic cramps.

Q. I'm thirty-five weeks and having some mild cramps, like when I get my period. Is this normal?

Symptom: Pelvic cramps.

Usual time of onset: Third trimester.

Cause: Braxton-Hicks contractions or real labor contractions. This may just be your uterus doing calisthenics as a warm-up for the big day—or it may be real labor. Remember: Braxton-Hicks contractions happen sporadically, they don't usually hurt, and you can sit, breathe, and talk through them. Another important difference—real labor contractions only last between a minute and a minute and a half. Braxton-Hicks contractions often last much longer—five minutes or ten minutes straight without going away.

Treatment: Rest. Drink lots of fluids. And notify your OB just so they can help decipher what is going on.

Red Flags:

- You feel your uterus getting hard with painful pelvic cramps.
- Vaginal bleeding and pelvic cramps.
- Watery fluid leaking from the vagina and pelvic cramps.
- Severe, constant abdominal pain or pelvic cramps.
- Painful urination and pelvic cramps.
- Vomiting and pelvic cramps.
- Fever and pelvic cramps.
- Diarrhea and pelvic cramps.

Q. I'm noticing quite a bit of discharge on my underwear. Is that normal?

Symptom: Vaginal discharge. You may have so much that you're forced to wear a panty liner every day.

Usual time of onset: Right from the beginning . . . all the way until the end.

Cause: There's more blood flow to the vaginal area, which leads to an increase in the normal vaginal discharge. The official name is "leukorrhea of pregnancy."

Treatment: Unfortunately, there is no treatment except childbirth. Bring a change (or two) of underwear with you each day so you can do a midday swap. Some women feel more comfortable wearing a panty liner every day. Caution: Daily panty liner use can lead to irritation of your outer genital area (vulva and vagina).

Red Flags:

- Itching and increased vaginal discharge.
- Burning and increased vaginal discharge.
- Painful urination and increased vaginal discharge.
- Abdominal pain and increased vaginal discharge.
- A change in the color or odor of your typical vaginal discharge.
- Bloody vaginal discharge.
- Watery vaginal discharge.

Q. I noticed a little bit of blood on the toilet paper when I was wiping myself. Is everything okay? I am panicking.

Symptom: Spotting or minimal vaginal bleeding.

Usual time of onset: Any point during the pregnancy.

Cause: Yes, this is scary to see when you are pregnant. Most of the time, it's not serious. It can be due to a broken blood vessel in the vagina or on the cervix, a yeast infection, recent intercourse, or a tiny bit of bleeding from the area where the placenta meets the uterus. You may also see blood from other places in the vicinity of the vagina—like from the urethra with a bladder infection or from the anus in the case of a hemorrhoid. You could also have a bit of spotting if you just had a recent exam by your OB provider or they used the transvaginal probe for an ultrasound.

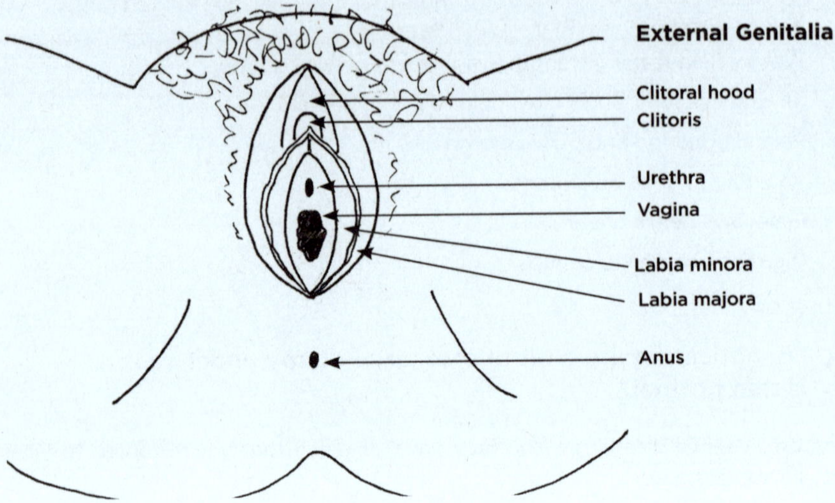

Treatment: Always talk to your OB provider. A little bit of blood with no other symptoms can wait until normal office hours—unless you are a high-risk pregnancy, in which case you should notify your OB provider at the time of bleeding.

Red Flags:

- A lot of blood (the same amount or more than a light period).
- Severe abdominal pain/cramping and spotting.
- Watery vaginal discharge and spotting.
- Painful urination and spotting.
- Fever/chills and spotting.
- Dizziness and spotting.
- Diarrhea and spotting.
- Known high-risk pregnancy and spotting.*

BOTTOM LINE: Even though there may not be a problem, you should always discuss any vaginal bleeding during pregnancy with your OB provider.

NEW PARENT-TO-BE 411:

Is Spotting in Early Pregnancy a Period?

Yes, you can have some spotting. No, it's not a period.

The word "period" (or ***menstrual period***) refers to the end of a monthly menstrual cycle when an egg is not fertilized, does not implant, and therefore a pregnancy does not occur. When a woman's body realizes it is not going to nurture a pregnancy, part of the ***endometrium*** (inner lining of the uterus) sloughs off, and some vaginal bleeding occurs for two to seven days.

If an egg is fertilized by a sperm and does implant, a period does not occur because the hormones change and the endometrium is needed to nourish and sustain the pregnancy.

That said, you can still have some spotting (a few drops of blood that stain a panty liner or undies) or light bleeding during a normal pregnancy. It's just not a period. If this occurs between week three and four, it is often due to ***implantation bleeding***, when the embryo finds a good spot and nestles into your endometrium. There are other causes of bleeding during pregnancy, but these are not periods, either.

*This refers to women with a ***placenta previa***, a history of preterm labor, ***chronic placental abruption***, ***subchorionic hematoma***, shortened cervix with or without a ***cerclage***, or those carrying multiples.

Q. My genital area feels swollen and tender. Did I do something wrong? Will there be any problems with delivery?

Symptom: Swollen ***vulva*** (the collective term for your external girl parts—labia, clitoris, outer part of vagina—see illustration on page 98).

Usual time of onset: Late second and third trimesters.

Cause: During pregnancy, more blood flows to the entire female genital tract, including the vulva. This makes the area swell. Some women may also get varicose veins in the labia (lips), and that makes things even more swollen and tender. Rarely do these issues cause a problem during delivery.

Treatment: Rest and wear a properly adjusted maternity belt. This lifts the uterus up and takes pressure off everything below it. Look for one with vulvar support if you have severe swelling or significant varicose veins of the vulva.

Red Flags:

- Itching and a swollen vulva.
- Burning and a swollen vulva.
- A change in your typical vaginal discharge and a swollen vulva.
- Vaginal bleeding and a swollen vulva.

DR. M'S OPINION

It may feel "like you've been punched down there," as a few of my patients have said.

DR. M'S OPINION

One of my patients was horrified after looking at her genital area with a mirror. She said the outside of her vagina looked like a baboon's backside. Look at your own risk, but I never think it's a good idea!

Q. I was sitting, and I started getting very sharp shooting pains in my vagina and rectum. They only lasted a few seconds, but they were very painful. Is that normal?

Symptom: Knife or lightning-like shooting pain in the vaginal and rectal area. It lasts a few seconds and is often repetitive.

Usual time of onset: Late second and third trimesters.

Cause: The baby puts pressure on the nerves that live in that area. A growing uterus and a moving baby conspire here as well.

Treatment: Get up and move around. That encourages the baby to move and (hopefully) alleviates the pain. Sitting or standing for long periods of time can trigger this pain. Try lying down on your side to see if that relieves the discomfort.

Red Flags:

- Pain that lasts more than a few minutes.
- Abdominal pain and shooting vaginal/rectal pain.
- Bleeding and shooting vaginal/rectal pain.
- A watery vaginal discharge and shooting vaginal/rectal pain.

Q. I often feel itchy down there, like when I have a yeast infection. Is that normal?

Symptom: External vaginal itchiness, known as garden variety ***vaginitis*** (inflammation and irritation of the vagina, but no infection).

Usual time of onset: Second and third trimesters.

Cause: Increased swelling of the vagina and increased vaginal discharge. If you used to shave or wax your pubic hair and now you've stopped, the hair is itchy as all heck as it grows back in. However, infection is still a possibility. Yeast loves pregnant women. There's more sugar in your vaginal discharge, so that means your vagina is a great place for yeast to grow.

Treatment: See your OB provider. They can take a look at your discharge with a pelvic exam and do a vaginal culture. Then they'll be able to tell you if there is an infection or not. If it's *not* an infection:

- Change underwear at least once throughout the day.
- Avoid wearing tight-fitting clothing, wearing underwear at night, bubble baths, and hot baths.
- Apply 1 percent hydrocortisone ointment to temporarily relieve the itching.

Red Flags: None.

Kidneys and Bladder

- **Increased urination, nighttime urination**
- **Lack of bladder control (incontinence)**

Q. I need to pee all the time. Do I have a bladder infection or diabetes?

Symptom: Frequent urination. You may get up at night once, twice, or even three times.

Usual time of onset: First and third trimesters, but often throughout.

Cause: Elevated hormone levels and the pressure of the ever-enlarging uterus on the bladder. The bladder literally sits right on top of the uterus, and as the uterus grows, the bladder is stretched. Once you enter your third trimester, you usually have extreme pressure on your bladder from your baby's head as well. Most pregnant women are very thirsty and pee all the time. This does not mean that you have diabetes.

Treatment: Because you need to be well hydrated during pregnancy, there isn't much you can do. Avoid drinking right before bed (we know, it's almost impossible because you are so darn thirsty all the time). Avoid caffeine. Empty your bladder just before getting into bed at night even if you don't have the urge to go.

Red Flags:

- Painful urination and frequent urination.
- Blood in your urine, frequent urination, fever, and back pain.

Q. Every time I laugh or cough, I leak a little urine. Will this end after pregnancy?

Symptom: Lack of bladder control. You may leak urine so often that you need to wear a panty liner for that and your vaginal discharge, too.

Your Body Organs

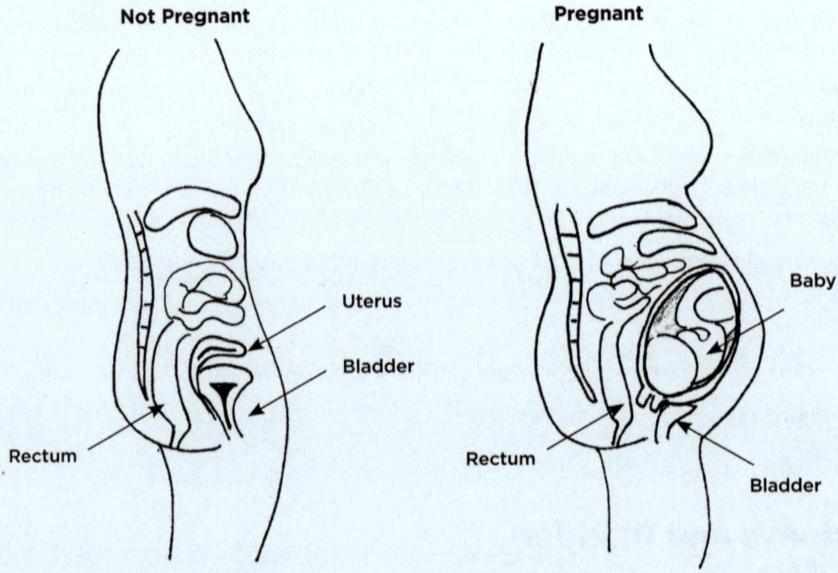

Usual time of onset: Late second and third trimesters. If this is not your first pregnancy, it may happen earlier. Sorry!

Cause: The pressure of the growing uterus on your bladder interferes with its ability to hold urine. Anything that increases your abdominal pressure (coughing, laughing, sneezing) will be the tipping point for your ***urethral sphincter*** (the muscle that prevents urine leakage until you decide it's time to release it). Your baby's kicking or moving can do it as well.

Treatment: Empty your bladder every two to three hours even if you feel like you don't have to go. Wear a panty liner or bring a change of underwear in your purse. This is temporary. (After you deliver, you'll exchange the undies for a baby diaper in your purse for the next three years!)

Red Flags:

- Leaking urine when you haven't been laughing, coughing, or sneezing.
- Leaking urine while at rest.
- Painful urination and leaking urine. If there is pain, make sure your doc confirms you don't have a bladder infection.
- You'll want to be sure that the leaking liquid is urine and not ***amniotic fluid***. This is especially true if it happens spontaneously.

Skin, Hair, and Nails

- Strange hair growth
- Hair and nail growth
- Glow
- Acne
- Black line (linea nigra)
- Stretch marks
- Itching
- Red palms and soles
- Skin tags and moles
- Chafing (intertrigo)
- Spider veins
- Varicose veins
- Sweaty
- Dark splotches (melasma/chloasma)

Q. I have hair growing in some strange places. Do I need to buy a trimmer?

Symptom: Hair growth, often involving your face, arms, belly, and around the colored part of your nipples (***areolae***).

Usual time of onset: Second and third trimesters.

Cause: Yes, once again the elevated hormone levels that are responsible for so many other fun things that happen to your body work their magic here, too.

Treatment: Shaving, plucking, and waxing are all okay. Steer clear of hair removal creams (for example, Nair) and laser removal, since we don't know if they are safe to use during pregnancy. Warning for waxers: Your skin may be much more sensitive to waxing right now. Ask your OB provider about applying a numbing cream (such as EMLA) before the wax job.

Red Flags: None, for the most part.

Q. My hair and nails are growing much faster than normal. Is this okay?

Symptom: Accelerated hair and nail growth. It's good news—your hair and nails may get thicker (temporarily).

Usual time of onset: Second and third trimesters.

Cause: Elevated hormone levels trigger most hair follicles to grow. Hormones also thicken nails and make them grow faster. Additionally, this may be the first time in your life that you are taking a multivitamin, extra calcium, and a DHA supplement. These can all aid in hair and nail growth.

Treatment: No treatment needed. Enjoy the new you! You can still get regular manicures/pedicures and see your hairstylist (see Chapter 10, "Self-Care," for dos and don'ts during pregnancy).

Red Flags: None. However, hair loss during pregnancy can be a red flag. See the New Parent-to-Be 411 box on page 104.

Reality Check

You get a beautiful mane during pregnancy because most of your hair grows all at once. However, that same hair is also lost all at once (instead of losing hair in phases, which happens when you aren't pregnant). About three months after you deliver (the range is one to five months), be prepared for a lot of hair to drop out in clumps both in the shower and your hairbrush. Yes, it is alarming—even Dr. M was alarmed when she saw what was falling out in the shower after her first pregnancy, and she does this for a living!

NEW PARENT-TO-BE 411:

Hair Loss During Pregnancy

As if pregnancy isn't enough to deal with, other health issues can crop up, too. If your hair is thinner, more brittle, or falling out during pregnancy, tell your OB provider. Thyroid disease, vitamin and mineral deficiencies, certain collagen vascular diseases (for example, lupus), and other rare disorders like alopecia areata can all cause hair changes. It's most concerning if you have bald patches, balding in the front (male-pattern baldness), or massive hair loss.

Treatment depends on what's causing the hair loss. But here are some general tips for everyone:

- Avoid chronic styling (and heating) of your hair with a blow dryer or curling/straightening iron.
- Avoid braids, weaves, or anything that pulls hair tightly and puts stress on the hair follicles.
- Use biotin-containing shampoos.
- Use a conditioner each time you wash your hair.
- Only brush your wet hair with a Wet Brush.
- Drink plenty of water, and eat fruits and vegetables (never a bad idea).

Q. I've always heard about having a pregnancy "glow." I haven't seen mine yet. Does it happen to everyone?

Symptom: A healthy-appearing shiny face and skin. Not everyone gets it, so no worries.

Usual time of onset: Second and third trimesters.

Cause: Elevated hormone levels get your oil glands revved up to make more oil. Plus, you also have 50 percent more blood volume compared to your non-pregnant friends—that blood circulation makes your cheeks and face look rosier and healthier.

Treatment: Enjoy it! If your face gets too oily you can switch to an oil-free daily cleanser and moisturizer. Try using an astringent occasionally (it can be drying if you use it too often).

Red Flags: Too much "glow" (oil) leads to acne. And although this is not a red flag from a medical standpoint, it can be a red flag from a personal and social standpoint! See details on acne next and in Chapter 10, "Self-Care."

Q. Help, I have acne!

Symptom: Acne. Unfortunately, not everyone is blessed with the pregnancy "glow"!

Usual time of onset: First through third trimesters.

Cause: Elevated hormones make the oil glands in your body secrete more oil. Oil clogs pores and causes acne. If you suffered with acne before pregnancy, it could get even worse now. But even women who have perfect complexions may see their skin change for the worse. You may be forced to face the world looking like a teenager again.

Treatment:

- Keep your skin clean with twice-daily washes.
- Avoid sleeping in makeup.
- Avoid certain foods with a high glycemic index like white bread, white rice, processed foods, sugary drinks, and snacks.[3] There's also some data suggesting milk may increase acne outbreaks, but the benefits of calcium intake during pregnancy probably outweigh the risk.
- Use topical acne medication sparingly, only on affected areas. Products containing salicylic acid, benzoyl peroxide, and finacea (azelaic acid) are safe to use in small amounts. Lathering them on can potentially lead to absorption into your bloodstream—don't do it!
- Proactiv is okay to use in severe cases (but always check with your healthcare provider first).
- Use a moisturizer that's made for oily skin.
- If you are having persistent, worsening acne, consult a dermatologist and together with your OB provider they can come up with a plan to help. Check out Chapter 10, "Self-Care," for details.

Red Flags: None.

Q. I have developed an odd, dark discoloration on my face. What is this?

Symptom: Melasma/chloasma/mask of pregnancy. These are splotchy dark areas on your face, most often on your cheeks and forehead. Up to 40 percent of pregnant women get it in varying degrees.

Usual time of onset: First, second, and third trimesters.

Cause: Increased melanin production that occurs during pregnancy. Exposure to the sun and UVA/UVB light makes it worse.

Treatment: Wear sunscreen (at least SPF 30) every day and avoid sun exposure on your face. Wear a hat and sunglasses, and stay in the shade. If your melasma does not fade after your pregnancy ends, see your dermatologist. Dermatologists have a few tricks to help remove or minimize dark areas on your face.

Red Flags: None. Melasma is completely harmless and may fade after your pregnancy ends.

Q. There is a dark line extending from my pubic bone up to beyond my belly button. What is it?

Symptom: ***Linea nigra*** (English translation: "black line"), a dark line extending from the pubic bone to the belly button and in some cases, above the belly button.

Usual time of onset: Late second and third trimesters.

Cause: There is something called the ***linea alba*** (which literally means "white line" in Latin) that is present in everyone, but it's invisible when you're not pregnant. It extends from the pubic bone to well above the belly button. When you are pregnant, the increased pigment (melanin) production can temporarily "stain" this line, making it darker. The darker your skin color to begin with, the darker this line becomes. Occasionally in some women who are very fair, there is no visible line at all.

Treatment: No treatment necessary. It almost always fades in the months following your pregnancy.

Red Flags: None.

Partner Tip

If you point out that new black line and call it the "Happy Trail," you might end up sleeping on the couch. Never call attention to new skin marks on a hormonal pregnant woman.

Q. I am so worried about getting stretch marks. How common is it to get them?

Symptom: Stretch marks. If you have them, you're in good company. Approximately 90 percent of pregnant women get them somewhere. They are pinkish, reddish, or purplish lines or streaks that occur most commonly on the breasts, abdomen, sides, buttocks, or thighs.

Usual time of onset: Late second and third trimesters.

Cause: Stretching of the skin, particularly if the stretching is due to rapid or dramatic weight gain. Genetic predisposition is also a cause. (If your mom has stretch marks, you may be more likely to develop them.)

Treatment:

- Keep your weight gain gradual.
- Exercise regularly.
- Moisturize, moisturize, moisturize. Use daily lotions/creams/oils/butters to keep your skin soft and moist.
- Most stretch marks fade after delivery to look like whitish-silver lines. If they bug you, laser therapy is an option. Talk to a dermatologist when you are done making babies. See Chapter 10, "Self-Care," for more details.

Red Flags: None.

Partner Tip

Pretend you don't see these marks, either.

Q. I'm itchy—all the time. What can I do?

Symptom: Itchiness.

Usual time of onset: Late second and third trimesters.

Cause: Your belly is growing. As it grows, the skin stretches and tightens. This can lead to dryness, stretch marks, and yes, itching.

Treatment:

- Use a moisturizer twice a day and immediately after a shower or bath.
- Use anti-itch creams like calamine lotion, 1 percent hydrocortisone cream, or diphenhydramine (Benadryl) cream.
- Avoid taking really hot showers, which can dry out your skin.
- Drink plenty of water to stay well hydrated.
- Try an oatmeal bath.
- Avoid long periods of time in hot weather or in the sun (which can make itching worse).

Red Flags:

- Nausea, vomiting, and itching.
- Severe fatigue and itching.
- Yellowing of your skin and eyes, particularly yellowing and itching on your palms and soles.
- Any rash and itching.

Reality Check

Nope, PUPPS is not a new show on Animal Planet. PUPPS stands for pruritic urticarial papules and plaques. They are intensely itchy, large, raised red patches on your belly that can spread to your upper thighs, lower legs, and arms. While it sounds kind of cute, PUPPS really irritates 1 in 150 pregnant women. See Chapter 17, "The Complicated Pregnancy," for details.

Q. My palms and soles are red. Any problem?

Symptom: Red palms and soles. This is totally normal.

Usual time of onset: Second and third trimesters.

Cause: Increased blood flow and circulation. Elevated estrogen levels.

Treatment: None.

Red Flags:

- Yellowing of palms and soles.

- Itching of only the palms and soles.
- Rash on palm and soles.

Q. I am noticing small growths of skin on my body, particularly under my arms and around my neck. What are these, and how do I get rid of them?

Symptom: Skin tags. These are small protruding growths of skin that usually show up on your neck, under your arms, on your breasts, or in your groin area. They are usually flesh-colored, although they can be a shade or two darker than your skin color.

Usual time of onset: Second and third trimesters.

Cause: Yep, you guessed it, elevated hormone levels.

Treatment: Skin tags may disappear after your pregnancy ends. If they don't, your OB (or a friendly dermatologist) can freeze or snip them off. There is nothing to do about them now, unless they are large or get in the way of your clothing (such as right where your bra strap sits) and bother you.

Red Flags: Tell your doc about any large growth on any part of your body, flesh-colored or not.

INSIDER SECRET:

Moles

Your moles may get darker or more prominent. While this is a common pregnancy phenomenon, your OB provider should always check out changing moles and refer you to a dermatologist if there is a concern.

Q. I've got rolls of skin I never had before. And some of those skin areas are now red and sore. What do I do?

Symptom: Chafing (***intertrigo***). These are red patches of skin usually in your armpits, under your breasts, and in other skin folds.

Usual time of onset: Second and third trimesters.

Cause: Elevated pregnancy hormone levels. Weight gain causing more skin folds than the Michelin Man. We know—it's depressing, but it's temporary.

Treatment: Keep the skin in these areas extra clean and dry. Because skin folds are usually moist, they're a setup for yeast and other skin infections. If it's not infected, your OB provider can give you the green light to apply 1 percent hydrocortisone cream.

Red Flags:

- Chafing that is getting worse.
- Foul odor and chafing.
- Burning and chafing.
- Excessive itching and chafing.

NORMAL?

Q. I have noticed a few patches of small bluish-purplish veins on my legs and feet. Do I need to worry about this?

Symptom: Spider veins on your lower extremities. They appear as broken blood vessels with a branching pattern on the skin's surface and are usually blue, purple, or red.

Usual time of onset: Second and third trimesters.

Cause: Elevated estrogen levels. You may be genetically predisposed. (It runs in families).

Treatment: Avoid crossing your legs when sitting down. Eating or drinking more vitamin C may help produce collagen and elastin, necessary to maintain healthy veins. After delivery, most spider veins fade in a few weeks to months. If yours remain (and they bother you), dermatologists and/or vascular surgeons can treat them with local injections or laser therapy. Ask your OB provider for a referral.

Red Flag: Pain or swelling and a large area of discoloration.

Q. My mother got varicose veins when she was pregnant with me. Will I be prone to them as well?

Symptom: Varicose veins. They appear as bluish-purplish tortuous veins usually seen on the legs, but sometimes on the tops of the feet, vulva, rectum (hemorrhoids), and buttocks. Sometimes they ache a bit.

Usual time of onset: Second and third trimesters.

Cause: Thank your genes. If someone in your family has them, you are more likely to get them during your pregnancy. Varicose veins also follow the laws of physics. When you are pregnant, the veins in the lower part of your body must work extra hard to return the blood back to your heart. Pretend your vein is a garden hose. Place a large boulder (the baby and uterus) in the middle of the hose. The part of the hose behind the boulder will bulge and possibly break as it tries to push the water against the boulder. This is what can happen to your veins during your pregnancy.

Treatment: The best treatment is prevention!

- Avoid sitting with your legs crossed.
- Avoid standing for long periods of time.
- When sitting, place your feet up on a few pillows so they are above the level of your body.
- Wear support stockings (they are far from sexy, especially in the summertime, but really help).
- Exercise.
- Take a vitamin C supplement.
- Avoid excessive weight gain during pregnancy.
- The good news: Many veins drastically decrease in size over the first few weeks to months after delivery. If you want permanent removal when you're done with childbearing, get a referral to a vascular surgeon.

Red Flags:

- Your entire leg is really painful.
- Swelling in one leg and varicose vein.

DR. M'S OPINION:

Varicose Veins

I recently delivered a patient who had one of the worst cases of varicose veins I had ever seen. Yet, at her two-week postpartum checkup, I told her that I wouldn't have recognized her if I hadn't seen her face. There was such a dramatic change, with 80 percent improvement in her varicose veins! The take-home message: Delivering the baby fixes many of these pregnancy maladies!

Q. I am hot and sweaty all the time despite sleeping without covers and having the air-conditioning on full blast. Will this last the whole pregnancy?

Symptom: Hot and sweaty 24/7.

Usual time of onset: Late second and third trimesters.

Cause: Elevated hormone levels make you and your menopausal mother feel the same way. View it as mother-daughter bonding. Carrying more weight around is also no friend to your thermostat.

Treatment: Buy a battery-operated fan, and take it with you everywhere. Dress in layers so you can easily adjust as the temperature changes throughout the day. Make sure you are drinking enough water. Freeze a water bottle every night so you have ice-cold water the next day.

Red Flags: None.

Partner Tip

Pregnancy may be the only time that you and your partner's body thermostat are aligned. You may be able to sleep in the same bed together without a down comforter and an extra blanket. That is if her fortress of pillows doesn't come between you.

Muscle, Bone, and Nerves

- Round ligament pain
- Groin pain
- Pubic bone joint (symphysis) pain
- Low back pain
- Sciatic pain
- Leg cramps
- Wrist pain (carpal tunnel syndrome)

Q. I am having pain in my belly. There is a pulling or tugging pain on one side more than the other. Should I be concerned?

Symptom: Round ligament pain. Sharp pain in your abdomen or hip area, on one or both sides. The pain may occasionally extend into the groin area. Pain is brief and typically only lasts a few minutes. There are no other symptoms.

Usual time of onset: Late first and early second trimester. It rarely occurs beyond that.

Cause: The rapidly growing uterus stretches the ligaments that attach the uterus to the sides of the abdominal wall. Any change in movement (like standing up or turning quickly) may also stretch this ligament(s) and cause pain.

Treatment: Unfortunately, there is no great treatment.

- Try to rest when it happens. Your body may be telling you that you're doing too much.
- Move and change positions more slowly.
- Try yoga or stretching exercises if round ligament pain happens regularly. Try this stretch: Place your hands and knees on the floor, while you lower your head to the ground and keep your tush in the air.
- Try using a maternity belt.

Red Flags:

- Constant, unrelenting abdominal pain.
- Vaginal bleeding and abdominal pain.
- Watery vaginal discharge and abdominal pain.
- Vomiting and abdominal pain.
- Diarrhea and abdominal pain.
- Fever or chills and abdominal pain.

DR. M'S OPINION

I used to tell my patients very casually, "Oh, it's just round ligament pain," until I experienced it with my first pregnancy. Wowsers! It's not serious, but it can be very painful.

Q. I am having pain in my groin. Do I have a hernia?

Symptom: Pain in the groin, particularly when walking or changing positions.

Usual time of onset: Second trimester.

Cause: Your pelvic and groin ligaments stretch, and this often causes pain. Your entire pelvic girdle (all the bones that make up your pelvis) is slowly opening in preparation for delivery, and this can cause all the bones to hurt (see question below). Your pubic bones can also hurt. Another source for groin pain: round ligament stretching (see previous question). It is rare for this pain to be caused by a hernia (when a body organ—usually your intestines—protrudes through a weakness in your connective tissue).

Treatment: A maternity belt can help.

Red Flags:

- Mass or bulge and groin pain.
- Severe, persistent groin pain.
- Severe abdominal pain and groin pain.
- Vaginal bleeding and groin pain.

Q. My pelvis and hip bones hurt! They seem to be out of sync. Should this be happening?

Symptom: Symphysis pubic dysfunction/pain. Your pubic bone hurts, or it hurts to stand or walk. At times, you may find it difficult to stand on one foot to wash the other one in the shower or even put on a pair of pants.

Usual time of onset: Late second and third trimesters.

Cause: In preparation for delivery, elevated hormone levels loosen the ligaments that hold your pelvic bones together. This loosens your joints and can cause the above symptoms. Some unlucky women have the same problem with their hips or their sacroiliac joint in the back (where the hip bone and backbone meet).

Treatment:

- Wear a pelvic girdle (you can be fitted for one at certain maternity stores).
- Wear tighter, more supportive garments like exercise pants or Spanx undergarments.
- Ask for a referral to a licensed massage therapist or chiropractor.
- Try yoga.

Red Flags:

- Painful urination and severe pubic pain.
- Blood in your urine and severe pubic pain.
- Vaginal bleeding and severe pubic pain.
- Abdominal pain and severe pubic pain.
- Any skin changes (such as redness) in the area of the pain.

Q. My lower back is really starting to hurt. Any way I can avoid having this discomfort?

Symptom: Low back pain.

Usual time of onset: Second and third trimesters.

Cause: As your pregnancy advances, the curvature of your spine changes. The added weight your body is carrying causes your center of gravity to shift. And loosening of ligaments (see above) contributes to back pain as well. Many pregnant women also suffer from sciatic pain because the sciatic nerve in their back is compressed. This feels like a sharp, shooting pain that goes from the lower back down to the legs. Not fun.

How to avoid it:

- Exercise.
- Avoid wearing high heels or completely flat shoes that do not offer any support.
- Squat to pick things up rather than bending over at the waist.
- Make a nest of pillows to get comfortable at night.
- Get enough rest.
- Work on your posture.

Treatment, once you've got it:

- Consider buying a maternity belt (around twenty-four to twenty-eight weeks). Get fitted at a maternity store.
- Wear shoes with good support.
- Sleep on your side.
- Place a pillow between your knees while sleeping.
- Get a massage from a licensed massage therapist or chiropractor who is well versed in pregnancy.
- Do stretching exercises upon waking and just before bed at night.
- Use a lumbar support pillow while sitting for long periods or driving.
- Use a heating pad.
- Take some acetaminophen (Tylenol) if all else fails.

Red flags:

- Painful urination and low back pain.
- Fever or chills and low back pain.
- Nausea or vomiting and low back pain.
- Abdominal pain and low back pain.
- Severe, constant low back pain that doesn't improve with any of the above treatments.
- Repetitive, rhythmic cramping pain in the back (concern: sometimes a sign of preterm or term labor contractions).

Fact Check

Lifting heavy objects will cause a miscarriage.

The truth: This is international folk wisdom. The story goes that lifting heavy objects can cause a miscarriage, the baby to get tangled up in its umbilical cord, or the baby to turn into a breech (bottom or foot/feet first) position.

All of these are false.

However, lifting heavy objects improperly *will* cause back pain. But you are more likely to suffer a back injury during pregnancy if you lift heavy things. We don't recommend that you carry around your thirty-five-pound toddler or rearrange furniture, even though we know it seems unavoidable. A word to the wise: no heavy lifting.

FEEDBACK FROM THE REAL WORLD:

Moving Furniture at Twenty-eight Weeks

You should have seen the look on my ex-husband's face when he saw me in my twenty-eighth week of pregnancy sitting in an entirely "redecorated" home office, complete with a new location for the desk and bookcase. It seemed like a good idea at the time . . .

Q. I've started having shooting pain on my left (or right) side going from my buttocks down the back of my leg. Is this something to be worried about?

Symptom: Sharp, shooting pain or burning on the backside of either leg. It may feel like "pins and needles" in the lower back or leg, and/or numbness in the leg or foot. It begins near the buttocks and travels down the back of the leg, sometimes all the way to the foot.

Usual time of onset: Late second and third trimester.

Cause: Sciatic nerve pain. Swelling in the tissues where the sciatic nerve exits the pelvis or pressure on the nerve by the enlarging uterus are the causes. It's also possible to reactivate an old injury, if you've had one before.

Treatment:

- Avoid walking up or down hills.
- Skip the high heels and ballet flats. Wear comfortable shoes with some degree of support. Although they aren't glamorous, a good pair of tennis shoes or clogs with rubber soles are perfect.
- Rest more and lie on the side that doesn't hurt.
- Limit how much you stand up.
- Avoid heavy lifting.
- Take a warm bath or place a heating pad on the area.
- Use acetaminophen (Tylenol) if necessary.
- Get a massage (by your partner or a professional).
- Buy a maternity belt.
- Get a physical therapy or pregnancy-chiropractor referral from your OB provider.

Red Flags:

- Severe, constant pain.

- A foot that drags or drops.
- Cannot walk.
- Swelling in one leg.

Q. I wake up in the middle of the night screaming because of cramps in my calf muscles. Do I need to take some vitamins or something?

Symptom: Severe leg cramps, most commonly occurring in the calves and at night, leading you to scream out profanities and scare your significant other half to death. Don't be surprised if your calf muscle is still sore a day or two after a middle-of-the-night attack.

Usual time of onset: Late second and third trimesters.

Cause: No one really knows why pregnant women have more leg cramps or why they happen more often at night. It's possible that your leg muscles are tired from carrying around all of your extra weight. And remember that your expanding uterus changes your blood circulation. Your leg muscles may not like this change.

How to avoid it:

- Don't sit with your legs crossed for long periods of time.
- Stretch your calf muscles before bedtime.
- Walk or exercise daily.
- Keep well hydrated.
- Wear support stockings.
- Take a warm bath.
- Get a bedtime leg massage from your partner.

Treatment:

- Keep a leather strap by your bedside, insert into your mouth, and bite down. (Just kidding—sorry, that's a bit of twisted OB-GYN humor.)
- Try this stretch: Straighten your leg by pushing out your heel first, then flexing your toes back toward your shin. This might not feel so great at first, but the spasm in your calf muscle will slowly ease.
- Apply local heat with a heating pad or warm washcloth.
- Try a calcium-magnesium supplement (if your OB provider thinks it's safe for you—check first). This won't treat the current cramp but may help prevent future episodes.

Red Flags:

- Muscle pain persisting for more than a day or two.
- Swelling or tenderness in the leg and severe leg cramps—this would require immediate medical attention. Pregnancy puts you at higher risk for a blood clot. They are rare, but they are serious.

If you have any of the above "Red Flag" symptoms, notify your OB provider immediately.

Q. My wrists and fingers have started to tingle and get numb. Why is that?

Symptom: Hand or fingers hurt or feel numb and tingle. But pain can also shoot up the forearm. It typically only involves the thumb, pointer, and middle fingers. This is called carpal tunnel syndrome (CTS). Symptoms are usually most intense at night and upon waking in the morning.

Usual time of onset: Late second and third trimester.

Cause: Swelling around your wrist puts pressure on the nerves and blood vessels that travel to your hand.

Treatment:

- Wear a wrist brace at night to relieve the discomfort.
- Limit your salt intake to decrease overall swelling.
- Avoid repetitive movements (like typing on a computer keyboard) that make it worse.
- Get a physical therapy referral.

Red Flags:

- Pain in your neck and shoulders with hand pain/numbness.
- Loss of sensation in your hands and/or fingers.
- Unable to hold objects in your hand.

Immune System

See Chapter 18, "Infections," for details on your body's immune system changes and answers to all your questions about preventing and treating infections during pregnancy.

But here is a brief summary of what you need to know: Your immune system is seriously suppressed during pregnancy because it has to be. Yes, this is the only time that you can have foreign DNA (husband's, boyfriend's, partner's, the sperm donor's, etc.) in your body and not reject it.

If you got a kidney transplant, you would need serious immunosuppressive medication in order to not reject the donated kidney. Your body does this on its own during pregnancy. But a lowered immune system means that you are more susceptible to everything . . . the common cold, cold sores, herpes outbreaks (if you have a history of these)—and everything your toddler brings home from preschool.

CHAPTER 6

Tests

"First the doctor told me the good news:
I was going to have a disease named after me."

—Steve Martin

What's in This Chapter

- **Standard pregnancy tests: when, why, and will it hurt?**
- **Additional tests**
- **The lowdown on ultrasounds**
- **Blood counts**
- **Infection screens**
- **First trimester genetic (chromosome) screening test**
- **Second trimester genetic screening test (AFP/spina bifida)**
- **Other genetic screening**
- **Diagnostic genetic tests (CVS and amniocentesis)**

Yes, you will have to endure many tests while you are pregnant. Good news: You don't have to study for any of them. But you may be curious as to *why* your OB provider needs a pint of your blood (okay, really a few tablespoons), makes you pee in a cup at what seems like every visit (because it is!), or, in certain cases, recommends testing that's a bit more intrusive (like putting a needle into your uterus).

That's why this chapter is here. It covers the tests you'll be taking, from A to Z.

As you'll discover, some tests are routine (usually blood and urine tests) and recommended for all pregnant women to help ensure a healthy pregnancy. If a test comes back other than normal, your OB provider can investigate further and will discuss other available tests or treatments to best protect you and your baby.

In contrast, other tests sometimes offered during pregnancy can be viewed as additional and are typically more useful for people at risk for more specific and less common problems or complications.

Our goal: This chapter aims to make you an empowered parent-to-be, armed with the information you need to make decisions about which of the tests that will be offered are appropriate and useful for you. We will do our best to explain it to you in English, in an organized fashion. We'll cover the tests in the order you will have them done or offered to you. And for each test, we'll note if it is routine or additional.

Before we get going, a word about tests and their limitations—science and technology have come a long way since our moms were pregnant with us. Yet, despite the sometimes dizzying array of tests on offer, none of them can guarantee your baby will be 100 percent perfect when born or in childhood. Nothing in life is guaranteed, and that rule applies here, too. Still, many of these tests can and will substantially lower the possibility that your baby will have one of the disorders that keep expecting parents up at night. It's also why your baby's pediatrician examines your newborn shortly after birth to make sure everything is as it should be.

Lots of Tests—Why and When

This table will give you an overview of all the tests that are offered during your pregnancy. They each fall into one of the following categories:

- **Routine tests.** These are screening tests recommended and routinely done on all pregnant women. Example: complete blood count (CBC).
- **Additional tests.** These are tests that may be useful for pregnant women whose individual medical history, age, or ethnic background puts them at risk for the disorders being tested for. They are done at your OB provider's discretion based on individual circumstances that arise during pregnancy. Example: Ashkenazi Jewish Genetic Screening Panel.
- **Chocolate tests.** These are tests involving the sampling of sixty-seven varieties of chocolate. (Just kidding!)

NEW PARENT-TO-BE 411:

Screening Tests Versus Diagnostic Tests

A ***screening test*** identifies a person to be ***at risk*** for a certain disorder or complication. A positive screening test only means that more specific and definitive testing needs to be done to see if a risk or diagnosis exists. A diagnostic test confirms that a disorder or diagnosis is actually present, in you or in the baby. For example, a pregnant woman who fails their one-hour glucola screening test does not necessarily have pregnancy-related diabetes. They will end up undergoing a diagnostic test—in this case, a fun-filled three-hour glucose tolerance test—which determines if they actually have the diagnosis.

First Trimester Tests

Blood Tests

Test	When It Is Done	Routine	Additional
Beta-hCG	First visit	✓	
Complete blood count (CBC)	First visit	✓	
Blood type; Rh/antibody screen	First visit	✓	
Hepatitis B testing	First visit	✓	
Hepatitis C testing	First visit	✓	
HIV testing	First visit	✓	
Syphilis testing	First visit and third trimester	✓	
Rubella immunity testing*	Before conception or first trimester	✓	
Varicella immunity testing*	Before conception or first trimester, unless you have had chickenpox	✓	
Cystic fibrosis screen (may be done with larger carrier screening panel)**	Before conception or first trimester		✓
Fragile X carrier screening**	Before conception or first trimester		✓
Hemoglobin electrophoresis**	First trimester	✓	
Ethnic carrier screening (such as Ashkenazi Jewish carrier diseases) or extended carrier screening**	Before conception or first trimester		✓
First trimester genetic screening: non-invasive prenatal screening (NIPS)/cell-free DNA screen for chromosome abnormalities	10–12 weeks	✓	

*Test is performed in a first pregnancy and not repeated with subsequent pregnancies if a person is immune.

**Test is performed in a first pregnancy only.

Urine Tests

Test	When It Is Done	Routine	Additional
Urine culture	First visit and when indicated	✓	✓ (when indicated)

Other Tests

Test	When It Is Done	Routine	Additional
Ultrasound, transvaginal (to check viability and size/dating)	First visit and later if indicated		✓

Test	When It Is Done	Routine	Additional
Pap smear (if you haven't had a recent one)	First visit	✓	
Cervical cultures (chlamydia/ gonorrhea)	First visit	✓	
First trimester fetal ultrasound (to check early anatomy and nuchal translucency)	10–14 weeks	✓	
Chorionic villus sampling (CVS) when indicated, for genetic testing, not screening	10–13 weeks		✓

Second Trimester Tests

Test	When It Is Done	Routine	Additional
Maternal serum AFP screening (for spina bifida)	16–20 weeks	✓	
Ultrasound, abdominal (fetal anatomy survey)	20–22 weeks	✓	
Ultrasound, transvaginal	When indicated		✓
Amniocentesis, when indicated, for genetic testing	15–20 weeks		✓
One-hour glucola (glucose challenge test for gestational diabetes)	24–28 weeks	✓	
Three-hour glucose tolerance test, if one-hour glucola test is elevated	24–28 weeks		✓
Fetal kick counts	26 weeks until delivery	✓	

Third Trimester Tests

Test	When It Is Done	Routine	Additional
Fetal kick counts	Now through delivery	✓	
Ultrasound, abdominal to assess fetal growth, possibly earlier if growth issues are present	32–36 weeks		✓
Repeat CBC	32–36 weeks		✓
Repeat vaginal/cervical cultures	32–36 weeks		✓
Repeat syphilis, HIV	32–36 weeks		✓
Non-stress test (NST)	28–42 weeks		✓
Biophysical profile	28–42 weeks		✓
Group B strep screening vaginal/ rectal swab	36-38 weeks	✓	

Tests Done at Every Visit

Test	When It Is Done	Routine	Additional
Urinalysis (U/A)	Every visit	✓	
Blood pressure	Every visit	✓	
Fetal heart tones	Every visit	✓	

Additional Specialized Tests

Test	When It Is Done	Routine	Additional
Toxoplasmosis and CMV antibody testing (screening when there is maternal illness or fetal concern)	Ideally before conception; for specific indications		✓
Herpes culture	First visit or if questionable lesion is present		✓
Parvovirus antibody testing	When indicated		✓

NEW PARENT-TO-BE 411:

True Positives Versus False Positives

Here's how to wrap your head around this concept.

Imagine a screening test is a fisherman's shrimp net. You want a net that catches all the shrimp ("true positive") and doesn't let them slip through the holes (that is, missing a true problem). But the net also picks up seaweed along with the shrimp. The seaweed is a "false positive" on a screening test. No screening test, by definition, can be perfect; otherwise, it would be diagnostic! But, when screening tests are designed and tested, the goal is to make sure the holes in the net are as small as possible, minimizing anxiety-producing false-positive results. This is an extremely important concept regarding screening tests: We typically start with them to avoid the potential annoyance, cost, or risk associated with some of the more definitive diagnostic tests, which provide the "true" results.

Q. There are so many additional tests, and many of them are expensive. How can I decide which tests I should do and which ones to skip?

Life was so much simpler when our parents were pregnant. As our moms like to remind us, they were never tested for diabetes nor did they have a single ultrasound during their pregnancies. They also casually mention that they didn't even put us in car seats when we were babies. We've come a long way, haven't we?

Today, there are so many tests it can make your head spin! While your gut says have every possible test done to check every possible thing, your pocketbook (or insurance company) may think otherwise.

The American College of Obstetricians and Gynecologists recommends certain tests in order to make sure all pregnant women get high-quality obstetric care. It's likely your insurance will cover the costs of all of those tests.

If you are delivering with a doctor, they will tell you which tests ACOG recommends. Other tests are your call.

Some optional tests are a good idea for all pregnant women. Other tests are most useful for members of certain at-risk ethnic groups or parents of certain ages. You should discuss these tests with your OB provider to find out which are most important for you. This chapter will help you consider your options.

Partner Tip

As you glance through this chapter, you'll notice a boatload of tests your pregnant other half will be enduring. Your job: Be there and be supportive. It's the little things that count: holding a hand, making a joke to distract from the needle, etc. And when test results are returned, be the rock. Your pregnant partner will need calm reassurance that everything will be fine.

There are also occasional tests that can or need to be done on both the pregnant woman and her male partner (screening for cystic fibrosis or other inheritable disorders, for example). Offering to do one or more of these tests will win you some mighty big brownie points. In addition, sometimes screening both of you is the only way to know if the pregnancy is at risk, so buck up!

First Trimester Tests

Routine Tests

Q. I had tubes and tubes of blood taken at my first prenatal appointment. Why?

There are certain tests that are recommended for every pregnant woman with every pregnancy, in order to identify potential health problems for mom and baby. The results of these tests are important to both your OB provider and your future baby's healthcare providers.

The standard tests include:

1. **Complete blood count (CBC).** This test identifies women who have ***anemia*** (see Complication #13 in Chapter 17, "The Complicated Pregnancy").

   People who are anemic carry less oxygen via their red blood cells to body tissues. There are many different causes of anemia, but it's most commonly due to iron deficiency.

   Your pregnant body requires more oxygen than your pre-pregnancy body. Plus, you will lose a good bit of blood during childbirth. So it's particularly important to detect anemia and treat it as soon as possible. For iron-deficiency anemia, treatment is pretty simple. Eat iron-rich foods and take an iron supplement.

   There may be other abnormalities detected on a CBC when people have inherited blood disorders involving the structure or production of hemoglobin (such as ***sickle cell disease*** and ***thalassemia***) that can potentially be passed on to the baby. These disorders can also lead to complications for you during the pregnancy. Both a CBC and hemoglobin electrophoresis (see more information below) help identify these inherited blood disorders.

The CBC also tells us your platelet count. Platelets are the cells that help your blood clot when it's supposed to. Certain conditions reduce platelet levels, so OB providers need to be aware of these as well (see Complication #17 in Chapter 17, "The Complicated Pregnancy").

2. **Your blood type and Rh.** Both your OB provider and your baby's pediatrician will want to know your blood type. This gets pretty technical, so buckle up.

   You've probably heard of blood types, but how are these determined? Well, your red blood cells have numerous proteins (antigens) that sit on the cell's surface. For the standard (letter) part of a blood type, there are two proteins: "A" and "B." You can have only one protein present (A or B blood type), both (AB), or no protein at all (O).

   Then, there is another group of proteins on the same crowded red blood cell that identify the Rh factor associated with a blood type (Rh stands for rhesus). If you have Rh proteins, you are Rh-positive. If you don't, you are Rh-negative; 85 percent of all people are Rh-positive.

   So, for example, if you have both an A protein and a Rh protein on your blood cells, your blood type is A positive. If you have no major blood type proteins or Rh proteins, your blood type is O negative.

   Now, let's tackle an important potential health issue involving Rh protein. If a pregnant woman's blood type is Rh-negative, their body could mount an immune response to their baby if the baby is Rh-positive (this is not a good thing). Long before delivery, the immune factors (antibodies) can cross the placenta into the baby's bloodstream and attack its Rh-positive blood cells. In these cases, the baby can develop severe anemia even before delivery. That's why if you are found to be Rh-negative, you will receive a standard, extremely well-studied injection called ***RhoGAM*** during your third trimester to prevent this response from occurring. The safety of this approach has been extensively established. The only exception to this protocol is if the baby's biological father is also Rh-negative and can produce a lab report to show it. In these cases, RhoGAM does not need to be given, since two Rh-negative parents can only make an Rh-negative baby. (More info on RhoGAM in Chapter 17, "The Complicated Pregnancy," Complication #14.)

   Separately, a different health issue can arise if your blood type is O and your baby is born with A or B blood type. (This can occur if the baby's biological father has A, B, or AB blood type.) A pregnant mother can potentially mount a response that destroys some of the developing baby's red blood cells, leaving the newborn at greater risk for jaundice in the first few days of life (***ABO incompatibility***). It's why your baby's doctor wants to know your blood type.

3. **Universal hemoglobinopathy testing.** The blood test called ***hemoglobin electrophoresis*** identifies people who are carriers or people with hemoglobinopathies such as sickle cell disease and thalassemia.

   Hemoglobin is a key protein that is found in red blood cells. Hemoglobin-

TESTS

opathy is a term used to describe all disorders involving abnormal hemoglobin, which could be due to either atypical structure or underproduction of the hemoglobin. These are genetically inherited disorders, and about one in sixty-six Americans have a hemoglobinopathy trait. When both parents have a trait, they are at risk for having a baby who has a hemoglobinopathy such as sickle cell disease or thalassemia. This is helpful for counseling for those who are at-risk about possible pre-implantation genetic testing and prenatal diagnosis. Because it is so common to have one of these traits, the ACOG recommends offering hemoglobinopathy testing to anyone who is interested in becoming pregnant or at the first prenatal visit if they have never been tested before.[1]

If you are interested in a deeper dive: Sickle cell disease is an inherited blood disorder where red blood cells are sickle-shaped (crescent-shaped) instead of round. This causes severe anemia, pain, and lack of blood flow to some organs and body tissues. It is more common in people of African, Central or South American (specifically Panamanian) descent as well as those of Caribbean, Mediterranean (Turkey, Greece, and Italy), Indian, and Saudi Arabian ancestry. One in twelve Black Americans is a carrier—one in every five hundred Black Americans has sickle cell disease.

There are two types of thalassemia—alpha and beta, depending on which protein abnormality is involved. Thalassemia disease can range from mild (thalassemia minor) to severe (thalassemia major). Most people with thalassemia minor lead normal lives and are usually symptom-free. The severe forms are treatable with frequent blood transfusions, but they can cause fetal death. People of Mediterranean (Italians, Greeks) and Middle Eastern ancestry (Iranians, Iraqis, Israelis) are more likely to be carriers of beta-thalassemia. Southeast Asian (Filipinos, Chinese, Vietnamese, Laotians, Cambodians) and African ancestries (African, Caribbean) are more likely to be carriers of alpha-thalassemia, although people of European ancestry can also carry the trait. For more detailed info see Chapter 17, "The Complicated Pregnancy," Complication #16.

4. **Infectious disease panel (HIV, hepatitis B, syphilis [RPR], rubella).** These diseases cause health problems for both the pregnant woman and the unborn baby. For example, a pregnant woman who had a previous hepatitis B infection but who didn't clear it is now a carrier and can pass it on to their baby. Those babies need two specific immunizations shortly after birth to prevent them from having a chronic hepatitis B infection. (For more information on vaccines, see "Vaccines," page 280.) Without those two shots, babies whose moms have chronic hepatitis B have a 90 percent risk of a long-term chronic infection themselves. With the shots, the risk goes down to 10 percent.

BOTTOM LINE: Knowing whether or not you have/had one of these infections is critical for both you and your baby. Check out Chapter 18, "Infections," for more details.

Q. My friends keep telling me about a blood test that can give me my baby's chromosomes and tell me the sex of my baby as early as ten weeks! Is that true?

OB and perinatal offices now routinely offer NIPS (non-invasive prenatal screening). It's also known as cell-free DNA (cfDNA) screening. These are screens for chromosome abnormalities that do not involve any risk to the pregnancy or fetus. Using new technology, this screen analyzes fetal DNA in a pregnant woman's blood.

This screening test is offered to pregnant women over the age of thirty-five, those who screened positive for a chromosomal problem using traditional testing, those with abnormal ultrasound findings, and those with a history suggestive of increased risk of certain chromosome abnormalities. This almost painless test (okay, blood draws can hurt a bit, but it's all relative!) can be done as early as ten weeks in a pregnancy with one or two fetuses.

If you were found to have triplets (and after you've gotten up off the floor), these tests are typically unreliable and not recommended at this time. If you begin pregnancy with twins, miscarry and lose a twin, hormones made by the second fetus and placenta can impact your NIPS results and increase the chance of a false-positive screening result.

These tests screen for ***Down syndrome***, trisomy 18, and trisomy 13 (three of the most common forms of chromosomal abnormalities). It can also give you the sex of your baby (XX or XY), and some can detect abnormalities in the sex ***chromosomes*** as well (missing or extra X or Y chromosomes, which are also associated with physical and developmental issues). The screening accuracy varies from 88 percent to 99.9 percent, depending on which abnormality is being assessed. Results come back in as few as ten days.

The downside? Cost. Yep, this screen is pricey (depending on what company you use), and most insurance companies do not pay for these tests.

Helpful Hint

ACOG does not recommend routinely testing for thyroid function. However, some doctors test their patients for this because altered thyroid function can lead to complications during pregnancy.

FEEDBACK FROM THE REAL WORLD:

Test Results

It's extremely important for medical providers to know the results of the routine prenatal lab work when your baby is delivered. The lab results should be on your chart when you are admitted to the hospital.

But just in case things don't go as well as planned, you should have a copy of your test results (or be able to access them on your medical practice's patient portal) to share with hospital staff when you are admitted in labor or for induction.

Q. Why is my blood pressure tested at every visit?

Your blood pressure is one of the most basic ways to assess your body's health—that's why doctors always check it whether you are pregnant or not. It's even more important to check your blood pressure during pregnancy because (as you know from reading the last chapter) you aren't living in the same body you were before this baby came along.

Some people experience pregnancy-induced high blood pressure that has to be monitored and occasionally treated (see Chapter 17, "The Complicated Pregnancy," Complications #20 and #21). And some people have high blood pressure *before* becoming pregnant. That needs monitoring and treatment, too.

OB providers check your blood pressure at the first office visit to make sure everything is normal. It is checked again at future visits to make sure it isn't getting too high.

By definition, 140/90 is high blood pressure (or ***hypertension***). But when you are pregnant, trends are also important.

DR. M'S OPINION

My doc radar goes on red alert if I have a patient whose blood pressure was 90/60 in her first trimester and is now 130/80 in the third trimester. This is a patient who must be followed very closely!

There's a wide range of normal. For example, "normal" for you may be 90/60 or it could be 120/78. What's not normal: 140 or higher for the systolic pressure—or 90 or higher for the diastolic pressure.

Helpful Hint

The first number (or the number on top) is the systolic (S) pressure, the force on the arteries when the heart is pumping. The lower number (the number on the bottom) is the diastolic (D) pressure, the force on the arteries when the heart is resting. Blood pressure is quoted as S/D.

Q. Why is my urine tested at every visit?

It is amazing what a few drops of urine can tell us about you!

First, ***bladder infections***. For non-pregnant women, detecting a bladder infection is easy—it hurts like the dickens to pee, and you have the urge to go every ten minutes. But many pregnant women with bladder infections do not have any symptoms at all. If this isn't treated, it can become a kidney infection, which in pregnancy can lead to a bunch of other not-so-fun things like pneumonia, an infection in your bloodstream, and preterm labor.

Next, we look for sugar (glucose), excessive fat breakdown (***ketones***), protein, and blood in the urine. These give clues as to whether you are taking in enough calories, are dehydrated, or possibly diabetic.

Now that you know why it's so important, just smile and nod every time the nurse hands you that plastic cup and says, "You know the drill. Use the towelette to wipe from the front to the back and then catch your midstream urine in the cup."

Reality Check

A word of prenatal etiquette—it's nice to wipe the outside of the cup with a paper towel before you hand it back to the nurse or leave it on the counter in the bathroom!

Q. Why do I need a Pap smear on my first pregnancy visit?

If you haven't recently visited your OB provider for well-woman care (a routine physical or checkup), you need a Pap smear. Your OB provider will be performing cervical cultures anyway, so it makes sense to screen for cervical cancer at the same time. Although it is relatively rare, about 3 percent of invasive cervical cancer is detected during pregnancy. Better to be safe and check it out!

If you have an abnormal Pap smear, your OB determines the next step based on the results, previous Pap smear results, your age, and if you have any other risk factors for cervical cancer. If there is a concern, you may need a simple procedure to look at the cells on the ***cervix***.

If everything looks okay, your doc will either repeat the Pap test in six months or may even wait until six weeks after delivery. In some cases, a vaginal delivery actually removes abnormal cells from the surface of the cervix and you might have a normal Pap afterward!

Q. Why do I need to be tested for sexually transmitted infections if my partner and I are faithful to each other?

You are correct that you are not at risk if neither you nor your monogamous partner currently has an infection. The problem is that women can have either chlamydia or gonorrhea without having any symptoms. It's technically possible for you to have a sexually transmitted infection and not know it. ACOG recommends that all pregnant women get this test done.

These infections can spell real problems for pregnancy and for a newborn whose birthing parent is infected. Chlamydia and gonorrhea can cause pelvic infections and other complications, including miscarriage. Babies born to women with active infections involving either chlamydia or gonorrhea are at risk for eye infections, blindness, and pneumonia. See Chapter 18, "Infections," for details.

BOTTOM LINE: Even though you don't think you need to be tested for sexually transmitted infections, it's worth doing it.

Additional Tests

Q. Will I have an ultrasound at my first visit?

Maybe.

Your OB provider may want to perform an ultrasound to confirm that your pregnancy is in the uterus and the due date is accurate.

But not every OB provider orders an early ultrasound. So don't be disappointed if you don't get to see your peanut at the first visit. And if your OB provider does order an ultrasound, don't be surprised if it is a *transvaginal* ultrasound.

Some women show up to their first OB visit with an excited grin, ready to see their bundle of joy on an ultrasound. That grin quickly turns to shock when they are told to take off their undies for the test.

In the early stages of pregnancy, everything is *really tiny*. A fetus at six weeks is actually only 4 to 6 *millimeters* in length. So a transvaginal ultrasound, which can get way closer to the uterus and the early pregnancy, is really the only way to see it and is usually the norm before nine to ten weeks of pregnancy.

To perform the exam, a thin ultrasound probe (we know it looks really scary, but it's not that bad) with a sterile protective sheath is inserted into the vagina, and voilà! The beauty of the female reproductive system is displayed on the screen.

After twelve weeks, the ultrasound images come from moving a different type of probe over a pregnant woman's belly (like you see on TV and in movies). Doctors only use transvaginal ultrasounds later in pregnancy for certain people who have high-risk conditions.

You'll find more info on ultrasounds in the second trimester section of this chapter.

Q. I just had a positive home pregnancy test and now have some bleeding. My doctor has asked me to come in for a blood test. Why?

Yes, some women have spotting during a normal pregnancy. But it can also be a sign of an ***ectopic pregnancy*** or a pregnancy that isn't developing normally.

In early pregnancy (before anything is visible on an ultrasound), your doctor can do a blood test to check rising ***beta-hCG*** levels to make sure your pregnancy is going in the right direction.

Your placenta makes beta-hCG, the pregnancy hormone. In most normal pregnancies, the amount of beta-hCG more than doubles (66 percent increase) every forty-eight hours until reaching its highest level at ten weeks gestation.

Beta-hCG levels decrease, stay the same, or rise at a slower rate with most (but not all) ectopic pregnancies and pregnancies that are developing abnormally.

FYI: Doctors can't see much on an ultrasound before five weeks gestation, even with a vaginal ultrasound. That's why the blood test is much more informative when there is spotting or bleeding early in pregnancy.

Q. My doctor offered genetic screening to me. What are these tests?

While there are many tests for this, we'll focus on four optional tests used to screen for genetic disorders (diseases caused by a defective gene). We will spare you the genetics lecture, but here is the general idea: Healthy people can be "carriers" for certain diseases. Carriers have one normal gene and one abnormal gene. People with the disease have two abnormal genes. If both parents are carriers, each of their children has a one in four chance of having the disorder.

Your OB provider or genetic counselor can advise you on which, if any, tests are worth doing with your ethnic background and family history, and on additional tests if you are carriers.

1. Cystic fibrosis (CF) carrier testing.

What is it? A disease affecting sweat and mucus production. It leads to chronic and serious problems with the lungs, pancreas, and digestive system. People with CF have a shortened life expectancy.

Who is at risk? Caucasians and Ashkenazi Jews are most likely to be carriers: the risk is about one in twenty-five. Other ethnic groups are less likely to be carriers: Latinos have a one in forty-six risk, Black patients have a one in sixty-five risk, and Asians have a one in ninety-four risk.[2]

What is the test? A blood test. If both parents are CF carriers, doctors can test the fetus for cystic fibrosis via an amniocentesis or ***chorionic villus sampling (CVS)***. As of this writing, a CF carrier test is covered by many insurance companies and is moderately priced for those who pay for it out-of-pocket.

How accurate is the test? CF can result from more than 1,000 known gene mutations, and the currently available tests can detect about 160 of them. So it is possible to have a negative screening test and have a baby with CF. Note: People of Asian and African descent have the least common CF mutations, so carrier testing is the least accurate in these ethnic groups. CF carrier screening can also be done by a newer technology called gene sequencing, which evaluates the CF gene at a much deeper level than a panel of set mutations. It is typically more informative for populations where CF is present but less common, and produced by less-common mutations.

CF screening is commonly included in larger extended carrier screening panels, which can use gene sequencing to identify if you are a carrier for more than 200 disorders (see item #4 on this list). You should discuss the pluses and minuses of single-test screening for CF or using a larger panel that includes CF screening. These extended panels typically use a grouping method that allows the cost for many tests together to be not much higher than screening for CF alone used to be.

Reality Check

In the United States, 1 in every 4,000 Caucasian babies is born with cystic fibrosis. The rate is 1 in 15,000 African American babies, and 1 in 32,000 Asian American babies.

2. Ashkenazi Jewish genetic panel (AJGP).

What is it? Test panels vary, but the panel Dr. M uses tests for carriers of up to twenty-two different disorders (including Tay-Sachs disease, Gaucher disease, Neiman-Pick disease, maple syrup urine disease, and Canavan disease). Note: Most AJGP tests include a cystic fibrosis carrier test because the risk of being a CF carrier is higher in this group. So be sure to ask what's included in the panel you are having done.

Who is at risk? These diseases are more common in Ashkenazi Jewish families who migrated from Eastern Europe—about 90 percent of Jewish Americans. One in every thirty Ashkenazi Jews is a carrier for Tay-Sachs disease. Tay-Sachs causes progressive neurologic deterioration and death in early childhood. For Jewish couples, I suggest doing this test. That's also true even when only one partner is

Jewish (although the risk is significantly lower of having a child with one of these diseases).

3. Fragile X carrier screen.

What is it? Fragile X syndrome is the most common inherited intellectual disability. It is named fragile X because the gene defect is located on the X chromosome. (This gene abnormality is different than the previous disorders discussed.) There is a broad range of symptoms. Some children have mild learning disabilities; others have autism spectrum disorder. Males with fragile X are more significantly affected because they have only one X chromosome, and it is abnormal. Females who have a fragile X defect are either unaffected or mildly affected, because they have two X chromosomes—one gene is normal and one is abnormal. The abnormal X chromosome is typically—but not always—inactivated, since only one normal chromosome is needed for normal growth and development in a female.

Who is at risk? A woman with a family history of autism spectrum disorder or undiagnosed intellectual disability is more likely to be a fragile X carrier. Testing is also helpful if either parent has a neurodevelopmental disorder or autism spectrum disorder.[3]

What is the test? A blood test. Fragile X screening is typically included in extended carrier screening tests (see below for more information). If you are a carrier (one of your X chromosomes has the mutation), there is a 50 percent chance that you will pass that mutation on to your offspring. CVS or amniocentesis can also determine if your baby is affected.

4. Expanded carrier screening (e.g., Inheritest).

What is it? Some commercial labs now offer very broad genetic screening panels covering more than ninety inherited diseases found throughout all ethnicities in the US population. Most of these commercial tests not only screen for diseases already discussed, such as for the genetic disorders that are more common among Ashkenazi Jewish parents, and for cystic fibrosis, but also screen for extremely rare disorders.

What is the test? If both partners are carriers of the same disorder, a test on the amniotic fluid or CVS specimen can determine whether the fetus is affected with that disease. The turnaround time for results is about ten to fourteen days. As you might expect, it's expensive. The cost depends on a person's insurance coverage, which varies by individual plan. As the technology improves, the overall cost for expanded carrier screening is becoming less pricey than one-by-one screening for individual disorders. These screens can be really useful, but we strongly recommend having genetic counseling *before* undergoing any genetic screening tests. Meeting with a genetic counselor prior to having any genetic screening tests not only allows for full explanation of the test and the possible results, but also gives you a point person to consult if results come back positive.

DR. M'S OPINION:

The Value of Testing

These screens have the potential to freak people out. If one parent-to-be turns out to be a carrier for such a disorder, it is a bit unsettling until both partners are tested. (Recessive inherited diseases require both parents to be carriers to produce a child with the disease.) Many people are carriers of autosomal recessive disorders, and in fact, it is rare to see someone who is not a carrier of any disease. More information is always better, so having both partners tested usually reveals that the disorder in question is not carried by both parents. And remember, a screening test is very different than a diagnostic test. Even if both parents carry the same autosomal recessive trait, only one in four babies will be affected with the disease.

Additional Tests

Q. Should I do any extra tests during pregnancy if I'm an "older mom"?

It's probably a good idea to at least discuss these with your OB provider and think about whether they'd be helpful for you. ACOG recommends that women who will be thirty-five or older at the time of delivery be offered prenatal *testing* (not screening) to diagnose (or far more likely, to rule out) Down syndrome and other chromosomal problems in the fetus.

And with modern medicine, not every pregnant woman who is thirty-five or older automatically needs to have an amniocentesis. There are less invasive, safer tests that are still very good at predicting (the usually low) risk of the more common chromosome abnormalities seen in pregnancy. See the next questions for more details. Take a moment to read up on chromosomes and the different test options in this category. We will pull it all together for you at the end of this section.

Note: Some tests are done in the first trimester and others are done in the second trimester. But for simplicity sake, all of them are covered here so you have a better feel for what your options are.

Q. Why would I want to test for chromosomal abnormalities if I am planning on having the baby no matter what?

Great question—and a very common one, we might add. Here are some things to consider:

- **It's nice to be prepared.** You can plan now for a baby that may need special medical attention after delivery and who may benefit from early intervention therapies as an infant. The doctor can also prepare to have all the necessary people ready at birth (the pediatrician, and in some cases a neonatologist or pediatric surgeon). It also helps you and your family prepare mentally, emotionally, and financially.

NEW PARENT-TO-BE 411:

Chromosomes

Chromosomes are very thin strands of DNA (deoxyribonucleic acid) that are found in almost all the cells in our body. A person normally has twenty-three pairs of chromosomes, for a total of forty-six. We get half of our chromosomes from our mother and the other half from our father. The first twenty-two are numbered. The last pair are the sex chromosomes, and they determine if we are male or female. In medical terms, genetic females have a chromosome reading (karyotype) of 46,XX, and males are 46,XY.

About 1 in every 200 babies will have some abnormality in the number or structure of their chromosomes. These occur when there is either an abnormal number of chromosomes or an abnormal amount of information on the chromosomes (such as when there is an extra or missing piece).

Trisomy means there are three chromosomes instead of two in a pair. The most common abnormality is Down syndrome (also called trisomy 21 because the twenty-first pair has three chromosomes). Trisomy 13 and trisomy 18 are also major chromosomal defects. Many fetuses with either of these two chromosome problems either miscarry early in pregnancy, result in fetal deaths in the second or third trimesters, or will pass away shortly after birth. Severe structural abnormalities are commonly seen in these fetuses or newborns; they often contribute to the life-limiting nature of these diagnoses.

Each abnormality has its own unique effects on a growing embryo/fetus/newborn, leading to varying degrees of intellectual impairment and birth defects.

How do these chromosome problems happen? There is usually an issue with the genetic material in either the egg or the sperm before conception even occurs. As women age, our chromosomes get "sticky." It is harder for them to separate after fertilization, and as a result, some early embryos get an extra chromosome in every cell as they divide, and some get too few. The older we are when we conceive, the higher the chances are that our eggs will result in embryos with abnormal chromosomes. Sad to say, but it is true that our egg quality declines with time. We are born with all the eggs we will ever have, and the older we get, the more likely our eggs will have issues. They are continually exposed to environmental dangers for all the years we've lived prior to pregnancy.

Guys are not off the hook, however, even though their sperm is "fresh" (meaning that new sperm are made every day). The older the guy, the more likely his sperm contains abnormal chromosomes (you can remind your guy of that if he chides you for your "advanced maternal age"). In fact, men over the age of forty have a five times greater risk of having a child with autism spectrum disorder, which is thought to be caused in part by several genetic abnormalities. Offspring of older dads, especially those over forty-five, are also at higher risk of having glitches in single genes, which can result in severe developmental abnormalities. Achondroplasia, or dwarfism, for example, is one of the more common diagnoses associated with single-gene abnormalities.

- **You might change your mind.** Some chromosomal abnormalities are, unfortunately, associated with very poor odds of newborn survival and can even be lethal after birth. It may be psychologically difficult to continue the pregnancy when you know the outcome. Your OB provider should discuss all options with you if there is an unexpected fetal test result, and also refer you to other consultants and specialists to help decide what is best for you.

Q. I'm over thirty-five and having my first baby. My doctor suggested that I have either a CVS (chorionic villus sampling) or amniocentesis. What are these tests?

Both a CVS and an amniocentesis are diagnostic tests—meaning that the results will accurately diagnose a chromosome defect in the fetus 99 percent of the time. Both tests can also diagnose some genetic disorders like cystic fibrosis and thalassemia.

Let's start with CVS, or ***chorionic villus sampling***—now you see why we call it "CVS" for short! A high-risk obstetrics specialist (also called a maternal-fetal medicine specialist) performs the test in the first trimester, between ten and thirteen weeks. Depending on the location of the placenta, either a very thin catheter (transcervical CVS) or a very thin needle (transabdominal CVS) is guided under real-time visualization on an ultrasound into the placenta to obtain a very small amount of placental tissue. In experienced hands, the risk of miscarriage with this procedure is small, and avoids the fetus completely.

The main advantage of CVS over amniocentesis is that it can be done earlier in pregnancy, so there is more time for a couple to make decisions if the results are abnormal. The slight disadvantage is that the procedure carries a slightly higher risk of miscarriage (1 in 700 to 800) than with amniocentesis (1 in 1,500). An ***amniocentesis*** (or amnio, for short) gives us the same information as a CVS, but it is done at a later point in pregnancy (around fifteen to twenty weeks). OB providers rarely do amniocentesis any earlier than fifteen weeks because the chance of complications caused by the test before fifteen weeks has been shown in a number of studies to be higher.

Your obstetrician or a maternal-fetal medicine specialist performs the amniocentesis. The doctor guides a very thin needle through the skin into the uterus (while watching its movement on an ultrasound) and withdraws a little bit of amniotic fluid for testing. About an ounce of amniotic fluid is obtained, which is less than 5 percent of all the fluid in the uterus in the second trimester. Since amniotic fluid is essentially

DR. M'S OPINION:

Does Amniocentesis Hurt?

Having had one of these myself, I'll tell you honestly. It's a combination of slight pain (like a pinch), a tickle, and the sensation of needing to pee all at once. The most common word my patients have used to describe it is "weird." But it's over very quickly, and you don't need anything more than a little Band-Aid to cover the area.

fetal urine (without the waste part), a fetus with normal kidneys will replace the fluid taken for an amnio within twenty-four hours.

Patients often worry that the needle will poke the baby during the procedure. Yes, it happens, but it is exceedingly rare (that's why we don't let your partner do the amnio, no matter how handy they swear they are). The doctor will be looking on the ultrasound to make sure the needle is in the right spot, away from the placenta and the baby. Very rarely, a fetus moves and bumps into the needle. And even if this happens, it's even rarer for something bad to happen as a result of this encounter.

The advantages of amniocentesis are that the procedure is a little safer, and the test, on occasion, eliminates some confusing results that rarely occur with a CVS sample (in less than 0.5 percent of CVS procedures a "mixture" of fetal and placental DNA is obtained). Otherwise, the accuracy of the two procedures is equivalent. Amniocentesis also checks the amniotic fluid for AFP levels, which screen for brain/spinal cord and stomach/intestine malformations. The disadvantage is that the procedure must be done later in pregnancy.

NEW PARENT-TO-BE 411:

CVS Versus Amniocentesis—Which Is the Better Test?

You are going to have to decide for yourself. But we'll give you the pros and cons to make the call.

CVS

Pros

- It can be done earlier, between ten and thirteen weeks.
- It allows decisions regarding termination to be made earlier in pregnancy.
- FISH (a high-tech molecular genetics test done on DNA obtained from either a CVS or amnio) typically gives preliminary results for the most common chromosome abnormalities in twenty-four to forty-eight hours.
- Final results are usually obtained within seven to ten days.
- It will definitively identify 99 percent of all chromosomal abnormalities.
- It can also test the fetus for certain inherited diseases, such as cystic fibrosis and thalassemia.

Cons

- It's an invasive test with a higher risk of miscarriage (1 in 700 to 800).
- There is a small amount of pain/discomfort involved with the procedure.
- It is expensive, although most insurance plans cover a portion or all of this procedure.

FYI: If you do an amniocentesis, you don't need a MSAFP test, because both tests screen for the same problems. (Read about second trimester screening below.) If you did a NIPS test in the first trimester and it came back low risk, you should discuss with your OB provider what additional information would be gained from doing an invasive test like a CVS or amniocentesis. Every pregnancy is different, and although in some cases it is safe to skip more invasive tests, an in-depth discussion with your OB provider will shed more light on what the best option is for you.

Reality Check

Does insurance cover these tests? Unfortunately, the answer for this varies by your state and insurance provider (most insurance policies cover needed tests during pregnancy). But, typically, insurers cover both CVS and amnio for birthing parents over the age of thirty-five, as they do for abnormal screening tests or fetal ultrasounds.

TESTS

- It is sometimes difficult to find an experienced physician to perform the procedure. There is less training for performing a CVS than for an amnio nationally, but this is changing.
- You need to rest for twenty-four to forty-eight hours after the procedure with restrictions on your activity for seven days.

Amniocentesis

Pros

- It is done between fifteen and twenty weeks. It is helpful for following up on an abnormality in a second trimester ultrasound once the window for CVS has passed.
- As with CVS, the FISH test gives preliminary results in two to three days.
- Final results are usually obtained within seven to ten days.
- It will definitively identify 99 percent of all chromosomal abnormalities.
- It can also test the fetus for different diseases, such as cystic fibrosis and thalassemia.
- AFP levels are tested in the amniotic fluid, which help detect neural tube and abdominal wall defects.

Cons

- It is an invasive test with a risk of miscarriage (1 in 1,500).
- There is a small amount of pain/discomfort involved with procedure.
- You will need to rest for twenty-four to forty-eight hours after the procedure with restrictions on activity for seven days.

Q. Are there any other non-invasive test options to diagnose fetal issues?

Yes, but only in the second trimester. The AFP blood test (alpha-fetoprotein) measures the level of AFP, a fetal blood protein, in the mom's blood. Higher levels of AFP are seen in pregnancies where fetal anatomy has not formed properly during development. These affected areas are typically the skull and the spinal column, as well as the abdominal wall. Major brain/spinal cord defects can be predicted with 80 percent accuracy with the AFP test, with even more severe skull and brain defects (***anencephaly***, where the skull has not developed at all) can be flagged with 97 percent accuracy. Abdominal wall and intestinal malformations can be identified by an elevated AFP level in 85 percent of cases.

Even if your NIPS test was normal, it's a good idea to do this test, as it screens for additional and completely different problems than the first trimester blood test can. And with the blood being drawn in the second trimester, there is enough time to do an amniocentesis if the AFP is elevated and additional information is desired. Even if you opt against an amniocentesis, with an elevated AFP test you will be referred for a high-level fetal ultrasound to get a better and detailed look at fetal anatomy overall.

NEW PARENT-TO-BE 411:

Chromosome Testing Options

How do you decide which chromosome testing you want to do? There are three options:

Option #1: NIPS (non-invasive prenatal screening)/cfDNA (cell-free DNA screening) and first trimester ultrasound

This blood test can analyze your fetus's DNA circulating in your bloodstream. These tests are highly sensitive in detecting fetal chromosomes and can detect the risk of trisomy 21, 18, 13, and a few more chromosomal issues in the fetus. It will also predict the sex of your fetus. There are a few on the market from different companies.

In addition to this blood test, a first trimester ultrasound screens for fetal malformations associated with chromosome abnormalities by looking at the development of the neck area (nuchal translucency) and early anatomy.

These tests are more sensitive than older screening tests that measured maternal hormone and protein levels to predict the risk of chromosome abnormalities in a pregnancy. The cfDNA test is currently the recommended first-line chromosomal screening option for all pregnant women in the United States.

Caution: cfDNA, while a much better screening test than most, is still a screening test. Different lab companies report their results differently. Some reports will read "negative" for trisomy 21, for example, but, as a screening test, the accuracy rate can never be 100 percent. Those that report results as "low risk" or "high risk" are getting the proper language to the patient. Most insurers

Here are a few reasons why you might get a positive AFP test result:

- Your dates are off. The test can only be done between fifteen to twenty weeks, and is most accurate between sixteen and eighteen weeks.
- You are carrying multiples and didn't know it.
- You have higher or lower amounts of certain hormones in your blood.
- You have a baby with one of the disorders mentioned above.

If your dates are solid and you aren't carrying multiples, you will be offered the option of doing more tests: an ultrasound, non-invasive prenatal screening, and/or amniocentesis.

This test may also throw you a curveball. Although your AFP levels may not suggest a specific disorder, the levels can indicate an increased risk of pregnancy-related complications. These include fetal growth restriction, preterm delivery, and ***preeclampsia***. See Chapter 17, "The Complicated Pregnancy" (see Complications #20 and #46). Your doctor will go over what additional monitoring you and your baby might need.

TESTS

cover these tests given that our national OB-GYN societies recommend them, but you should check with your insurance carrier to see whether they have preferred in-network testing companies, and how much the out-of-pocket costs might be.

Dr. M's opinion: If available to you, cfDNA is a more accurate screening test than what we've had in the past and something to strongly consider if you are over the age of thirty-five.

Option #2: Chorionic Villus Sampling

This is the better choice if you want definitive testing early on in your pregnancy. Your doc may recommend it if you had a previously abnormal fetus, had multiple miscarriages, or have other risk factors that place you into the "high-risk" category.

Pro: Testing provides a definitive answer in the first trimester.

Con: There is a small risk of miscarrying from the procedure.

Option #3: Amniocentesis

Just as with the CVS, you will know your fetus's exact chromosomes. The test is performed between fifteen and twenty weeks (but usually between sixteen and eighteen weeks).

Pro: Testing provides a definitive answer. Amniocentesis also offers additional screening for certain malformations. The risk of miscarrying from the procedure is slightly lower than with CVS.

Con: There is a small risk of miscarrying from the procedure, and it has to be done later in your pregnancy.

Helpful Hint

Carrying twins can make test results for the second trimester screening a bit tricky to interpret (because multiples will increase the levels of AFP, one of the substances tested). And the test is inaccurate if a woman is carrying a multiple pregnancy greater than twins (triplets, quads, etc.).

So it's a good idea to know if you are carrying more than one baby before signing up for this test.

Reality Check

It is important to realize that although the words "positive" and "negative" are typically used when discussing test results, what you actually get is a risk assessment. For example, a positive screen may say that the risk of having a baby with Down syndrome is one in seventy-five. But look at it this way: The odds of having a normal fetus are seventy-five times greater than having a fetus with Down syndrome.

Second Trimester Tests

Routine Tests

Q. What is an ultrasound anyway, and how does it work?

An ultrasound is a machine that uses sound waves to form pictures of internal body structures. Denser structures (like bone) look bright white on the screen, and liquids (like urine, amniotic fluid, and blood) look black.

Yes, it is safe when a skilled ultrasonographer or OB provider is doing it for a medical reason. There is no radiation risk to the baby with an ultrasound.

Fetal ultrasounds have been performed for more than forty years now, and to date, no significant health concerns have popped up. If you do a quick internet search on this topic, you'll see speculation that ultrasounds cause lower birth weights or left-handedness. But there's no quality research to back up these claims.

However, both ACOG and the American Institute of Ultrasound in Medicine (AIUM) only recommend ultrasounds for medical purposes. Doing an ultrasound only for personal reasons (keepsake pictures, or 3D "glamour shots," for example) is not standard practice.

Q. What can you see on an ultrasound?

Doctors can see lots of things. But you'll think your doctor is making it up, because to the untrained eye, the images resemble fuzz on an old black-and-white TV!

Early in pregnancy, doctors can see:

- whether the pregnancy is in the uterus.
- the number of fetuses in the uterus.

- abnormalities like an ovarian cyst.
- the length of the cervix.

By mid-pregnancy, doctors can see:

- all major organs of the fetus.
- the placenta, thriving and in a good position.
- whether there is an adequate amount of amniotic fluid.
- the sex of the baby!

In late pregnancy, doctors can see:

- fetal position—what direction the baby is facing in the pregnant woman's pelvis.
- baby's size (give or take a little).
- volume of amniotic fluid.
- placental health.
- baby's overall well-being.

BOTTOM LINE: Remember . . . if you don't want to know the sex of your baby, tell anyone who is caring for you, has access to your chart, and gives you test results that you want to be surprised!

Q. How accurate is the ultrasound?

When it comes to the baby's age and size, it depends on when it is done. First trimester ultrasound exams can accurately determine how far along your pregnancy is and your actual due date. It's less accurate as the pregnancy progresses. The same goes for size. An ultrasound exam can more reliably predict a baby's weight at twenty-five weeks than at forty weeks.

Ultrasound is very good at detecting some major abnormalities, but it can't identify every structural birth defect. Ultrasounds are amazing but not perfect. The humans performing the exams aren't perfect, either. For instance, an ultrasound may not always pick up a ***cleft lip***, ***cleft palate***, or even some heart defects. Ultrasounds also cannot screen for disorders that affect body function and not structure—like ***cerebral palsy*** or autism. But *most* of the time, ultrasounds identify *most* major structural defects.

If you only have one ultrasound exam, the ultrasound done between twenty and twenty-two weeks is most useful. This ultrasound is performed to see all of your baby's anatomy in detail. At this point, most problems involving the major organs are detectable.

In a few cases, however, they will be missed or will develop later on in pregnancy after most ultrasounds have already been performed. So, although it is rare, it is possible to deliver a baby with a problem that wasn't detected on any of your earlier ultrasounds.

Q. How often will I have an ultrasound?

It depends on your OB provider and whether or not you have a high-risk pregnancy. If you are carrying multiples, or have a history of preterm labor or diabetes, you will undoubtedly have more ultrasound exams than your low-risk preggo friends.

Some OB providers do not perform *any* ultrasounds. Some will do two to three throughout the pregnancy. Others will do more. An ultrasound is not absolutely necessary if you have a low-risk pregnancy. But ultrasounds do provide reassurance, as well as some pretty useful information.

No matter what the frequency, you probably won't have an ultrasound at every office visit!

DR. M'S OPINION

I think it's helpful to do at least two to three ultrasounds for a low-risk pregnancy. But every doc has their own opinion.

Here are the typical times for ultrasounds and the reasons why:

- **First prenatal visit:** to confirm that your pregnancy is in the uterus, that your dates are accurate, and to detect the presence of a fetal heartbeat.
- **First trimester (10–14 weeks):** to assess early fetus anatomy and to measure the thickness of the fluid-filled space that is the fetus's developing neck area (nuchal translucency). Nuchal translucency measurements screen for Down syndrome and some other chromosomal defects.
- **Second trimester (20–22 weeks) fetal anatomy survey:** to look at all of baby's internal/external body parts.
- **Third trimester (28–32 weeks):** to assess fetal growth, confirm or follow up on the location of your placenta, and assure an adequate amount of amniotic fluid.

Helpful Hint

If your doctor doesn't do ultrasounds, you can request one. ACOG policy says your doctor should honor that request and make a referral.[4]

Q. What happens if an abnormality is found on an ultrasound?

Remember our analogy comparing false positives and shrimp nets? Most of the stuff an ultrasound identifies is seaweed.

In this case, the seaweed is either a normal variation in fetal development, one that resolves on its own . . . or one that you or your baby would never know about if you didn't have an ultrasound.

The first thing to do is relax. Second, listen carefully to everything your doctor tells you. Third, ask questions. And call your doctor the next day if you come up with twenty-two more questions once you have had time to absorb it all.

What happens next depends on what the abnormality is, when it is found, and where it is found.

Partner Tip

Remember at the beginning of this chapter when we said it was your job to be there to support your pregnant half? Well, here is where the rubber meets the road: If an abnormality is found on an ultrasound, you have to help calm the waters. It is your job to take notes and organize questions. Calm and cool is your mantra.

Q. All of my friends are getting 3-D and 4-D ultrasounds of their babies. My doctor only does 2-D ultrasounds. Is that okay?

Yes.

A three-dimensional (3-D) or four-dimensional (4-D) ultrasound can help rule out certain defects, like a ***cleft lip*** or ***cleft palate***. However, an experienced doctor can often identify birth defects and problems in pregnancy with a conventional 2-D ultrasound.

FYI: ACOG does not find any clear advantage of using 3-D or 4-D ultrasound routinely over 2-D.

Yes, it is pretty cool to see what your baby really looks like inside your womb with one of these fancy 3-D or 4-D ultrasounds. Fun, yes. Necessary, no.

TESTS

DR. M'S OPINION:

Keepsake Ultrasounds

Like ACOG, I believe that ultrasounds should be done for medical reasons only. I discourage you from going to a pregnancy spa and getting a glamour shots-style 3-D or 4-D ultrasound.

Why? First of all, you don't know whether the technician has received proper training. And you don't know if the technician's supervisor has had any medical training. Or if the ultrasound machine is properly maintained.

And some of these "photo shoots" can last three to four hours. It's not worth the risk of exposing your baby to several hours of sound waves and excess heat.

Bottom line: Medical ultrasounds, okay. Keepsake ultrasounds, not okay.

Reality Check

Your OB provider can print out some pictures of your medical ultrasound if you want a keepsake for your baby book. Your OB provider or ultrasonographer may also allow you to snap some pictures or take video during your ultrasound—but it's best to ask permission first.

Q. What is the one-hour glucola test?

The one-hour glucola screening test identifies those at risk for diabetes during pregnancy (***gestational diabetes***). It is usually done between twenty-four and twenty-eight weeks. But people who have risk factors for gestational diabetes may have this test done as early as the first visit. It tests how efficiently your body handles sugar.

We know what you are thinking. You don't have a history of diabetes or any symptoms. No one in your family has diabetes. But despite all of that, being pregnant is a risk factor in and of itself, so everyone—yes, you, too—gets screened. The only people who don't get this test are those who already have diabetes and know it.

Here's how the test works: An hour before your lab appointment, you drink eight ounces of a sugary liquid that tastes like an extra sweet, flat soda. If you're lucky, you get to pick the flavor. One tip: Chill the drink. It tastes better that way.

Some doctors will request you fast before drinking the cocktail; some don't.

The key part: You must drink the whole thing in about five minutes, *exactly* an hour before having blood drawn. It's best to be on the safe side and arrive a little early for your appointment. Why? If you are late, your blood can't be drawn and (yep, you guessed it) the test has to be repeated on another day. So if you are stuck in traffic and will be two hours late, call your doctor's office to reschedule (and get another sugar drink).

DR. M'S OPINION:

Glucola Taste Tests

I tried the orange glucose drink with my first pregnancy and the lemon-lime with my second. I came to the following scientific conclusion: If you are a 7UP or Sprite fan, pick the lemon-lime flavor. If you like orange soda, go for the orange one.

Common risk factors for gestational diabetes include:

- history of gestational diabetes with a previous pregnancy
- family history of diabetes
- obesity
- ethnicity (Latino, African, Native American, South or East Asian, or Pacific Islands ancestry)
- over the age of thirty-five
- history of previous stillbirth
- history of having a large baby
- other endocrine problems such as thyroid disease

If you *aren't* pregnant and have diabetes, your body does not make enough insulin—or does not respond to the insulin it does make. Insulin is a hormone that tells your body to process sugar (glucose) you eat and turn it into energy. Excess sugar is stored for later use. Diabetes *during pregnancy* (gestational diabetes) is usually due to a completely different issue. The culprit: a hormone made by the placenta (human placental lactogen or hPL). This hormone impairs the pregnant woman's body's ability to use insulin.

Reality Check

If you had gestational diabetes with a previous pregnancy, you have a 33 to 50 percent chance of having it with any subsequent pregnancy.

Q. My glucola test was abnormal. What does that mean?

It means your blood sugar level was higher than what it should be.

According to ACOG, an abnormal test result is anything above 140.

FYI: Many OB providers are being more conservative with this test, especially for moms-to-be who already have other risk factors for diabetes. In these cases, test results in the 120s or 130s may be flagged as abnormal. As a rule, a cutoff of 135 to 140 is standard, and lower or higher cutoffs are now common practice.

Of course, there is a downside to this conservative approach: More women who *don't* have diabetes have to endure additional testing.

If the glucola test is abnormal, your OB provider will ask you to do another test to see if you really have gestational diabetes. This is called a ***three-hour glucose toler-***

INSIDER SECRET:

Carb Loading Before Your Three-Hour GTT

If your one-hour glucola screening test came back abnormal (that is, you might have diabetes), the natural tendency after hanging up the phone is to go into starvation mode. You'll be tempted to cut out those foods you think might worsen blood sugar, like pastas, breads, sweets, fruits, etc.

This is not the right thing to do!

Ironically, if you skip the carb loading for at least three days prior to your next test (three-hour GTT), you are more likely to falsely elevate your blood sugars. Then you will get a false positive diabetes test . . . and be treated like a diabetic for the remainder of your pregnancy. You may want to consider using a continuous glucose monitor. Otherwise, you'll endure daily finger pricks to check your sugar levels upon waking in the morning and after meals. Yes, that's 200 to 400 needle pricks during the rest of your pregnancy!

Our advice: Just follow your doctor's directions and enjoy carb-loading prior to your three-hour GTT. Your doctor typically will provide you a list of foods; we have also included one below.

Eat at least ten servings of foods each day, such as bread, fruit, and milk. Here is an example of ten servings:

1 cup milk
1 slice bread
1 dinner roll
⅓ cup cooked pasta
½ cup black beans
1 tortilla
1 cup berries
1 small apple/orange
½ cup corn
3 cups popcorn

ance test (GTT). Personally, we think this test should be named the glucose torture test . . . it's no fun.

Here's how the test works.

- You eat an unrestricted diet with at least 150 grams of carbohydrates per day for at least three days before the test (your OB provider will provide a list of good carb choices; see the box on the previous page).
- You fast after midnight.
- You show up at your doctor's office or lab first thing in the morning.
- You get your fasting blood drawn.
- You drink another yummy glucose drink, one with twice the amount of sugar as the first test.

Then, here comes the really fun part. Wait for it . . .

- You sit in the office or lab for *three* hours and get your blood drawn each and every hour.

Sorry, you can't run errands in between. Getting up and running around affects your metabolism and how your body uses sugar (glucose)—thus ruining your test results. Bring your laptop or favorite book.

Q. My three-hour GTT was abnormal. My doctor said I have gestational diabetes. Now what? Will my baby be okay?

An abnormal test means that at least two of the four glucose levels came back elevated. Don't panic. Most people who develop gestational diabetes control their sugar levels with diet and exercise alone. With excellent control of sugar levels, your baby will be fine.

Here is the key issue: Because of the placenta and the process of diffusion, your unborn baby has the same sugar levels as you do. If your blood sugar levels are high, so are your baby's. So you and your baby benefit from keeping your blood sugars under control.

Your OB provider may refer you to a diabetic educator or nurse. That person will teach you about your diet and optimal blood sugar levels. They will also instruct you how to check your own blood sugars (yes, unfortunately, that means you need to poke your fingers a few times a day or opt for a continuous glucose monitor instead) and record your glucose values throughout the day. Although we know it is a pain in the butt (or finger), you need to follow your diet and monitor your sugar levels closely.

You will discuss your sugar levels with your doctor at each visit. Occasionally, glucose levels remain elevated despite a patient following a strict diet. If this is the case, you may need injectable insulin.

If you need more inspiration, read more about gestational diabetes in Chapter 17, "The Complicated Pregnancy," Complication #26.

Q. My doctor talked to me about "fetal kick counts." What are they? Do I really have to do them every day?

A healthy baby is a baby that moves around. Most babies have certain times during the day and night (four a.m. is a popular time) that they are most active, and that varies from baby to baby. When you are active, you probably won't notice your baby moving until you come home and sit down at the end of the day.

Fetal kick counts are one way to make sure your baby is healthy. We usually recommend starting to do kick counts at about twenty-six weeks. Before this time, fetal movement is pretty random. You might go for days without feeling movement that you once noticed before.

So how do you count the kicks? If you follow the textbook method for fetal kick counts, you should sit down for one hour during each twenty-four-hour day to count how many times your baby moves. Ten kicks during one hour is the standard for a healthy fetus.

Of course, most of us don't have an hour a day to sit there and do nothing but write down how many times our baby is moving. And what if the baby only moves eight or nine times? Should one panic? Rush off to the hospital? The answer is no.

A more realistic approach to fetal kick counts: Be aware of fetal movement every day. Do not go more than twelve hours without feeling some movement.

If you don't have a reassuring count, call your OB provider to investigate things further. Continue doing these all the way until the day you deliver.

TESTS

Reality Check

Most women pregnant with their first babies are aware of movement somewhere between eighteen and twenty-two weeks. Women pregnant with their second or third child are often aware of fetal movement much earlier. At first, early fetal movement feels like little bubbles inside your belly, and women often mistakenly think they have gas!

Q. I haven't felt my baby move all day. What should I do?

Here are a few tips if you notice a decrease in or absence of your baby's movement:

- Drink and eat something (preferably something with sugar in it).
- Lie on your left side.
- Place your hands on either side of your belly and gently "move" your baby.
- Count how many times your baby moves in the next hour or two.

Usually, you will feel your baby moving around and breathe a sigh of relief. If you still feel very little movement (the baby moves once in two hours, for example) or no movement at all, you should contact your OB provider immediately.

It could mean many things, and most of them are nothing to panic about. Most commonly, you have been moving around all day and although your baby has been moving, too, you have been unaware of it. Sometimes babies have very long sleep cycles, lasting up to ninety minutes. If you are trying to do your kick counts during a sleep cycle, there won't be too much kicking. Sometimes babies are just resting and are lazy, for lack of a better word.

In some situations, however, decreased fetal movement means that a fetus is not getting what they need. Lower levels of amniotic fluid can cause less fetal movement. Fetuses that aren't getting enough oxygen, nutrients, or blood from the placenta often have decreased fetal movement.

Studies have shown that pregnant women often perceive decreased movement days before a fetal death.[5] Obviously, this is a situation everyone wants to prevent. That's why you need to call your OB provider pronto if you notice a sudden decrease in movement.

Third Trimester Tests

Routine Tests

Q. What is Group B strep?

Group B streptococcus (GBS), or *Streptococcus agalactiae,* is a bacteria that normally lives in harmony in your gastrointestinal tract (the gut/bowels).

The GBS that lives in your intestinal tract can easily spread to the vagina. As women, we have three body cavity openings sitting in a line, one above the other: the urethra, the vagina, and the rectum. That makes it pretty easy for bacteria to spread from one area to the next no matter how clean you are. This happens in up to 30 percent of healthy women.

Usually, the GBS just hangs out in the vagina without causing any problems. Occasionally, GBS causes bladder infections, an infection of the amniotic sac (***chorioamnionitis***), or an infection in the blood.

The key concern for pregnancy and GBS: A newborn can be "colonized" with GBS as they pass through the birth canal, which means that the bacteria get onto their skin, and into their body through the mouth, the nose, and the eyes. Not all colonized babies will become infected, but only colonized babies get sick, and newborn GBS infection is a very serious event. So while a pregnant woman may just be a carrier of GBS without any problems (docs call it being "GBS-positive"), her baby may get very sick if they get the infection.

Your OB provider does a vaginal/rectal swab at thirty-six to thirty-eight weeks and sends it to the lab for a GBS test.[6] Yes, that means your vagina and rectum are swabbed. Although the thought may make you want to run and hide, the collection procedure itself takes about two seconds. And your doc will distract you by talking about baby names or something. So it's not really as bad as it sounds.

The only time this test is not done is if:

- GBS was already found in your urine during your pregnancy, or
- you've already had a baby with a GBS infection. In that case, docs assume you are persistently colonized with higher levels of the GBS bacteria and treat the condition preemptively during labor.

If you go into labor or need to be induced *before* thirty-six weeks and haven't had a GBS test yet, you automatically get treated with preventive antibiotics in case you are GBS positive. Preterm newborns whose moms are GBS colonized are at least ten times more likely to have a serious infection if antibiotics aren't used during labor to temporarily get rid of the GBS in the vagina. The risk is high enough that we don't do a GBS swab and wait for the results to come back if someone is going to deliver prematurely—the risk of missing an opportunity to prevent infection in the newborn is just too high.

Q. What precautions are taken if I am GBS positive?

If you are GBS positive, the goal is to give you at least one full dose of intravenous (IV) antibiotics during labor, at least four hours before delivery.

You will also be on IV antibiotics if you have one of these issues:

- You have not yet had a GBS culture done before you go into labor.
- Your water has been broken for more than eighteen hours.
- You go into labor earlier than thirty-six weeks.
- You have a fever greater than 100.4°F.

If you have a planned ***C-section***, you don't have to worry about this stuff since your baby isn't going through the birth canal . . . unless you go into labor or have your water bag break prior to your scheduled C-section. In those scenarios, you'd need antibiotics to treat GBS prior to your C-section.

It is standard protocol *for the newborn* to get a complete blood count and blood culture if mom is Group B strep positive and didn't get pretreated with at least one dose of antibiotics (which happens with quick labors). Ditto when the baby is born earlier than thirty-six weeks gestation or if a baby starts misbehaving (temperature instability, labored breathing, stealing the car keys, etc.). These tests help tell the pediatrician if the baby may have been infected with GBS.

Q. Will it hurt the baby?

Group B strep can cause infection in the blood, pneumonia, and meningitis in newborns. All newborns are watched closely, but those babies with moms who test positive for Group B strep are watched even more closely. Babies born before thirty-seven weeks are the most likely to get a GBS infection if a carrier mom is not treated.

That's why there is a standard protocol to test all pregnant women for GBS and to treat GBS positive women with antibiotics when they go into labor. In fact, routine screening and treatment of GBS during labor has cut the rate of newborn GBS infections by two-thirds in the past twenty-five years.

BOTTOM LINE: Don't be too alarmed if you carry Group B strep. This does not mean you are Typhoid Mary. Remember, most babies with GBS positive mothers do not get sick and do absolutely fine.

Q. I tested positive with my first pregnancy, and negative this time. Should I still be treated?

Nope. GBS colonization comes and goes without notice, like a teenager. In fact, two-thirds of women who are positive in the first part of pregnancy are not near the end. The same goes for women who have been positive in previous pregnancies (the risk of being colonized in a subsequent pregnancy is about 50 percent). Assuming your baby did not develop a GBS infection (in which case you would automatically be treated during this pregnancy), you should only be treated if you have tested positive in the current pregnancy or fit one of the other criteria mentioned earlier.

Reality Check

If you are GBS positive, you won't pass it to your partner. GBS is not a sexually transmitted infection. But (there's a butt here) if you engage in anal intercourse, you should always use a condom and should never go from the rectum to the vagina. This is a very easy way for bacteria to spread!

Additional Tests

Q. I let my doctor know that my baby wasn't moving around like usual, and now I need to come into the office for a non-stress test. What is that?

A non-stress test (NST) is one of the ways to reassure both doctors and patients that the baby in question is not in any distress. It is sort of like an EKG for baby—specific heart rate patterns and tells your doc that the placenta is doing what it's supposed to do to support a growing baby.

This is a pain-free test for you and your baby. How does it work? First, two monitors are strapped on the outside of your belly. One monitor helps to pick up uterine contractions, while the other one tracks your baby's heartbeat. The doctor evaluates both uterine activity and fetal heartbeat on a display.

By evaluating many different aspects of your baby's heart rate, docs determine whether your baby is fine or if further testing is needed. Sometimes, especially when there is little fetal movement, an ultrasound is performed to measure the amount of amniotic fluid around the baby.

NSTs are also used to monitor fetuses in pregnant women with high-risk pregnancies, such as those with high blood pressure, diabetes, certain clotting disorders, and multiple pregnancies (twins, triplets, etc.).

Q. My friend starting getting NSTs at thirty-two weeks and now has them twice a week. I haven't had one yet. Why?

Certain people with high-risk pregnancies need NSTs once or twice a week. These are pregnancies that have a higher-than-average risk of the baby getting sick or being stillborn. Your friend is likely getting tested frequently because they have one of a number of high-risk conditions.

If you have what your doctor considers a low-risk pregnancy, you may never have an NST during your pregnancy, unless you happen to go past your due date or another unforeseen condition arises.

Q. Why would I need a non-stress test?

This is a useful test for a variety of conditions. Here's a list of them:

Examples of maternal conditions requiring non-stress tests

- High blood pressure (***hypertension***)
- Diabetes
- Severe asthma

- Certain clotting disorders
- Seizure disorders
- Poorly controlled thyroid conditions
- Certain blood diseases such as sickle cell anemia, thalassemia, hemoglobin S disease
- Chronic kidney disease
- Lupus
- Certain types of heart disease
- Pregnancy over the age of forty

Examples of fetal or pregnancy-related conditions requiring non-stress tests

- Small size (***fetal growth restriction***)
- Decreased fetal movement
- Too little amniotic fluid (***oligohydramnios***)
- Too much amniotic fluid (***polyhydramnios***)
- Post-term pregnancy (a pregnancy that extends past forty-two weeks)
- Immune response to Rh factor (***isoimmunization***)
- Previous stillborn
- ***Preeclampsia***
- ***Gestational diabetes***, poorly controlled or on insulin
- Multiples

Q. My doctor told me "everything looked great" with my NST. But they said it must be done again next week. Why?

Most of the time, it's highly reassuring to have a normal NST. A normal test means that there is less than a 0.5 percent chance of having a stillborn in the next seven days. This is why doctors usually repeat the test once a week.

In certain very high-risk conditions, however, the test is done *twice* weekly.

Q. What is a biophysical profile (BPP)?

This is yet another non-invasive test that docs use to gain valuable information about your baby's well-being. It involves doing an NST (as described above) in conjunction with an ultrasound. In recent years, this test has replaced the contraction stress test as the most popular way to seek reassurance about your unborn baby.

The ultrasound looks at four different parameters: fetal movement, breathing, fetal tone, and the amount of amniotic fluid present. A score is given from zero to ten (you get two points for each of the components of the ultrasound tests and the NST). The total score helps doctors determine whether:

- your baby is okay and can be observed
- more testing is needed, or
- immediate intervention is needed.

The biophysical profile (BPP) is considered more reassuring than an NST alone because it provides more information about a fetus and their environment. A normal score on a BPP indicates there is just a 0.1 percent chance of having a stillbirth in the next seven days.

PART TWO

Life Goes On

You've adjusted to the shock and awe of pregnancy, and now reality sets in. What do you need to eat for a healthy pregnancy? What environmental hazards should you avoid? What about exercise during pregnancy? Sex? Travel? Work? Smoothies? This section covers it all, plus answers to whether it is safe to color your hair, whiten your teeth, get your nails done, and more.

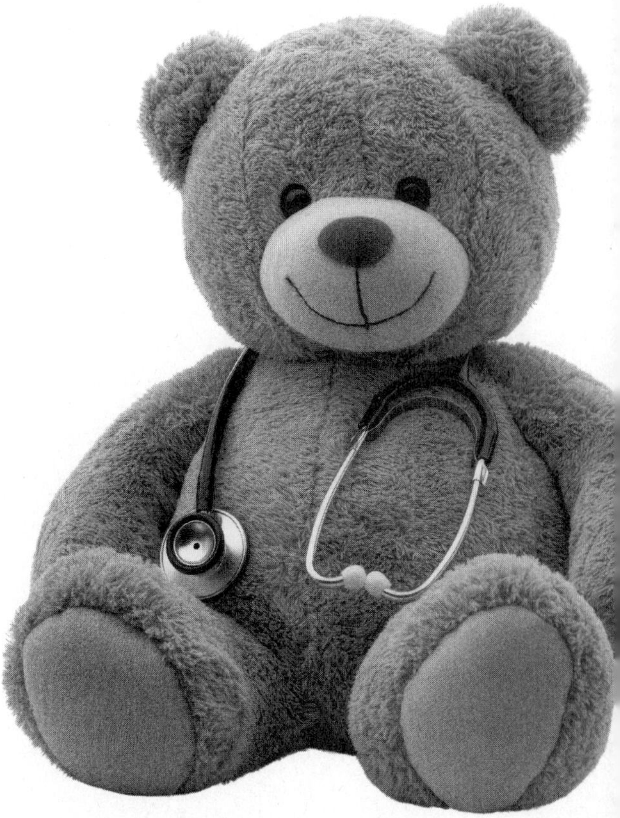

CHAPTER 7

Nutrition

"The perfect lover is one who turns into a pizza at four a.m."

—Charles Pierce

What's in This Chapter

- **Nutritional needs**
- **DHA supplements**
- **Vitamin D**
- **Counting calories**
- **How much weight should I gain?**
- **Advice for dieters**
- **Pregnancy after gastric bypass**
- **Special diets: vegan, lactose intolerant**

Stop us if you've heard this before: When pregnant, you're eating for two.

But what does that mean in the real world? How does what you eat affect your baby? Can you take herbal supplements? How much water should you be drinking?

This chapter covers everything you wanted to know about nutrition and your baby.

Yes, you are eating for two—literally. That doesn't just mean that you clean your plate and then poach what's left on your partner's. It means that what you eat, your baby eats, too. And that second person growing inside you only needs about 300–400 calories a day, starting in the second trimester. They need about 600 calories daily in the third trimester. If you are carrying twins, double those numbers.

If you've picked up some unhealthy eating habits, now is the time to begin changing your lifestyle. You have the perfect motivation!

We know change is hard—but your own meals are the meals you are serving to your growing fetus right now. The nutrition your baby gets in the womb actually does impact their later health. For instance, we know that excessive weight gain during pregnancy is associated with a baby's risk of neural tube defects, impacting the development of the brain and spinal cord.[1] And we know that good fetal nutrition reduces the risk of obesity later in your baby's life.[2]

And once the baby is born, you need to keep up the healthy diet that you may have started in pregnancy. Why? Because your child relies on you to buy the groceries. You and your child both eat what is in your pantry. For those of you who like to count carbs or calories and squeeze into those skinny jeans, it's time to change your mindset! We're not recommending that you head to the all-you-can eat buffet for every meal, but you need to be realistic.

For now, eat what you need to eat and read on. Being pregnant is a beautiful thing.

Your Nutritional Needs

Q. What do I need to eat during my pregnancy?

In general, you need more calories, protein, iron, and folic acid than you did pre-pregnancy. And it wouldn't hurt to crank up your fiber intake to save you from wonderful pregnancy constipation. If you do not eat meat, you also need a B12 supplement. Otherwise, if you didn't have any nutritional deficiencies prior to pregnancy, you should be able to reach your nutritional goals with a well-balanced diet and a prenatal vitamin.

Here is a list of nutrients you should aim to get each day of your pregnancy (okay, *most* days, because we won't count the days when all you feel like eating is a bean and cheese burrito).[3]

Nutritional Needs During Pregnancy

MACRONUTRIENTS

Nutrient	Benefit for Mother and/or Fetus	Amount (RDA)*	Where to Find It
Protein	Makes blood and energy stores for you and body tissue for your fetus.	10–35 percent of total daily calories 71 grams	3 ounces chicken breast (27 grams) 3 ounces fish (21 grams) 1 cup cottage cheese (28 grams) 1 cup low fat yogurt (11 grams) 1 cup skim milk (8 grams) 2 tablespoons peanut butter (8 grams) ½ cup black beans (7.5 grams) 3 ounces tofu (7 grams) 1 egg (6 grams) 1 ounce almond (5 grams) ½ cup green pea (4.5 grams)
Carbohydrates (includes fiber)	Provides energy for mother and fetus. You will want more fiber than your usual daily intake to help you poop.	Total carbohydrates: 45–65 percent of total daily calories, 175 grams (grams); fiber: 28–36 grams of total daily intake; added sugars: less than 10 percent of total daily carbohydrate intake	1 cup skim milk (12 grams) 1 cup low-fat yogurt (46 grams) ½ cup black beans (22 grams) 1 apple (32 grams) 1 banana (28 grams) 1 cup orange juice (24 grams) ½ cup potatoes (26 grams) ½ cup green beans (4 grams) 1 large bagel (48 grams) 1 cup Raisin Bran cereal (46 grams) 8 saltines (17 grams) 1 cup pasta (40 grams) 1 cup brown rice (45g)

MACRONUTRIENTS

Nutrient	Benefit for Mother and/or Fetus	Amount (RDA)*	Where to Find It
Fats (includes linoleic acid, known as omega-6,** and linolenic acid, known as omega-3 or ALA**)	Some fats are needed for fetal brain and vision development.	20–35 percent of total daily calories; saturated fats: less than 10 percent of total daily fat intake; omega-6: 13 grams daily; omega-3: 1.4 grams daily	1 cup whole milk (8.2 grams) ¼ pound hamburger (21 grams) 3 ounces chicken breast (3.8 grams) 1 egg (1.6 grams) 1 ounce peanuts (14 grams) 1 ounce almonds (16 grams) 2 tablespoons avocado (5 grams)

VITAMINS

Nutrient	Benefit for Mother and/or Fetus	Amount (RDA)*	Where to Find It
Vitamin A (should be in the form of beta carotene)	Helps with fetal growth, bones, skin, vision, and immune function.	770 mcg	3 ounces organ meats (1,500–9,000 mcg) ¾ cup carrot juice (1,700 mcg) 1 sweet potato (1,000 mcg) ½ cup carrots (670 mcg)
Vitamin D	Helps with fetal bone and tooth development. Deficiency may increase risk of preeclampsia.	600 IU	1 tablespoon cod liver oil (1360 IU) 3.5 ounces salmon (360 IU) 1 cups fortified milk (100 IU)
Vitamin E	Antioxidant that protects cells from damage. Note: Excessive intake may lead to congenital heart defects.	15 milligrams	1 ounce almonds (7 milligrams) 1 ounce sunflower seeds (6 milligrams) 1 tablespoon sunflower oil (5.6 milligrams) 2 tablespoons peanut butter (3 milligrams)
Vitamin K**	Helps with blood clotting for mother and newborn.	90 mcg	½ cup cooked broccoli (110 mcg) ½ cup spinach (444 mcg) ½ cup cooked asparagus (46 mcg)
Vitamin C	Antioxidant that protects cells from damage. Helps body use iron. Helps with connective tissue production and the development of gums, teeth, and bones.	85 milligrams	1 cup fresh orange juice (124 milligrams) 1 cup strawberries (85 milligrams) 1 orange (70 milligrams) 1 mango (60 milligrams)
Thiamin (B1)	Helps with nerve conduction.	1.4 milligrams	3.5 ounce pork chop (0.9 milligrams) 1 ounce sunflower seeds (0.6 milligrams) 1 cup cooked pasta (0.3 milligrams) 2 tablespoons brewer's yeast (2.3 milligrams)
Riboflavin (B2)	Supports energy metabolism.	1.4 milligrams	3.5 ounces beef liver (4 milligrams) ½ cup almonds (0.8 milligrams) 1 cup yogurt (0.5 milligrams)

VITAMINS

Nutrient	Benefit for Mother and/or Fetus	Amount (RDA)*	Where to Find It
Niacin (B3)	Helps with energy metabolism.	18 milligrams	3.5 ounces beef liver (14 milligrams) ½ cup peanuts (10.5 milligrams) 3.5 ounces salmon (8 milligrams) 1 packet corn grits (7 milligrams) 1 cup Cheerios (5 milligrams)
Vitamin B6	Helps with amino acid (protein) metabolism, and red blood cell formation.	1.9 milligrams	3.5 ounces beef liver (1.4 milligrams) 1 cup oatmeal (0.7 milligrams) 1 banana (0.7 milligrams) 3.5 ounces salmon (0.7 milligrams)
Folic acid (also called folate; called vitamin B9 when synthetically made)	Supports fetal development and placenta. Deficiency can cause neural tube defects in fetus (spina bifida).	600 mcg	1 cup breakfast cereal (100 mcg) ½ cup orange juice (100 mcg) ½ cup asparagus (130 mcg) ½ cup lentils (180 mcg)
Vitamin B12	Works with folic acid in cell formation. Supports nervous system. Deficiency causes anemia, fatigue, neurological issues.	2.6 mcg	3.5 ounces beef liver (112 mcg) 3.5 ounces steamed clams (99 mcg) 3 ounces crab (9 mcg) 3.5 ounces trout (5 mcg)
MINERALS			
Choline**	Helps with brain and spinal cord development in fetus.	450 milligrams	3 ounces salmon (187 milligrams) 1 egg (169 milligrams) 3 ounces beef (116 milligrams)
Calcium	Helps fetal bone, cartilage, tooth growth, nerve conduction. It may help prevent preeclampsia.	1,000 milligrams	1 cup yogurt (350 milligrams) 1 cup milk (300 milligrams) 1 ounces cheese (200 milligrams) 3 ounces salmon (180 milligrams)
Iron	Lowers the likelihood of developing anemia for mother and potential prematurity and low birth weight in baby.	27 milligrams	1 cup kidney beans (5.2 milligrams), white beans (6.6 milligrams), or soybeans (9.1 milligrams) 3.5 ounces steamed clams (22 milligrams) ½ cup tofu (6.7 milligrams) ½ cup spinach (3 milligrams) ¼ pound hamburger (3 milligrams)
Magnesium	Helps with energy metabolism, muscle contractions, nerve conduction.	350 milligrams, ages 19–30; 360 milligrams, ages 31–50.	¼ cup pumpkin seeds (303 milligrams) ½ cup almonds (240 milligrams) ½ cup cashews (150 milligrams) ½ cup tofu (130 milligrams) 1 cup yogurt (40 milligrams)

MINERALS

Nutrient	Benefit for Mother and/or Fetus	Amount (RDA)*	Where to Find It
Phosphorus	Supports bones, teeth.	700 milligrams	¼ cup pumpkin seeds (665 milligrams) ¼ cup sunflower seeds (380 milligrams) 1 cup yogurt (350 milligrams) 3.5 ounces salmon/trout (260 milligrams)
Potassium**	Helps maintain electrolyte balance in cells and fluids.	2900 milligrams	1 banana (425 milligrams) ¼ cup dried apricots (378 milligrams) ½ papaya (390 milligrams) 1 kiwi (240 milligrams)
Sodium	Helps maintain electrolyte balance, heart and muscle health.	2300 milligrams	Everywhere
Zinc	Helps with metabolism, growth, and development. Deficiency may increase risk of prematurity and low-birth-weight baby.	11 milligrams	3.5 ounces cooked oysters (39 milligrams) 3.5 ounces ground beef (5.5 milligrams) 3.5 ounces turkey (4.5 milligrams) 1 cup yogurt (2 milligrams)
Iodine	Helps make thyroid hormone, which regulates body growth and energy use. Needed for fetal brain development.	220 mcg	2 slices whole wheat bread (276 mcg) 2 tablespoons nori seaweed (116 mcg) ¾ cup Greek yogurt (87 mcg)

*RDA stands for recommended daily allowance.

**Nutrients with values that are considered adequate intake (AI), not RDA.

Source: U.S. Department of Agriculture and U.S. Department of Health and Human Services, *Dietary Guidelines for Americans, 2020–2025*, report, 2020, https://DietaryGuidelines.gov.

Applies to people of childbearing ages nineteen to fifty years of age.

Macronutrients

Q. How much food is 71 grams of protein? Must I eat carbs? And what kind of fats are healthy? What does this all mean in the real world?

Even though there are several food groups, they all boil down to three *types* of essential nutrients, or macronutrients, that your body recognizes and utilizes in different ways: proteins, carbohydrates, and fats. Here's a look at each.

1. **Protein.** Why do we need protein? Our bodies break protein down into amino acids. These amino acids then make different proteins for our body. In pregnancy, that extra protein you eat becomes the basis for your baby's cells and tissues.

Yes, you need a little more protein in your pregnancy diet. But what's the difference between 45 grams of daily protein you were getting pre-pregnancy and the 60–80 grams you need now? It may mean noshing on a high-protein snack and adding one glass of milk a day. Just take a look at the amount of protein in some typical foods in the Nutritional Needs During Pregnancy chart above. It takes remarkably small amounts to meet your additional protein needs.

BOTTOM LINE: You need 5.5 to 6.5 ounces of meats/poultry/fish (or nuts/legumes) a day and three cups or servings of milk/dairy products a day to reach your protein goal.

Fact Check

Avoiding peanuts during pregnancy will keep my child from developing a food allergy.

The truth: Current pediatric research shows that infants who are exposed to high allergy foods earlier in life may actually have a lower risk of developing a food allergy. Feel free to have a PB&J while you read this chapter.

2. **Carbohydrates.** What's so special about carbs?

   With the exception of fiber, our bodies break down most carbs to become sugar (glucose), our main energy source. You need glucose, your placenta needs glucose, and your baby's growing brain needs glucose.

   There are simple sugars, like honey and some fruit. And there are complex carbohydrates, called starches, found in grains, legumes, and vegetables. Finally, there are indigestible complex carbohydrates, better known as fiber. These are found in vegetables, beans, seeds, citrus fruits, berries, oats, wheat, and barley. Fiber is not broken down by our body's digestive enzymes, so it heads to our large intestines intact. Soluble fiber dissolves in water, forming a gel. It is beneficial for sugar metabolism, cholesterol lowering properties, and support of the gut microbiome. Insoluble fiber absorbs water, leading to softer and bulkier poop. You don't need to track your fiber intake based on these categories—they are both necessary. Plant-based foods have a combination of soluble and insoluble fiber (bonus!). High-fiber foods go in and come out of our bodies virtually undigested without breaking down into sugar.

   You don't really need more carbohydrates during pregnancy than in pre-pregnancy. About 45 to 65 percent of your daily intake should be in this category. But, because it is currently popular to eat a low-carb diet, you may not be eating as much as your pregnant body needs. You will also do your bowels a favor if you eat more fiber. That's one reason we suggest making whole grains at least *half* of the grains you eat.

   What does "45 to 65 percent" of your daily intake really look like? Well, that depends on how many calories you need to eat a day. And that total calorie goal depends on your pre-pregnancy weight, height, and level of activity dur-

INSIDER SECRET:

The Most Beneficial Carbs

Warning: Casually browsing just about any online wellness site may cause your head to spin. Whole grains, refined versus unrefined, low glycemic index? We aren't going to give you an entire nutrition lecture here, but we will give you the facts you need to know to make some healthy choices.

"Whole grain" means that a food product is made from the entire grain seed. Grains that get "refined" lose many of the good nutrients—fiber, vitamins, minerals—in the manufacturing process. Manufacturers may enrich these grains after refining to add back some of the lost nutrients.[4] In short, whole grains are more nutrient-rich than refined grains. Refined grains have the hull removed, which is the outside layer containing both color and fiber, kind of like a grain's "jacket."

Whole grains as well as fruits and vegetables are unrefined.

Try to make at least half of your grains whole grains. Eating a diet rich in whole grains may reduce cholesterol levels, and thus lower the risk of heart disease. Added bonus: They're loaded with fiber so they'll make you poop.

So where are these whole grain foods lurking? Look for products made with whole wheat flour. Or choose brown rice or wild rice instead of white. Other options include: whole grain bread, oats/oatmeal, whole grain corn, popcorn, whole rye, whole grain barley, buckwheat, triticale, bulgur, millet, quinoa, sorghum.

Yes, you now have an excuse to eat popcorn.

And some carbs are better than others. This is where the terms "simple" versus "complex" carbs and "low glycemic index" and "glycemic load" enter the picture. Your body quickly digests simple carbohydrates (such as white bread and white rice), causing a rapid rise and fall of glucose and insulin. It's better for you to eat carbohydrates that your body digests more slowly, causing a more gradual rise and fall of insulin levels. Complex carbohydrates and foods that metabolize sugars more slowly are considered low on the glycemic index (GI). The glycemic load is a calculation that reflects a truer picture of how a certain carbohydrate is metabolized. If you are at risk for gestational diabetes, your healthcare provider will probably discuss the glycemic index as well as the glycemic load in more detail. Here are some examples of more complex, slow-digesting carbohydrates and low glycemic index foods:

Fruit/Vegetables	Beans/Legumes	Nuts	Dairy	Bread/Grains
Apples Carrots, raw Grapefruit Orange Peaches Pears Pumpkin Sweet potatoes	Baked beans Chickpeas Kidney beans Lentils Peanuts Soybeans	Cashew nuts	Skim or soy milk Yogurt	Buckwheat Bulgur Millet Oats Quinoa Rice, brown Whole-wheat pasta

ing the day. But for simplicity sake, most pregnant women need roughly 175 grams of carbohydrates per day.

See the nutrient table above to take a look at serving sizes and carb content. Aim for six to eight ounces a day of grains, three cups a day of vegetables, and two cups a day of fruit. And try to have a variety of fruits and veggies to round out your diet.

3. **Fat.** Why do we need fat? Your body uses fat for energy, brain, and nerve function, and your unborn baby needs it for their developing nervous system (which includes their brain).

   So which fats are better than others? Here's an overview:

   - **Monounsaturated fats:** These are the great fats for your heart. They lower both your *total* cholesterol and bad (LDL) cholesterol. Look for them in nuts, olives, avocados, and olive oil.
   - **Polyunsaturated fats:** These fats are good because they lower cholesterol and may reduce the risk of heart disease. They also promote your baby's overall growth as well as brain and vision development. Essential fatty acids (omega-6 and omega-3) are long-chain polyunsaturated fats and necessary in our diets because our bodies do not produce them. There are three types of omega-3 fatty acids: ALA (alpha-linolenic acid), EPA (eicosatetraenoic acid), and ***DHA*** (docosahexaenoic acid). ALA is plentiful in walnuts, flaxseed, sunflower seeds, and chia seeds, whereas DHA and EPA are plentiful in fatty fish such as salmon, mackerel, and herring. Omega-6, or linoleic acid, is plentiful in pumpkin seeds, some nuts, and vegetable oils (including seed oils). While polyunsaturated fats have health benefits for both the pregnant person and the growing fetus, consuming the right ratio is important. The recommended daily allowance of omega-6 and omega-3 in pregnancy is 13 grams and 1.4 grams, respectively.[5] We'll discuss more about essential fatty acids later in this chapter, as well as the buzz about seed oils in Chapter 8, "Environmental Health."
   - **Saturated fats:** In general, some saturated fats raise your body's LDL cholesterol, which can lead to strokes and heart disease. You'll find saturated fats mostly in animal products (red meat, pork, lamb, veal, eggs, butter, cream, any dairy product made from whole or 2 percent milk) and a few plants (coconut, coconut oil, palm oil, and palm kernel oil). But saturated fats are not all bad. Some specific saturated fats can have positive health effects.
   - **Trans fats:** Almost a decade ago, the FDA banned synthetically made trans fats that were used extensively in processed baked goods and snacks. However, there are naturally occurring unsaturated trans fats that are found in ruminating animal (cow, sheep, goat) products such as whole or 2 percent milk, cheese, butter, and meat. Trans fats raise your bad LDL cholesterol and lower your good HDL cholesterol. There is no data to say what effect it has on your unborn baby, but what it does to your body is probably enough to limit your intake.

   How much fat do you need? Fats should make up less than 30 percent of your daily food intake. However, this depends on your pre-pregnancy weight and how active you are. But in real world numbers, that's about 40 to 70 grams a day. Preferably, that's mostly from good fat, not the stuff that clogs your arteries!

The American Heart Association (AHA) recommends that less than 7 percent of your daily fat intake come from saturated fats. The majority of fat intake should be from mono- and polyunsaturated fats.

Here's a shocker: Americans eat more fat than recommended. And as a pregnant woman, you can reach half your daily fat intake with just two tablespoons of oil.

Helpful Hint

Just take a look at your hand.

A three-ounce serving of meat or fish is about the size of your palm. A half-cup serving of rice or pasta is what you could place in your rounded hand. A serving of fruit or vegetable is the size of your closed fist.

Reality Check

Eggs are having a moment. Not only are they a good source of fat and protein, but eggs are also an excellent source of choline, a key nutrient that supports development of the fetal brain and nervous system.

NEW PARENT-TO-BE 411:

Cholesterol

Now that you've got the skinny on fats, what about cholesterol? Cholesterol is needed by your body to make cells and hormones. The problem: An excess of cholesterol piles up, clogging your blood vessels. That makes your heart work extra hard to pump blood through those vessels. It also clogs the arteries that provide blood flow to the heart and the brain. Bottom line: Those clogged pipes leave you at risk for a heart attack or stroke.

There are three types of cholesterol:

- **LDL** (low-density lipoprotein) is bad cholesterol. It clogs your arteries. Your body makes some LDL naturally, and genetics puts some folks at risk because they make too much LDL. Of course, eating fats that raise LDL levels doesn't help the situation.
- **HDL** (high-density lipoprotein) is good cholesterol. Instead of allowing cholesterol to collect in your arteries, HDL carries it to your liver, where it is broken down and eliminated. That's a good thing!
- **Triglycerides** are fats that your body makes. People who smoke, don't exercise, overindulge with alcoholic beverages, and overeat carbs tend to have high triglycerides. High triglycerides usually go hand in hand with high LDL and low HDL (a recipe for a heart attack).

Other Key Nutrients

Q. Are there any other nutrients I need to be certain to get while pregnant?

Yes. Calcium, folate/folic acid, and iron. And while it is technically not a nutrient, per se, water is also a critical part of your daily intake. Here are some details about each of these:

1. **Calcium.** Technically you don't need *more* calcium during pregnancy. But most Americans don't consume enough calcium, pregnant or not. You need 1,000 milligrams a day in divided doses—three cups of milk would do it. If you are pregnant and younger than eighteen years of age, you need 1,200 to 1,300 milligrams/day (4 cups of milk).
2. **Folic acid.** This key nutrient prevents brain and spinal cord (neural tube) defects. We've known for decades that having adequate folic acid in pregnancy reduces the risk of spina bifida by 70 percent. That's why some fortified cereals, pastas, breads, and grains in the United States have been enriched with folic acid (a synthetic form of folate) since before the turn of the century. Most prenatal vitamins have 800–1,000 micrograms (1 milligram)—which covers your daily dietary needs. While some dietary supplements contain a methylated form of folic acid called 5-MTHF (5-methyltetrahydrofolate), this product has not been proven to prevent neural tube defects to any greater degree than regular or normal folic acid. See the Insider Secret below for more info.

INSIDER SECRET:

Folic Acid Supplements

As we have discussed, folic acid helps the developing brain and spinal cord (neural tube) form properly. Researchers are also investigating a potential association between folic acid deficiency in pregnancy and risk of autism spectrum disorder, although studies thus far have failed to demonstrate a clear link.[6]

This is why it is so important to take a folic acid supplement. But which supplement should you take? The official recommendation from ACOG and other health professionals worldwide is to take a standard folic acid supplement because there is extensive research on both safety during pregnancy and prevention of neural tube defects. But there is an alternative product you might hear about. That supplement is called methylated folic acid.

Warning: There is a deep dive ahead on genetics.

We all carry two copies of a MTHFR (methylenetetrahydrofolate reductase) gene that produces an enzyme needed for certain metabolic functions, one of which is processing folate in foods and folic acid supplements.

About 30 percent to 50 percent of the population carry one copy (heterozygous) that is a genetic mutation of this gene. Because it is a recessive trait, one needs to have two copies of the mutated gene to be affected by it. Far fewer people, about 5 percent, have two copies (homozygous) of this genetic mutation. People are not routinely screened for this genetic mutation because even those who are homozygous may not suffer any health consequences because of it. To date, current evidence suggests that people with a homozygous MTHFR mutation should still take standard folic acid supplements, and they will have adequate levels needed for a healthy pregnancy.[7,8]

But there is still some discussion about whether people with homozygous MTHFR mutation can properly metabolize standard folic acid. Supplements containing a methylated form of folic acid, called L-methylfolate or 5-MTHF (5-methyltetrahydrofolate), is a more bioavailable form, so the body does not need to metabolize it. However, only standard folic acid has been proven to prevent neural tube defects.

Bottom line: If you are planning a future pregnancy, it is a good idea to maintain a healthy weight and take a standard folic acid supplement at least one month before getting pregnant. If you have questions about what specific folic acid supplement is right for you, ask your healthcare provider.

3. **Iron.** You need almost 40 percent *more* iron in your pregnancy diet. Here are a few practical tips:
   - Eat more lean meat—if you're not a vegan! Your body absorbs iron from animal sources (like meat) the best. It absorbs iron from plant sources (like spinach) the least.
   - But don't have a glass of milk with your steak. Calcium prevents the absorption of iron—so avoid eating iron-rich foods or taking your iron supplements with calcium-rich foods (dairy products, milk).
   - Do eat iron-containing foods or supplements with vitamin C (fruit, orange juice). Vitamin C helps the body absorb iron.

Q. How much water do I need to drink?

Water is the ideal beverage for everyone, but it's especially perfect for pregnant women. Staying well hydrated helps decrease your risk of ***bladder infections***, dehydration, preterm contractions, and dizziness. Water also ensures that your baby is cushioned by an adequate amount of ***amniotic fluid***.

Do you really need to drink at least 64 ounces (eight full glasses) of water a day? Not only should you, but remember that your water intake increases with your weight. A good rule of thumb is to take your weight in pounds and divide it by two. That's how many ounces of water you should be drinking in a day. And chances are you'll want to! You will be thirstier as you get further along in your pregnancy.

This extra water helps to create amniotic fluid, increases your blood volume to be twice the amount of normal, and helps ensure breast milk production.

If that isn't enough, water helps prevent constipation. By the end of the first trimester, you'll be willing to drink an ocean to prevent that!

Reality Check

Salt is not your friend when you are pregnant.

You don't have to cut it out completely, but you should watch your intake. That means you need to be aware of how many chips you are inhaling at your favorite Mexican food joint or how much soy sauce you are putting on your rice and tempura at the Japanese restaurant.

A higher intake of salt can lead to some serious swelling during pregnancy. You may have already noticed this. A word to the wise: Don't overdo the salt!

Special Diets

Q. I am a vegetarian. What should I add to my diet to be sure my baby gets what they need?

If you eat eggs, legumes (such as beans or lentils), tofu, and milk, you have a variety of options for your protein needs. However, you will need a source of iron and B12. Ask your OB provider if you need to take a B12 supplement.

Q. I am a vegan. Any special precautions?

If you don't eat any meat, milk, or eggs, it could be challenging to meet your protein needs. Nuts and legumes are great sources of protein, so load up! But your pregnant body also needs a variety of protein sources, not just a particular amount. Making a smoothie and putting a scoop of plant-based or whey protein in will give you between 25 and 35 grams—mix in some fruit, spinach, ice, and oat or almond milk and you have a very healthy, tasty treat!

You will also need to be creative with finding food sources for iron, calcium, and vitamin D. You will likely be asked to take a calcium supplement during both pregnancy and breastfeeding (lactation), so find one with vitamin D in it as well. And you will probably need a B12 supplement, as that vitamin is only plentiful in animal food sources.

Talk to your OB provider about your dietary restrictions. You may also want to consult a registered dietitian.

Q. I am lactose intolerant. What should I eat to replace what I am missing in milk and dairy products?

A quick primer on lactose intolerance: This means that you have trouble digesting the sugar that is found naturally in milk, called lactose. It does not mean you are allergic to milk. People with a true milk allergy are allergic to milk *protein,* not sugar.

You need the calcium and vitamin D in milk products during your pregnancy. In this case, you can eat dairy products that are lactose-free (there are many lactose-free milks, cheeses, and yogurts). Or you can take a lactase digestive enzyme supplement before eating dairy.

As a side note, some people who are lactose-intolerant find that they can eat cheese or yogurt, but cannot tolerate drinking straight milk. If you have never tried this, it might be worth it to do a little experiment.

Q. I have a milk protein allergy. Any advice?

For those with true milk protein allergies, a calcium and vitamin D3 supplement is likely in your future. There are also fortified plant-based milks, which contain calcium and vitamin D3, and non-dairy sources of calcium such as tofu, green leafy vegetables, seeds, and beans.

Q. I am on a gluten-free diet. Any advice here?

If you follow a gluten-free diet, like those with celiac disease, it's a great idea to get the help of a dietitian. Gluten-free diets can be low in iron, B vitamins, and fiber. A professional can help you find creative solutions to get these nutrients in your diet.

Vitamins and Nutritional Supplements

Will your diet alone be enough to fulfill your body's nutritional needs? For many nutrients, the answer is yes. But all pregnant women need prenatal vitamins, almost all need calcium supplements, and some need additional supplements to sustain a healthy pregnancy.

Prenatal Vitamins

Q. What type of vitamin supplements do I need to take?

You need a daily prenatal vitamin (a multivitamin made especially for pregnancy) and, most likely, a 500- or 600-milligram calcium supplement—even if you are a healthy person who actually eats from all the food groups! Your body has a lot of work to do to grow that baby. Additionally, many people are vitamin D deficient and need to take a vitamin D supplement. Talk to your OB provider about whether they feel you need to take one during your pregnancy.

You will also need to take an iron supplement if you begin pregnancy anemic or become anemic during pregnancy.

People with preexisting medical conditions, such as celiac disease or a history of weight-loss (bariatric) surgery, often need additional supplements (such as vitamin B12). People who follow vegetarian diets also need a B12 supplement.

While it would seem to make sense to have one prenatal supplement that includes all the nutritional needs of a pregnant person, there are practical reasons why that supplement does not exist. Calcium competes with other nutrients for absorption in the body, which would reduce the benefits of other ingredients—like iron, magnesium, and zinc—if it was in one supplement. Supplemental calcium is also very big in size, so adding it to a standard prenatal vitamin would make it too large to swallow.

INSIDER SECRET:

Tips on Calcium Supplements

Most pregnant women need an additional calcium supplement beyond what's found in a prenatal vitamin because they don't drink enough milk or eat enough dairy products to achieve their daily needs. Most experts recommend a supplement of 250–500 milligrams for a total daily intake of about 1,000–1,200 milligrams in populations of women getting a well-balanced diet. In higher risk populations, 1,500–2,000 milligrams is recommended. Much of this can be found in food, but here are some key tips to maximize the benefits of taking calcium with your other supplements and daily food intake. Talk with your OB provider to see what is recommended for you.

- Take your calcium supplement at a different time of day than your prenatal vitamin to optimize absorption of important nutrients like iron, magnesium, and zinc. Ideally, take them at least two hours apart.
- Take your calcium supplement in divided doses, twice daily. Your body can't absorb all the calcium at once.
- Take your calcium supplement (or glass of milk) at a different time of day than sitting down to eat an iron-rich meal. Again, calcium and iron compete for absorption in the body, so try to separate the calcium and the iron by at least two hours.

Q. Are prenatal vitamins and iron supplements available over the counter? Or do I need a prescription?

Yes, you can buy over-the-counter prenatal vitamins (as well as calcium, vitamin D, and iron supplements) and these are often less expensive than the prescription options. Consult with your OB provider to be sure the supplement has the right amount of nutrients.

Reality Check

Fifty percent of pregnancies are unplanned. By the time you know you are pregnant, your baby's future brain and spine (neural tube) have already developed. So it makes sense to just take prenatal vitamins throughout your childbearing years!

Q. I'm at the drug store and there are several types of prenatal vitamins. Is there any major difference among them?

Most prenatal vitamins are created equal, but there are some things to look out for. These pills vary in size—although none of those pills would ever be classified as "small"!

Some over-the-counter vitamins contain more iron than others, and some contain a stool softener (which is usually a welcome treat in the first trimester, as constipation is a frequent side effect of pregnancy). Many prenatal vitamins also contain DHA (an omega-3 fatty acid), which is a good idea—we'll discuss that later in this section.

There are also prenatal vitamins available by prescription. Most prescription prenatal vitamins now have lower amounts of vitamin A, vitamin A as 100 percent beta-carotene, and some have none at all. The reason? Most women get enough vitamin A in their diet, and too much vitamin A in pregnancy is not a good thing.

Until your first visit with your OB provider, take any over-the-counter prenatal vitamin that looks appealing. Most are just fine, assuming there is at least 400 mcg of folic acid and the vitamin A level is less than 5,000 IU (International Units). When you get to that first appointment, ask your OB provider what they recommend and share which brand you're taking.

DR. M'S OPINION:

Watch Out for Vitamin A

Many over-the-counter prenatal vitamins contain too much vitamin A. As of today, most prescription prenatal vitamins no longer contain vitamin A, have decreased amounts of vitamin A, or have vitamin A in the form of beta-carotene, which is safe. Too much vitamin A can be associated with some birth defects.

Q. My prenatal vitamins nauseate me. Any suggestions?

You're not alone. This is a very common complaint.

Here's our advice: Don't follow the instructions that tell you to take them on an empty stomach—unless, of course, you want to vomit. It's best to take them with some food. We suggest taking your prenatal vitamin on a full stomach, with your biggest meal of the day.

You can also crush your vitamin into a powder form and mix it with a spoonful of peanut butter or applesauce. This is easier said than done, and you may actually need a mortar and pestle to accomplish this task. There are also some chewable prenatal vitamins on the market.

And yes, many prenatal vitamins leave a terrible "vitamin taste" in your mouth, which may make you nauseated just thinking about taking another one. There are some newer vanilla-coated prenatal vitamins just for those of you with a discriminating palate.

Finally, if nothing else works, and you are so sick you just can't stand it, ask your OB provider about the option of taking individual supplements (folic acid, iron, and calcium in particular) or taking two children's vitamins (gummy or Flintstones Vitamins). Do be sure to let your OB provider know if you plan to take children's vitamins, because they do not contain iron and you'll need to take an additional iron supplement.

DR. M'S OPINION

I've had patients who have had severe nausea with one vitamin but none with a different brand. So keep trying until you find one that stays down.

Q. I'm a vegetarian. Are there any prenatal vitamins that do not contain animal products?

All prenatal vitamins are animal product–free, except those that contain DHA, which is often derived from fish. Nordic Naturals sells prenatal vitamins, and one variety has DHA from a plant source. New Chapter vitamins also contain DHA from a plant source. Needed is a brand that is created for vegans. So if you don't do fish, these may be the vitamins for you.

Omega-3 DHA Supplements

Q. What are omega-3s, and do I need them?

Omega-3s are long-chain polyunsaturated fatty acids that provide essential nutrients for heart health, as well as brain, eye, and nervous system development. There are three types of omega-3s used by the human body: DHA, ALA, and EPA. DHA is the most common—we'll discuss this next. And yes, you need them.

Q. Do you recommend I take omega-3 DHA supplements?

Yes.

DHA (docosahexaenoic acid) is an omega-3 fatty acid that helps in fetal brain and eye development. These long-chain polyunsaturated fatty acids have health benefits to mother and baby with very low risk (except for fish burps if yours comes from a marine source). While there is no question that omega-3 fatty acids are essential for nervous system development of a growing fetus, the data on whether taking omega-3 dietary supplements during pregnancy will make your baby smarter is pretty mixed.[9] But there is strong evidence that omega-3 supplementation of at least 350 milligrams of DHA (or DHA and EPA) reduces the risk of preterm births.[10,11]

> DR. M'S OPINION
>
> *With so many potential health benefits, there's really no downside to taking an omega-3 DHA supplement.*

Here's the catch, however (pun intended): Fatty fish is the most common source of DHA in our diets. And because of the high levels of mercury in certain types of fish, pregnant and nursing women are told to limit their intake of some fish. As a result, the average American pregnant person consumes less than 100 milligrams/day of DHA. ACOG recommends 350–400 milligrams/day for pregnant and nursing people.

So it makes sense to pick a prenatal vitamin that contains DHA. It's unlikely that you will get that much in your diet.

Q. How much DHA do I need a day? How do I get this in my diet?

ACOG recommends 350–400 mg of DHA per day.

Your body absorbs vitamins and minerals best in a food source. Eating fish high in DHA is helpful for getting part of the weekly recommendation and relying on your prenatal vitamin for the rest.

Here's a look at foods with the most DHA:

Omega-3 Content of Foods[12]

Food Source	Omega-3 Content (Milligrams)
Salmon, Atlantic, 3 ounces	1,825
Salmon, pink, canned, 3 ounces	1,400
Whitefish, 3 ounces	1,400
Sardines, oil-canned, 3 ounces	800
Mussels, blue, 3 ounces	700
Fish sticks, 3 ounces	680
Chia seeds, 1 tablespoon	2,500
Walnuts, ¼ cup	825
Edamame, ¼ cup	140

FEEDBACK FROM THE REAL WORLD:

Better Tasting DHA Supplements

Which DHA supplements are the least "fishy" tasting? Our readers suggest Gummy Omega-3 Naturals from Costco and Nordic Naturals, sold in natural foods stores (nordicnaturals.com).

Reality Check

Is there mercury in fish oil supplements? No. Consumer advocate groups tested the top forty brands of fish oil supplements and have found no significant levels of mercury. This is most likely because mercury collects in fish meat and not the oil, and the fish used to produce oil are lower on the predator fish food chain.

If you are really nervous about mercury levels in fish oil supplements, find a brand that lists "pharmaceutical grade" on the packaging. It means that the fish oil has been processed and contains no other substances.

Fact Check

Fatty acid supplements like DHA increase your risk of bleeding during pregnancy.

The truth: There is no valid evidence to support this theory. Hence, you can take DHA supplements all the way up to delivery.

Vitamin D Supplements

Q. I've heard a lot about people not getting enough vitamin D. Is there any risk to me or the baby if I have a deficiency?

Yes, you need vitamin D. It works with calcium to build both your and your baby's bones during pregnancy and breastfeeding.

There is a strong association between vitamin D deficiency and a type of high blood pressure (***preeclampsia***) that can occur during pregnancy.[13]

Vitamin D deficiency is more common than you would think, even for people who eat a healthy diet. Our bodies make most of our vitamin D when our skin is exposed to the sun. But since many of us avoid sun exposure to prevent skin cancer (hats, sunglasses, sunblock, and shade), we aren't letting our skin manufacture vitamin D! So it's a catch-22.

Unfortunately, most adults don't get enough vitamin D from a typical diet, either. Milk is an obvious source, since it is fortified with vitamin D. You can get most of your daily vitamin D needs if you drink three cups a day, but most adults don't drink that much milk.

You can also get quite a bit of vitamin D from a teaspoon or two of cod liver oil, but, seriously, how many of us would actually guzzle this stuff? Salmon, mackerel, and tuna are about the only other foods that contain high levels of vitamin D.

It's a great idea to get your vitamin D level checked prior to getting pregnant. If it is low, begin supplementation. Most calcium supplements include vitamin D. You can take 2,000 IU a day unless your OB provider recommends taking more based on your blood work

Helpful Hint

Make sure you are taking vitamin D3. D3 is a form of vitamin D that is more easily absorbed and utilized by the body more efficiently than D2.

NEW PARENT-TO-BE 411:

Too Much of a Good Thing

Vitamin supplements are good for you and your baby. But going above and beyond the standard recommended intake is not a good thing. In fact, it may even do some harm. Here are some ugly examples of why more is not necessarily better:

- **Vitamin A:** High doses of vitamin A (greater than 10,000 IU/day) can cause birth defects. This is why many vitamin companies have removed vitamin A from their prenatal vitamins altogether.
- **Vitamin E:** Excessive vitamin E levels are associated with congenital heart defects.[14]
- **Folic Acid:** Most prenatal vitamins contain one milligram (more than double the dose needed to prevent neural tube defects). In higher doses, it can hide the symptoms of a rare type of anemia in a pregnant person and thus delay treatment.

Iron Supplements

Q. My iron supplement makes me constipated. Any suggestions?

You have a few options.

Over-the-counter slow-release iron supplements (like Slow Fe) are often less constipating. You can also ask your pharmacist to make a liquid iron formula, which may help.

Make it a goal to get more iron from food in your diet. This iron is more easily absorbed. Foods such as dried apricots, raisins, lentils, eggs, chicken, red meat, liver, kale, and spinach are high in iron. Remember that your body absorbs iron from animal sources most effectively.

If you have tried it all, nothing is working, and you still need to take an iron supplement, eat a ton of fiber and take a stool softener, or ask your OB provider about an IV iron infusion.

Herbal Supplements

Q. Can I take herbal supplements?

With all the supplements stocked at your local natural food store, it may be tempting to sneak one of these into your diet. But are they safe?

Short answer: There is little scientific research on most supplements. That means we have *no idea* how they may affect pregnancy and breastfeeding.

We'll discuss the most common supplements in Appendix B, "Complementary Medicines and Therapies."

BOTTOM LINE: Ask your OB provider about particular supplements *before* taking them. Don't take anything on the sly!

Q. I keep hearing that smoothies are a great way to get my daily protein and vitamins during pregnancy, but there are so many things that can be added into them. I'm confused regarding what's safe and what isn't.

Smoothies are a great way to ensure good nutrition during pregnancy, and Dr. M often recommends them to her patients. It can be confusing standing in line at Kreation, Erewhon (for those of you in the Los Angeles area), or even at your local grocery store, deciding if chlorella, lion's mane mushroom, and spirulina, to name a few, are okay to put in your protein smoothie. So we've listed the most common additives to a smoothie and whether or not they are safe for your little one. Keep in mind they should be purchased from a trusted source and should be taken in moderation.

Smoothie Ingredient	Safe for Pregnancy?
Chlorella	Yes
Spirulina	Yes
Lion's mane mushroom	No
Chia seeds	Yes
Flax seeds	Yes
Cacao powder	Yes
Spices (cinnamon, nutmeg, ginger, cardamom)	Yes
Maca root	No
Acai powder	Better to use the fruit itself than the concentrated powder
Creatine powder	Very limited data in pregnancy, best to avoid

Protein Supplements

Q. Can I still use protein powder?

Yes. In fact, it's a great way to meet your daily protein needs, as one scoop of most powders has between 20 and 30 grams of protein. It doesn't matter if the protein source is whey-, plant-, or pea-based, as long as the main ingredient in any protein powder should be just that—protein!

Note that protein powders, like all supplements, are not regulated by the FDA. Since individual manufacturers are in charge of their own regulation, it's recommended to look for a protein powder that has undergone third-party testing, thus verifying the quality and safety of the ingredients.

Q. Are protein shakes okay?

Yes.

Just read the nutrition facts to see how much protein is in your drink. During pregnancy, you need 60 to 80 grams of protein each day. If you aren't getting enough in your diet, protein shakes are an excellent way of getting more. Inadequate protein intake in pregnancy is linked to growth problems in the fetus, so try to meet your body's needs.

Probiotics

Q. What about probiotics? Are they safe? Is there any benefit in taking them?

Yes, probiotics are safe to take during pregnancy. Known to promote healthy digestion, probiotics are also touted to boost immune function, inhibit the growth of harmful bacteria, and increase resistance to certain infections and disease-causing bacteria. While the jury is still out on some of these claims, there is enough scientific evidence on probiotics to say they are helpful. And the benefits of probiotics highly depend on the strain.

Pregnant people have more digestive issues than anyone on the planet (the nausea, vomiting, heartburn, belching, gas, constipation—need we continue?). Probiotics help keep your gastrointestinal tract functioning normally. They also prevent recurrent vaginal infections, such as yeast infections and ***bacterial vaginosis***.

Despite all the good things we can say about probiotics, always check with your OB provider first before adding any new supplement to your diet during pregnancy.

NEW PARENT-TO-BE 411:

PRObiotics and PREbiotics

Probiotics and prebiotics are touted to have numerous potential health benefits. But what are they?

What are PRObiotics?

These are "good germs" (bacteria or yeast) that help the body digest food. They can be found naturally in yogurt, kefir, kombucha, tea, miso, tempeh, and sauerkraut. You can also buy them in capsules or powder form. Note: The good germs are only present when you ingest them. So once a person stops taking them, the benefits go away.

What are PREbiotics?

These are complex starches or polysaccharides in food that help the gut grow the good bacteria mentioned above. This is what sustains the healthy gut environment. Prebiotics are found naturally in whole grains, honey, bananas, garlic, onions, leeks, and artichokes. Other food and beverage products are fortified with them. Note: Prebiotics basically provide the food for probiotics. So even if someone doesn't take prebiotics every day, the benefits have longer lasting effects.

What It Takes to Grow a Human

Q. How much weight should I gain?

The amount of weight you should gain during pregnancy depends upon your pre-pregnancy weight. Check with your doctor to help you determine if you are starting out at a healthy weight, underweight, or overweight.

Once you have figured this out, you can see how much weight you will need to gain to have a healthy pregnancy. The National Academy of Medicine offers pregnancy weight gain guidelines listed below, based on women's pre-pregnancy ***Body Mass Index (BMI)***.[15] Note: The ACOG acknowledges these basic guidelines but emphasizes that patients should consult with their OB providers for an individualized pregnancy care plan.[16]

Category	Body Mass Index*	Recommended Total Weight Gain (in Pounds)	Recommended Weight Gain Range (in Pounds) in Second and Third Trimesters
Underweight	Less than 18.5	28–40	1–1.3
Normal weight	18.5–24.9	25–35	0.8–1
Overweight	25–29.9	15–25	0.5–0.7
Obese	Over 30	11–20	0.4–0.6

*To calculate your BMI, go to nhlbi.nih.gov/calculate-your-bmi and plug in your height and pre-pregnancy weight. It's confidential, so no cheating!

Reality Check

Sixty-six percent of American women of childbearing age experience overweight, and 35–40 percent live with obesity.

Q. How much weight should I gain in each trimester?

This is a tough question to answer, because all of us are different.

We will give you a rough idea of average weight gain by trimester, but remember this is only a guideline. It is not something to obsess over.

Okay, that's easy for us to say. We realize it is common to get freaked out after seeing your weight at your OB provider's office—is it too much? Too little? Again, take a deep breath—remember your OB provider is tracking your weight and will let you know if there are any concerns. If your doc isn't worried, you shouldn't be!

Healthy Weight Before Pregnancy

Trimester	Estimated Weight Gain (in Pounds)
First trimester	3–5
Second trimester	1/week
Third trimester	1/week

Underweight Before Pregnancy (Talk to Your Doctor)

Trimester	Estimated Weight Gain (in Pounds)
First trimester	5–8 depending on your starting weight
Second trimester	1–2/week
Third trimester	1–2/week

Overweight or Obese Before Pregnancy

Trimester	Estimated Weight Gain (in pounds)
First trimester	1–2
Second trimester	Less than 1/week
Third trimester	Less than 1/week

Reality Check

If you are getting really depressed about how much weight you are gaining, don't look at the weigh-in!

Partner Tip

If you value your life, don't talk about your partner's weight gain. Remember, you are also at risk for gaining a few extra pounds during pregnancy.

Q. How many extra calories do I need?

Fewer than you think.

Even though you are growing a baby and the accessories that go with them, you only need about 400 extra calories a day. That's the equivalent of some cheese and crackers and a one-ounce bag of almonds. Or it's one very small milkshake indulgence.

So you don't need to clean your plate and your partner's to meet your calorie needs. It may just mean you add in a couple of healthy snacks throughout the day.

BOTTOM LINE: Don't go overboard on counting calories and checking your weight on a daily basis. Just make wise food choices.

Q. What happens if I don't gain enough weight?

Your OB provider keeps an eye on your overall weight gain. That's why you have to suffer through a weigh-in at every visit. There are two key reasons your doc tracks weight gain:

- You need enough calories to maintain your changing body. Your organs get bigger, and your nutrient stores decline.
- If you don't eat, neither does your baby. Your fetus may not grow properly if you don't gain enough weight.

If your weight gain is not what it should be, your OB provider will probably tell you to do some of the following:

- Keep a food diary to make sure you are eating enough.
- Eat whole milk dairy products instead of low-fat options.
- Add snacks in between meals.
- Have a protein shake or smoothie instead of lower calorie snacks.
- Add nuts to your diet.

DR. M'S OPINION:

Stressing About Weight

I have seen so many patients come in and really stress over the fact that they have gained six pounds in a month . . . or lament that they have only gained two pounds during that same time period. It is okay. As your OB providers, we keep a close watch on overall trends and will let you know if you are gaining too much or too little.

INSIDER SECRET:

Where Does All the Weight Go?

The good news is that if you gain between twenty-five and thirty-five pounds during your pregnancy, only about seven to eight pounds is actually fat tissue. In general, the rest is as follows:

Where It Goes	Weight in Pounds
Baby	7–8
Uterus	2
Placenta	1–2
Amniotic fluid*	2
Extra blood volume	4
Increase in other body organ size	1–2
Breast tissue	2
Extra fluid in maternal tissue	4

*This is why your doctor is covered in waterproof attire at the time of your delivery!

Q. I've been a chronic dieter for most of my adult life. I am currently on a low-carb diet. Will this be safe to continue during my pregnancy?

Short answer: NO.

Long answer: A growing fetus requires a constant supply of glucose (from carbohydrates) to grow normally. Low-carb diets don't provide enough carbs for a growing baby.

Glucose is the fuel for developing the brain and nervous system. If a pregnant woman's diet does not provide carbohydrates for her fetus, her body tries to use fats and protein for energy. Fat cannot be broken down into glucose. Instead, it breaks down into something called ***ketones***.

Normally, a small amount of ketones float around in the blood. But if a pregnant person continually deprives themself of carbohydrates, large amounts of ketones accumulate. Ketones can and do cross the placenta. High amounts can result in fetal

ketoacidosis, which can lower the baby's blood pressure and increase the baby's heart rate.

Low-carb diets also promote water loss. When the body breaks down proteins instead of carbs, water is lost. Important body electrolytes, like sodium and potassium, are lost with the water.

This all spells danger for the fetus. Many studies show elevated ketone levels stress the fetus (changing fetal vital signs) and put the baby at risk for health problems later in life, such as high blood pressure, heart disease, and diabetes.[17]

DR. M'S OPINION

This is the one time in your life that you need to put your dieting aside and do what is best for your little one.

Q. What happens if I gain too much weight?

If you gain too much weight (but had a normal BMI prior to pregnancy), your OB provider will watch you a little more closely, looking for any potential health risks. Examples: gestational diabetes and high blood pressure (***preeclampsia***). See Chapter 17, "The Complicated Pregnancy," Complications #26 and #20. It may also make delivery a bit more difficult as increased weight gain in pregnancy is often associated with bigger babies—and bigger babies are tougher to get out!

If all goes well with pregnancy and delivery, you've just got a few extra pounds to work off afterward.

Q. I have battled obesity all my life. I am now eight weeks pregnant—what risks do I face?

If you are already overweight and then you gain more than you need to during pregnancy, there are some potential health risks to both you and your baby. Your job is to do the best you have ever done in your life to watch what you eat, how much you eat, and be physically active.

The key health concerns for you: potential gestational diabetes, high blood pressure (***preeclampsia***), impaired immunity to fight infections, and an increased risk of having a cesarean delivery. The key health concerns for your baby: potential birth defects, increased risk of miscarriage/stillbirth, bigger birth weight (increasing risk of complications and cesarean delivery), future risk of diabetes, obesity, and heart disease.[18] Scary, we know. Be assured that your OB provider is looking out for all these issues to try to prevent them or treat them early if they arise.

Reality Check

Obese women face additional health risks during pregnancy, including a higher risk of miscarriage, gestational diabetes, preeclampsia, and primary C-section. About one-third of overweight women end up having a C-section.

Q. What can I do to make sure I am getting the right kind of nutrition during my pregnancy?

Eat well and spare the calories. Here are some relatively easy food swaps to avoid gaining too much weight during pregnancy. Whenever possible, choose low-fat and low-sugar options.[19]

Food	Serving Size	Fat content in Grams	Calories
Cheese			
Regular	1 ounce	6	114
Low-fat	1 ounce	1.2	49
Ground Beef			
Regular (25 percent fat)	3 ounces, cooked	6.1	236
Extra lean (5 percent fat)	3 ounces, cooked	2.6	148
Milk			
Whole	1 cup	4.6	146
1 percent fat	1 cup	1.5	102
Ice Cream	½ cup	4.9	145
Frozen yogurt	½ cup	2	110
Butter	1 teaspoon	2.4	34
Margarine spread	1 teaspoon	0.7	25
Chicken			
Fried leg	3 ounces	3.3	212
Roasted, skinless breast	3 ounces	0.9	140
Fish			
Fried	3 ounces	2.8	195
Baked	3 ounces	1.5	129

Helpful Hint: Banish the Four Cs

Sometimes it's hard to resist temptation because it's simply too easy to access junk food. Don't get us wrong, we need our chocolate fix, too, every once in a while.

Our point: If it's not in your pantry, it's much more likely to be a treat. If it's in your pantry, it's a staple. So consider banishing the Four Cs: cola, candy, chips, and cookies. These are empty calorie foods. Just eliminating the temptation to snack on these foods and drinks will go miles in helping you maintain a healthy pregnancy weight.

Partner Tip

Got to have those potato chips but your pregnant other half has banned them from the house? Our advice: Partner up! Be supportive and suffer together. You will both be healthier as a result!

NEW PARENT-TO-BE 411:

Managing Weight Gain

Three tips for people who were overweight before they got pregnant:

- See a registered dietitian when you realize you are pregnant.
- You still need to gain weight during pregnancy. But it should be no more than 11 to 20 pounds.
- Incorporate exercise into your daily routine (always check with your OB provider first before beginning any exercise program).

Three tips for people who were underweight before they got pregnant:

- You need to gain between 28 and 40 pounds during your pregnancy.
- Remember, don't get freaked out by those large numbers on the doctor's scale—your baby needs that extra weight.
- Make sure you are eating a balanced diet with enough caloric intake. Keeping a food diary is helpful.

Q. Does food "program" your baby's health?

Does what you eat during pregnancy set up your baby for a lifelong health? Or chronic disease? There is a scientific theory (the "thrifty gene" or Barker hypothesis) that suggests poor pregnancy and newborn nutrition permanently changes a child's metabolism. In other words, nutrition while in the womb "programs" a baby's metabolism for life. This alteration might lead to obesity and diabetes, which subsequently leads to heart disease.

While there are certainly other risk factors that may cause disease later in life, this is one very good reason to eat healthy during pregnancy!

Q. How quickly will I lose my pregnancy weight?

You will lose ten to thirteen pounds shortly after birth, but you won't see it on the scales until a week or two later. That's because you will initially have quite a bit of fluid retention. Here's an important fact: *Only 28 percent of women are back to their pre-pregnancy weight within six weeks.*

So don't compare yourself to celebrity newbie moms flaunting their post-pregnancy bikini bodies on the cover of *People*. Most normal women (without twenty-four-hour chefs and trainers on call) lose their weight in three to six months after delivery.

Bariatric Surgery

Bariatric surgery refers to the surgical procedures used to aid in weight loss. There are two primary types:

- Gastric banding places a fluid-filled band around the stomach to reduce its volume. This makes patients feel full faster and decreases total food intake.
- Roux-en-Y gastric bypass uses a loop of your intestine to bypass the lower portion of your stomach and upper intestine. This decreases stomach capacity and food absorption.

Q. I have had the gastric banding procedure and want to get pregnant. How long do I have to wait to conceive?

Most experts recommend waiting twelve to twenty-four months after bariatric surgery before conceiving. The reasons: to avoid exposing the fetus to all of the metabolic changes that occur when rapid weight loss happens; and to allow patients to achieve their full weight loss goals before becoming pregnant.

Q. I had gastric bypass surgery eighteen months ago and am pregnant. Am I at risk for any additional complications?

Yes.

Many patients remain obese after undergoing bariatric surgery. If you haven't reached your maximum weight loss goal, you may still be obese. Hence, you will be at risk for all of the previously mentioned complications.

With bariatric surgery, your risk of needing a C-section increases by 62 percent, according to the latest research.[20]

Also: You should be watched closely for complications due to the bariatric surgery itself (bowel obstruction and severe bleeding from your stomach or intestines). Tell your OB provider if you have any abdominal pain during your pregnancy.

Reality Check

If you have lost the excess weight after bariatric surgery, terrific! Then you have lowered your risk of gestational diabetes and high blood pressure (***preeclampsia***).

Q. Is my baby at risk if I've had bariatric surgery?

If you have lost weight after having your procedure, then your baby is actually much better off. Fetuses born to women who have had this procedure are more likely to be of normal weight. The risk of stillbirth and birth defects also decreases.

Q. Are there any special tests or consultants needed during my pregnancy because of my history of bariatric surgery?

Yes.

Your pregnancy medical team should include an OB, a maternal-fetal medicine or high-risk pregnancy specialist, as well as the surgeon who performed your bariatric surgery.

People who are followed by their bariatric team during pregnancy are able to manage their weight much better than those who are followed by an OB alone.[21]

You also have some special nutritional issues. If you had a Roux-en-Y procedure, there is an increased risk of protein, iron, vitamin B12, folate, vitamin D, and calcium deficiencies. Your OB provider will check for these and will recommend supplementation if necessary.

If you had a gastric bypass procedure, you won't be able to do the standard glucola screening test for gestational diabetes. You may have a severe reaction if you take 50 grams of glucose. So you may need to have your fasting blood sugar checked and pass these numbers on to your doc for review.

Lastly, if you are still obese, you may need non-stress tests (NSTs) in your last month of pregnancy to assess the well-being of your fetus.

GLP-1 Medications

Q. I've been on a semaglutide for six months and have lost twenty pounds. I just found out that I'm pregnant. Do I need to stop?

Yes. GLP-1 drugs, such as semaglutide (brand names: Ozempic, Wegovy) and tirzepatide (brand names: Mounjaro, Zepbound), are medications used to treat type 2 diabetes and have recently been used in larger amounts for weight loss. They work by mimicking a naturally occurring hormone called glucagon-like peptide-1 (GLP-1). They stimulate GLP-1 receptors in the body, which leads to increased insulin production, reduced appetite, feeling full sooner, and slower emptying of your stomach. There are no studies suggesting any harm, but we have physiologic data that it's not recommended in the first trimester when all of your baby's organs are forming. And since we don't have data for use in the second or third trimesters, we can't say it's safe here, either. So if you are taking a GLP-1 drug and find out you are pregnant, it's best to stop, notify both your OB provider and the physician giving you the medication to help come up with a plan for your pregnancy.

CHAPTER 8

Environmental Health

"The only way to keep your health is to eat what you don't want, drink what you don't like, and do what you'd druther not."

—Mark Twain

What's in This Chapter

- **Food and drink**
- **Caffeine**
- **Mercury and fish**
- **Cheese**
- **Sushi**
- **Lunchmeat**
- **Bad habits**
- **X-rays and the microwave**
- **Surgery**
- **BPA, phthalates, and microplastics**
- **Pets**

Your baby's placenta acts as a great barrier to the outside world—but it doesn't block the passage of *everything* to your unborn baby. Germs (viruses, bacteria), drugs, and certain toxins that circulate in your bloodstream can go right to your developing baby. Some of these items have well-known adverse health effects. For others, the jury is still out.

Scary fact: More than 100 environmental chemicals are found in umbilical cord blood. That means your developing baby is exposed to the same daily toxins you are. And a growing fetus is likely more vulnerable than adults to adverse health effects from these pollutants because the exposures occur during critical periods of their human development.[1] Environmental exposures can permanently interfere with how organs and body systems develop.

This chapter will cover things you may never have considered before—how the air you breathe, the food you eat, the house you keep, and some of the bad habits you have affect you and your unborn baby. But don't let this chapter alarm you. The goal is to open up your eyes to the world you live in.

No book or expert has all the answers on what is safe or acceptable exposure, because environmental health is an emerging science. Compared to other fields, scientists have only just started to look at the effects of natural and human-made environmental exposures. Most of the evidence we have about toxins and their potential damage comes from animal studies; the effects on humans are guesswork. There simply isn't enough research on many of these issues to tell which toxins are most dangerous to humans. Until we have more answers, it makes sense to limit or avoid potential environmental hazards when it is practical to do so.

NEW PARENT-TO-BE 411:

Hazardous to Your Health?

Environmental toxins can be broken into six basic categories:

- **Carcinogens.** These agents are known to cause cancer. (Examples: arsenic, tobacco, solvents like benzene.)
- **Mutagens.** These agents increase the rate of change (mutation) in genetic material. This can lead to defective cells and cancer. (Example: ionizing radiation.)
- **Teratogens.** These agents alter a fetus during development in the womb. Abnormalities are present at birth. (Example: alcohol.)
- **Neurotoxins.** These agents damage or interfere with nerve/brain function. (Example: lead, methylmercury, polychlorinated biphenyls or PCBs, organophosphate pesticides.) The scary part: There is a spectrum of neurotoxicity. Severely affected people will have obvious symptoms. Those with lower amounts of exposure may have more subtle symptoms such as a shorter attention span or slightly lower IQ.
- **Endocrine disruptors.** These agents mimic the body's natural chemical messengers (hormones) and can potentially interfere with body responses in the reproductive system and thyroid gland. (Example: phytoestrogen.)
- **Irritants and allergens.** These agents cause allergic responses in the airway and/or the skin. (Example: volatile organic compounds or VOCs.)

How do these toxins affect a fetus developing in the womb? It depends on the toxin and when the exposure occurs. For instance, a significant toxin exposure in the first two weeks of pregnancy might result in miscarriage. The same exposure during the fifth or six week might cause a birth defect. Exposures after the first trimester might result in low birth weight.

An important caveat: The brain is sensitive to injury during the *entire* pregnancy.

Food and Drink

Alcohol

Q. Can I drink at all during my pregnancy?

The most recent studies say no. Even small amounts of alcohol during pregnancy can affect your unborn baby.

Fetal alcohol syndrome disorders (***FASD***) is the fancy name for health effects from alcohol exposure in the womb. These disorders share common issues: behavioral, learning, and physical problems. *Fetal alcohol syndrome (FAS)* is the most severe form. Children with FAS have lifelong neurological and physical disabilities.

We know that 40 to 60 percent of pregnant people who binge drink or have chronic alcohol intake (five to seven drinks per day) have babies with FAS. But the latest research shows that much smaller amounts (one to two drinks a day) may adversely affect a child's birth weight, attention, behavior, and IQ.

BOTTOM LINE: Don't drink alcohol during pregnancy. If you are drinking, so is your baby. Most people actually lose their taste for alcohol during pregnancy, so you probably won't be craving a margarita with Mexican food anyway.

Q. I had some drinks before I realized I was pregnant. Is this going to harm my baby?

This is one of the top ten most-asked pregnancy questions.

In a perfect world, people would abstain from alcohol while attempting to become pregnant. In reality, however, most have a few alcoholic drinks before they know they are pregnant.

If you discover you are pregnant after being late for a period and doing a home pregnancy test, four or more weeks may have gone by while you were pregnant, didn't know it . . . and visited the local happy hour.

So should you be freaking out now? Answer: no.

It may sound harsh, but there is an "all or nothing effect" for alcohol (as well as other toxin) exposure in the early part of the first trimester. If enough damage is done to a growing fetus, a miscarriage happens. If your pregnancy continues, most of the time your baby will be just fine.

BOTTOM LINE: Once you know you are pregnant, stop drinking. Your baby should be fine as long as you do this.

Q. Why is alcohol risky for babies?

Let's be blunt: Alcohol affects the brain. Exposing a rapidly growing brain to alcohol is just a bad idea. And alcohol is not only a neurotoxin, but both hypophilic and lipophilic, meaning it can enter into every single cell in our adult bodies and certainly into a developing fetal body.

Fetal alcohol syndrome is the number one *preventable* cause of intellectual disability. A child with FAS has a misshapen face, a small head, poor growth, kidney and heart problems, hearing and vision problems, as well as behavioral and learning issues.

Although FAS is the most severe end of the spectrum, *any* alcohol-related birth defect is devastating . . . and avoidable.

Q. What about the amount of alcohol in cough and cold meds?

There is a negligible amount of alcohol in these products. Don't worry unless you are downing large amounts of the stuff for days on end. If you have specific concerns, check with your OB provider.

Caffeine

Q. I admit it. I have to have my coffee in the morning. Can I have any caffeine during my pregnancy?

Caffeine is a stimulant that increases heart rate and blood pressure. Caffeine is also a diuretic, causing your body to lose water.

When caffeine crosses the placenta, your baby's developing metabolism can't quite handle the caffeine jolt the way you do.

So what does the science say on caffeine and pregnancy? There are no conclusive studies in humans showing that caffeine consumed during pregnancy causes birth defects. Some studies in animals, however, have shown decreased fertility, birth defects, preterm delivery, and an increased risk of low-birth-weight babies.[2]

Despite the lack of clear-cut science on this issue, the general consensus among OB-GYNs is to limit caffeine intake during pregnancy.

What does that mean in the real world? Well, unfortunately, there is no science that says 200 milligrams is safe, more than 300 milligrams is dangerous, etc. Despite the lack of evidence, ACOG,[3] March of Dimes, Health Canada, and the UK Food Standards Agency all recommend limiting caffeine intake to 200 milligrams a day during pregnancy.

DR. M'S OPINION

If you can abstain from caffeine altogether, great. If you can't, limit your intake to one caffeinated beverage a day.

Our advice: No more than one (or on rare occasion, two) caffeinated drinks a day. By one beverage, we are referring to an *average*, 200 milligrams of caffeine, eight-ounce cup of coffee (sorry, that venti Starbucks counts as nearly three drinks). And if you are having some caffeine, make sure you stay well hydrated (with water or fluid-replacement drinks such as Gatorade) to prevent dehydration.

Reality Check

When researchers study caffeine's effects on pregnancy, they are looking at high levels, which generally mean more than 300 milligrams a day. As you can tell from the chart on the next page, one Starbucks can put you over that limit.

The Daily Buzz: The Amount of Caffeine in Food and Drinks

Remember that caffeine isn't just in coffees and teas, but also in sodas, chocolate, and some over-the-counter headache medicines (such as Excedrin).

Source	Serving Size	Amount of Caffeine in Milligrams
Starbucks "Venti" coffee	20 ounces	415
Starbucks "Grande" coffee	16 ounces	330
Starbucks "Tall" coffee	8 ounces	260
Celsius Energy drink	12 ounces	200
Standard home-brewed coffee	8 ounces	200
Red Bull	12 ounces	111
Coffee ice cream	1 cup	60–75
Excedrin	1 capsule	65
Black tea	8 ounces	50
Coca-Cola	12 ounces	34
Green tea	8 ounces	30
Chocolate candy bar	1.5 ounces	10

Herbal and Non-Herbal Teas

Q. What is the difference between herbal and non-herbal teas?

Non-herbal teas come from leaves of tea plants, and there are three types: black, green, and oolong. They contain different amounts of antioxidants, as well as caffeine. Examples of black tea include English breakfast, Earl Grey, and Orange Pekoe. Oolong teas are a combination of black and green tea.

Herbal teas are made from seeds, berries, roots, flowers, and a variety of other plant parts, not from actual tea leaves. True herbal teas do not contain caffeine. These teas often claim to have medicinal uses.

Q. Can I have non-herbal tea during my pregnancy?

Yes. Non-herbal teas may offer health benefits, thanks to antioxidants found in the tea leaves.

But remember that the average cup of non-herbal tea contains between 40 and 50 milligrams of caffeine. Caffeine crosses the placenta and enters your baby's circulation. So drink it in moderation.

Q. Can I have herbal tea during my pregnancy?

Yes, if you stick to commercially made herbal teas.

Commercially made herbal tea (such as Celestial Seasonings, Pique, Tazo) are regulated by the FDA and are presumed safe.

Of course, there are many other herbal teas sold online and in health food stores. Some folks make their own herbal teas from herbs they collect from a garden or farmer's market.

Non-commercial herbal teas may have varying (sometimes excessive) amounts of herbs or herbs known to be dangerous during pregnancy (such as nettle). And there isn't much research or safety data on these teas and developing fetuses.

Our advice: Avoid non-commercially made herbal tea products, unless you are using them under the supervision of your doctor or midwife. Some herbal teas, like red raspberry leaf, are safe in pregnancy. Midwives and some OB-GYNs often use this tea to decrease the length of labor, help with blood loss after delivery, increase milk production, and decrease nausea.

Herbal teas are naturally caffeine free.

Reality Check

While we are on the subject of herbs . . . many herbal supplements are off-limits during pregnancy. But it is certainly fine to cook with herbs and spices, such as garlic, nutmeg, and cinnamon.

Artificial Sweeteners

Q. What are artificial sweeteners, and can I use them during pregnancy?

Artificial sweeteners are sugar substitutes created by chemicals in a lab. They add sweetness to different foods and drinks, such as sodas, juices, desserts, chewing gum, certain candies, and pastries. They are also used as tabletop sweeteners for coffee and tea, taking the place of sugar.

Although there is ongoing research and the FDA[4] has approved several artificial sweeteners (aspartame, sucralose), they are, in short, chemicals, devoid of any nutritional value. Additionally, Sweet'N Low (containing saccharin) does cross the placenta and remains in fetal tissue for long periods of time.

BOTTOM LINE: It is probably safer to avoid artificial sweeteners while pregnant.

Q. Is high-fructose corn syrup safe?

No. High fructose corn syrup (HFCS) is found in many processed foods, from soda to pancake syrup. Over the years, HFCS has replaced many other types of sugar in foods for one simple reason: It's cheap.

At the same time, however, concerns have been raised about HFCS: Is it contributing to our nation's obesity epidemic? Well, too much sugar is never a good thing. But HFCS may lead to metabolic dysfunction. Specifically, it may impact the body's response to insulin and raise triglyceride levels, potentially leading to diabetes and liver disease. Animal studies suggest that a pregnant person's HFCS intake may negatively impact the fat metabolism and liver composition of the growing fetus.[5]

BOTTOM LINE: You should avoid or limit HFCS in your diet. And since HFCS is found mostly in processed foods, it is more nutritious to stick with fresh foods for better overall health for you and your growing baby.

Q. Are seed oils safe?

Short answer: yes.

Long answer: Seed oils are the catchy term used to describe vegetable oils derived from plant seeds, such as canola, sunflower, and soybean. There have been many podcasts devoted to the evils of seed oil and gut inflammation. While it is true that these oils are frequently used in fast food and fried foods, and are heated to very high temperatures (also not ideal), they have become the target of the wellness industry without good science to support those claims.

On the flip side, these oils contain linoleic acid (omega-6 fatty acids), a polyunsaturated fat that lowers bad cholesterol and can reduce the risk of heart disease and strokes. According to the American Heart Association, "There's no reason to avoid seed oils and plenty of reasons to eat them."

As we discussed in Chapter 7, "Nutrition," the key is to have the right balance of long-chain polyunsaturated fatty acids in your diet and in any nutritional supplements you may take. So while you do not need to avoid seed oils and other sources of omega-6 fatty acids like walnuts and pumpkin seeds, it's wise to increase your consumption of omega-3 fatty acids found in foods such as fish, chia seeds, and edamame.[6]

Cheese

Q. My friend has completely freaked me out—she said I shouldn't have eaten Brie at that dinner party last night! Is this true? Why? Are there other cheeses I should avoid?

Here's the basic rule: Avoid unpasteurized cheese and dairy products during pregnancy. Why? In a word, listeria.

Listeria is a bacteria that's found in certain imported, *unpasteurized* soft cheeses, among other things. Listeria can cross the placenta and may cause an infection in your fetus, which can sometimes lead to miscarriage.

Here's a list of soft cheeses that raise red flags:

- Brie
- Blue-veined cheeses
- Camembert
- Feta
- Gorgonzola
- Mexican cheeses (such as queso blanco and queso fresco)
- Roquefort

Avoid these cheeses unless they clearly state that they have been pasteurized or made with pasteurized milk. This advice goes for all dairy products. Unpasteurized products are commercially available in the United States, so don't assume cheese is pasteurized because it is sold at the grocery store or natural foods mart. When in doubt, ask.

If you are out at a restaurant, check with the waiter or kitchen before ordering any dish with soft cheese. For more info on listeria, check out Chapter 18, "Infections."

Fish and Shellfish

Q. I am dying for sushi. Why is my doctor telling me I shouldn't have any?

Two words: food poisoning.

Don't get us wrong, we are both huge sushi fans. However, when pregnant, you need to think of yourself as immune-compromised. This means that you and your partner can eat the same food, but you are the only one who gets sick.

As an OB-GYN, I see this all the time—patients who end up with severe food poisoning from eating just one piece of sushi, a medium rare steak, or that seared (but still rare) ahi tuna.

As we've discussed before, your immune system is temporarily suppressed during pregnancy (so you don't reject that foreign DNA growing in your uterus). This means you are much more susceptible to getting sick from both viruses and bacteria.

Most sushi contains raw fish or fish eggs (roe). Raw or undercooked fish (just like any other meat) may be contaminated with multiple types of bacteria, including salmonella, shigella, and toxoplasmosis. Not only can you get extremely sick from these germs, but your baby can get infected, too. Infection can cause miscarriage as well as multiple birth defects, including intellectual disability.

Have some celebratory sushi on your first date night with your partner *after* the baby is born. For now, you'll have to get your sushi fix by eating vegetable sushi or sushi with cooked fish such as imitation crab or shrimp tempura. Just be certain that the chef doesn't prepare it on the same cutting board with the same knife that is being used for all of the other uncooked sushi.

Q. Which fish are safe to eat during pregnancy? How much can I eat?

Fish is good for you and your developing baby. You just have to choose the *right* fish. The big concern with some fish: methylmercury contamination. Fish can absorb methylmercury from coal-fired power plant waste that ends up in nearby rivers, lakes, and oceans.

Developing fetuses whose pregnant parent eats diets high in fish contaminated with methylmercury are at risk for developmental delays, intellectual disability, learning issues, and attention problems. Predator fish (example: swordfish) have the highest levels of methylmercury, so those are the ones to avoid. See the handy table below for more info. You can also see how much methylmercury is in fish at this website: fda.gov/food/consumers/advice-about-eating-fish.

Highest Mercury Levels: Steer Clear

Bass	Marlin
Bluefish	Orange roughy
Croaker	Shark
Grouper	Sea trout
Halibut	Swordfish
Lobster (American/Maine)	Tilefish
Mackerel	

ENVIRONMENT

Medium Mercury Levels: Have Fewer Than Three Six-Ounce Servings per Month

- Carp
- Cod
- Crab (blue and snow)
- Herring
- Mahi Mahi
- Monkfish
- Perch (seawater)
- Skate
- Snapper
- Tuna (canned, chunk light)
- Tuna (fresh Pacific albacore)

Low Mercury: Have Two Six-Ounce Servings per Week

- Anchovies
- Butterfish
- Calamari (squid)
- Catfish
- Caviar (farmed)
- Clams
- Crab (king)
- Crawfish/Crayfish
- Flounder
- Haddock
- Hake
- Herring
- Lobster (spiny/rock)
- Oysters
- Perch (ocean)
- Pollock
- Salmon
- Sardines
- Scallops
- Shad
- Shrimp
- Sole
- Sturgeon (farmed)
- Tilapia
- Trout (freshwater)
- Whitefish

Q. I'm confused about canned tuna. I've heard that some is safe and some is not. Is that true?

Yes, it is confusing. There is not an easy answer here. Methylmercury levels vary in tuna based on the *type* of tuna and where it was caught. Experts agree that chunk light tuna contains less methylmercury than white albacore tuna. The most recent FDA guidelines say that canned chunk light tuna is relatively safe during pregnancy.[7] But food safety advocates fear that the amount of methylmercury in each can varies widely, and this broad recommendation may not be applicable for a pregnant person. They argue that pregnant people should avoid all tuna completely.

BOTTOM LINE: If you are a canned tuna fan, choose chunk light tuna (packed in oil or water is fine) and limit your intake to an occasional five-ounce can every week or two.

Q. What about smoked seafood?

It's a no-no.

Even refrigerated, smoked seafood (such as lox, Nova Scotia style or jerky) may contain public enemy number one, listeria.

On the bright side, it's okay to eat if this type of seafood is an ingredient in a *cooked* dish, like a casserole.

Q. I am on a camping trip with my family. Is it okay to eat the fish we catch?

Nope.

Unfortunately, some of our lakes and rivers are contaminated with industrial pollutants that may be a health hazard to developing fetuses. You can contact your local health department or the EPA (epa.gov) to figure out which lakes/streams/rivers are polluted.

Even if a local river or lake is deemed safe, we'd still err on the side of caution and not eat any fish caught during a camping trip.

Q. What about raw shellfish?

Sorry, you can't eat uncooked oysters, clams, or mussels. Even if you're not pregnant, these are high-risk items for food-borne illnesses. You are welcome to eat shellfish if you cook it. But save the oyster shooter for that glass of champagne you will have after delivery.

Meat

Q. Can I eat deli meat?

No, unless it is heated or cooked. Since deli meat can be contaminated with listeria, either avoid it altogether or reheat the meat until it is steaming to kill off any potential bacteria.

So if you crave a pastrami sandwich on rye, just order it *hot.*

Q. What about raw or seared meat?

No—for the same reason you can't eat sushi. Again, you are temporarily immune-compromised. Undercooked or uncooked meat/poultry/seafood may contain Salmonella, toxoplasmosis, and other bacteria (like *E. coli*) that can make you sick. Cook all meat thoroughly before you eat it.

Eggs

Q. I love eating cookie dough. Is it okay to eat raw eggs while pregnant?

No.

Salmonella is the big risk with any food containing raw eggs. Examples include:

- Homemade ice cream
- Custard
- Freshly made Caesar salad dressing
- Hollandaise sauce
- Homemade mayonnaise
- Homemade eggnog

Commercially made ice creams, dressings, and mayonnaise are safe because they use pasteurized eggs. Typically restaurants use pasteurized eggs, but ask if there is any doubt. The eggnog you buy in the grocery store has so many preservatives it's probably safe to drink until next Christmas! There are some stores that sell pre-made, pasteurized cookie dough for eating and not baking, and despite being pretty expensive, those are actually okay to eat.

DR. M'S OPINION

I commiserate with you. I would rather eat an entire batch of cookie dough than eat the actual baked cookies! But this is a dangerous thing to do, especially while you're pregnant.

Other Food and Drink

Q. Are freshly squeezed juices okay?

Yes, if you are the one freshly squeezing them. Unpasteurized fruit or vegetable juices, or even ones that are "flash" pasteurized and sold at natural food stores may contain bacteria you and your baby don't want to encounter.

And if you are on the juice-pressing bandwagon (there seems to be a new place popping up on every corner here in Los Angeles), go to a reputable place that washes their fruits and vegetables thoroughly. And drink the juice right away. Letting freshly squeezed juice sit around can lead to bacterial or parasite problems.

Q. Am I taking any risks eating at a salad bar during my pregnancy?

We love that you want to eat salad, as it can be such a great source of so many vitamins and nutrients needed for your growing baby. However, be very cautious eating from salad bars where the individual ingredients are sitting out in the open in trays or containers. Many items are not refrigerated and sit out for long periods of time. You are also counting on the fact that all of the veggies and leafy greens were washed thoroughly and properly. And last, all that food is subject to germs (viruses in particular but bacteria, too) that other people may unknowingly be spreading through coughing, sneezing, and improper handwashing. Our advice would be to have the salad, but order one off the menu or make it at home yourself, and skip the line at the salad bar.

Reality Check

Raw bean sprouts and alfalfa sprouts can also be sources of food-borne infection, particularly listeria and should be avoided during pregnancy.

FYI: We will cover the debate on pesticides in foods (organic versus conventional produce and milk) in the "Household Exposures" section later in this chapter.

Bad Habits

Smoking

Q. I was smoking before I knew I was pregnant. Is this going to harm the baby?

Probably not—if you find out that you are pregnant between four and nine weeks *and* you quit smoking right then and there.

Truth is, many folks indulge in bad habits (alcohol consumption, tobacco) before they know they are pregnant. The key is to stop once you know you are expecting.

Reality Check

Smoking during pregnancy increases the risk of having a child with asthma. Nicotine seems to impair fetal lung development, resulting in asthma after birth.[8]

Q. I am still smoking. Is this going to harm the baby?

Short answer—yes.

A pregnant person who smokes has less circulating oxygen in their body and thus so does their unborn baby. This is called ***fetal hypoxia***. There is also less blood flow to the uterus and placenta, and therefore to the baby. Lastly, nicotine goes right through the placenta and circulates in the bloodstream of the fetus.

So how do all of these things affect your baby?[9] There's an increased risk of:

- Having a small fetus who doesn't grow properly
- A placenta that implants over the ***cervix (placenta previa)***
- A placenta that pulls off the wall of the uterus prematurely (***placental abruption***)
- Breaking your water bag early (***premature rupture of membranes***)
- Preterm delivery
- Low birth weight (less than five pounds)
- Stillbirth and newborn death
- Sudden infant death syndrome (SIDS) in infancy
- Asthma, colic, and obesity in infancy and childhood

We know it sounds grim, but it's the truth. There has really never been a better time to quit.

Q. I am smoking, but I want to quit. I've tried before and have been unsuccessful. What should I do?

Good news: There are many options. The best advice is to have a detailed conversation with your OB provider. You can create a plan that works best for you, discussing what symptoms you may have during withdrawal and how to cope with them.

To get started, figure out what situations increase your desire to smoke. Do you smoke with meals? After meals? At the end of the day? Before bed? While driving? Once you identify your triggers, change or eliminate them.

Next, create a smoke-free home. It really helps to have a quitting buddy who can support you. If your partner smokes, this is a great time for *both* of you to stop. Having other people in your home who smoke can make the process of quitting extremely challenging, to say the least.

Your OB provider should have a list of resources to help educate you about the risks of smoking and, most importantly, strategies on quitting. But here are a few great places to start:

- HelpPregnantSmokersQuit.org
- Truthinitiative.org/exprogram
- SmokeFree.gov
- National Quitline Network (800-QUITNOW): Check for local services in your state.

Although quitting in the first trimester is the best thing for your baby, it's beneficial to quit at any point. Even if you quit before the third trimester, you will greatly lower the risk of harm to your baby.

You can do this . . . for you and your baby.

Q. Is it safe to use a nicotine patch or gum?

Ideally, the safest way to quit is to . . . just quit. There is zero health risk in support groups, counseling, or group therapy. All of these things can help you change your behavior.

Doctors can't say with 100 percent certainty that nicotine replacement products (like gum, lozenges, patches, and inhalers) are safe during pregnancy or in breastfeeding women. But the American College of Obstetricians and Gynecologists says if you have failed at quitting, the benefit of stopping smoking outweighs the risks potentially associated with these the products.

If going cold turkey doesn't work, trying a nicotine replacement product is the next step. Most OBs (me included) recommend trying nicotine gum or an inhaler first. These products offer nicotine in intermittent doses. Nicotine patches are the last choice because they administer nicotine continuously. If you must resort to the patch, remove it at night to decrease nicotine exposure to your fetus.

Q. My doctor is recommending an antidepressant to help me quit. Is that okay?

Yes. Some medications have multiple uses!

Bupropion (Wellbutrin) is an antidepressant, which, in certain doses, helps reduce withdrawal symptoms in people trying to quit smoking. Taking this medication is almost certainly safer than smoking. For more on medications and pregnancy, see Appendix A, "Medications."

Q. If I smoke after I give birth, are there any risks to the baby?

YES. *A parent's smoking habit is one of the key risk factors for sudden infant death syndrome (SIDS).*

If the risk of SIDS isn't enough to convince you to stop smoking, parental smoking increases a child's risk of asthma, ear infections, infantile colic, and obesity.[10]

If you weren't able to quit during your pregnancy, it's never too late to try.

Reality Check

Nicotine also passes through breast milk. Studies show that nursing parents who smoke have babies who sleep less than their peers. The higher the dose of nicotine, the less they sleep.[11] When you realize how little sleep you get as a new parent, this may also inspire you to quit smoking!

Cannabis

Q. I smoked marijuana before I knew I was pregnant. Have I done anything to harm the baby? Is it a problem if I continue to smoke during pregnancy?

The research on this issue is limited but clear. There are no studies that show that any level of cannabis use during pregnancy is safe. And ACOG is very clear as well, advising against recreational or medicinal use of cannabis in pregnant or breastfeeding women.[12] The active compounds in marijuana, such as THC (tetrahydrocannabinol), cross the placenta and is found in umbilical cord blood after birth. There is also a slightly higher risk of miscarriage, fetal growth restriction (having a smaller baby), and stillbirth.

Regular marijuana use in pregnancy (loosely defined as four to six times a week) increases chances of preterm delivery. And since THC crosses the placenta, your baby is also getting it. Babies born to women smoking marijuana regularly are at risk for withdrawal-like symptoms, including excessive crying, trembling, and irritability.

What we don't know is how your marijuana use affects your baby in the long term. Some studies show no long-term problems in children, and others have found an increased risk of neurodevelopmental disorders like autism spectrum disorder and attention deficit hyperactivity disorder (ADHD).[13]

The most important thing to do (as with all other drug use) is to quit now. If you have trouble quitting, ask your OB provider for a referral to an addiction medicine specialist, a substance abuse treatment center, or a counseling group.

Q. What about edibles? Do they have the same effects on my baby as smoking marijuana?

Whether cannabis is smoked, vaped, taken orally, or mixed with food or beverages, it is still being absorbed into your bloodstream and therefore is able to cross the placenta and enter into your baby's circulation. So although adults may have different effects based on how they ingest cannabis, babies get exposed no matter what.

Q. Are cannabis-derived products that don't have THC (like CBD products, for example) safe to use?

No, they aren't. ACOG and the FDA strongly advise against products that contain cannabis (THC and/or CBD). Although there has been much more research focused on pregnancy and the effects of THC on the fetus, the few human studies we do have, as well as many animal studies, show that CBD does cross the placenta and enters the fetal brain. While there, CBD interacts with serotonin and potassium receptors, which are important for proper neurodevelopment.

Speak with your provider regarding your reasons for wanting to use CBD and ask for a list of alternative options that are pregnancy-safe.

Cocaine

Q. I used cocaine before I knew I was pregnant. Have I done any harm to the baby? Are there any health risks if I continue to use it occasionally during pregnancy?

Possibly.

Cocaine is a powerful stimulant that, without any doubt, affects most major organ systems in developing fetuses. Cocaine has the biggest impact on the developing nervous system, including the brain. So even if a person only uses cocaine before discovering they are pregnant, damage to the fetus has most likely already happened. Long-term studies show that cocaine-exposed babies may have behavior and conduct issues even into adulthood.[14]

If you continue to use cocaine, your health risks include a greater chance of miscarriage, preterm labor and preterm delivery, placental abruption, high blood pressure (hypertension), and stroke.

Experts don't know the exact amount of cocaine that triggers the above problems. But even if an adult uses cocaine *once*, they can have a heart attack or stroke. The same is probably true for your baby.

The safest thing to do is to stop using cocaine once you find out you are pregnant. If you need help, ask your OB provider or contact the National Drug Help Hotline by texting or calling 988.

Methamphetamines

Q. I have been using methamphetamine prior to pregnancy. I am now pregnant and just can't stop. What are the risks to me and my baby?

Methamphetamine is a stimulant that elevates your heart rate, as well as your baby's. Meth causes problems similar to cocaine when used during pregnancy. Risks include miscarriage, preterm delivery, low-birth-weight babies, and placental abruption.

Methamphetamine crosses the placenta into your unborn baby's bloodstream, so babies that are born to women using methamphetamine are also likely to suffer withdrawal symptoms, including tremors, sleeplessness, feeding difficulties, bonding issues, and muscle spasms.

Children who were exposed in the womb may have behavioral issues and learning disabilities.

NEW PARENT-TO-BE 411:

Prenatal Substance Use and the Law

Drug use is not only unhealthy during pregnancy, but it's also considered child abuse or a criminal act in some states. The Child Abuse Prevention and Treatment Act requires Child Protective Services (CPS) to investigate when a newborn tests positive for exposure to drugs, alcohol, or controlled substances. In some cases, parents could lose custody of a baby exposed to drugs.[15]

Opioids

Q. What about heroin? Can my addiction be treated during pregnancy?

Yes, you can and should be treated. Heroin is an extremely addictive drug and, like other drugs, it crosses the placenta. Your baby may be born premature, with low birth weight, low blood sugar (which can lead to seizures), breathing problems, and bleeding into the brain. And some heroin-exposed babies die.

Heroin is so addictive that even an unborn baby can become dependent on the drug and suffer severe withdrawal symptoms at birth. Newborn withdrawal symptoms are similar and often just as severe as those seen in adult heroin users. They include irritability, convulsions, diarrhea, fever, joint stiffness, and sleeping difficulties. Note: A pregnant person who uses IV drugs also puts themself *and* their unborn child at risk for HIV and hepatitis B and C infections.

This is a very tough addiction to treat. Start by talking to your OB provider. They will likely refer you to an addiction medicine specialist for help. You may need to take methadone, buprenorphine, naltrexone, or suboxone as part of the treatment program. While not an ideal medication, methadone is much better for you and your baby than the ongoing use of heroin, especially if you are injecting it.

The best thing you can do is quit, no matter how far along you are in your pregnancy.

Q. **I am addicted to a prescription opioid pain medication (Vicodin, Vicoprofen, Percocet, Darvocet, Tylenol with codeine). What are the health risks to me and my baby during my pregnancy?**

Prescription opioid pain medications are among the most commonly abused substances. Examples include Oxycontin (oxycodone), Vicodin (hydrocodone), morphine, codeine, and Demerol (meperidine).

You can take some of these medications safely during pregnancy if the need arises—like when you need a root canal or some equally unpleasant medical procedure.

But there is a difference between appropriate use and misuse. Taking these medications in larger doses than prescribed, at more frequent intervals than prescribed, and for reasons other than what it was prescribed for is considered misuse of the drug and is *not* safe for your developing fetus.

These medications cross the placenta and impact your baby. They can lead to preterm delivery, low-birth-weight babies, withdrawal symptoms, and difficulty breathing.

Household Exposures

Insecticides/Pesticides

Q. **Is it okay to use insect repellent while I am pregnant?**

Yes!

All Environmental Protection Agency–registered insect repellents are safe to use at recommended doses during pregnancy. That includes products containing these active ingredients: DEET (N, N-diethyl-m-toluamide or m-DET), picaridin (KBR 3023), and lemon eucalyptus oil.

Studies of insect repellent (even in toxic doses) and pregnancy showed no increase in birth defects, preterm labor, stillbirth, or growth restriction. The benefit of using insect repellents is far greater than any theoretical risk of using one of these chemicals.

Zika virus, an infection that spreads mostly by mosquito bites, can lead to serious birth defects if a pregnant person becomes infected. Luckily, the rates of Zika infection have dramatically dropped over the last few years. As of the publication of this book, there have been no confirmed cases of Zika reported in any of the US territories and no local transmission within the United States.[16] Other mosquito-borne diseases include infections such as West Nile Virus and dengue, which can be serious for a pregnant person or the developing fetus.[17]

BOTTOM LINE: Bug spray is safe. Protect yourself from mosquitoes and mosquito-borne diseases.

Reality Check

Pregnant people are mosquito magnets. Mosquitoes like things that put out heat. We don't need to tell you that pregnant people emit more heat than other people because you know how hot you are right now! You also exhale more carbon dioxide with each breath, which makes you very attractive to a mosquito.

It's never fun getting a thousand mosquito bites, especially when you are pregnant, itchy, and uncomfortable anyway. So it's smart to either stay inside or spray up!

Q. I live in an agricultural area, and I constantly smell pesticides as they are sprayed on neighboring crops. What should I do now that I am pregnant?

If possible, avoid agricultural pesticide exposure during your first trimester.

During this time, your baby's nervous system is rapidly developing, so you definitely want to avoid *any* type of contact with pesticides that can lead to brain/spinal cord defects.

Numerous studies have looked at pesticide/insecticide exposure during pregnancy, and there are definite associations between *agricultural* pesticides and miscarriage as well as birth defects (particularly ***cleft lip/palate***, brain/spinal cord, heart and limb defects). Pregnant people living within a quarter mile of agricultural crops seem to be at highest risk.[18]

Before you decide to move to Antarctica, most experts believe that you need *prolonged* and/or *intense* exposure to be at risk. Unless you are the one flying the crop duster, you should be fine.

To err on the side of safety, however, we'd advise leaving an agricultural area with heavy pesticide use, particularly during the first trimester, if you can. We know this is much easier said than done.

Q. Is it okay to have the exterminator come over to spray the perimeter of my home?

It's best to avoid home pesticides, if possible.

The timing and the frequency of home pesticide exposure both prenatally and early in life has been linked to childhood cancers such as soft tissue sarcomas, leukemias, and cancer of the brain.[19] Some studies have found an association between organophosphate pesticides and lymphoma and leukemia, but others have not.[20] Some research suggests a possible link between home pesticide use to neurocognitive and behavioral issues in children.

If you must use pesticides outside, try to wait until after your first trimester. Stay out of the area for at least twenty-four hours (a good excuse to take a spa retreat!) and avoid direct contact with anything that has been sprayed outside your home. You can also talk to your exterminator about less toxic options or hire a company that uses organic or "green" methods of pest control. These aren't completely safe, either, but they can be less toxic than the alternatives.

It's also a good idea to avoid doing routine pesticide treatments on your lawn. Pregnant people exposed to household gardening pesticides have an increased risk of delivering babies with ***cleft palates*** and neural tube, heart, and limb defects.

Q. I love to garden, but my roses need spraying. What should I do?

Avoid gardening for seven to ten days after the pesticide was applied. When you do resume gardening, wear protective clothing to help avoid contact with plants that have been sprayed.

Helpful Hint

Whether you use pesticides or not, you should always wear gloves when gardening. Gloves help reduce your risk of toxoplasmosis exposure, which can be present in soil.

Q. What about indoor pesticides?

It's best to avoid indoor pesticides completely. The pesticide residue will collect on upholstery, rugs, and carpeting. Only treat for pests when there is a problem. Skip scheduled or routine pesticide applications. And opt for non-chemical options and use the least toxic products. Think roach paper or traps.

Why? Fetuses who are exposed to higher levels of indoor pesticides have a higher risk of developing leukemia in childhood.[21]

The highest risk appears to be exposure during the first trimester or when a professional pest control service is used.

So you may be wondering, what exactly is a "higher level" of pesticide? Unfortunately, researchers didn't quantify that.

Q. What about organic or natural pesticides during pregnancy?

Almost all chemicals used in pesticides are compounds that are naturally present in plants. Although they may sound healthier, the terms "organic" and "natural" do not mean "better" or "safer." All of these chemicals, including natural chemicals, are toxins and have the potential to cause harm if you don't handle them properly.

Read the warning labels on all pesticide and insecticide packages before handling them.

BOTTOM LINE: Although occasional exposures are probably okay, it is best to avoid all household, pet, and garden pesticides and/or insecticides (conventional or organic) during pregnancy and when you have children living in your home . . . or maybe never use them.

Reality Check

Children are more vulnerable than adults to pesticides.[22] The World Health Organization has concerns regarding both the amount and timing of pesticide exposure. There are potential links to certain types of cancer, endocrine issues, and reproductive health.[23]

Q. Should I eat organic fruits and vegetables to reduce my exposure (and my baby's) to pesticides?

Well, the latest outcomes data on pesticide exposure is definitely concerning. Long-term studies assessing participants from birth to young adulthood (called a birth cohort study) demonstrate that children who are exposed to higher levels of a pesticide (organophosphates) in the womb score slightly lower on IQ tests and have more behavioral and mental health issues than less exposed peers.[24]

While it would be ideal to be able to access and afford a completely organic diet, we realize that is aspirational and unrealistic in the world today. Also, it is important to note that "organic" does not mean a product is pesticide-free. Pesticides are in both water and soil. There will be some in just about anything we and our children eat or drink (including breast milk and, yes, organic products).

But it makes sense to limit pesticide exposures when it is practical to do so and not cost-prohibitive. For more information on ways to reduce pesticide exposure, see the tips in the following Insider Secret box.

INSIDER SECRET:

Six Ways to Reduce Pesticide Exposure from Foods

Don't want to spend your entire paycheck on organic groceries? Here are some tips to reducing pesticide exposure:

1. Scrub produce with a brush under running water to get rid of any obvious residue.
2. Peel whatever produce you can. (FYI: This often removes the main fiber source, though.)
3. Don't eat the outer leaves of leafy vegetables (e.g., lettuce, kale).
4. Grow your own garden and don't use pesticides.
5. If you are buying imported produce, only purchase produce that can be peeled.
6. Buy produce that is in season.[25]

Unfortunately, these tips don't eliminate all the pesticides, but they help.

Q. Should I drink organic milk?

Well, no major medical organization recommends organic milk over the regular stuff. We'll share some facts here, and then you can decide for yourself.

Organic milk promises to be chemical-free, but because chemicals remain in the soil for so long, even organic milk may contain pesticides. Organic farmers may also use organic pesticides. Compared to, say, apples, the pesticide residue in milk products is rather low.

All milk products are screened for antibiotic residues. If residue is detected (which happens in about 1 in 1,000 tankers of milk), the milk is rejected for sale. Hence, conventional milk should also be antibiotic-free. The concern here: Even though the finished product is antibiotic-free, antibiotic use in livestock is contributing to antibiotic resistance. Doctors have tried to limit antibiotic overuse in humans; it is time to reduce use in animals, too. Your grocery store purchases drive the marketplace.

BOTTOM LINE: While there is probably no antibiotic residue in milk, buying organic milk encourages milk manufacturers to avoid using antibiotics.

Q. Should I buy organic meat?

There are plenty of reasons to choose organic meat, but the key health issue is antibiotics.

Antibiotics are given to healthy animals to prevent disease and improve growth. In fact, at least 40 percent of the antibiotics used in the United States are used in animals that are destined to become our next meal. Antibiotics used in the food industry are indirectly a problem for humans because they allow antibiotic-resistant bacteria to evolve.

So, while there is no direct health hazard from eating conventional meat, there is an indirect health risk. If you want to buy antibiotic-free meat simply on principle, look for meat labeled "USDA Organic."

Q. Is it safe to eat genetically modified foods?

A quick primer on genetically modified foods (GMOs): Humans have been genetically modifying foods since the beginning of time. As technology has advanced, scientists have been able to splice genes of seeds to make plants resistant to drought, disease, and so on. This has provided an abundance of food at a very low cost. That's the good news. Opponents of GMOs, however, are concerned with the potential long-term health impacts of GMO foods and want mandatory labeling of GMOs in foods.

So what does the science say? The American Cancer Society says bioengineered foods are safe to eat. The potential health concern is that most genetically engineered crops are created to survive the herbicide farmers use as weed killer. The main ingredient in the herbicide is glyphosate, which is potentially carcinogenic.[26] The American Academy of Pediatrics has expressed concerns about the safety of glyphosate.[27] And those herbicides are sprayed all over the crops that eventually make it to our kitchen tables.

BOTTOM LINE: The evidence is lacking on the health risks of GMOs themselves, but the benefit of non-GMO foods may mean less exposure to glyphosate. Like all environmental health issues, it's wise to limit exposures whenever possible.

Q. What are forever chemicals or PFAS, and should I worry about them?

PFAS stands for perfluoroalkyl and polyfluoroalkyl substances, which are a diverse group of thousands of chemicals used in various products in packaging, processing, cookware, clothing, and carpeting, to name a few. These chemicals have been used since the 1950s, and they do not break down very well. As a result, we are exposed to them in the water, food, soil, and air, so it is hard to avoid them. And these "forever chemicals" also stick around in our bodies . . . forever.

So, unfortunately, we probably should worry about them as they may be harmful to our health. PFAS exposure has been linked to decreased immune system function, altered growth and development, impaired endocrine function, elevated cholesterol levels, and risk of some cancers.[28] While there are blood tests to screen for PFAS, they are not offered at standard laboratory facilities and are not covered by insurance. But, truthfully, knowing the levels in one's bloodstream cannot predict any future health consequences from exposure. There is also no treatment to remove PFAS from our bodies.

You can assume that everyone, including our babies, will have PFAS exposure. The best thing to do is limit exposures. Here are a couple of suggestions:

- Run your tap water for a couple of minutes in the morning before using it.
- Consider getting a water filter certified to remove PFAS.
- Use PFAS-free bottled water.

Q. Is it worth it to get a water filtration system?

It depends on your water supply. It can be an expensive investment. Those little filters that attach to faucets aren't going to do very much. Tap filters may remove lead and other toxins, but not excessive fluoride or PFAS (forever chemicals). And if you don't take care of them properly and replace the carbon filters regularly, bacteria will end up growing in the filters.

One easy first step: Run your tap water for two minutes in the morning before you use it—that flushes any lead out.

Reverse osmosis filters do remove both toxins, PFAS, and fluoride—but these are much more expensive and need to be installed housewide.

Here's our recommendation: Get your community's water quality report (most are posted online on water company home pages) or go to ewg.org/tapwater/. If your community has a serious problem with contamination or PFAS, then a whole-house reverse osmosis filter would be a useful investment. The same is true if you are relying on well water: Get it tested and treat it if necessary. The Environmental Working Group has tested and rated their favorite water filters if you want a few options.

Household Cleaning Products

Q. I'm worried about using cleaning products during pregnancy. Should I have someone else clean my house?

Household cleaning products are safe, but there are many options for conventional cleaning liquids and sprays that are less toxic, like Mrs. Meyer's, Koala Eco, and Seventh Generation.

Pregnancy is an excellent excuse to accept help from others or call in a cleaning crew. Between the awkward positions that leave your back aching and fumes that only worsen your nausea, cleaning is not an easy task. Unfortunately, many of us get hit with that "nesting phenomenon" and cleaning is not just a necessity but an obsession.

If you can call in help (your partner, a cleaning service), do so. If you are going to do all the dirty work yourself, try to use a brand mentioned above if cleaning regularly yourself.

Here are a few suggestions:

- Minimize contact with chemicals: Wear long sleeves, gloves, and a mask (particularly for cleaning small spaces like ovens).
- Read all instruction labels.
- Never mix cleaning products with each other or with other chemicals.
- Try to keep the area you are cleaning well ventilated with open windows and/or a fan.
- Have your partner do some/most/all of the cleaning if possible.

Q. I just can't bring myself to use my normal cleaning products while pregnant. Is there anything else I can use?

You have a few options. You can dilute many products with water to decrease the intensity of fumes. You can use more natural products, such as those mentioned above. You can also use baking soda or vinegar to clean most things. Check out Eartheasy (eartheasy.com) for an extensive list of options and homemade recipes.

Fumes

Q. Is it okay to paint the house?

Yes, with a few precautions.

Like many eco hazards, there isn't much research on this subject to suggest what the health hazards are for you or your fetus. But here are some commonsense suggestions:

- If possible, get someone else to do the painting for you and remove yourself from the area until the project is complete.
- Do not use oil-based paints. They contain organic solvents whose fumes can be irritating.
- You can't buy any lead- or mercury-based paints. Since 1978, the Consumer Product Safety Commission has required paints to have less than 0.06 percent lead. The Environmental Protection Agency banned mercury levels above 0.06 percent in latex paint decades ago. The bad news? Lead-based paint was commonly used before 1978. If you live in a house built before 1978, *do not* scrape or remove the old paint (or perform any other do-it-yourself home renovation projects)! Consult with your local health department for a list of certified professional lead remediators. See the "Get the Lead Out" box on page 207 for more details.
- Minimize exposure to paints that contain ethylene glycol ethers and biocides (pesticides/antimicrobials). Ethylene glycol ethers are associated with miscarriage.

- Consider using paints labeled "zero-VOC." VOC stands for volatile organic compounds. VOCs can cause nasal congestion, eye irritation, headache, nausea, and vomiting. They are also possible carcinogens (cancer-causing agents). Zero-VOC is the same paint, without the toxic compounds and smell. Many paint brands, such as Dunn-Edwards and Benjamin Moore, carry this type of paint.

If you must paint the nursery yourself, there are a few precautions that we suggest:

- Talk to your OB provider before beginning a project.
- Protect yourself by wearing long sleeves, long pants, gloves, and an N-95 mask or similar.
- Make sure the room is well ventilated with open windows and/or a fan.
- Absolutely avoid scraping and sanding old paint. This releases chemicals into the air, which increases the risk of inhaling them.
- Work in small bursts of time, and take frequent breaks to go outside and get fresh air.
- Keep all food and drinks away from the area you are painting.
- Avoid spray paints, as the mist increases the amount of chemicals that you might inhale.
- Stop painting if you begin to feel lightheaded, nauseated, dizzy, short of breath, or experience chest pain. Contact your OB provider.

FEEDBACK FROM THE REAL WORLD:

Painting the Nursery

Painting the nursery is often a rite of passage for new parents—myself (Dr. M) included. The hardest part: picking the right color. It took me, four grandparents, and three neighbors to select the perfect hue for my first child's nursery (lemon yellow). The nursery color for our second child (sage green) took less than two minutes at the hardware store while my ex-husband was looking at power tools.

Q. What if I have already been exposed to paint/paint fumes when I didn't realize I was pregnant?

Don't sweat it. There are no studies that indicate any harm to a fetus from accidental paint exposure during pregnancy.

However, recreational use of paint (yes, there are people who sniff or inhale paint solvents to get high) exposes fetuses to much higher levels of chemicals, and there is definite potential for miscarriage, birth defects, and intellectual disability.

Q. Can I get new carpeting installed in my home?

Yes, but we recommend that you leave the house while installation is going on. And get someone to open the windows and run the fans before you return home.

New carpeting, as well as the padding and adhesive that goes under it, can release VOCs (volatile organic compounds). VOCs can irritate the eyes, nose, and/or throat, as well as cause coughing or trouble breathing. The health risks of VOCs depend on the type of VOC, the duration of the exposure, and the amount of exposure. Currently, there aren't any specific health risks associated with typical exposure in the womb to new carpet fumes.

Reality Check

In addition to paint and carpets, other sources of VOC exposures include dry cleaning fluid, hobby and craft supplies, photographic solutions, permanent markers, printer ink, and smog. The best you can do is limit exposures where possible.

Heavy Metals

Q. I'm worried about mercury exposure during pregnancy. How can I limit exposure?

The short answer: Limit your intake of high-methylmercury-containing fish (as discussed earlier in this chapter).

The long answer: It's nuanced. We have long cautioned pregnant people to be mindful of their seafood intake, based on research on children's neurodevelopment in communities whose pregnant parents consume fish every day.

One leading research team has been studying families in the Republic of Seychelles, a group of islands in the Indian Ocean, for the past thirty years. These islanders eat about ten times more fish than Americans do. The most recent findings of the Seychelles Child Development Study state there are no adverse outcomes in children's neurodevelopment! Any low levels of mercury exposure are significantly outweighed by the benefits of a seafood-rich diet that is high in omega-3 fatty acids and other micronutrients. One of the principal researchers, Gary Myers, MD, feels that fish consumption advisories can be "overly cautious and counterproductive" because they discourage fish intake and the nutrients in seafood support the developing brain.[29]

Q. I have dental fillings and heard that they contain mercury. Do I need to do anything about them?

Dental fillings (amalgams) contain mercury. However, if you already have amalgams in your mouth, they do not have to be removed. If you have a cavity that must be filled during pregnancy, talk to your dentist about your options (there are several mercury-free alternatives).

Q. I'm worried about lead exposure. Is there any way to reduce my exposure?

Good question. We know a great deal about lead exposure during pregnancy and early childhood—and what we know is scary.

Pregnant women exposed to lead have:

- A greater risk of preterm labor
- Low-birth-weight babies
- Babies with brain/spinal cord defects

The risk of preterm labor is three times greater even with mild exposure to lead (officially, that is a lead level over five micrograms per deciliter).

Any level of lead exposure can have subtle but permanent effects on the brain.[30]

So what can you do to reduce your lead exposure? Here are five tips:

1. Do not eat out of lead-glazed ceramics.
2. Do not drink out of lead-crystal glassware (it is particularly important not to store liquids like juice in lead-crystal containers, as lead may leach into the beverage as it sits).
3. Avoid DIY home improvements if you live in a home built before 1978. (More on this in the box below.)
4. If you live in a home built before 1986, run your tap water for two minutes in the morning before drinking. Older homes have lead solder in the water pipes.
5. Get tested if you work in a job where you might be exposed to lead (such as a lead refiner, automobile finisher, typesetter, spray painter, printer, pottery, ceramics, rubber/plastic products maker, brass/bronze products maker, etc.).

NEW PARENT-TO-BE 411:

Get the Lead Out

If you live in a home built before 1978 and want to do some home repairs or painting, don't watch some online videos and think you can tackle this project yourself. You can inhale a significant amount of lead dust by tearing up the house or even just scraping off old paint. Here is our advice:

- Call in an expert. Your local or state health department should have a list of certified home lead inspectors and contractors who specialize in lead renovation work. Yes, there are DIY home lead test kits, but each kit only tests one small area. They aren't going to save much money because you'll end up buying several test kits.
- If the old lead-based paint is in good condition, you should paint over it. Do ***not*** scrape it or sand it off.
- The biggest problem areas are windows and other areas that rub and create dust. These areas need to be cleaned thoroughly as they will be where your future baby/toddler perches to look out the window and gets dust on their little fingers (which then go into their mouths).
- If it is necessary to do a lead remediation, you should leave the house and not return until both the job and the cleanup are done.

For more info, check out the Environmental Protection Agency (EPA) at epa.gov/lead/lead-renovation-repair-and-painting-program.

Plastics

Q. I've heard about certain plastics causing health problems in babies. What should I know, and do I need to avoid exposure to them?

Yes. Our overarching advice is to avoid or limit exposures when it is practical and possible to do so. Let's nerd out on plastics for a bit and cover the biggest concerns: microplastics and phthalates.

1. **Microplastics.** Many plastic bottles and containers are made of polypropylene. We know that polypropylene releases microplastics (tiny plastic fragments), especially when the food or liquid is heated and shaken.[31] We know that we all ingest plenty of microplastic particles on a daily basis, and we also eliminate some in our poop. But what is the long-term health impact of microplastics? Only time will tell. But given their tiny size and ability to accumulate in the body, there are concerns about the impact on several organ systems, especially those that are developing.

   Here are a few relatively easy and inexpensive ways to reduce your exposure to microplastics:

   - If you own plastic containers, do not wash them in the dishwasher with harsh detergents.
   - Do not microwave plastic food containers. Plastics may break down from repeated use at high temperatures.
   - Eat less canned food. Opt for fresh or frozen foods.
   - Use glass, porcelain, or stainless-steel containers, particularly for hot food or liquids. Silicone is also an option for water bottles.

2. **Phthalates.** Phthalates are plasticizers that make plastic soft and durable. The health concern? Phthalates are considered endocrine disruptors, chemicals that can mimic the actions of actual hormones found in our body, even in low doses. Phthalates mimic weak estrogens and block our body's androgen receptors, which can impact glucose metabolism, thyroid function, reproductive organs and hormones, and possible carcinogens. There is also concern that phthalates can affect male genital development in the fetus.[32]

   Phthalates are used just about everywhere. For example, you'll find them in plastic cling wrap, plastic food packaging, shampoos, creams, and, for future reference, toys. Phthalates can be both ingested and absorbed through the skin. Babies have been found to eliminate the breakdown products of phthalates in their urine.

   The good news: Both the United States and Canada require toys and products that are intended for use in the mouth (pacifiers, teething toys, bottles) to be phthalate-free. And newer US federal legislation has tighter restrictions on phthalate use.

   Our advice: If you want to reduce phthalate exposure, minimize or eliminate use of plastic utensils, plastic water bottles, plastic storage bags and Tupperware, and use a napkin or paper towel when you heat food in the microwave.

Pets

Q. I have a cat. I've heard they can carry a disease that can be harmful to the fetus. Can I still play with them?

The concern with cats is toxoplasmosis.

This is a parasite that lives in the soil. As a result, it can be found in unwashed produce, undercooked meat, and cat poop. Cats can become infected with toxoplasmosis by eating infected prey, like birds or rodents, or just by burying their poop in outdoor soil that is contaminated. Cats don't usually have any symptoms when they are carriers of the parasite, although sometimes they have soft poop or diarrhea. Outdoor cats and kittens are more likely to be carriers than indoor cats.

You can be exposed with a cat bite, scratch, or just by cleaning the litter box.

About 15 percent of American women are immune to toxoplasmosis, and it's more likely if you are a long-time cat owner.

If you are immune to toxoplasmosis before pregnancy (determined by a simple blood test), then the baby is safe. If you are not immune, you can play with your cat, but be very careful. Toxoplasmosis is not something you want to get while pregnant. Contact your doctor if you are scratched or bitten. And don't change the litter box!

For a more detailed discussion of toxoplasmosis, check out Chapter 18, "Infections."

Q. Why do I have to avoid changing the litter box?

The parasite is in the cat poop. And even stirring up some dust while you are cleaning the litter box can expose you to it.

Ask, barter, or pay your spouse, partner, or friend to do the dirty work. If you live alone and absolutely must do it yourself, move the litter box outside while cleaning it, wear a mask and gloves, and wash your hands thoroughly afterward.

DR. M'S OPINION:

Testing for Toxoplasmosis Immunity

I test all of my cat-owning patients (either attempting conception or at the first prenatal visit) to see if they are already immune to toxoplasmosis.

Q. I was cleaning the litter box during my first trimester before I knew I was pregnant. Is that okay?

The best advice is to stop cleaning the litter box once you know you are pregnant.

There is a chance that you are already immune. So relax.

If you get infected for the first time between ten and twenty-four weeks, your newborn has a 5 percent chance of having serious problems. See Chapter 18, "Infections," for the details.

If you get infected during the third trimester, your fetus can still get sick, but the risk of damage is much less since most of your baby's organ development has already occurred.

If you think you may have been exposed to toxoplasmosis, ask your OB provider to test you. The blood test will tell if you already have immunity or if you have had a recent infection.

Q. Do I have to give up my cat while I am pregnant?

No, you don't. Follow the safety guidelines listed in the following New Parent-to-Be 411 box, and talk to your OB provider if you have any questions or concerns.

NEW PARENT-TO-BE 411:

Toxoplasmosis Safety Tips

Where Do You Get It?

1. Cats. They are symptom-free (usually) carriers of the parasite.
2. Unwashed/poorly washed fruits and vegetables from contaminated soil.
3. Undercooked meats.

How to Prevent It

1. Don't clean the cat litter box. Have someone else change it daily.
2. Feed your cat commercial cat food (not undercooked meat).
3. Wash all fruits and vegetables thoroughly.
4. Cook meat thoroughly—use a food thermometer to measure the internal temperature of cooked meat.
5. Beef, lamb, veal roasts, and steaks should be cooked to at least 145°F throughout.
6. Pork, ground meat, and wild game should be cooked to 160°F.
7. Whole poultry should be cooked to 180°F in the thigh.
8. Freezing the meat for several days before cooking is another way to greatly reduce the chance of infection.
9. Do not get a new cat during your pregnancy, and avoid stray cats and kittens (as cute as they may be).
10. Speak to your veterinarian about whether your cat can be tested for toxoplasmosis. For more details, see Chapter 18, "Infections."

Q. My friend's cat just scratched me. What should I do?

Contact your OB provider so you can be tested for immunity or to see if you've had a recent infection. Clean the area well to prevent infection.

FEEDBACK FROM THE REAL WORLD:

Cats in the Cradle

How do you keep your cat out of your baby's crib? Cats love warm spots, and a crib is a cozy place. Simple advice: Keep your nursery room door closed when baby is sleeping or the room is unoccupied. That will keep your cat from converting your baby's crib into their favorite nap spot.

Q. I have a dog. Is there anything I have to worry about during my pregnancy?

Dogs pose no significant infection risk to you or your unborn baby.

If you have a big dog, just keep them from jumping on your belly. And exercise extreme caution if you are the one who walks the dog. As your belly gets bigger and your center of gravity begins to shift, you are much more likely to fall after getting twisted in the leash or after man's best friend goes chasing the neighborhood cat. Falling when you are pregnant can be dangerous for your baby, so take care to avoid it.

Q. My partner didn't tell me they just treated our dog for fleas, and I have been playing with them all afternoon. I'm panicked! What should I do?

First of all, don't panic. The real risk here is *long-term* or *intense* exposure to chemicals. Your dog's flea bath presents a *very* small risk to your unborn baby—especially if you are out of the first trimester.

Red Flag: Pesticides

Call your poison center at (800) 222-1222 and OB immediately if you inhale or swallow a pesticide, or your skin comes in direct contact with a pesticide. The poison control experts will want to know the specific ingredients, so have the pesticide container nearby to reference when you call.

Q. Will my baby be prone to allergies if we have a cat or dog in the house?

Actually, the opposite is true.

Early exposure in the first year of life to cats and dogs may prevent allergies. It's called the hygiene hypothesis. It goes like this: If your body is busy fighting off germs (like the ones the cat or dog carries), it doesn't have the desire to mount an allergic response to things (like cat dander).

Kids who grow up on farms have significantly fewer problems with allergies, presumably because they have constant exposure to animals and the germs they carry.[33]

INSIDER SECRET:

Introducing Fido to the New Family Member

Many couples get a dog as their first test of parenthood. If your dog is your first child, how do you introduce them to the first human baby of the house?

Here are some things you can do to help make the transition easier:

- Prepare your dog for the baby ahead of time. Follow routines that will be commonplace after the baby arrives. You can even pretend using a baby doll.
- Once the baby is born, bring home an article worn by your baby (hat, shirt) for your dog to sniff before the baby arrives. Introduce them as soon as you bring the baby home, but keep your dog on a leash and supervise initial interactions.
- Teach your dog the difference between their toys and the baby's toys. Make sure you keep baby's and dog's toys in separate locations so that there aren't any jealousy issues.
- Always keep an eye on your baby/child when they are with your dog, and never leave the two of them alone.
- Remember that your dog may act like an older child and become jealous of all the attention lavished on a new baby. Make sure you pay extra attention to your dog, and if appropriate, include your dog in play with the new baby.
- Keep the dog's food bowl away from the baby. Once your baby is crawling, the baby may either a) try to eat it or b) get into a fight with your dog who wants to defend their territory.
- Ask your OB, pediatrician, and veterinarian for more suggestions!

Note: Babies and young children are the most frequent victims of dog bites. Children are curious and will poke, pull hair, and scare dogs. Sometimes this innocent play can lead to a dangerous bite by a startled dog.

Q. I live on a farm. What concerns should I be aware of?

Farm animals carry certain germs (salmonella, listeria, campylobacter, and cryptosporidium) that can pose a risk to you and your fetus. Since you can't exactly vacate the farm for nine months, here are a few things you can do to help prevent infection:

- Never drink untreated water. If you have well water, have it tested for nitrates and bacteria, as well as other possible contaminants.
- Only eat or drink pasteurized dairy products.
- Do not handle stillborn animals.
- You should not be present when animals are fed with food stored in a silo.
- Wear gloves if possible when feeding or handling the animals.

- Always wash your hands with soap and water after any contact with animals or their living quarters.
- If you believe you have come in contact with an infected animal, contact your OB.

Q. I have a pet turtle (lizard, iguana, frog, snake, etc.). Any health risks to worry about?

Although pet turtles (as well as other reptiles and amphibians) are fun, they can pose a health risk for you during pregnancy. The problem: salmonella.

These animals may carry the bacteria salmonella, which comes out (guess where) in their poop. (We aren't afraid to talk about anything in this book, including turtle poop!)

Direct or indirect contact with your pet's poop can lead to infection in you and your baby.

Our advice: It's probably best to give up Mr. Turtle (or any other reptile or amphibian pet) when you learn you are pregnant. Even after delivery, your baby is at risk becoming ill from a salmonella infection.

If you and your little guy are inseparable, take these precautions to reduce the risk of infection with pet turtles, lizards, and the like:

- Wear gloves when handling the pet or its cage.
- Wash your hands with warm water and soap after handling the animal.
- Do not have your pet on or near any area where food preparation may occur.
- Do not wash the pet or its cage in the kitchen sink. Ideally, have someone else do it, and do it outside your house.
- Do not let your pet roam freely in your house.
- Consider screening your exotic pet to see if they are a carrier for salmonella. One of our readers (who works for Texas Parks and Wildlife and handles snakes for a living) tells us it costs less than fifty dollars to test each snake. Try searching online for "exotic pets vet" to find a provider who can offer testing in your area.

Q. I have a pet bird. Is it okay to keep it during pregnancy?

Birds may carry germs that can infect humans, including salmonella, campylobacter, some protozoal infections, and chlamydiosis (we know what you are thinking: not the same as the sexually transmitted chlamydia!).

Our advice: A healthy bird is fine to keep around during pregnancy. Take your bird to see a veterinarian for a well-bird visit and make sure.

Here are some bird safety tips:

- Always wash your hands with soap and water after handling your bird or bird cage.
- Some birds (especially cockatoos) are very dusty. You may want to consider getting an air filter. This could be especially helpful when the new baby comes home.

FEEDBACK FROM THE REAL WORLD:
Pet Iguanas

I have had more than one baby patient get a salmonella infection long before they were old enough to eat steak tartare. Example: One baby got sick after their uncle's pet iguana roamed freely on the kitchen counter (near washed baby bottles). Another baby was infected after their grandmother prepared chitterlings (pig intestine) in the kitchen sink before the baby took a bath there. Truth is sometimes stranger than fiction!

Q. I was bitten by a _______________ (fill in the blank). Are there any health risks?

No matter what bites you, call your OB provider. Some animal bites (such as dog bites) are only dangerous because of the risk of skin infection, assuming there is no rabies.

Other bites, however, can be much more dangerous, such as those from a cat infected with toxoplasmosis or a wild animal, like a squirrel or raccoon.

Wash the area immediately with soap and water, then seek medical advice.

Noise

Q. Can I go to a concert during my pregnancy?

Yes. Just make sure you are not in the front row.

At about sixteen weeks, your developing baby can hear noises; by twenty-seven to thirty weeks, the ears are fully formed and they will begin to respond to many sounds.

These sounds include blood rushing through the vessels in your body, the sound of food moving through your intestines, as well as the sound of your voice.

Your baby doesn't hear sounds as clearly as we do. The ***amniotic fluid***, uterus, and your body act as barriers that help muffle external sounds and noises. Additionally, the baby's eardrum and middle ear can't amplify sounds like ours do, so loud sounds to us aren't quite as loud to them.

However, we still don't want to expose fetuses to really loud noises for prolonged or repeated intervals. Babies can suffer hearing loss in the womb, but that typically results from conditions such as working an eight-to-ten-hour workday next to a chainsaw or lawnmower (85 to 100 decibels). Extremely intense sounds (over 140 decibels), such as a jet engine or noise from a concert speaker, can also cause similar problems.

Here are some sources of loud noises to avoid during pregnancy:

- Standing near jet engines.
- Being at a firing range or firing guns yourself.
- Being in the front few rows of a concert.

- Working at a job that subjects you to constant, loud noise (above 80 decibels for many hours a day, day after day).

Q. What about my hair dryer?

Using a hair dryer during pregnancy is fine.

Helpful Hint

The national MotherToBaby program offers free evidence-based guidance on environmental exposures and medications during pregnancy and while breastfeeding. Check out their website here: thegenesisfoundation.org/programs-services/mothertobaby/.

Odds and Ends

Electromagnetic Fields

Some quick definitions here: Electromagnetic fields (EMFs) are invisible lines of force created by electric charges. Power lines, electric appliances, cell phones (and towers), the earth's magnetic field, and even humans emit these EMFs.

Low- to mid-frequency electromagnetic fields are non-ionizing radiation. Most experts believe they do not emit enough energy to damage DNA. These include small appliances, cell phones, and MRI scanners.

High-frequency electromagnetic fields are ionizing radiation. Large exposures can damage DNA. These include X-rays, CT scans, and UV rays from the sun or tanning beds.

Q. I worry about exposing my growing baby to electric and magnetic fields. Should I worry about my cell phone or laptop?

While there is some conflicting data, most experts contend that low-frequency fields don't have enough energy to cause damage to you or your baby's DNA or organs.[34] Hence, your hair dryer, coffee maker, and microwave are probably safe. But researchers continue to look at possible connections between EMFs (including cell phone use) and brain tumors and certain types of leukemia. At this time, many experts believe that cell phones do not emit enough energy to damage human DNA. While some studies do suggest a link, the overall evidence is not conclusive, and the World Health Organization (WHO) and National Cancer Institute (NCI) have not found a clear association. The greatest concern is the distance of the body organ (example, the brain) from the EMF source (say, the cell phone).[35]

Even so, it's not a bad idea to use a Bluetooth headset, earbuds, or a temporal headphone device instead of holding a cell phone to your ear for hours on end. And trying to keep your laptop off your lap while working is always a good idea.

Q. Are hair dryers safe?

Yes. But it's best to dry your hair in a well-ventilated place so you don't get too hot.

Q. Can I use a microwave?

Yes, it is absolutely safe to use a microwave during pregnancy. Just move away from the microwave while it is on and don't open the door until the microwave has completely stopped.

Q. How about the X-ray machine at the airport?

It's safe. For starters, you actually don't walk through an X-ray machine. It's a glorified metal detector, and the machine can't hurt your baby, no matter how far along you are in your pregnancy.

Q. What about those full-body scanners at the airport? Are they safe?

Yes. These scanners use non-ionizing radiation to see under your clothes. Since the scanners use a technology that doesn't penetrate the body's organs, experts say they are safe. To get a harmful dose from a full-body scanner at an airport, you'd need to be screened 2,500 times in a year.[36]

Or you can opt for the pat-down by airport security instead! Good times.

Q. Why do they always ask if you are pregnant before an X-ray?

There are two concerns with X-rays: developmental abnormalities (***teratogenic effects***) and cancer risk (***carcinogenesis***).

High levels of ionizing radiation early in pregnancy can lead to miscarriage, growth restriction, small head size, and intellectual disability. Fetuses between eight and twenty-five weeks (especially eight to fifteen weeks) are the most susceptible.

Before you worry, let's discuss how experts come up with these risks . . . and what defines "high levels" of radiation (that's at least 20 to 50 rad). The studies on this issue are all from animals and pregnant women unlucky enough to be present and survive an atomic bomb explosion. Even if you have multiple diagnostic X-ray procedures, you still won't reach these levels of exposure.

A pregnant woman has to be exposed to a large dose of radiation (more than 5 rads) to have an increased risk of having a miscarriage, a baby with birth defects, intellectual disability, or growth restriction. No diagnostic procedure has this much radiation (see the chart below).

While it is unclear if a fetus exposed to radiation while in the womb puts them at increased risk for leukemia, there is enough concern to avoid it if possible.[37] Ultrasounds and MRIs are safer choices than standard X-rays or CT scans during pregnancy.

But there are certain situations when these tests are necessary (for example, when a pregnant woman is injured in a car accident).

BOTTOM LINE: If you have an X-ray done only to find out later that you were pregnant, don't sweat it. Better yet, if there is a chance you may be pregnant, take a home pregnancy test the day before your procedure. If it is positive, notify your OB provider and radiologist immediately.

Amount of Radiation Used in Imaging Studies

Imaging Study	Amount of Radiation in Rad or Millirad*
Chest X-ray	0.02-0.07 mrad
Abdominal X-ray	100 mrad
Intravenous pyelogram	Over 1 rad
Hysterosalpingogram	1 rad
Hip X-ray	200 mrad
Mammogram	7–20 mrad
Barium enema	2–4 rad
CT scan (head or chest)	Less than 1 rad
CT scan (abdomen or spine)	3.5 rad
CT scan (pelvis)	3.5 rad

*Note: "Rad" stands for radiation absorbed dose; "mrad" stands for millirad, which is 1/1000 of one rad.[38]

Q. Is it okay to get X-rays or dental X-rays?

It's best to avoid all X-rays if possible.

Of course, it is extremely important to take care of your teeth during pregnancy. You need regular visits and regular cleanings. And if necessary, you can have fillings or even a root canal.

If your dentist feels that X-rays must be done, try to postpone them until after the first trimester. Make sure your neck *and* your belly are completely covered with a lead apron.

As for X-rays of other body parts, avoid them as well. But if you are in a car accident and need an X-ray to rule out a broken bone, do it, but have a lead apron draped over your belly.

If there is ever a question, get your OB on the phone. The dentist, orthopedist, or any other medical personnel taking care of you can discuss a plan of care with your OB provider. Getting one or two diagnostic X-rays during pregnancy does not pose a significant risk to your fetus, in our opinion (we'll discuss this more below).

Reality Check

Try to wait until after your first trimester to have a routine dental cleaning. Your gag reflex is at an all-time high, and watching your breakfast land on the lap of the hygienist is not fun!

Q. Is it okay to have a CT scan during pregnancy?

Only if you absolutely have to (which is rare).

CT scans (computerized tomography) emit ionizing radiation, which has potential risks for you and your developing fetus. In most cases, a safer MRI (magnetic resonance imaging) would work just as well (see below for details).

There are rare situations that require a CT scan instead of an MRI, such as assessing for a blood clot in the lungs. And some trauma centers do not have an MRI scanner immediately available.

CT scans emit differing amounts of radiation, depending on what body part is involved (see the chart on page 217).

Q. Is an MRI safe?

Yes. An MRI uses a magnetic field and radio waves instead of ionizing radiation to produce the images and can usually provide your medical provider the information they need.

An MRI can help rule out appendicitis or make the diagnosis when a pregnant woman has chronic, severe abdominal pain or severe headaches.

People who are claustrophobic (even those who aren't) may be scared of the very narrow tunnel and the loud buzzing of the machine as it takes pictures. But from a pregnancy standpoint, you don't have to worry. They are safe and there are no concerns for adverse effects on a fetus.

So if you need an MRI, do it.

Q. Is it safe to use radio-opaque dye and contrast agents during pregnancy?

It's best to avoid both if you can.

In the little research done on contrast agents and pregnancy, there is some concern about risks of miscarriage, bone defects, and other birth defects. The studies were done on animals that received two to seven times the normal dose of contrast agents given to humans. So you should only have an imaging study with a contrast agent if the potential benefit outweighs the risks to the fetus.[39]

Radioactive dyes (like radioactive iodine) easily cross the placenta and can affect the fetal thyroid gland, particularly after ten weeks. These are absolute no-nos during pregnancy. If you require diagnostic imaging of your thyroid during pregnancy, ask your doctor and radiologist about using Technetium Tc 99m instead of radioactive iodine.

Q. Is it okay to have ultrasounds done?

Short answer: yes. See Chapter 6, "Tests," for a detailed discussion.

Q. Is it safe to work at a radiology office while I am pregnant?

Yes, just take some minor precautions.

Previously, many workplaces just reassigned a pregnant employee's duties to avoid any possible exposure. Workplaces feared legal action if the employed person delivered a baby with any sort of birth defect.

Today, medical offices now use the "Principle of ALARA" (ALARA stands for "as low as reasonably achievable") to devise radiation protection measures for pregnant workers.

If you are a radiology tech, radiology nurse, physician-in-training, or radiologist, the easiest way to decrease exposure to your fetus is to restrict the type of work you are doing and to limit the number of times you perform a particular task. Tell your employer that you are pregnant as soon as you find out so that the two of you can review your exposure history and discuss possible new work assignments.

Procedures involving fluoroscopy and portable X-rays do not put your fetus at an increased risk. Radiology techs and radiologists can continue their work in stationary radiography, portable radiography, fluoroscopy, and other special procedures throughout pregnancy. You should wear a lead apron during all procedures and monitor your film-badge readings.

BOTTOM LINE: The levels of radiation are so low that experts conclude there is no significant risk to the fetus. Otherwise, there wouldn't be people of childbearing age ever working in radiology offices!

Surgery

Q. If I need a surgical procedure done, can anesthesia be used? Or do I need to wait on the operation until after I am no longer pregnant?

Yes, for emergency surgery. No, for elective or cosmetic surgery.

Docs would rather not expose your fetus to general ***anesthesia*** unless it's necessary. Appendicitis and broken bones that poke through the skin are examples of surgical emergencies that simply won't wait. When the benefit outweighs the risk, you need the operation and the general anesthesia.

The "best" time to operate on a pregnant person is in the second trimester because it puts their fetus in the least danger of miscarriage (first trimester) or preterm delivery (third trimester). For urgent, but not emergency, situations, it's optimal to delay surgery until the second trimester if possible.

Q. My dentist says I need a root canal. Is it safe?

Short answer: Yes.

However, your dentist and your OB provider need to chat with each other. They can discuss the procedure as well as pain medications and antibiotics that are safe to use in pregnancy.

It's common to have dental problems during pregnancy. Pregnant people are more likely to suffer from cavities and oral infections than non-pregnant people. Be sure to take care of all dental problems!

Medications

We'll cover common concerns in Appendix A, "Medications."

CHAPTER 9

Lifestyles

"Note for new mama: Falling asleep during sex?
It's forgivable."

—*Haiku Mama* by Kari Anne Roy

What's in This Chapter

- **Exercise 411 and reasons not to exercise**
- **Swimming**
- **Sex: All you wanted to know but were afraid to ask**
- **Travel**
- **Work: When to tell the boss**

Your life still goes on, despite being pregnant. You want to feel like you are a normal human being, and we'd like you to feel that way as much as possible!

This chapter will walk you through activities of daily living and adventures along the way. We cover both work and play in this chapter—exercise, sex, travel, and more.

Exercise

We know, we know—you are nauseated, bloated, and so exhausted that there is no way in the world you are getting off that cozy sofa to go work out. But your mind, your body, and your developing baby need to get through the next nine months together—and exercising helps all of these aspects of pregnancy. Yes, it is *that* important to make exercise part of your *daily* routine. ACOG recommends thirty minutes of exercise a day. If you have no medical reasons or pregnancy complications (see "What are the reasons not to exercise?," page 222), your goal should be thirty minutes a day of aerobic exercise.

Here are some reasons if you need convincing (or sheer motivation) to take off your fuzzy slippers and put on running shoes.

Overall, exercise helps decrease weight gain, improve body image, decrease stress, and reduce your chances of having low back and pelvic pain. Exercise throughout pregnancy helps to reduce labor and delivery time, as well as delivery complications.

In the first trimester, exercise can reduce nausea and fatigue. As exhausted as you are, that thirty-minute walk outside is worth the effort. You will feel better in the long run and also have *more* energy than your non-exercising preggo friends.

In the second and third trimesters, exercise helps decrease the risk of gestational diabetes. If you do have diabetes, it can help treat it.

Exercise also benefits your baby. Babies born to pregnant parents who exercised moderately during pregnancy tolerate the stress of labor better, and they are more alert and less irritable as newborns.

One added bonus: Over 90 percent of pregnant people who exercise during pregnancy will continue to do so afterward—leading to a healthier lifestyle and quicker weight loss after pregnancy ends.[1]

BOTTOM LINE: We recommend daily exercise even if you didn't do this prior to getting pregnant. But be sure to talk with your OB provider before beginning any exercise regimen.

Q. Which forms of exercise are safe during pregnancy?

In general, skip any activity that is a contact sport, high-speed, or has a high risk of falling.

The Good: The Best Exercises for Pregnancy

- Yoga
- Aqua-aerobics
- Swimming
- Pilates
- Resistance training with light weights
- Aerobics
- Walking/hiking
- Stationary bike
- Tennis
- Stairmaster/elliptical machine

The Bad: The Exercises You Should Definitely Avoid

- Sumo wrestling
- Powerlifting
- Rugby
- Waterskiing
- Surfing
- Horseback riding
- Ice skating and ice hockey

- Rock climbing
- Kickboxing
- Lacrosse
- Scuba diving
- Snow skiing
- Skateboarding
- Beach volleyball
- Rollerblading
- Gymnastics

Red Flags: Exercise

Stop exercising if you experience any of these symptoms. Then call your doctor.

- Lightheadedness
- Headache
- Chest pain
- Feeling overheated
- Calf pain or swelling
- Vaginal bleeding
- Shortness of breath before you really exert yourself
- Shortness of breath that does not resolve if you stop exercising
- Overall feelings of severe fatigue
- Contractions

Partner Tip

Want to do something to help your baby-carrying mate? Exercise together. Find an activity you both can do and enjoy (okay, you may need to make some concessions here) and spend some healthy, quality time together.

Q. What are the reasons not to exercise?

These are legitimate medical reasons to avoid aerobic exercise. Yes, we can all come up with a million lame excuses, but these are legit!

- Heart disease that alters blood circulation
- Lung disease limiting the air volume breathed in
- ***Cervical insufficiency*** with or without a ***cerclage***
- Multiple babies at risk for preterm labor
- Persistent second- or third-trimester bleeding
- ***Placenta previa*** or ***vasa previa*** after twenty-six weeks gestation

- Premature labor
- Ruptured membranes
- ***Preeclampsia*** or pregnancy-induced hypertension (***gestational hypertension***)
- Severe ***anemia***
- Abnormal heart rhythm that has never been evaluated (cardiac arrhythmia)
- Chronic bronchitis
- Poorly controlled preexisting diabetes
- Extreme obesity
- Extremely underweight (BMI < 12)
- History of extremely sedentary lifestyle
- Fetal (intrauterine) growth restriction
- Preexisting bone, joint, or soft tissue problem
- Poorly controlled high blood pressure
- Poorly controlled seizure disorder
- Poorly controlled thyroid disorder
- Heavy smoker
- Your OB provider has placed you on bed rest

We discuss many of these medical conditions in Chapter 17, "The Complicated Pregnancy."

Q. I've heard I shouldn't be flat on my back during my exercise regimen. Is that true? Why?

That's true—for pregnant women after about twenty weeks. Why? Because this position lowers your blood pressure, which can lead to dizziness and fainting.

Your uterus lies on top of your major blood vessels (the vena cava and aorta) that take blood to and from your heart. After twenty weeks, when lying on your back, the increased size and weight of the uterus can cause a relative blockage of blood flow. Less blood returns to your heart and so less blood leaves your heart, hence, lower blood pressure.

What does that mean for your baby? Less blood goes to your uterus and to the baby. What does that mean for you? Less blood goes to your head. You feel dizzy or faint.

BOTTOM LINE: After twenty weeks, don't lie on your back for long periods (more than five minutes) during exercise.

Q. Can I still continue to do my normal exercise routine? Do I have to monitor my heart rate?

Yes, and maybe. Assuming your exercise routine doesn't involve something that is not on the list of exercises you should definitely avoid during pregnancy on page 221 and you do not have a high-risk pregnancy, you can continue your usual routine of exercise.

Whether it is jogging, swimming, using a stationary bike or elliptical machine, tennis, yoga, Pilates, etc., you can continue your routine with a few caveats: Always clear your routine with your OB provider, keep your routine to less than sixty minutes, and watch for red flag symptoms (see the Red Flags list on page 222).

If you experience any of these symptoms, stop exercising immediately.

You will likely have to alter the type and duration of your exercise routine as your pregnancy progresses.

If you have been exercising regularly prior to pregnancy and plan to continue your usual routine, a heart rate monitor is not necessary.

Q. What exactly do you mean by "light weights"?

There is no agreed upon definition of what light-weightlifting means. What I tell patients is you can lift lighter weights (think five pounds, eight pounds, etc.) to keep fit, but this is not a time to increase the weights you are lifting, push yourself, or break records.

If you are used to resistance training with a certain set of weights (e.g., squatting with a thirty-pound weight), you can continue doing that until about twenty weeks, which is when many physiologic and anatomic changes happen to your body. After twenty weeks, although resistance training can continue, it should consist of even lighter weights.

Q. We are going on vacation to the mountains. Can I exercise at higher altitudes?

Yes, up to certain altitudes.

Altitudes up to 6,000 feet above sea level appear to be safe. But even at these altitudes, you may feel out of breath faster. You may need to shorten the length of your workout and stop if you have any of the Red Flag symptoms mentioned on page 222.

Above 6,000 feet in altitude, exercise can lead to altitude sickness, dizziness, fainting, shortness of breath, and chest pain. So it is best to avoid exercise at these altitudes.

If you live at elevations above 6,000 feet, check with your OB provider before beginning any exercise regimen.

Q. Can I swim in a chlorinated pool?

Yes.

Don't let the prospect of wearing a pregnancy bathing suit scare you away. Swimming is a great form of exercise during pregnancy, even if you weren't a swimmer beforehand.

Chlorine kills germs, and that's a good thing. An adequately chlorinated pool will prevent the spread of viruses (like enterovirus and hepatitis A). So yes, you *want* to swim in a chlorinated pool.

Q. Can I swim in a freshwater lake or stream?

Sorry, but the germ factor makes freshwater lakes and streams off-limits.

Everyone (including non-pregnant swimmers) faces *some* risk when they swim in fresh bodies of water. But as you become an infectious disease expert with this book, you know that germs and pregnant people are often risky business.

Here are the three bugs (bacteria and parasites) that can bug you when swimming in freshwater lakes and streams: giardia, leptospirosis, and amebiasis. All of them can cause horrible cramps, diarrhea, and potentially miscarriage and preterm labor.

The safest thing to do when you are pregnant is to use the pool or sit in the shade and enjoy some alone time reading while everyone else is in the water!

Q. Can I go waterskiing or scuba diving?

No. These are two activities that are better left for days without a baby in your belly.

Waterskiing can be dangerous, particularly during a fall. The impact of a fall can cause extreme jolting, which could lead to a separation of the placenta from the wall of the uterus (***placental abruption***).

Scuba diving is another activity that's not recommended. First, you have to strap on some serious gear. This can be uncomfortable, especially as you get bigger. Second, you descend to depths that can decrease oxygen levels in your bloodstream and therefore baby's bloodstream. Finally, divers have to decompress as they return to the surface. Developing babies may have difficulty decompressing.

While there is no solid scientific evidence, there is a concern for potential birth defects and preterm delivery among women who go scuba diving during pregnancy.[2]

Although we know we are taking all of your fun away, stick with a virgin daiquiri on the beach while the rest of the crew heads down below. You can return to all these activities about six weeks after having the baby, with your doctor's blessing.

Reality Check

Placental abruption can even happen with low-impact falls or accidents. That's why it's a good idea to avoid any activities that cause sudden or abrupt jolts.

Q. I went diving during my last vacation and didn't know that I was pregnant at the time. Is that a problem?

Probably not.

There's no evidence that diving around the time of ***conception*** leads to miscarriage. Pregnant women were diving for years before docs started advising against it. And there was no significant health impact to the mother or the developing baby.

Experts don't recommend it anymore because of the theoretical risk and some research that suggests concern.

Q. Will exercising really make my labor and delivery go more smoothly?

It would be nice to say that exercise would shorten labor and make delivery smoother . . . but there are no guarantees.

What we can tell you is that it reduces your overall weight gain and chances of gestational diabetes—both of which can complicate labor and delivery.

And continuing the exercise routine that you start during pregnancy will help you lose those pregnancy pounds afterward and improve your overall health. Daily exercise also gives you more muscle tone and stamina to endure labor and delivery.

Q. I am an avid runner. Can I still run a marathon while I am pregnant?

Can you continue to run? Yes. Should you run a marathon? No.

Studies show that runners who continue exercising during pregnancy gain less weight, have leaner babies, and shorter labors. Running a marathon, however, is a tremendous strain on a non-pregnant body, let alone a pregnant one.

If you have any pregnancy complications, your OB provider will probably tell you to stop jogging. Otherwise, keep up the jogging, with a few precautions:

- Stay well hydrated.
- Exercise for a maximum of sixty minutes.
- You should base your workouts on something called rate of perceived exertion (RPE). RPE is how hard you feel your body is working. This means that you can continue exercising as long as you aren't experiencing any physical symptoms such as chest pain, shortness of breath, or dizziness.

Ask your OB provider about specific advice for you.

Truthfully, most runners stop running in the second trimester as the weight of their belly becomes uncomfortable when bouncing up and down. They usually trade in running for the elliptical machine, swimming, hiking, or something less jarring.

Q. I love riding my bike outside for exercise. Is it safe to continue doing that for my entire pregnancy?

Riding a bike is an excellent way to give yourself a good workout and be outdoors. And it is safe, up to a certain point. Once you are out of your first trimester, your fourteen-week uterus is no longer a pelvic organ; it's considered an abdominal organ. What that means is that it is no longer protected by the bones of your pelvis, and any abdominal trauma could potentially be pretty dangerous for your baby. Although those who ride bikes routinely are very good at it, accidents happen. As your pregnancy progresses, your center of gravity changes as does your balance. A fall onto your belly means risk of a placental abruption, and that is a very dangerous condition for your baby. So once you enter into your second trimester, its best to have a picnic outside, but stay on an indoor/stationary bike for exercise.

Q. I regularly go hiking, and I'd hate to give this up while pregnant. Any advice here?

Hiking is an excellent form of exercise and is not as tough on the body as running. Hiking can be done for your entire pregnancy with a few precautions—never go alone, take more water/electrolyte solution than you think you need, bring a fully charged cell phone and a portable charger, avoid strenuous hikes with a lot of elevation change, take bug repellent with you, and (you'll hear us say this frequently) don't push yourself. You really have to listen to your body and rest, slow down, and hydrate when your body tells you to do so.

NEW PARENT-TO-BE 411:

Seven Rules for Exercising While Pregnant

1. Wear comfortable clothing.
2. Consume lots of water to keep well hydrated.
3. Walk with a friend or bring a cell phone.
4. Take frequent breaks. (Some of you will feel like you aren't even breaking a sweat with all the restrictions, but now is not the time to train for a marathon.)
5. If you are new to an exercise regimen, periodically check your pulse, and if it is persistently over 140 beats/minute, slow down. The easiest places to find your pulse are your neck (just under your jaw bone on either side) or the inner part of your wrist. Count how many times you feel a beat in fifteen seconds and then multiply that by four. That equals your pulse (how many times your heart beats in a minute).
6. Do not lie flat on your back for long periods of time after twenty weeks.
7. Do notify your trainer, instructor, or gym that you are pregnant.

Reality Check

Pregnant people get all sorts of advice about what exercise is kosher—and what to avoid.

The problem: It's impossible to do a study that shows exercise X leads to birth defect Y. Or that exercising with a target heart rate of 140 is more dangerous than 130. That's why most OB providers follow the precautionary principle—better to be safe than sorry, even in the absence of scientific proof.

Here is the concern: When a person is exercising, blood flow is diverted away from the abdominal organs (intestines, spleen, and in pregnancy, the uterus) and diverted toward the skeletal muscles. Decreased blood flow to the uterus means less oxygen goes to the fetus. But does this significantly impact a growing fetus? Studies show conflicting results. There is also a risk of the pregnant person's core body temperature increasing as their heart rate goes up. We know that a pregnant person's body temperature above 101.5°F in the first trimester can be associated with birth defects.

Ask your OB provider for specific advice on exercise options. Your exercise regimen should be tailored to your physical conditioning and general health. There is not one target heart rate for everyone. While their opinion may vary a bit from your friend's OB, they will both probably tell you not to run the New York Marathon or swim the English Channel (although pregnant people have accomplished both of these feats!).

Q. After I deliver, when can I start exercising again?

The textbook answer is six weeks, if you had an uncomplicated pregnancy and delivery.

Occasionally, OB providers might give the green light a little earlier to a patient who had an uncomplicated vaginal delivery. But "green light" means a person can do some light walking before six weeks—not a triathlon.

Always check with your OB provider first before starting or resuming any exercise program after delivery. We know six weeks seems like a really long time, but it's important to listen to your OB provider and to your body.

FEEDBACK FROM THE REAL WORLD:

Exercising Too Soon

I had a patient who was determined to get back on the treadmill after a **C-section**. I told her that *after* her six-week postpartum visit, we would decide when she could go back to exercising.

She decided that she felt great at two and a half weeks. She returned to my office with her previously closed surgical incision now gaping open. She had to wait another month to have the wound surgically repaired.

Q. I have a high-risk pregnancy. Am I still able to exercise?

It depends on what makes your pregnancy high-risk.

For example, if you have gestational diabetes, then yes, you can and should exercise during your pregnancy.

But if you have a ***placenta previa*** and have had two episodes of vaginal bleeding, then the answer is no, you should not exercise during your pregnancy.

Again, always check with your OB provider about what is right for you.

Sexuality

Here's the section you (and your partner) have been waiting for. Do you have the green light to continue your sexual relations? Will you want to? Will your partner want to? And what do you do if only one member of your party is ready to party? Read on.

Q. Will I die if I have oral sex?

No. Oral sex is considered safe during pregnancy.

A popular pregnancy book warns women about fatal oral sex, so we are here to allay your fears.

Medical journals from decades ago reported on a few extremely rare cases of fatal air embolism in pregnancy from forcefully blowing a lot of air into a woman's vagina during oral sex.[3,4]

How could this happen? Well, pregnant women have engorged, enlarged blood vessels in their pelvis. When pushed forcefully, those vessels are more likely to allow water or air to enter.

If you look at the millions of women enjoying oral sex during pregnancy (okay, that's an optimistic assumption but quite possibly true) and you compare that to a few fascinating cases in the medical literature, having a fatal air embolism is far-fetched. In fact, you are 1,000 times more likely to get into a car accident during your pregnancy than die from oral sex. And most people don't forcefully blow air into the vagina during oral sex anyway—so the risk here seems very remote. (If this is something you practice, please write to us and explain why this would be a desirable thing to experience.)

In fact, the medical journals indicated you have to force so much air into a vagina to cause a problem there probably isn't a concern here . . . unless your partner is a professional balloon animal artist.

BOTTOM LINE: Oral sex is safe during pregnancy, and many pregnant people find it more pleasurable than vaginal intercourse.

Q. Is it normal to not be in the mood?

Absolutely, and you are not alone.

Although some people have an increased sexual desire during pregnancy (see below), most do not. You have tender breasts, you are exhausted, your hormones are running amuck, and you are most likely self-conscious about your weight gain (not to mention the fact that in the later stages of pregnancy you can't see your legs, let alone shave them).

Even if you are not in the mood, make sure to take some time for intimacy during your pregnancy. Being intimate does not always mean having intercourse. Kissing, holding hands, bathing together, massaging each other, and hugging are all forms of intimacy.

We cannot overemphasize the importance of talking to your partner about this issue. Lack of communication can lead to dysfunction and hurtful feelings in your relationship.

Partner Tip

Are you up and your partner isn't? Yes, you may resort to masturbation. That may take the stress off both of you! By the way, it is safe for your baby-carrying partner to perform oral sex on you. Although beware, pregnancy can worsen one's gag reflex.

Q. Is it normal to be excessively horny?

For a few pregnant people, yes.

The physiologic changes happening to your body may increase your sexual desire. Your breasts are larger, your nipples are more sensitive, and you have more blood flow to your vagina and vulva. These changes often lead to increased desire.

You'll also be naturally lubricated (with all that lovely vaginal discharge), which enhances the intercourse experience. In fact, some people experience orgasms for the very first time during pregnancy.

If you are one of the lucky ones experiencing an increase in sexual desire (and you have your doctor's blessing), go for it!

DR. M'S OPINION:

Staying Connected

Yes, it might be stating the obvious, but you probably won't have intercourse as often as usual during pregnancy (and even beyond that). Maybe you're not in the mood as often as your partner is. Or maybe you have a high-risk pregnancy that requires you to temporarily stop sexual relations. And maybe (okay, more than maybe), you are apathetic about sex for a while *after* you deliver, too, while your body heals and you have to deal with newborn-parent sleep deprivation.

Whatever the case may be, it's mission critical to maintain your loving relationship beyond friendship and just being roommates. So make a plan together to keep your relationship on course.

Q. What will happen to my sexual desire, trimester by trimester?

Everyone is different, but here is a rough guideline on what may happen to your sexual desire as your body changes throughout pregnancy:

- **First trimester:** Most people are fatigued beyond belief and many experience some degree of morning sickness—or really, all-day sickness. Even if you aren't truly nauseated, you may feel queasy or have an upset stomach, which usually doesn't make anyone feel sexy. Breast sensitivity is worst in the first trimester—to the point where some people can't even tolerate a sheet or water in the shower touching their nipples and breasts. You may find this very uncomfortable and may not want your breasts touched during intercourse. Or, like others, you may find extreme pleasure in your larger and more sensitive breasts during foreplay and lovemaking.

- **Second trimester:** Good news, you are over the fatigue and nausea. But you'll probably be more uncomfortable with low back pain and continued soreness around the breasts and nipples. You may continue to have low libido, or you may have a peak in sexual desire. This is due to increased blood flow that causes the vulva and vagina to swell.
- **Third trimester:** The third trimester is tough, no matter how you look at it. You are bigger, more uncomfortable, and you may feel your baby move around after having an orgasm. (This is not a problem, but it might be a real mental leap for you to overcome.) As the baby's head moves lower into the pelvis, you could also be more uncomfortable with vaginal intercourse. For most pregnant people, and their partners, the third trimester is a time when sexual desire is at an all-time low. (Yes, there will be a point when your partner doesn't want to have sex with you, either.)

Q. My clitoris seems to be more sensitive now. Is this permanent?

You now have a supersized clitoris. And no, it's not permanent.

Because of that increased blood flow, your entire pelvic region is completely engorged and swollen—especially during the second and third trimesters.

This can be good or bad. Some people find that it heightens their sensation and so they have really easy, great orgasms. Others find this sensation rather uncomfortable.

This is not a permanent change, and the size of your clitoris will go back to normal after delivery. So either enjoy it now or relax knowing you will have your regular body back soon.

Q. Is it normal for my partner to be uninterested in sex?

Yes.

Some partners are less interested in sex for a number of reasons. They may feel extra stress from the impending birth and becoming a parent. Or there may be fear of potentially harming you or the baby during intercourse. (You can assure a partner that having vaginal intercourse will not poke the baby's head!)

Again, it is extremely important to talk with your partner about their fears and concerns. Don't be shy about bringing up this topic at one of your prenatal visits. You and your partner will have a sense of relief if you discuss this subject with your OB provider. They can reassure you that all is normal and offer helpful suggestions.

Q. Is it normal for my partner to have an increased sex drive during my pregnancy?

Yes.

Some partners may be more aroused by your fuller breasts and rounded figure, the chance to try new positions, and the fact that contraception is a non-issue.

And believe it or not, impending parenthood can be a turn-on! The concept of becoming parents together often strengthens the relationship bond and increases sexual desire between two people.

NEW PARENT-TO-BE 411:

Doctor's Orders

FYI: Your doctor may put you on bed rest or pelvic rest during pregnancy, and in both cases, it means no intercourse. Here's a brief description of each:

- **Bed rest:** Resting and reclining 24/7, likely with brief bathroom breaks and trips to the shower and kitchen.
- **Pelvic rest:** No sexual intercourse, no tampons, no douching . . . nothing in the vagina.

Q. What happens if I go on bed rest? Can I still have an orgasm, even if we can't have intercourse?

It all depends on why you are on bed rest.

Orgasms can cause uterine contractions. Although contractions usually don't put people with uncomplicated pregnancies into labor, they can worsen preterm labor or increase bleeding if there is a ***placenta previa***.

If your OB sidelines you for the remainder of your pregnancy (which is very rare), ask for detailed instructions on sexual restrictions.

Q. Can an orgasm cause a miscarriage or hurt my baby?

No.

An orgasm will make you have a contraction, though, and you will feel it. Your uterus is simply flexing its muscles for a moment. This will not hurt the baby.

Once intercourse and your orgasm are over, the contraction should stop. If you feel like you are continuing to have contractions for more than sixty minutes following an orgasm, contact your OB provider.

Q. Can my partner hurt my baby?

Nope. Your baby is well protected.

In fact, your baby has several layers of protection. They sit inside an amniotic sac, which sits inside the thick, muscular walls of your uterus, which sits within the bones of the pelvic cavity. The ***cervix*** and the ***mucus plug*** within the cervix are also barriers between your baby and the outside world of the vagina.

The penis does not come into contact with the fetus during sex. This could only happen if your cervix was dilated (like it can be at the end of pregnancy) or you were having intercourse during labor, which you shouldn't be doing anyway!

Q. Why does my baby move so much during and after sex?

Some couples feel weird about having their unborn baby participate in their lovemaking. Don't let this get to you!

Think about it. Babies are human beings, albeit tiny ones. They are simply responding to stimulation and touch. When their little home (your uterus) starts rocking and rolling with an orgasm-induced contraction, it's going to make them move around.

And because you have an adrenaline rush when you have an orgasm, so does your baby. Medically speaking, your body releases a large volume of adrenaline into your bloodstream and a little bit of that also goes into your baby's system.

Don't worry about any of this, because it is safe (assuming you have your doctor's blessing). Your developing baby has no idea what the two of you are doing. When they are old enough to understand, make sure you have a lock on your bedroom door!

Q. I've heard that sex can trigger labor. Is that true?

This falls into the "I'll try anything to go into labor" category. People hear that spicy food or long walks will induce labor. Unlike those myths, this one actually has some truth behind it. Yes, if your partner has a penis, vaginal sex can make you go into labor if your body is ready to go.

When your partner has an orgasm, *semen* (also called seminal fluid) is released. That fluid contains sperm as well as the hormone *prostaglandin*. And prostaglandin is the same ingredient in many of the medications docs use to help soften the cervix and help start labor. So your partner's "natural" prostaglandin has the potential to do the same thing.

Before you demand that your partner make love to you, know that there probably isn't enough prostaglandin in semen to induce labor. The odds go up slightly if you were ready to go into labor even without this contribution. Most women will just have a few contractions after intercourse, and that's it.

If you are at high risk of going into labor early, however, your doctor may want to restrict any activity that increases the motion of your uterus. That may mean no orgasms, nipple stimulation, or sexual intercourse at all. Be sure to get details from your doctor.

Reality Check

If you do decide to demand your partner make love to you when you are nine months pregnant, they may not be as excited as you'd like (or need them to be). It's a lot of pressure! You may want to inform him that you will be off-limits for six weeks after delivery, so their chance to enjoy it is now.

Q. What happens if my partner has herpes? Do I need to take special precautions?

Yes, you do need to take special precautions if your partner has herpes and you don't.

The reason? You really don't want to get herpes for the first time while you are pregnant. It's miserable for you and dangerous for your unborn baby (see more info on herpes infections in Chapter 18, "Infections").

Here are your options:

- Abstain from all intercourse.
- Have intercourse, but always make your male partner wear a condom.
- Abstain from all intercourse if your partner feels like an outbreak is imminent or there are visible lesions.

Talk to your doctor about a preventive medication for your partner. Your partner can take a daily antiviral medicine (such as acyclovir) that reduces the chance of shedding the herpes virus and spreading it to you.

BOTTOM LINE: Even if your partner does not have any visible lesions, there's a 1–3 percent chance on any given day that they are shedding the herpes virus without any symptoms. And that means there is a 1–3 percent chance that you can get it from them. Having your partner take antiviral medication reduces those chances.

NEW PARENT-TO-BE 411:

Seven Reasons Why Your Doc Won't Let You Have Sex

1. History of premature labor or birth.
2. Ruptured membranes.
3. Unexplained vaginal bleeding.
4. ***Placenta previa*** or low-lying placenta.
5. Cervical insufficiency with or without ***cerclage.***
6. Dilated cervix.
7. Sexually transmitted disease in you or your partner.

Q. Are there any positions that are more comfortable than others?

That's a trick question, because *no* position will be really comfortable toward the end of your pregnancy. You will be uncomfortable just sitting or standing, let alone twisting like a pretzel during intercourse.

But if you are still game, we have some suggestions for you. We'll start with the old standby, the missionary position. But you will probably find that options two, three, and four below are more comfortable for you.

- **Missionary position.** Lying on your back with your partner on top. After about twenty weeks, you should not be lying flat on your back for long periods of time. But if this is the most comfortable intercourse position for you, put a small pillow under your pelvis to tilt yourself to the left a bit. This will take most of the weight of the uterus and the baby off your major blood vessels.

- **Doggie style.** You bend over and lean on your hands and knees, with your partner behind you. If you have never tried this position, now may be the time. It allows easier access without your belly coming between the two of you.
- **Spooning.** You lie on your left side and your partner enters behind you. This is a popular pregnancy lovemaking position for the same reasons as doggie style. It requires less energy than doggie style since you are lying down.
- **You on top.** You straddle on top of your partner, who lies beneath you. This gives you more control over your belly and how your bodies move together.

Q. Can I have anal sex during pregnancy?

Yes, but we don't recommend it.

Hemorrhoids are common during pregnancy. You could have internal hemorrhoids even if you can't see any on the outside of your anus. Anal sex can flare up hemorrhoids and cause them to bleed. Proceed with caution!

If you decide to give it a try, you should always use a condom, lubrication, and have your partner be very careful. If having anal sex and vaginal sex, it's best to start with vaginal sex to minimize bacterial contamination.

Q. Can I use sex toys during pregnancy?

Yes, as long as you are careful.

It's safe to use a vibrator externally on the clitoris. You need to be very careful using other toys *in* the vagina. Any high-risk condition that makes sexual intercourse off-limits means these toys are off-limits, too.

Make sure you clean all toys appropriately after using them.

Q. Are there any other sexual behaviors that are not safe during pregnancy?

Yes.

Do *not* have intercourse with anyone who has a known sexually transmitted infection (STI) or HIV, or with anyone whose sexual history is unknown to you.

You and your unborn baby can both get sexually transmitted infections such as HIV or hepatitis B or C.

Red Flags: Sex During Pregnancy

Call your doctor if:

- You aren't sure if sex is safe for you.
- You experience unusual symptoms after intercourse such as severe or persistent pain, vaginal bleeding, or abnormal discharge.
- You have contractions that continue after sex.

Travel

Many people have a last fling before they take on the rigors of having a newborn in the house. This is a good idea, because you won't get another vacation without kids for a very long time (unless you can persuade the grandparents to babysit). We want you to have fun, but here are a few considerations to keep in mind.

Q. What special preparations should I take before traveling?

Prepare for the unexpected—travel delays, flight cancellations, or a medical issue that might be related or unrelated to your pregnancy. Travel with more medication than the number of travel days (and a few extra pairs of socks and underwear) and take your medical records with you. Ask your obstetrician if there are any special precautions for your travel destination, such as receiving any vaccinations or avoiding unpasteurized dairy products or undercooked meat. Identify an obstetrician and hospital at your destination, before you go—hopefully just for peace of mind. And, while you may have never purchased travel insurance before in your life, now might be a good time to do so.

Q. I'm traveling internationally. What precautions do I need to take to avoid getting sick?

If you are going somewhere outside the continental United States for a babymoon, be extra certain you do your homework.

- Be cognizant of unpasteurized dairy products and undercooked meat in many European countries.
- Consult your family practice doc and/or OB provider regarding vaccine recommendations.
- If you are headed to a tropical destination, bring pregnancy-safe mosquito repellent and sun protection.
- Purchase travel insurance in case your OB provider decides it isn't safe for you to travel. Although the rise of Zika virus–carrying mosquitoes in the Americas was of concern a few years ago, your travel options today are not as limited. There is currently no local transmission of Zika virus in the United States, and the CDC does not have any active Zika travel health notices. We highly recommend that you go to cdc.gov/travel and check out the risks of your potential travel destination.

Q. How far along in my pregnancy can I continue to travel by car?

There are no restrictions, except that you probably don't want to be more than forty-five to sixty minutes away from your OB provider and delivery/birthing center in the final weeks of your pregnancy.

Sitting around for long periods of time in a car puts you at risk for forming a blood clot in your legs (***deep venous thrombosis or DVT***). Long flights carry the same risk. So be sure to take frequent breaks to walk around (you'll probably need to take several potty breaks anyway). Always clear travel with your doctor.

Q. Is it okay for me to drive up until the end of my pregnancy?

Yes.

You can get behind the wheel up until the end of your pregnancy. Just adjust your seat so that you are comfortable and there is some distance between your belly and the steering wheel. That way, the airbag can properly deploy in an emergency.

Helpful Hint

As your pregnant belly expands, the bottom portion of your seat belt should go *under* your belly, not across it.

FEEDBACK FROM THE REAL WORLD:

Driving and Bed Rest

We should point out that it's okay to drive, assuming you are *not* on bed rest! True story: A fellow OB colleague was placed on bed rest at twenty weeks for preterm labor with her first child and was bored out of her mind. While her husband (also an OB) was at work, she snuck out of the house to run a few errands. When she ended up in a car accident and went to the nearest hospital for evaluation, she sheepishly called him and said, "Hi, honey, I'm being taken to the hospital because I got into a car accident." His response was, "You must have mistaken me for someone else, because my wife is on strict bed rest, so it's absolutely impossible for her to have been in a car accident!"

I don't think we really need to point out the moral of the story here!

Q. How far along in my pregnancy can I travel by plane?

ACOG says thirty-six weeks. Dr. M says thirty-four weeks. Your doc may say something different.

Barring any medical complications, it is safe to fly in the first twenty-eight weeks of your pregnancy. It gets riskier with each subsequent week after that. Your OB provider may tell you to stop flying at twenty-eight weeks or thirty-two weeks, even though ACOG's cutoff is thirty-six weeks. And if you have a high-risk pregnancy (such as carrying multiples), your OB provider will have their own set of rules. Ask before you book those nonrefundable tickets to Hawaii.

Airlines, especially international carriers, vary with their own policies, so you'll need to check with them as well. You may need a letter from your doctor in order to travel by air on some carriers late in pregnancy.[5]

Helpful Hint

This may be the one time that it is worth it to purchase travel insurance for your trip. You may be a low-risk pregnancy when you book the trip but confined to bed rest when it comes time to travel.

Q. I have a high-risk pregnancy. Can I still fly?

In most cases, the answer is no.

You should not be flying on a plane if you have preexisting medical or obstetric complications. Emergency situations happen without warning in obstetrics, and being on a plane over the Atlantic is one of the last places you want to be. You do not want to be in preterm labor as the captain asks via the overhead speaker if there is a doctor on the plane, and the only person who raises their hand is a podiatrist.

Here are just a few examples of pregnancy conditions where you should avoid air

NEW PARENT-TO-BE 411:

Tips for Air Travel During Pregnancy

1. **Go gas-free.** Don't drink or eat any gas-producing items (carbonated beverages, refried beans, etc.) before or during your flight. Entrapped gas expands at higher altitudes and can give you a stomachache.[6] Avoiding these foods also prevents burping and gas passing next to a stranger who can't escape!
2. **Prevent air sickness.** If you are still in the morning sickness phase of pregnancy, air travel may make things worse. Consider asking your OB provider for an anti-nausea medication to take with you.
3. **Take a walk.** You should not be immobilized for long periods of time. Being pregnant means you are at higher risk of developing a blood clot in your leg (deep venous thrombosis, or DVT), which can potentially travel to your lungs. Stretch your calves periodically while you are seated and walk the aisle once an hour if you are on a long flight.
4. **Book an aisle seat.** It's easier access for your hourly walks and trips to the restroom.
5. **Support stockings.** Some OB providers recommend that you wear support stockings to increase circulation and help prevent a blood clot from developing in your leg.
6. **Drink water.** You'll feel better by being well hydrated. It also helps prevent those blood clots. Take an empty water bottle with you in carry-on luggage and fill it up after you get through security.
7. **Wear your seat belt.** Since air turbulence is unpredictable, it's wise to wear your seat belt when you are seated. The seat belt should rest as low as possible under your belly, not across the top.

travel: preterm labor, high blood pressure, poorly controlled diabetes, and sickle cell disease or trait (which can flare up with high altitude). However, although someone with gestational diabetes is considered to have a high-risk pregnancy, flying would be okay in this case.

Always check with your OB provider first.

Fact Check

Pregnant people shouldn't fly because of radiation risk.

The truth: All available data says that the amount of cosmic radiation is negligible and not a health concern for pregnant air travelers.

Q. How far along in my pregnancy can I take a cruise?

The cutoff varies between twenty-three and twenty-seven weeks.

Just like the airlines, every cruise line has its own policy. Many require your doctor to fax a note prior to the day you board. Even if it isn't required, we recommend that you take a note from your doctor and a copy of your prenatal medical records with you.

Some cruise lines do not have a doctor on board. That may impact which cruise line you decide to take—check this before booking. As long as you have a low-risk pregnancy, it is perfectly safe to take a cruise vacation. Just chat with your OB provider before you set sail. And consider purchasing medical evacuation insurance (example: Medjet Assist, medjetassist.com).

INSIDER SECRET:

Seasickness and Morning Sickness

If you are already suffering from morning sickness or get seasick even when you aren't pregnant, be prepared for motion sickness. If you are prone to puking, you might want to wait on that cruise vacation until after the first trimester.

Here are a few things you can try to avoid getting green around the gills:

- Book a cabin in the middle of the ship.
- Book a cruise on a larger ship with better stabilizers (you'll appreciate it on rough seas).
- Spend more time outside on the deck.
- Exercise.
- Eat frequently (that's easy). Choose non-greasy meals or bread and crackers.
- Pack an emergency supply of acupressure wristbands or medication prescribed by your doctor.

Q. Are there any special things I should bring on my cruise?

Yes. Remember to bring enough of any medication you are currently taking as well as prenatal vitamins. Ship pharmacies may not carry everything you need.

Wear a hat and lots of sunscreen, especially on your face to help prevent ***melasma***. And if there is any chance you may become seasick, talk to your doctor about possible medication. It's better to have it with you, just in case.

Q. Will the ship have a life preserver that will fit me correctly?

Yes.

Since most cruise lines do not allow you to travel after twenty-four weeks, you are still small enough to have a life preserver fit you correctly.

If you actually need a life preserver beyond the routine drill on the first day, ask for assistance.

Q. What are the restrictions on amusement park rides?

Basically, any ride that causes a jarring motion or abnormal force is off-limits for you.

Most amusement parks, including Busch Gardens, Disney parks, Six Flags, and even local fairs and carnivals have warning signs directed at pregnant people.

Admittedly, we don't have any studies showing that they are dangerous, but we also don't have any demonstrating they are safe. The big concern is the potential for damage to the placenta, and therefore the fetus. Vigorous movements (similar to a car accident) can cause a separation of the placenta from the uterine wall, which compromises the fetus's blood flow and oxygen supply (***placental abruption***).

Although plenty of pregnant people have ridden on roller coasters and other thrill rides without serious complications, it's wise to avoid them.

Q. If I go camping, can I use insect repellent?

Yes! You can and should use bug spray. See Chapter 8, "Environmental Health," for detailed information.

Work

Whether you work outside the home or inside the home, it's an important aspect of your life to discuss with your OB provider. Pregnant moms-to-be working outside the home in offices, operating rooms, retail stores, classrooms, or anywhere else may have possible exposure risks, physical limitations, or other concerns. If you are a pregnant woman working in the home (the hardest job of all, in our opinion!), you should share this with your OB provider, too. There are things to think about here as well, like the physicality of maintaining a home and caring for other children at home, as well as possible infection risks from your other rugrats.

Q. When do I need to stop working?

It depends. There are no hard and fast rules here.

Certain occupations and workplaces set their own restrictions (examples: pilots and flight attendants). Most employers, however, will let you continue to work as long as you are low-risk, comfortable, and have the okay of your OB provider.

Some people work up until the day before they deliver (it's not easy, let us tell you), whereas others need to stop at some point in the third trimester due to severe low back pain, sciatic pain, or pregnancy complications.

Q. I have a high-risk pregnancy. Do I need to stop working?

This depends on the nature of your high-risk pregnancy as well as the nature of your job. If, for example, you are a tennis instructor and you are a gestational diabetic, you can continue working. But if you are a tennis instructor and are in preterm labor, you'll need to stop running around on the courts.

Sometimes OB providers limit what a pregnant person can do at work without needing them to stop working altogether. Talk to your doc about possible accommodations instead of having to completely stop working.

FEEDBACK FROM THE REAL WORLD:

Dr. M's Experience of Working During Pregnancy

Working during pregnancy certainly is not a walk in the park. I almost fainted twice in the operating room and got such severe backaches from delivering babies (the last one I delivered was two days before I had my first child!) that I almost requested an epidural for myself. But the beauty of working up until the end was that I wasn't at home lamenting about all of my discomfort. I was distracted and in the good company of many other pregnant women who were experiencing the same things as me.

Fact Check

Heavy lifting causes miscarriages.

The truth: While heavy lifting is not recommended for any pregnant person, it doesn't cause miscarriages.

Q. My job requires me to do some heavy lifting. What are my restrictions?

You should avoid all heavy lifting.

The curvature of your spine changes during pregnancy, and you are much more likely to strain the muscles of your back and create a serious injury.

So what is heavy lifting? Anything over fifteen to twenty pounds. If you need to lift items at work that weigh less than this, wear a maternity belt and stop lifting altogether if you experience back pain.

Astute readers may notice the fifteen to twenty pound limit above and wonder about lifting a toddler that weighs that much—after all, if this is your second pregnancy, odds are you are also lugging around a toddler who tips the scales at more than twenty pounds. Is this safe? The answer: The same advice goes for lifting a toddler as for work-related lifting. Avoid it if you can, wear a maternity belt if you can't, and stop if you experience pain. We understand that it is nearly impossible to stop lifting a toddler, and as your pregnancy progresses, they often become clingier. Lift with caution. Have your toddler jump up onto something higher than ground-level and slowly pick them up from there. Again, if you are experiencing any pain, please stop lifting.

If you have a high-risk pregnancy, consult with your OB first regarding any lifting.

Q. My job requires quite a bit of walking. What are my restrictions?

None.

Walking during pregnancy is not only okay, but it is good for you! Again, consult with your doctor first, but if you are a low-risk pregnancy, it is fine for you to walk during work all the way up until the time you deliver.

Q. My job is very stressful. Do I need to quit?

Probably not.

It takes extreme amounts of stress to affect your pregnancy. By extreme, we mean divorce, death of a family member, loss of income, or loss of home by fire. The day-to-day stresses of a job or home life that most of us experience are not enough to worry about.

However, we all process stressful situations differently, and there is a growing body of evidence that pregnant people under stressful situations (at work or at home) are at risk for preterm birth and low-birth-weight babies. So if you have a highly stressful job, it's worth discussing it with your OB provider. You two can come up with a plan to help decrease your stress.

DR. B'S OPINION:

Making a Baby and a Living

As someone who was pregnant with my first baby during my senior year of pediatric residency, I can attest that it is no cake walk to work eighty hours a week and grow a baby. It's definitely possible, but I don't really recommend it! If you have a stressful or exhausting career, be sure to recharge whenever you have the opportunity to do so.

NEW PARENT-TO-BE 411:

Six Ways to Help Decrease Stress During Pregnancy

1. Exercise.
2. Get regular massages (your partner should be a pro by now).
3. Consider acupuncture.
4. Get enough sleep.
5. Have a good support system around you . . . family, friends, neighbors, healthcare providers, pregnancy and new parent groups.
6. Speak with a therapist.

Q. I work as a pilot/flight attendant. How long can I continue to work?

Most airlines restrict pregnant workers from flying after twenty weeks.

Some commercial airlines even restrict pilots from flying once pregnancy is diagnosed, even though there is no increased risk of miscarriage or pregnancy complications.

Q. When should I spill the beans to my employer?

Short answer: It makes sense to tell your boss at the same time as you let the rest of the world know. Unless you have a completely private life outside of work and no social media connections to your co-workers, the word will get out.

Long answer: Here are some tips to make your pregnancy life at work at bit smoother:

1. **Give your employer a heads-up.** Tell your employer about a pregnancy at the same time you announce it to friends and family.
2. **Be honest.** Most employers understand that there may be times in which it is difficult for you to work. They will appreciate it if you communicate openly.
3. **Offer solutions.** If you are not able to work on a day, make suggestions for ways in which you can complete your work. Employers prefer to hear solutions to issues rather than problems.
4. **Find out about FMLA.** Not all employees are eligible for Family Medical Leave Act (FMLA); however, most companies are willing to allow for some time off for childbirth and recovery.
5. **Stay in touch during maternity leave.** Communicate to your employer if an issue arises requiring more time off than you planned.
6. **Make a financial plan.** If you qualify for FMLA, you are eligible for twelve weeks of time off, but it does not guarantee that the time off will be paid. In fact, most

employers will allow you to take as much accumulated vacation or sick time as needed, but the remaining time will be unpaid.

7. **Inquire about short-term disability.** Check with your employer to see if you have a short-term disability plan. Some employers offer this as a benefit perk. A few states require it. Most of these plans will enable you to receive a portion of regular pay during your time off. This is a good way to supplement your finances until you return to work. Note: The paperwork required for a claim is extensive. Get going on this early in your pregnancy.
8. **Give your OB provider a heads-up.** Usually, you need your OB provider to complete a portion of disability paperwork. Give them ample time to do it.

NEW PARENT-TO-BE 411:

Your Rights Regarding Work During Pregnancy

Let's take a look at the law and pregnancy when it comes to work. This may become relevant if you end up on bed rest or cannot perform certain functions at work due to your pregnancy. Find out what your state laws are, as well as your individual company's disability policy. Here are the basics:[7]

- You should be able to continue performing your job if you are able to.
- If you are unable to perform your job due to pregnancy, your employer must treat you like any other partially disabled employee.
- If a partially disabled employee is able to take leave with or without pay, that is the same option you have.
- If you have to discontinue work for a period of time due to a pregnancy-related issue and you recover, you should be able to return to work.
- There should be no predetermined length of parental leave that requires you to stay out of work for that period of time.
- Employers must hold your job open during your parental leave for the same period of time as employees out on sick or disability leave.
- The Family and Medical Leave Act entitles you to a maximum of twelve weeks off for certain medical or family reasons within a twelve-month period. It only guarantees *unpaid* leave. If you have a difficult pregnancy (for example, bed rest), that time can be counted toward the twelve weeks. To qualify for this legal benefit, you must have worked at the employment site for at least twelve months for 1,250 hours, and there must be at least fifty employees of the company within seventy-five miles.

For more information, go to the websites of the US Equal Employment Opportunity Commission (eeoc.gov/pregnancy-discrimination) or the US Department of Labor (dol.gov/general/topic/benefits-leave/fmla). It's also wise to check laws that may be applicable in your state.

9. **Be kind about quitting.** Some new parents decide not to return to work after the birth of a child. If you decide that you are not going to return to work, the more notice that you can give to your employer, the easier it will be to find a replacement. You will also want to check in with your human resources manager about any loss of benefits or repayment due should you decide to permanently leave your job.

BOTTOM LINE: The birth of a child is a special moment, and most employers will share in this joy with you. However, your employer needs to do some planning in order to make it work. Communicate honestly throughout your pregnancy and parental leave.

Q. Can my healthcare provider sign off on disability or FMLA forms?

Yes. And you have to submit these forms in writing to your employer thirty days in advance of your leave. Talk to your company's director of human resources regarding employee leave benefits. Sometimes there is a ton of paperwork. It's nice to fill in as much as you can for your OB provider so they only have to fill in their part.

Drop the paperwork off well in advance of when it is due because it often can't be filled out in full at the time of your visit. Ask your OB provider to have everything ready in a few days—then you can come back to pick it up or have it mailed to you.

In addition to the forms you may receive from your work, there are also state disability forms that can be filled out and sent depending on your occupation. Check with your OB provider for details. Most OB providers have them in the office to hand out to patients.

Q. What are my partner's rights for parental leave?

Paid parental leave is an employee benefit, not a federally mandated law.

Parental leave, however, is part of the Family and Medical Leave Act. A parent is eligible if they are employed for at least one year, have worked over 1,250 hours, and work in a US company that employs at least fifty people. All parents, including those accepting a child for adoption or foster care placement, are eligible for FMLA.[8]

Reality Check

Find out what you can use to piece together a decent parental leave. You may be able to use vacation time, personal days, sick leave, or even short-term disability. FMLA only guarantees that you will have a job after taking twelve weeks off. It doesn't guarantee any income while you are out. State laws vary regarding family leave benefits.

CHAPTER 10

Self-Care

"Maintenance is what you have to do just so you can walk out the door knowing that if you go to the market and bump into a guy who once rejected you, you won't have to hide behind a stack of canned food."

—Nora Ephron

What's in This Chapter

- Hair
- Teeth
- Face
- Body and skin
- Tattoos
- Nails
- What's safe and what's not

You are beautiful, and we hope your partner tells you that every day—because it's true. But we know you won't look at your pregnant body and always feel that way. As fellow women, we know you may be tempted to try some services and treatments while you're pregnant. Admit it, your body deserves to be pampered right now!

A nice massage could be just the cure for those aches and pains, or you may want to treat yourself to a pedicure (since you can't see, much less reach, your toenails toward the end of your pregnancy).

This chapter will walk you through a variety of aesthetic treatments and daily care products that you may be tempted to try. We'll discuss whether they are safe, not safe, or questionable based on the latest research.

We'll cover these topics head to toe and point out safety concerns (if any) during certain stages of pregnancy. Check out the handy table at the end of the chapter for a recap of the thumbs up or down for each treatment.

Hair

Q. Can I color my hair while I am pregnant?

Short answer: Highlights are fine in all trimesters. Wait to dye your hair until after the first trimester.

Long answer: You can highlight your hair at any point during your pregnancy because the chemicals don't touch the scalp. However, hair dye (that is, applying color to the roots of your hair) is more controversial. That's because product placed directly on the scalp has the potential to get absorbed into your body (and thus, into your baby's body through the placenta).

Of course, there are no credible scientific studies that show hair dye is harmful to babies. That's because researchers can't find 100 pregnant women to volunteer to see if this (or any) chemical causes birth defects . . . as you might guess.

Since there is a ton of blood flowing to the scalp (just think about how much it bleeds when cut!), doctors are concerned the chemicals in hair dye (ammonia, peroxide) may be absorbed through the scalp, so it's probably safest to wait until after the first trimester to dye your hair. We know this may be hard medicine to swallow, because many of us are having children in our thirties and forties and gray hair is no stranger to our heads.

Our advice: If you must dye those roots in the first trimester, use a vegetable-based dye that doesn't contain ammonia or peroxides. You can also use a henna product, since it is completely plant-based. Alternatively, you could also use a gray root touch-up pen to help you in those first few weeks.

BOTTOM LINE: If you can wait to dye your hair until after the fourteenth week (the end of the first trimester), that's the safest.

Q. Can I get a relaxer, a keratin treatment, or a Brazilian blowout?

Nope, and you may want to reconsider using chemical straighteners at all. Do we have your attention?

Most of these hair products are applied directly to the scalp, which raises the same red flags discussed above, because they can be absorbed through the scalp and get into your bloodstream, the placenta, and your developing fetus. These chemicals include formaldehyde, formalin, methylene glycol, and phthalates.[1,2] They are known ***carcinogens*** and endocrine disruptors and are associated with an increased risk of hormone-sensitive cancers including breast and ovarian cancer.

Recent studies suggest that there is also an increased risk of uterine fibroids and uterine cancer in people who regularly use chemical relaxers and chemical straightening products.[3]

Permanents and body waves use different chemicals, but they are still applied to and absorbed by the scalp. If these procedures are an absolute must for you, try to wait until after the first trimester.

From a practical standpoint, many expecting moms report a less than satisfactory result from these treatments. Why? Your hair, just like your skin, is a different animal during pregnancy. Don't expect the same results you got pre-pregnancy.

Helpful Hint

Here's one more reason to avoid hair chemicals in the first trimester: They stink! Many pregnant people are sensitive to odors (and get queasy) in the first trimester. Have a trash can nearby if you are that determined to sit in your hair stylist's chair for a couple of hours.

Reality Check

A lot of pregnant women wake up to find "I have hair where?!" Increased hair growth on the head is a welcome side effect of pregnancy for most of us. However, many pregnant women also find hair growing in other not-so-welcome areas, such as the face, around the nipples, lower belly, and the ever-expanding bikini area.

Q. What's the safest way to get rid of unwanted hair while I'm pregnant?

Shaving.

Yes, we know that trying to reach your legs may be difficult, but it is the safest strategy that won't bother your skin or potentially affect your baby. This may sound like a no-brainer here, but we recommend that you sit down while shaving your legs during pregnancy. Standing like a flamingo with a new center of gravity on a wet tile floor is not an acrobatic feat you should attempt.

Helpful Hint

Many spas now cater to pregnant women—from pregnancy massages to pedicures. Ask your local spa if they have a special menu for parents-to-be.

Q. Can I use wax or have threading to remove unwanted hair?

Yes . . . but your skin will be much more sensitive during pregnancy, making waxing more painful than usual.

Q. Can I use hair removal or bleaching creams?

No.

We don't recommend using these products because they can be absorbed through your skin and into your body. Again, we don't have solid research to prove that these products are harmful to the baby, but as we've mentioned, we know there are chemicals found in the umbilical cord blood of unborn babies and that means the potential risk is there.

Q. Can I do laser hair removal while I'm pregnant?

No. Laser hair removal is not recommended during any trimester.

Pregnant skin is much more sensitive and responds differently than non-pregnant skin. Laser hair removal is not only extremely painful, but it can cause pigmentation changes (dark spots called ***hyperpigmentation*** or light spots called ***hypopigmentation***) on the skin where the hair is removed.

Our advice: Wait until after pregnancy to start or continue laser hair removal.

Q. What about electrolysis?

No. It's not recommended during pregnancy.

There are two types of electrolysis: galvanic and thermolysis.

- **Galvanic electrolysis** uses an electrical current passed down a needle to the unwanted hair follicle. The current sets off a chemical reaction to destroy it. Because your unborn baby is surrounded by ***amniotic fluid*** that can potentially conduct electrical current, having a procedure done with galvanic current is a bad idea.
- **Thermolysis electrolysis** uses an alternating current that produces heat to cauterize an unwanted hair follicle. We don't recommend this method either because a) there isn't enough safety info on this procedure and b) it may leave a dark discoloration on your sensitive pregnant skin, just like laser hair removal. We think it's better to be temporarily hairy than permanently blotchy!

Q. Can I dye my eyebrows or eyelashes or get a lash lift or brow lamination?

Yes, after the first trimester.

Only a small amount of dye is placed over a small segment of skin for a very short amount of time, so it's fairly safe to do.

Teeth

Q. Is it okay to get my teeth whitened?

No.

There's no proof that these products are safe during pregnancy. The American Academy of Cosmetic Dentistry currently recommends waiting to whiten your teeth until you're done with pregnancy and lactation.

Elevated hormone levels during pregnancy increase tooth sensitivity and can cause gum swelling. The bleach in teeth whiteners can aggravate this condition.

Face

Q. Can I get a facial?

Yes. But tell your aesthetician that you are pregnant. Your skin may be more sensitive now and may react differently to previously used products. All new products should be tested on a small area of skin (such as behind the ear) prior to use. Absolutely avoid products containing:

- Retinol or Retin-A
- Accutane
- Large amounts of salicylic acid

Q. I've been using a topical retinol cream at night before getting pregnant. Should I stop now?

Retinol and Retin-A products contain a large amount of vitamin A. Research shows that more than 10,000 IU per day of vitamin A can cause birth defects. And we just don't know how much of these products gets absorbed through the skin. Small amounts of substances containing retinol are theoretically safe, but most OBs agree that it is best to steer clear of these products during pregnancy.

Q. Am I allowed to use topical salicylic acid?

Small doses of salicylic acid can be used during pregnancy since so little is absorbed through the skin. The reason it's considered a potential problem is that salicylic acid is related to aspirin. Aspirin in full doses should not be routinely used in pregnancy. In large doses, it can cause miscarriage, problems with the placenta, and heart problems in the baby.

That said, don't panic if your OB provider prescribes a low-dose baby aspirin for a specific medical reason. Baby aspirin is often used to help prevent certain conditions during pregnancy.

We'll talk about using small amounts of products containing salicylic acid in the section on acne later in this chapter.

Q. Can I have extractions or chemical peels done with my facial?

Yes, with a few exceptions.

Your pregnancy skin may revolt if you have an extraction-happy technician. Heavy-duty pore extractions can traumatize your sensitive skin. Just ask your aesthetician to be kind to you.

Superficial peels that use glycolic acid, trichloroacetic acid (TCA), or lactic acid are fine during pregnancy. Test out a small area first before trying it out on your entire face. However, you should steer clear of frequent salicylic acid peels for the reasons discussed above.

Q. I've got acne. Help!

Yep.

We know, we know, you thought you were done with acne years ago. Instead of that healthy pregnancy glow you hear about, you've got zits.

You can treat the affected areas with products containing salicylic acid, benzoyl peroxide, and finacea. They are all safe to use in small amounts. However, slathering them on night after night can potentially lead to absorption into your bloodstream. Limit your application to small areas.

As discussed previously, you need to avoid products that contain large amounts of salicylic acid because they can cause complications for you and your baby. But it's okay to use these products sparingly when you are spot treating a zit or two.

Q. Are prescription antibiotics safe to use for my acne?

It depends on the medication.

We'll give you the full rundown on medications in Appendix A. But in general, clindamycin taken by mouth or applied to the skin is okay to use. Erythromycin-based creams and gels are also safe.

However, tetracycline, doxycycline, and minocycline are off-limits because they can adversely affect your unborn baby's teeth. Because these antibiotics interfere with calcification, exposed fetuses can end up with discolored teeth, cavities, and poor enamel development.

Q. Okay, nothing is working and I still have acne. What now?

You can try using a steroid cream.

Steroid creams are safe to use while you're pregnant, and they might help reduce the redness and irritation surrounding a resilient pimple. You can try over-the-counter 1 percent hydrocortisone cream. Or your doctor can prescribe a slightly higher strength cream.

Q. Can I still use my anti-wrinkle cream?

Look at the ingredients and then make the call.

Most anti-wrinkle creams contain vitamin A or one of its derivatives, like retinol. Since these are off-limits during pregnancy, so are most anti-wrinkle creams.

Q. Can I do Botox?

Skip it during pregnancy and wait until you are done breastfeeding.

First, let's talk about what Botox and other neuromodulators, like Dysport or Xeomin, actually are. The key ingredient in all of these wrinkle relaxers is a protein product (botulinum toxin type A) from the bacteria *Clostridium botulinum*. The toxin blocks nerve signals in tense facial muscles responsible for those unwanted wrinkles. Injecting the toxin into the muscle makes those little wrinkles relax for about four months (until you have to do it again).[4]

That's the positive. The negative: *Clostridium botulinum* is also the same player that causes botulism (a form of horrible food poisoning). We know we are starting to sound like a broken record, but there just aren't studies on safety and pregnancy. There is limited safety data in humans.[5]

What we do know is based on animal research, however, and it's not pretty. There is a risk of low birth weight, delayed bone development, other malformations, and miscarriage.[6] So we can't recommend using Botox or any other neuromodulator during pregnancy for cosmetic reasons.

There are a few cases of pregnant women exposed to botulinum toxin with no ill effects to their fetuses. If you happened to get Botox before you realized you were pregnant, you can relax (especially since that little worry line between your eyes is banished for a few months), but put your next appointment on hold.

You'll need to wait until you are done breastfeeding to resume your sessions. With any Botox treatment, a tiny amount of botulinum toxin passes through the bloodstream, which can potentially enter breast milk. For this reason, it's wise to avoid it while breastfeeding.

After saying all this, there are some women who need Botox injections for medical reasons. For example, if Botox is the one thing that helps you with debilitating migraine headaches, the benefit may outweigh the potential risk. Just have the doctor administering the Botox discuss it with your OB provider first.

Q. Can I use facial fillers?

Nope.

Restylane, Juvéderm, and other facial fillers have warning labels advising against use by pregnant and nursing people. No studies. No green light.

Body and Skin

Q. Is it safe to get a massage? I could really use one right now!

Yes.

A massage is a welcome and often needed treat during pregnancy. It is important, however, to have a few ground rules:

- Select a massage therapist who is comfortable with and has experience in prenatal massage.
- After about eighteen to twenty weeks, pregnant people should not be flat on their backs for prolonged periods of time; the weight of the uterus can compress the blood vessels in the body, preventing adequate blood flow to both the pregnant person and baby. Most therapists have either table cut-outs to allow room for a pregnant belly or know how to position someone on their side with pillows.
- It is very important to stay hydrated when at the spa or even if you're just getting an hour massage at home.

Here are the absolute no-nos during a massage:

- No warming or electric blankets.

FEEDBACK FROM THE REAL WORLD:

The Pregnant Nose

Some of the wonderful fragrances a massage therapist uses may not smell so wonderful to your pregnant nose in the first trimester. I still can't bring myself to smell lavender, a fragrance used by many massage therapists and one that threw me for a loop during my first pregnancy.

- No massage of the inner or outer ankle bones or the webbing between the thumb and index finger as these are acupuncture points that might lead to stimulation of the uterine muscle.
- No cedarwood, chamomile, eucalyptus, juniper, rosemary, or frankincense essential oils. These oils may have the potential to cause bleeding.

Q. I'm in my second trimester and am already starting to have low back and hip pain. Can I see a chiropractor?

Chiropractors who are properly licensed can be very helpful for both pregnant and non-pregnant people. But, when you're pregnant, you need to be 100 percent certain that the chiropractor you choose to see is well educated in prenatal care. Check to make sure they are certified and have a basic DC degree (Doctor of Chiropractic degree) and are licensed in your state. Each state has an online site where you can check to see if someone is currently certified. Once you know they are certified in basic chiropractic medicine, look for a certification such as one from the International Chiropractic Pediatric Association's Perinatal Certification Program (ICPA) to know they are certified to work on your body while pregnant.

Q. Is it safe to have acupuncture done?

Yes. Just be sure you use an acupuncturist who is comfortable treating pregnant people.

Your acupuncturist needs to avoid areas that might trigger uterine contractions. Those are the inner or outer ankle bones or the webbing between the thumb and index finger.

I recommend acupuncture to many of my patients who suffer from chronic headaches, low back pain, nausea, and discomfort in their pelvic bones. And anecdotally, some have found great relief.

Helpful Hint

Acupuncture may be useful to help turn breech babies into the normal head-down position needed for a vaginal delivery.[7]

Q. Is it okay to sit in a hot tub or sauna?

A *warm* tub is okay. A *hot* tub is not.

Saunas, Jacuzzis, and steam rooms all fit into the hot category. The concern here is twofold:

1. **Neural tube defects.** Neural tube refers to the beginnings of your baby's spine, skull, and brain. In the early part of pregnancy (usually before six weeks), high heat exposure that increases your body temperature over 101°F can disrupt development of your baby's neural tube. That can cause birth defects called ***neural tube defects*** (***spina bifida***, ***meningocele***, and ***myelomeningocele***). FYI: The neural tube closes after four weeks, so the concern over hot tubs in the second or third trimesters focuses on risks to the pregnant person (see #2 below).

2. **Dehydration.** You are more likely to get dehydrated, which can lead to dizziness, fainting, and preterm contractions. Anything lukewarm is fine (under 99°F). We know it's not fun to take a lukewarm bath, but it's better than passing out in the tub.

Q. Can I have a mud bath, seaweed wrap, or paraffin treatment?

No.

As tempting as mud baths, seaweed wraps, paraffin treatments, and hot baths sound, they should all be avoided during pregnancy as they can significantly raise core body temperature.

Q. Can I take hot showers?

Absolutely, as long as you limit your time. Your body isn't submerged in water when you're in a shower, so you are less likely to overheat. Just limit your shower time or turn down the water temperature after a few minutes.

Q. Can I take a bubble bath?

Yes, with a few caveats.

If you are going to treat yourself to a warm bath, make sure the water temperature is under 100°F to avoid potentially overheating yourself and your baby (see discussion above).

And bubble bath solutions often irritate the vagina and vulva (your outer genitalia). Many of us have learned this lesson in our own childhood. Although it looks like fun to immerse yourself in bubbles, it's not fun later when you have an itchy vagina.

Our advice: Take a warm bath with candles, dial up a little Michael Bublé on the stereo, and skip the bubbles.

Q. I started doing cold plunges prior to getting pregnant. Is this something I can continue?

Unfortunately, no. Cold plunging has many proven medical benefits with the release of cold shock proteins and lessening cortisol responses to stress in the body. However, this shock on the system is not great for pregnancy. Cold plunging can interfere with hormonal feedback loops and, on rare occasions, can lead to irregular heart rhythms.

Q. Can I spend time outside in the sun?

Yes.

While it is important to avoid direct sunlight on your face (see the following Reality Check), this shouldn't prevent you from enjoying a day at the beach. Being pregnant is about being smart, not crazy. Just use good judgment. Wear sunblock and a hat or visor to protect your face.

Reality Check

Keep your face out of direct sunlight during pregnancy. It helps prevent ***melasma***, a pregnancy-related discoloration of the face. (More on this in Chapter 5, "Is This Normal?") However, be sure to get your vitamin D from food sources or multivitamins, since you won't be absorbing it through your skin.

Q. Can I lie in the sun during my pregnancy?

Yes, with caution.

Good news: There's no direct damage to your baby from sunbathing. Bad news: There's risk of potential skin damage for you. You are more likely to develop ***melasma,*** a darkening of your skin. It happens on your face and it can be permanent. And as we are all aware, sitting in the sun can certainly increase your risk of skin cancer. So if you must get your sun time in, shade your face with a hat and use lots of sunscreen.

You can also get overheated and dehydrated from lying in the sun too long. Make sure you are drinking lots of water. Avoid the sun when it is at its hottest, between the hours of ten a.m. and four p.m.

Fact Check

Sunscreen is dangerous, especially for pregnant women.

The truth: Unprotected sun exposure is an actual health concern.

Q. What's the deal with sunscreen?

Sunscreen is having a moment on social media. Some influencers have sparked a debate about the theoretical health concerns surrounding the body's absorption of the chemicals in sunscreen and its environmental impact (coral reef damage and microplastic pollution).

Here's what the science says: It's true that there are safety concerns about oxybenzone, avobenzone, and octinoxate ingredients in sunscreen. These chemicals are absorbed through the skin and may be endocrine disruptors, though it is unclear if these chemicals have detrimental hormonal effects.[8] And those same chemicals have absolutely been shown to be toxic to coral reefs and marine life in general. (Growing up on Maui and having much of my family still living there has made me acutely aware of this.)

But you do have other options. Use a mineral-based, reef-safe sunscreen containing zinc oxide or titanium dioxide, which is what most dermatologists currently recommend anyway.

Buy products that have broad spectrum coverage for both UVA and UVB protection. Both UVA and UVB sunrays can cause skin damage and cancer.

Apply sunscreen liberally (at least a half ounce each time) and reapply frequently (every two hours and after swimming or sweating).

BOTTOM LINE: Whether you are pregnant or not, please protect your skin from the sun! There are several safe and effective options.

Q. Can I use any tanning alternatives, like spray-on tans or tanning beds?

Yes to the sprays and creams. No to the tanning bed.

Spray-on tans use a sugar-based product called ***DHA*** (dihydroxyacetone). It acts by temporarily staining the surface of your skin (and any clothing you wear afterward). This is safe.

Self-tanners are also safe to use. Just do a patch test first on your inner thigh or wrist since your pregnancy skin may react differently from your expectation.

We don't recommend tanning beds—whether you are pregnant or not. During pregnancy it's a particularly bad idea because, like the sun, UV rays can cause skin discoloration (***melasma/cholasma***; more in Chapter 5, "Is This Normal?").

Even if you aren't pregnant, tanning beds are still a bad idea, as numerous studies have linked their use to skin cancer including basal cell carcinoma, squamous cell carcinoma, and melanoma.[9] Melanoma is the most aggressive form of skin cancer. It's also one of the few cancers that can spread across the placenta to an unborn baby.

Q. Is there anything I can use to prevent stretch marks?

No, because you can't select your own mom.

The likelihood of getting stretch marks is based on whether or not your mom did.

Here's the skinny on stretch marks. During pregnancy or whenever someone loses or gains weight quickly, the skin stretches and can disrupt one of the layers of skin called the dermis. In pregnancy, stretch marks can appear over the lower part of your belly, your breasts, and your inner thighs.

There is really only one thing you can do to reduce your chances of stretch marks: watch your diet. There are many reasons to eat healthfully during pregnancy, and this is one of them. If you don't gain weight rapidly, you may be able to fool Mother Nature's destiny for you. We make no guarantees, mind you, but it doesn't hurt to try.

You may hear that creams and oils prevent stretch marks. They definitely keep the skin moist, which could prevent *some* stretch marks. And asking your partner to do a nightly massage to apply them certainly has its benefits. But there are no guarantees here, either!

Q. Can I get a tattoo while I'm pregnant?

No. It's not recommended due to both health and cosmetic reasons.

First of all, remember that your pregnant skin is more sensitive. So getting a tattoo could be much more painful. There are also cases of people contracting hepatitis B, hepatitis C, and HIV from tattoo parlors that don't take precautions with sterilizing equipment. Those aren't diseases you want during pregnancy (or ever!).

Also, you may not be pleased with the results. Most people gain at least twenty-five pounds during pregnancy and certain areas of your body will change dramatically (particularly your belly, breasts, and buttocks). Your cute butterfly ink may end up looking like an eggplant after it has been stretched out.

BOTTOM LINE: It's not worth taking the health risk for you and your unborn baby. And who wants an eggplant on their butt anyway?

DR. M'S OPINION:

Bikini Line Tattoos

A popular place to put tattoos is below the belt/above the bikini line . However, this makes doing a ***C-section*** (if one is needed) a real cosmetic challenge for your doc. I remember a case where a patient of mine had a huge sunflower right in the spot where the incision for her C-section had to be made. It took a really long time to put that incision back together as I painstakingly matched up each petal and leaf on the top to its counterpart on the bottom!

We realize you were probably not thinking of the potential of having a C-section (much less being pregnant) when you got that tattoo there. However, having a misshapen tattoo may be one of the many sacrifices you make as a parent.

SELF-CARE

Q. What about permanent makeup. Is that okay?

No.

Although it would be amazing to wake up from just a few hours of sleep looking like a million bucks with eyeliner and pink lips, there isn't enough data to indicate whether permanent makeup is safe. Therefore, just like most of the other things in this chapter, if there isn't any data on safety, we have to recommend waiting until pregnancy and breastfeeding are over.

Q. Can I have a body piercing done while I am pregnant?

No.

Body piercing is not recommended for people who are trying to conceive or are already pregnant. Again, the skin is more sensitive, so this equals more pain. Second, as the skin stretches with the pregnancy, incomplete healing can occur leading to larger holes, infection, and scarring. Last, and probably most important, although most places are clean and use sterilized equipment, there is always a risk of localized skin infection, as well as more serious infections such as hepatitis B, hepatitis C, and HIV.

Q. What about the piercings that I had prior to getting pregnant? Do I need to take any special precautions?

Short answer: yes.

If you have a piercing in your nipple, navel, or genitals, the smartest thing to do is to remove the jewelry. Why? It can catch on clothing more often as pregnancy advances and leave you at risk of injury. Replace any jewelry with either a flexible bar or a flexible space holder made of PTFE (polytetrafluoroethylene).

For specific piercings, here are our suggestions:

- **Nipple piercings.** As you might expect, there is a risk of getting a breast infection (***mastitis***) if you've got a pierced nipple. The good news is that most women with piercings can breastfeed. You'll need to remove any jewelry before you nurse. Jewelry can potentially injure the baby's mouth or, worse, create a choking hazard, should it become dislodged.

- **Navel piercings.** As your innie becomes an outie, your piercing may get uncomfortable, and it will certainly look and fit differently. Although it's not absolutely necessary, you may want to remove it for a few reasons. As we've already mentioned, it may catch and pull more on clothing. Also, as your skin stretches (I know, this is a scary thought), it may pull your piercing so that the hole stretches and enlarges. If you need a C-section, the piercing definitely has to be removed. No, not because your incision is up by your navel. The reason: An electrocautery device is used to clot off blood vessels during surgery. Any metal in its vicinity can redirect the electrical current and burn the skin. (That's probably more than you wanted to know.)
- **Genital piercings.** Yes, the ***clitoral hood*** (see the diagram on page 98 in Chapter 5) is a new popular place to pierce. If you've got one of these, you should remove the jewelry once your pregnancy test comes back positive. This shouldn't be a newsflash, but you have many pelvic exams and pelvic ultrasounds in your future. Besides potential discomfort for you, the jewelry (or even a space filler) may get in the way. Your entire genital area (***vulva***) will also get swollen as your pregnancy progresses. And some women are unlucky enough to get varicose veins in their genital area during pregnancy. Having clitoral jewelry through this experience is extremely painful, and that's why it's a bad idea. But if you choose to keep it around through your pregnancy, it definitely needs to go before you go into labor.
- **Tongue piercings.** While tongue piercings do not interfere with your growing body parts, they are potentially a problem if you need to have a C-section or another surgical procedure that uses electrocautery to clot off blood vessels during surgery. Hence you may need to remove any tongue piercing during labor and delivery.

Nails

Q. Can I get a manicure or a pedicure?

Yes, just take a few precautions.

During your pregnancy, you'll notice that your hair and nails grow at a freakishly fast rate. That's normal, as you are in metabolic overdrive. And you may want to treat yourself to a manicure or pedicure. Go ahead, you deserve it. Tell your partner we said so.

Here are a few helpful tips to do it safely:

- **Make sure the room is well ventilated.** Other customers who are getting services done like silk wraps can create pretty strong fumes that you shouldn't be inhaling.
- **Go to a licensed salon.** While having a current license from a state health department doesn't guarantee a risk-free experience, it helps.

- **Use sterile instruments.** Look for a clean salon that uses sterilized instruments . . . or better yet, bring your own. Dirty instruments or wash basins can put you at risk for dangerous (even life-threatening) infections. Infections in the nail beds can be more difficult to fight off during pregnancy—especially in people with chronic medical conditions, like diabetes.
- **If you've got open cuts or wounds, skip it.** Again, don't put yourself at risk for an infection.
- **Don't shave your legs the day before.** That is, if you can reach them. Shaving may cause microscopic cuts in your skin that can leave you at risk for infection.
- **Use a nontoxic nail polish.** Most major nail polish brands including OPI, Essie, and Sally Hansen are "toxic trio free" or "three-free," meaning they do not contain phthalates, formaldehyde, or toluene. While there is no confirmed evidence of harm, manufacturers have voluntarily phased out these ingredients.[10] Some brands go a step further and remove additional chemicals and fragrances. They market themselves as five, seven, or ten-free formulations. It makes sense to avoid nail polish containing the top three chemicals of concern because it is relatively easy to limit environmental exposures here. You'll need to decide on the other questionable ingredients in nail polish.

Q. What about gel nails? Can I still get that done during my pregnancy?

Gel nails, like acrylic nails, are artificial nails. First, a gel substance made up of a monomer liquid and a polymer powder is brushed onto the nail bed. Then the nails go under UV light for a few minutes to dry and harden the gel into a resin.

The benefit is that the color lasts much longer and does not chip, which is why gel nails have become so popular. We lack any studies on the safety of gel nails during pregnancy. Since the process is odorless (unlike acrylic nails), it is probably safe during pregnancy. Note: There is potential for underlying nail damage if gel nails are applied for long periods of time.

Q. Can I have acrylic nails applied?

Yes. The nails themselves are okay. It's the really intense fumes that can be problematic. Get your nails done in a well-ventilated area.

Other Assorted Body Parts

Q. Can I use a heating pad?

Yes. It's just wise to avoid placing a heating pad directly on your belly. Using one for low back pain and to help ease the muscle pain in your calf after that excruciating middle-of-the-night charley horse is okay.

Q. Can I douche?

No.

Douche is French, meaning "to wash" or "to soak." Women take a mixture of fluids—usually water with vinegar, baking soda, or iodine—and squirt it up their vagina with a spray bottle or tube.

It's no longer trendy for women to douche after having sex or having their periods to "clean" themselves, but some women still do it.

OB-GYNs do not recommend douching for most women. Douching can alter the normal balance of good bacteria that live in your vagina—which then leads to various vaginal infections.

Douching can also potentially cause pelvic infections by pushing bacteria from the vagina through the ***cervix*** and into the uterus and fallopian tubes. Contrary to what other pregnancy books may say, douching won't cause a fatal air bubble to enter your bloodstream and kill you. However, because of infection risk, douching is just a bad idea—pregnant or not.

Q. Can I have a colonic?

No. A better question is, do you really want one?

Colonic irrigation or colon hydrotherapy is an alternative medicine practice that involves flushing the colon with warm water. The colonic supposedly removes a buildup of waste, which supporters of the practice believe is harmful for digestive and general health.

A colon hydrotherapist inserts a sterile, single-use speculum (attached to tubing) into the patient's anus. The colon is gently flushed repeatedly with warmed water, which loosens feces stuck in the colon and filters it out through a tube. This practice, when done occasionally, is supposedly not harmful to healthy people.

In pregnant women, there are a few reasons to avoid this practice. First of all, it's really uncomfortable . . . even if you don't have hemorrhoids the size of Texas, which most of us do at some point. Second, the elevated progesterone levels during pregnancy slow down the entire intestinal tract (leading to all the fun GI symptoms of pregnancy, like nausea, vomiting, heartburn, excessive belching, gas, and constipation). This means doing a colonic probably won't solve your preggo-related gas. And your body and your colon may respond differently to this procedure while you're pregnant.

Finally, there have been complications during these procedures leading to excessive bleeding, infection, and surgery.

Q. After delivery, is vaginal rejuvenation something I might need?

Short answer: It depends on what kind of delivery you had, what size baby you had, and if you plan on having any more children.

For the long answer, check out Chapter 15, "Postpartum: What's Next?"

Is It Safe?

HAIR

Treatment	Safe During Pregnancy?	Safe During Breastfeeding?
Highlights	Yes	Yes
Dyeing	Yes, second and third trimesters only	Yes
Perms	No	Yes
Relaxers/chemical straightening	No*	No*
Laser hair removal	No	Yes
Waxing	Yes, but painful	Yes
Hair removal cream	No	Yes
Electrolysis	No	Yes
Brow/eyelid dye	Yes, second and third trimesters only	Yes

*There are safety concerns for everyone, pregnant or not.

TEETH

Treatment	Safe During Pregnancy?	Safe During Breastfeeding?
Whitening	No	No

FACE

Treatment	Safe During Pregnancy?	Safe During Breastfeeding?
Facial	Yes*	Yes
Anti-wrinkle cream	Mostly no, check ingredients	No
Botox	No	No
Facial fillers	No	No

*No Retinol or Accutane.

BODY

Treatment	Safe During Pregnancy?	Safe During Breastfeeding?
Massage	Yes	Yes
Acupuncture	Yes	Yes
Mud bath	No	Yes
Seaweed	No	Yes
Paraffin treatment	No	Yes
Bubble bath	No, baths okay under 100°F	Yes

Treatment	Safe During Pregnancy?	Safe During Breastfeeding?
Hot tub	No	Yes
Sauna	No	Yes
Sun exposure	Yes, avoid direct sun on face	Yes
Sunscreen	Yes, use mineral-based products	Yes, use mineral-based products
Sunless tanners	Yes	Yes
Tanning beds	No*	No*
Tattoos	No new ones	No
Permanent makeup	No	No
Body piercings	No new ones	Yes, but not on nipples

*Safety concerns for everyone, pregnant or not.

NAILS

Treatment	Safe During Pregnancy?	Safe During Breastfeeding?
Manicure/pedicure	Yes	Yes
Acrylic/gel nails	Yes	Yes

OTHER

Treatment	Safe During Pregnancy?	Safe During Breastfeeding?
Douching	No	Yes, if you must
Colonics	No	Yes, if you must

PART THREE

Getting Ready for the Big Event

Prepping for parenthood is more than picking out a crib. You also have to stare down a myriad of decisions: Bank your baby's cord blood? Circumcision? Expanded newborn screen? And how do you pick a pediatrician? This section covers it all. We'll look at going back to work (and how to compare childcare options), feeding your newborn, and a key hot topic: vaccinations for your child. Finally, we'll cover the home stretch: getting ready for delivery, childbirth classes, how to tell if you are in labor, and more.

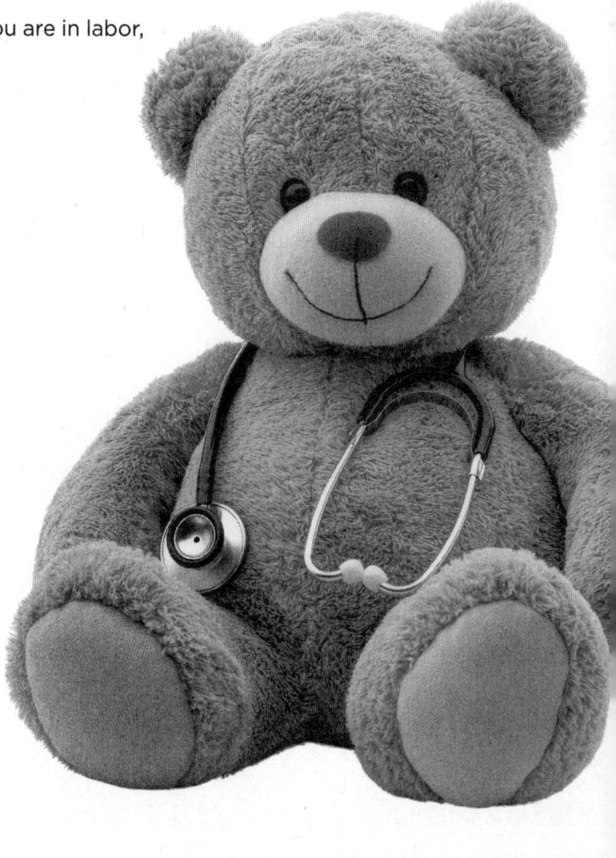

CHAPTER 11

Parenthood Prep

"Diaper backward spells repaid. Think about it."

—Marshall McLuhan

What's in This Chapter

- **Routine treatments after birth**
- **Cord blood banking**
- **Circumcision**
- **Expanded newborn screening**
- **Picking a pediatrician**
- **Childcare options**
- **Vaccines**

Your pregnancy is nearing an end, but you are also approaching the beginning of the enormous number of responsibilities and decisions you have as a parent. It's time to start thinking about your baby's life outside the womb.

During pregnancy, people spend a great deal of time learning about and, occasionally, ruminating about their upcoming childbirth experience. Here's a little secret: It's just one day (albeit a very long and important day). It will happen, and then it will be over. It's important to start spending time learning about how to take care of your newborn and the rest of your life as a parent.

While you are up at all hours of the night trying to get comfortable, you might as well make good use of your time. Start thinking about what you will do with your baby after they arrive because that encompasses Day 1 until eternity.

This chapter covers topics you are certain to have questions about like routine eye ointment and a vitamin K shot after birth, cord blood banking, circumcision, newborn screening, picking a pediatrician (baby doctor), parental leave, childcare, feeding your newborn, and vaccines. Some of these issues require decisions to be made ahead of your due date, so let's go!

NEW PARENT-TO-BE 411:

New Parent Anxiety

It's okay to admit that you are scared to death of becoming a parent.

Helpful Hint

The topics discussed in this chapter often overlap with *Baby 411*. Since a detailed discussion of these topics is beyond the scope of this book, you can find a more expanded discussion in *Baby 411*.

Routine Screenings and Treatments After Birth

Q. Why do all babies have eye ointment applied after birth? Can I refuse this treatment?

Having a baby is messy. Some mothers carry bacteria that can lead to serious eye infections in the baby. To avoid this horrible infection, treating every baby immediately protects every baby. Antibiotic ointment has low risk with great benefit. While some countries have stopped routinely using eye ointment and moved toward screening mothers for infection at delivery, it is still the norm and standard of care in the United States to simply treat all newborns. While you can refuse this treatment, we highly recommend that you accept this safe and easy treatment to protect your little one.

Q. Why do all newborns get a shot of vitamin K? Can I refuse it?

The short answer: One in sixty newborns are born with a vitamin K deficiency, leaving them at risk for a life-threatening condition if they do not get vitamin K replacement immediately.

The long answer: Vitamin K is essential for blood clotting. Most newborns have a deficiency in vitamin K because it does not efficiently cross the placenta while fetuses are in the womb. Babies who are born with a severe vitamin K deficiency can have significant bleeding into vital organs (such as VKDB or vitamin K deficiency bleeding, which causes bleeding in the brain) within the first two to fourteen days of life. Late onset bleeding can occur anytime in the first six months of life. Since time is of the essence, it makes more sense to give all babies vitamin K than to test them all and find out too late who really needed it.

A small number of parents decide to decline the vitamin K shot for their baby. Why? Podcasters and social media influencers have spooked them, casting suspicion on the vitamin K shot and questioning the additives (aluminum) in the shot. While that sounds scary, this topic is a much more nuanced than the sensational way it is presented in these health and wellness forums. First of all, aluminum is ubiquitous, as it is in our water, soil, and air. This is not a good thing, but it is a reality. Several biologic products contain trace amounts of aluminum to keep the medication stable or enhance its efficacy. There is a minuscule amount (about 0.05 mcg in a single dose of vitamin K), it is rapidly excreted out through the urine, and there is more aluminum (about 1 mcg per ounce) in breast milk. It's also important to look at risk versus benefit. About one in sixty newborns are deficient in vitamin K, and VKDB has a mortality rate of 20 percent. And 50 percent of those who survive VKDB suffer permanent brain damage.[1]

Pediatricians highly recommend the vitamin K shot and have been recommending it since 1961—there can be serious consequences if you skip it. Vanderbilt University Medical Center reported five babies in Nashville needlessly experienced brain hemorrhages when their parents opted out of this extremely safe and simple vitamin injection.[2] No, the shot does not cause leukemia, autism, or any other malady.

What about giving the vitamin K dose orally? Giving an oral vitamin K supplement is not an effective alternative to prevent this potentially tragic problem. It takes several months of taking oral vitamin K to treat a vitamin K deficiency.

So while you can refuse the vitamin K shot, we do not recommend doing so.

Q. What is the newborn screening test?

The first newborn screening test dates to 1961, when Dr. Robert Guthrie discovered a way to diagnose a newborn with a genetic metabolic disorder called phenylketonuria (PKU) using a little dried blood on some filter paper.

This was a huge deal because babies with PKU weren't ordinarily diagnosed until at least six months of age . . . after they were permanently neurologically impaired.

Newborn screening has come a long way since then. Every state in the United States now requires an extensive panel of blood tests on every newborn—done with just a few drops of blood on filter paper.

Most of the tests detect "inborn errors of metabolism." Translation: These are diseases caused by a failure of the body to break down (metabolize) certain products. If these products are not broken down, they start to build up in the body and create problems—heart enlargement, intellectual disability, and even death. Other tests screen for hormone abnormalities, blood disorders, and cystic fibrosis.

Q. Do all babies get tested for metabolic diseases?

Yes. Every state in the United States performs a panel of blood tests on every newborn. All states test for thirty-one to thirty-five standard "core" disorders in the recommended uniform screening panel.

There are also tests for twenty-six additional disorders. These other diseases are very rare and there's no treatment, even if a diagnosis is made in the first weeks of life. That's why some states don't require these additional tests. To find information on required screenings in your state, go to Baby's First Test (BabysFirstTest.org).

Q. Are there more newborn metabolic screening tests available other than those required by the state?

Yes. If you live in a state that only tests for core disorders, you can get your baby tested for many more disorders on your own dime. Private laboratories and academic institutions offer a low-cost expanded test that screens for more than sixty metabolic disorders.

When blood is drawn for the state-mandated screening test (shortly after birth or at the two-week well check), additional blood can be used for these optional tests. The cost varies, but you probably spent at least as much on a diaper bag. For more information on supplemental newborn screening, check out Revvity (Revvity.com/category/Stepone-test) or Mayo Medical Laboratories (MayoMedicalLaboratories.com).

Keep in mind that disorders tested for in the optional screen are quite rare (about 1 in 56,000). That's why some states weigh the cost of testing, the low number of abnormal results, and the lack of treatment, and opt to test only for the more common disorders.

Our opinion: In an ideal world, there would be one national standard for newborn screenings. But that just isn't reality today.

BOTTOM LINE: Although most metabolic diseases are rare, early detection is very important.

Cord Blood Banking

Q. What is cord blood banking?

The era of modern medicine has given us the opportunity to collect and store the blood and tissue from your baby's umbilical cord.

Why is this a cool idea? Well, that blood is loaded with the "seeds" (hematopoietic stem cells) that later grow into white and red blood cells. These very special cells are also found in the bone marrow of all humans.

As a result, the umbilical cord blood/tissue can be used like a bone marrow transplant. These cells are currently used to treat some genetic and blood disorders and certain types of cancer. One of the advantages of using a cord blood transplant as opposed to bone marrow transplant is that you don't have to find a perfect genetic match to the recipient and there may be less risk of transplant rejection.

Q. Does cord blood contain embryonic stem cells?

No.

The cells in cord blood come from your baby's blood after birth, not from an ***embryo***. The only similarity here is that both cord blood cells and embryonic cells are considered "stem" cells because they can develop into mature cells. Stem cells from cord blood are considered "hematopoietic" (blood) stem cells because they can become white blood cells, red blood cells, or platelets. To make things even more confusing, umbilical cord tissue contains mesenchymal stem cells that have the ability to grow into other cell types, raising the possibility of additional medical uses. The placenta is also rich in stem cells, which is why some private cord blood banks offer placental storage options.

Q. What can cord blood be used for?

Cord blood transplants are now used to treat several diseases, and there are more potential therapeutic uses in the pipeline.

Note: Your baby may not be able to use their own stem cells for certain diseases, though. For example, if your baby ends up having leukemia, their frozen stem cells cannot be used to treat it. Those stem cells may already have pre-cancerous changes in them.

But here is the good news: Your healthy baby's stem cells could be used for another family member (sibling, parent, etc.) who has a disease treatable with cord blood.

Q. Are there options for storing the cord blood?

Yes. There are two options for banking your baby's cord blood: private and public.

With a private or "family" bank, you pay a company to store your baby's cord blood for potential personal use. If you bank your blood privately, only your family or loved ones who need it and are an acceptable match can use it.

Public banks are donation programs, where families contribute cord blood for use by the general public. If you donate cord blood to the public bank, anyone who needs it can use it. Every day, 6,000 patients worldwide are looking for a match in the national donor registry to treat their leukemia, lymphoma, or other disease with a bone marrow or cord blood transplant.

A limited number of US hospitals participate in the public cord donation program, but it is possible to collect the blood and have it shipped to a regional, centralized public banking facility. For more information go to the National Marrow Donor website at www.NMPD.org.

DR. B'S OPINION

Don't let potentially life-saving cells go to waste. Donate them if possible.

If you want your baby's cord blood to go to the National Marrow Donor Program, you just need to pass some screening questions before the program accepts the donation. You should contact these folks before thirty-four weeks of gestation if you want to donate. We'll discuss private cord blood banking next.

INSIDER SECRET:

Cord Blood Banking for Two?

If you have twins (or more), you cannot donate to the National Marrow Donor Program. The reason? With two or more umbilical cords, there is the potential of the cord blood being mixed, making it too risky to use.

Q. Is it worth the money to privately store cord blood?

And you thought selecting a crib was a major decision . . .

Here's some information to help you decide if you want to open an account at the local blood bank.

What are the odds you or a family member will need to use the cord blood? The estimates vary from 1 in 400 to 1 in 200,000.[3] The odds are a bit of a moving target because no one can look into a crystal ball and predict the potential uses of umbilical cord blood in the future. If you already have a family member with a disease known to be treatable with cord blood, the likelihood of ever needing it goes way up.

The stem cells may have great potential to treat many diseases, but many of the treatments are experimental at this point. The chance you'll use it will depend on a variety of factors, such as scientific advances and if the blood specimen is still viable when you are seventy. At this moment, these potential uses are being tested in the research labs of academic medical centers and pharmaceutical companies. If your family has a genetic disorder, banking might be worth it for you.

Here are the costs: There is an initial enrollment fee, then there is an annual storage fee. Those fees are just for cord blood; there are additional fees to store umbilical cord and placenta tissue, both of which have promise to treat medical disorders in the future.

Some banks charge a one-time, lump-sum fee to store the cord blood "forever." (With current technology, banks can freeze and utilize cord blood for at least twenty years.)

Here are some factors to consider when choosing a bank:

- Be sure to use a company that processes and stores cord blood in their own facility. Why does that matter? Some companies subcontract the storage to another company. Even if you identify a company you trust, you may not know the track record of the company that is storing your cord blood.
- If a company you're interested in does other lab work besides cord blood banking, make sure their storage facilities are intended for long-term use. Special cryogenic techniques are required to make sure the blood is stored properly.
- Ask about the bank's storage method. Studies show that cord blood can be preserved and used for at least twenty years. Virtually all American cord blood banks store the blood in multi-compartmental bags to prevent contamination.
- Most obstetricians are experienced in cord blood collection. It is imperative that the blood be collected quickly (within ten minutes) and that enough blood is collected (at least 40 milliliters). If you don't get enough cord blood, the specimen cannot be stored. Multiple births and low birth weight reduce the chance of getting enough blood. Most companies offer training resources for doctors. Obstetricians will charge a fee to collect the cord blood, even if it is for donation. Be sure to find out this cost in advance.
- Even if the blood is properly collected and stored at a reputable cord blood bank, the specimen may not be viable for use.

Helpful Hint

Some companies offer discounts to families serving in the military, repeat customers, and those having twins or who have a first- or second-degree relative with an existing disease treatable with cord blood. Do your homework and ask questions.

Q. What happens to cord blood if it isn't saved or banked?

It clots in the umbilical cord and gets sent to the pathology lab with the placenta. Ultimately, it gets disposed of in a biohazard bag.

If you don't authorize it to be publicly or privately banked, the blood is discarded.

Q. If I want to privately bank my baby's cord blood, which company should I choose?

There isn't one company we recommend over all others—we advise you to check out ParentsGuideCordBlood.com. This is an excellent nonprofit website with tips and advice on evaluating cord banks. They offer an easy, up-to-date comparison of private cord blood banks that are accredited by the American Association of Blood Banks (AABB.org).

Q. Are there any official recommendations?

The American Academy of Pediatrics (AAP) supports donating umbilical cord blood to the national donor bank.[4]

The American College of Obstetricians and Gynecologists also supports public cord blood banking. ACOG advises its physicians to provide balanced and accurate information about the benefits and limitations of both public and private cord blood storage. The most recent guidelines state, "The routine collection and storage of umbilical cord blood with a private cord blood bank is not supported by the available evidence . . . [but] . . . Private umbilical cord blood banking may be considered when there is knowledge of a family member with a medical condition (malignant or genetic) who could potentially benefit from cord blood transplantation."[5]

Helpful Hint

Make sure the bank you select follows the standards set by the Foundation for the Accreditation of Cellular Therapy (factglobal.org).

Q. How is the cord blood collected?

After your baby is born, two clamps are placed on the umbilical cord and then it is cut. Your OB provider then places a needle into the umbilical cord vein (the part of the cord still attached to the placenta—not your baby) and draws blood into a collection bag or syringe. An adequate specimen volume is two ounces, or even better, about ½ to 1 cup.

If you are privately banking the cord blood, you will need to call a toll-free number on the side of the box to tell the bank your specimen is ready (your labor and delivery nurse will usually package everything up and remind you to make the call). Then a medical courier magically appears at your birthing facility to ship the blood to the processing and storage facility.

Q. What if there isn't enough blood in the specimen?

It happens. Sometimes in certain conditions (***placental abruption***, for example) the placenta detaches early, and very little blood can be collected.

Some private blood banks offer a service called cell amplification in the hope of using the reduced specimen volume someday. No one can promise that those cells will be viable should the need ever arise. But the scientific research is encouraging. You'll just have to make your own call on this one.

Circumcision

Before we delve into this hot topic, we have a major disclaimer. Discussing circumcision provokes very strong reactions in some people. And like other parenting decisions, the pendulum swings back and forth.

We realize no matter how objectively we present this information, some readers will not be happy (believe us, we've tried). Even a discussion of pros and cons of circumcision is considered blasphemy—the Intactivist Movement (anti-circumcision group) believes circumcision should not be an option at all. They argue that the studies showing medical benefits of circumcision are flawed and biased.

The goal for this section is to let you hear both sides so you can make an informed decision on your own. Honestly, what you decide to do with your child's penis is up to you (or your child).

Q. What is a circumcision anyway?

Circumcision is the surgical removal of the foreskin of the penis. It's been done as a religious ritual for centuries.

The practice of circumcision (surgical removal of foreskin) became common in the United States in the late 1800s for hygienic reasons, and it was also thought to reduce masturbation (ha—didn't work, did it?).

Although the use of circumcision has declined in recent years, about 60 percent of American newborn boys are circumcised. Rates vary among geographic and ethnic groups.[6] Other countries and cultures have varying viewpoints on circumcision.

Q. When do I need to make this decision?

Circumcision procedures can be performed at any time, but there is a reason you should consider the options right now. Doctors typically perform the procedure before a baby goes home from the hospital, or within the first week or two of life in the doctor's office.

When a circumcision is part of a Jewish religious ceremony, it is done at eight days of life. Circumcision for an older child or adult is a much bigger ordeal. And there are some advantages to performing it earlier in life (see info below).

Alternatively, you can wait and let your child decide the fate of their penis.

Q. What are the arguments for circumcision?

In a nutshell, it lowers the risk of HIV, sexually transmitted infections, hygiene problems, and cancer.

1. **Reduced risk of HIV.** Why? In uncircumcised men, the area under the foreskin makes a nice spot for the HIV virus to set up shop. A landmark study in South Africa found that circumcised men were 60 percent less likely to acquire HIV from infected female partners.[7] Based on this and additional research, the Centers for Disease Control created new guidelines about making an informed choice about this procedure.

2. **Reduced risk of other sexually transmitted infections.** Besides HIV, circumcised men are also 30 to 45 percent less likely to become infected with nasty little germs like genital herpes (HSV-2).[8]
3. **Better hygiene.** Compared with a circumcised penis, it is harder to keep the uncircumcised penis clean. The foreskin can get infected and swell (called balanitis). Although balanitis doesn't occur often, it really hurts. The foreskin can also get stuck in a pulled-back position (called paraphimosis)—ouch!
4. **Fewer bladder infections.** Bladder infections (see ***urinary tract infection [UTI]***) occur more frequently in girls. However, boys who are uncircumcised may have ten times greater risk of infection than their circumcised friends.[9] This risk is greatest in the first six months of life. This again is due to hygiene reasons. In general, boys have about a 1 percent risk of getting a bladder infection.
5. **Less risk of cancer.** Again, the foreskin of an uncircumcised penis can harbor germs. When it comes to cancer risk, the issue here is a virus called human papillomavirus (HPV). HPV infection can lead to cancer of the penis, anus, throat, and ***cervix***. (Note: Oral, vaginal, and anal intercourse allow HPV virus to spread to these areas.) Circumcised men have a 30 percent lower risk of being infected with cancer-causing strains of HPV. They have a lower risk of developing cancer of the penis, and their female partners could have a lower risk of developing cervical cancer.

Reality Check

The HPV vaccine is universally recommended, so your children can significantly reduce their risk of HPV-related cancer simply by being vaccinated. The argument for circumcision is relevant for about 30 percent of HPV cancer-causing strains that are not included in the vaccine.

Q. What are the arguments against circumcision?

Here are the top five reasons:

1. **Lack of medical necessity.** While circumcision lowers the risk of HIV infection in men, and transmission of HPV to female partners, so does abstinence and safe sexual activity (using a condom every time, etc.). So if we could wave a magic wand and eliminate risky sexual behavior, there would be fewer medical arguments supporting circumcision.
2. **Surgical risks.** Circumcision involves cutting the foreskin away from the head of the penis. As with any surgical procedure, there is a small chance of bleeding (1 in 3,000 risk) or infection (1 in 1,000 risk).
3. **Penile adhesions.** Occasionally, the skin between the shaft and the head of the penis will get stuck together due to a collection of sticky, cream cheesy stuff called smegma. The penis will look like it is uncircumcised. Minor adhesions will resolve on their own. But if the adhesions are really tight, they may need to be treated by using a steroid cream, having a doctor pull the skin back, or having another surgical procedure (circumcision revision).

4. **The hidden penis.** It sounds like a concealed weapon, doesn't it? Chubby babies have a fat roll above their genitals. It causes the circumcised penis to get sucked inward. The penis looks normal as the boys grow up, but it's always concerning to parents. See our other book *Baby 411* for details on the "Hidden Penis" and penile adhesions. Bottom line: If your son is circumcised, learn how to clean it properly afterward.
5. **Reduced sexual pleasure.** Some concerns have been raised about the removal of sensitive nerve fibers in the foreskin when a male is circumcised. Anti-circumcision groups contend that circumcision is genital mutilation. So what's the latest science on this subject? Studies that address this question report conflicting results. Some studies show a decrease in sexual pleasure; others show heightened sensitivity and orgasm after circumcision. The data is based on men who were circumcised as adults who subjectively rated their sexual pleasure before and after circumcision.[10,11,12]

Q. What do medical organizations say about this subject?

The World Health Organization supports circumcision in countries with high HIV rates to reduce the risk of HIV in men. The American Academy of Pediatrics policy statement also acknowledges that the health benefits outweigh the risks of circumcision. Should families choose it, they say the benefits justify doing the procedure.[13] The American Urological Association has a neutral stance, but feels that circumcision "should be presented as an option for health benefits."[14] As of this writing, the CDC recommends that parents, teenage boys, and adult men should make an informed choice. In short, healthcare providers should explain the risks and benefits . . . like we just did here.

Ultimately, you have to make the call.

Q. We've decided to have our newborn son circumcised. When is this done?

In most cases, a newborn boy may have a circumcision performed after at least twenty-four hours of age and the pediatrician has done a complete exam. It is performed before the mother and baby are discharged home.

The doctor needs to make sure the genitals formed correctly before doing a circumcision. A baby with an abnormally formed penis (hypospadias) will need surgery later in infancy that utilizes the foreskin in the repair, so the circumcision is delayed and performed at that time. A pediatric urologist typically does this surgery.

In babies who are premature or ill, havng a routine circumcision may be delayed until they are healthy.

Ceremonial/religious circumcisions are often done on the eighth day of life, unless there are medical issues.

Q. Where is it done?

When a physician performs a routine circumcision, it is usually done at the delivery hospital before discharge home. Some physicians will perform them in their offices.

For Jewish families, a mohel performs a *brit milah* usually in the family's home or place of worship.

Beyond the newborn period, it is a day surgery procedure that is done with general ***anesthesia*** in an outpatient surgery center.

Q. Who performs the circumcision?

Most often, your obstetrician performs the circumcision procedure just before your baby leaves the hospital. But family OB providers or pediatricians may also do it. As long as the person has been trained to do the procedure, it does not matter what the doctor's specialty is.

Why the obstetrician? Many pediatricians do not perform any surgical procedures—for good reason. (You wouldn't want to see the way Dr. Brown slices Thanksgiving turkey!) Obstetricians have surgical training and are already at the hospital taking care of mom. Ask your OB first what the usual protocol is.

Urologists can also perform a circumcision on your baby. This requires special arrangements, however. Urologists do not generally come to the hospital to perform routine circumcisions. You'll need to do some homework if you choose this option.

Q. Is any pain medication used during the circumcision?

Yes. Every doctor has their own approach. You can ask your doctor what they feel comfortable doing. Here are the options:

1. Injecting numbing medicine directly into the area (nerve block)
2. Applying topical numbing cream one hour before the procedure
3. Giving the baby sugar water just prior to the procedure

BOTTOM LINE: The whole procedure is relatively brief. Yes, it hurts—but pain medication minimizes most of the discomfort. Most babies will go to sleep afterward as a stress response and wake up happy to see you. Check out our companion book *Baby 411* for details on how to care for a healing circumcision.

DR. B'S OPINION:

It's Your Decision

Circumcisions are done more for social, cultural, and religious reasons than for medical necessity. This is a very personal decision.

Picking a Pediatrician

While you have bonded with your OB-GYN by now, it's time to start thinking about a new doctor in your life: your baby's pediatrician. You'll be spending some serious quality time with this person over the next several years, so it's important to find the right one.

You'll want to begin your selection process in your third trimester, since you never know exactly when you will deliver! You don't want to be shopping for a pediatrician while you are recovering from labor! The pediatrician will see your newborn at the hospital or at the first office visit between three and five days of life.

An early start also gives you time to ask your baby's healthcare provider about decisions you will make prior to delivery or just afterward.

Ask your OB and your friends for recommendations and contact the baby's doctor before delivery to make sure they are accepting new patients and your insurance plan.

The sequel to this book, *Baby 411,* has detailed questions to ask your baby's potential doctor.

Q. Do I need to select a pediatrician before the baby is born? If so, why?

Yes. It's helpful to meet a pediatrician (at a prenatal consultation or meet-and-greet event) before the baby is born. Here are three reasons:

1. **It gives the pediatrician a chance to review any medical problems** during your pregnancy or with your family members that could affect the baby. (The doctor appreciates being prepared.)
2. **You can get advice** regarding medical decisions you'll be making in the first few days of your baby's life. (You'll appreciate being prepared.)
3. **You will be more relaxed** knowing who is examining and advising you in those first days after your baby is born—yes, your pediatrician's job begins right after delivery.

Q. What general questions should I ask at a prenatal consultation?

Just about every pregnancy guide has a list of questions to ask at your prenatal visit. Here is some advice: Ignore those cookie-cutter lists and make your own, based on the issues that are important to you.

1. **Ask questions about topics you are wondering about.** You may be so overwhelmed, you can't come up with specifics, and that's okay—just pick the topic and we can fill in the details. Example: allergies. You might discuss how to avoid food allergies or the history of allergies in your family.
2. **Ask open-ended questions.** You want to get a feel for how you and the doctor communicate. Questions with "yes" or "no" responses don't lead to conversation.
3. **Ask questions about how the practice flows.** It's helpful to learn about the office as well as the healthcare provider. You need to be an informed consumer. Medical care has changed dramatically since you were a kid.

BOTTOM LINE: Ask questions to see if this is someone you can be real with, have honest conversations with, and trust to steer you in the right direction.

Q. How do I decide which doctor is right for my child?

Go with your gut instincts. Think to yourself, "Will I feel comfortable asking this person some really embarrassing questions? Can I trust this person to guide me on this scary journey?" If the answers are yes, go for it.

Pediatricians develop important relationships with both you and your child. Doctors enjoy being a part of your family and watching your child grow with you.

Finding Childcare

If this is your first pregnancy, you are probably working outside the home while you are pregnant.

Should you drop your current career and make raising your child your new career? Can you carve out some creative combination of working part-time and staying at home with your little one? Or will you return to the daily grind and make the most of your family time when you are able? Raising a family is one of life's major crossroads that makes you ponder which path to take. These decisions weigh heavily on the minds of working parents.

No doubt, this choice can be very stressful and laden with guilt. Whatever you decide to do, your child needs a loving and attentive caregiver who attends to their needs and provides developmentally appropriate activities during the day.

Assuming you will choose to (or need to) go back to work, here are some things you may want to think about now.

Q. Why do I need to sign my unborn baby up for childcare now? That's crazy.

Yes, we agree, but childcare is very competitive. Your pals in prenatal class are also looking for childcare and the highest quality programs fill up fast. Many daycares will ask for your baby's due date (instead of their birth date) on the waiting list application.

Some programs require a deposit; others don't. Even if you aren't sure of your work plans (and childcare needs) after your delivery, get on waiting lists that don't require a deposit.

Q. Why is my selection for childcare so important?

Your baby is the most precious gift in the world to you. And you want to give your baby the best childcare you can find.

Studies have consistently shown that the first three years of life are critical times in your child's development. This is when your baby learns to trust others, function independently, problem-solve, and learn the boundaries of acceptable behavior. The person/people you choose to care for your baby are incredibly important.

Q. What are my options for childcare?

Your baby stays at home with someone, goes to someone else's home, or goes to a licensed childcare facility. Let's go over these options so you can get moving on this one.

1. **Parent at home.** Your childcare cost is the loss of one parent's salary—which may be significant unless you already have a single-earner household. Think of your parenting job as a career change. Full-time parenting is hard work and an admirable profession. (We have great respect for stay-at-home parents! Our jobs as doctors are much easier than our jobs at home.)
2. **Family caretaker.** This is when a grandparent or some other willing family member cares for your baby while you go to work.

   It is a great alternative if you have someone who is able and willing. It lets you pay the bills while your baby is at home with someone you can trust. Not only is family childcare often free, but your child develops a special relationship with a family member.
3. **Nanny/au pair.** You hire someone to care for your child in your home.

   This is a great way to have a consistent caregiver. Your child will have a special relationship with another caring adult. Because you are paying this person and they aren't your mother-in-law, you can set up the parenting guidelines you have in mind. If your child gets sick, you don't need to miss work. You'll only have a problem if your provider gets sick, needs to take a vacation, or (yes, it happens) quits.

   And it is the most expensive form of childcare. Some parents fear that they cannot trust someone (other than a family member) alone with their child. This option requires good instincts from both the parents and the provider.
4. **In-home daycare.** A parent has a license to care for a few children (in addition to their own kids) in their home.

   It can be great. Your child will be around different ages of children. Often, older kids enjoy playing with the little ones. Your child may get lots of love and attention and may also see these kids as role models. Sick child policies with in-home daycare tend to be less rigid than those in licensed daycare facilities, so you may be able to go to work even if your child is ill. The cost is moderate, but if your child gets sick, you may need to take off work.
5. **Licensed daycare facility.** This is the option chosen by many working families. You may have a sense of security knowing that providers are licensed professionals (and you can catch a glimpse of your little one during your workday on their webcams). It's one of the least expensive options for childcare, but there is a hidden cost that centers don't put in their promotional brochures—increased sickness. Factor several missed workdays and doctor bills into your budget equation.

This is just a brief overview to help you consider your choices.

Helpful Hint

You won't need a Nest or home surveillance system to check on your caregiver, although many parents use one. An infant will tell you if they are uncomfortable with someone—they won't be happy to see that person. You need to do an extensive background check on a nanny before you hire them.

Q. How do working parents do it all?

If you are a two-parent household, decide what is truly important to you as a family and how—as a couple—you will accomplish those goals. Real talk: It's not a cakewalk, people. Be prepared for some tension and arguments as you adapt to your new normal. The best advice we can give you is to have periodic honest, open discussions with your partner about the division of labor and everyone's role in sharing the mental load of parenthood—and keep those communications lines open!

If you are a single working parent, recruit and accept help from loved ones and friends to get things done. Being a parent is a continuous balancing act.

Reality Check

We know there is always a pang of guilt when it comes to going back to work after having a baby. A key point to consider: Quality time is more important than the sheer number of hours you spend with your child. Research shows that children do best when their parents focus their attention, engage, and respond to them.[15]

DR. B'S OPINION:

Work Versus Family

You can do it all, but you can't do it all at the same time. You will have to make some sacrifices/delays with your career path to accommodate your new full-time job as a parent. But I promise you that you won't ever regret the time you spend with your baby or child.

DR. M'S OPINION:

Work Versus Family

People often say to me that I must be really proud of the fact that I have accomplished so much in my career, spending all those years in school and now having the privilege of taking care of women. They are right. But no matter how much I love my job (and I do!), the best thing I have ever done with my life is being a mommy to my kids.

Vaccines

If you think the topic of circumcision is controversial, do a quick internet search for "vaccines" in your spare time.

Better yet, don't.

When it comes to vaccines, the web is full of info that is good, bad . . . and ugly. But this is not the only place you will hear about vaccines. Whether you are at the grocery store or at a local playground, your baby bump will attract those folks who think it is their duty to warn you of the evils of vaccines. It's probably best to offer these folks a polite smile and move on to the produce aisle.

Vaccines are a hot topic that has reached a boiling point as we go to print with this book. To be fair, the subject of childhood vaccines has pitted the quiet majority of believers against the vocal minority of disbelievers at family Thanksgiving dinners and playgroups for a couple decades now. But we live in very divisive times, and the silent majority of parents who believe in vaccinations are far from silent. And sadly, skepticism surrounding the COVID-19 vaccine and public health has spilled over to all vaccinations in general.

A heads-up: Since there is so much false information out there on vaccines, you need to be armed with detailed, accurate facts. And like the rest of this book, that is what you will get in this section. The guidance we provide is based on scientific evidence and solid peer-reviewed research. Remember our mantra: Show us the science! Your child is too precious to make such important decisions on anything less. This section is not based on personal anecdotes, conspiracy theories, or provocative podcasters.

First, let's discuss the key truth about vaccines: ***Vaccines are one of the most important things you can do to protect your child from serious and life-threatening infections.***

DR. B'S OPINION:

Ask Your Doc About Their Kids

As parents, our job is to protect our kids as best we can. I get it. I am a parent, too. And I certainly understand that after browsing online and hearing parent chatter you may have questions and concerns about vaccinations.

At the end of the day, you've got to put your trust in someone to help guide you in some of those decisions. I hope you and your baby's pediatrician have a good relationship and this person can answer questions that concern you on any topic. Our job is to advocate for and protect your child. If I ever had any doubt about vaccines, or anything else that might harm your child, I guarantee that I would be the first to stop doing it. I treat my patients like my own children. So I suggest asking your doctor the most important question you can ask regarding vaccines: Did you (or would you) vaccinate your own children?

I vaccinated both my children and would do it again without hesitation.

There are many myths and misunderstandings about vaccines—we'll discuss these next, as well as the most common questions and concerns about immunization. While this section is meant as a short primer on the topic, you may want to read the expanded section on vaccinations in *Baby 411*. Reputable sites like HealthyChildren.org from the American Academy of Pediatrics and chop.edu/vaccine-education-center from Children's Hospital of Philadelphia are also helpful resources for vaccine information.

And, of course, please talk with your baby's doctor before making any decision on this topic. It's what we are here for—to help you! Your child's life is too precious to base vaccine decisions on falsehoods and myths.

Q. What is the standard vaccination schedule?

The routine childhood immunization schedule is listed in the chart below. Don't worry if you don't understand it right now. It's here to give you the big picture. You can read all the details about the diseases and vaccines in *Baby 411*.

<table>
<tr><th>Birth</th><th>1 month</th><th>2 months</th><th>4 months</th><th>6 months</th><th>12 months</th><th>15 months</th><th>18 months</th><th>2 years</th><th>3 years</th><th>4–6 years</th></tr>
<tr><td colspan="5">RSV antibody (0–8 months)</td><td></td><td></td><td></td><td></td><td></td><td></td></tr>
<tr><td>Hep B #1</td><td colspan="2">Hep B #2</td><td></td><td colspan="4">Hep B #3</td><td></td><td></td><td></td></tr>
<tr><td></td><td></td><td>DTaP #1</td><td>DTaP #2</td><td>DTaP #3</td><td></td><td colspan="2">DTaP #4</td><td></td><td></td><td>DTaP #5</td></tr>
<tr><td></td><td></td><td>Hib #1</td><td>Hib #2</td><td>Hib #3</td><td colspan="2">Hib #4*</td><td></td><td></td><td></td><td></td></tr>
<tr><td></td><td></td><td>PCV #1</td><td>PCV #2</td><td>PCV #3</td><td colspan="2">PCV #4</td><td></td><td></td><td></td><td></td></tr>
<tr><td></td><td></td><td>IPV #1</td><td>IPV #2</td><td colspan="4">IPV #3</td><td></td><td></td><td>IPV #4</td></tr>
<tr><td></td><td></td><td>RV #1</td><td>RV #2</td><td>RV #3**</td><td></td><td></td><td></td><td></td><td></td><td></td></tr>
<tr><td></td><td></td><td></td><td></td><td></td><td colspan="2">MMR #1</td><td></td><td></td><td></td><td>MMR #2</td></tr>
<tr><td></td><td></td><td></td><td></td><td></td><td colspan="2">Varicella #1</td><td></td><td></td><td></td><td>Varicella #2</td></tr>
<tr><td></td><td></td><td></td><td></td><td></td><td colspan="2">Hep A #1</td><td colspan="2">Hep A #2</td><td></td><td></td></tr>
<tr><td></td><td></td><td></td><td></td><td colspan="7">Annual Flu</td></tr>
<tr><td></td><td></td><td></td><td></td><td colspan="7">COVID-19***</td></tr>
</table>

*Whether a fourth Hib dose is needed depends on the brand.

**Whether a third rotavirus dose is needed depends on the brand.

***COVID-19 is routine for children under twelve months of age, previously unvaccinated children, and immune-compromised children.

Source: American Academy of Pediatrics.[16]

Reality Check

While parents are asking more questions, they are still choosing to vaccinate their kids. The most recent National Immunization Survey showed 98.8 percent of US children at two years of age are vaccinated. Despite all the hype on social media, only a tiny fraction of parents—1.2 percent—are choosing to forgo vaccinations completely.[17]

Q. Is it safer to delay or space out vaccines?

Easy answer: no. Timing matters. Any "alternative" vaccination schedule is more appropriately termed "delayed vaccinations"—because it truly is a delay in getting protected.

Many, many doctors, scientists, and researchers work together to decide what is the best timing to give shots. The goal: protect babies as soon as it is safe and effective to do so. This schedule was not created out of thin air.

The immune system learns and responds to vaccines in a particular way, and both the frequency of giving a particular vaccine as well as timing with giving other vaccines is well studied. If you were to pick your own vaccine schedule, no one really knows how your child would react and respond to the vaccines.

It is also difficult to prioritize which vaccine-preventable disease is more important than another. One form of deadly bacterial meningitis is not less important than another, nor is polio or measles.

I know it is hard to watch your child getting several shots on the same day. But know that it is safe to do so. It's less stressful for your baby to endure several shots and deal with potential post-vaccination fussiness if it gets done in one visit (instead of three or four visits). There is also no benefit to spacing vaccines out, only risk.

There is no difference in how your baby will feel afterward in the short or long-term. We understand that having control and choice makes parents feel better about the process. Our goal is to protect your child.

Sketchy anti-vax online influencers, collectively called The Disinformation Dozen, often cry "too many shots, too soon." They also conveniently sell vitamin "immune-boosting" product lines as an alternative to vaccinations, by the way. But it makes new parents wonder if it would somehow be safer to wait on shots altogether or stagger them out.

Here's the truth about spaced-out vaccination schedules: There is absolutely no research that says delaying certain shots is safer.

In fact, studies have shown there is absolutely no difference in children's development whose vaccinations are delayed compared to children who receive their shots on time.[18] Studies also show that giving numerous shots at the same time and giving the recommended vaccination schedule has no impact on a child's risk of autism.[19]

As a pediatrician, I'd much rather follow a schedule that has been extensively researched for both safety and effectiveness by experts in the field of infectious diseases.

What we do know about alternative vaccination schedules is that delaying shots is playing Russian roulette with your child. The simple truth is that you are leaving your child unprotected, at a time when they are the most vulnerable.

Parents who choose to delay or opt out on vaccines are not bad parents. They are scared parents. The fear you *should* have is of the diseases that vaccines prevent. If you are on the fence about vaccinations, please take the time to research the diseases.

BOTTOM LINE: Many experts who are tops in their fields created this vaccination schedule. And there is a specific reason for the timing, spacing, and offering of certain vaccines.

Q. If I want to space out my baby's shots, how should I do it?

Set up a consultation with your pediatrician to discuss what both of you feel comfortable with doing. Remember, the ultimate goal is to have your child vaccinated in a timely manner.

Pediatricians are passionate about protecting their littlest patients. It's our job to protect kids, and we will be your child's fiercest advocate. Following the recommended schedule is the best way to do that. Many of us refuse to deviate from the recommended schedule just to appease a nervous parent. But we do want families to get their questions answered and their concerns addressed. Building a trusting relationship and having an open dialogue with your child's doctor provides reassurance and confidence in immunizations and all aspects of your child's healthcare.

DR. B'S OPINION:

Delayed Vaccination Schedules

Virtually all pediatricians are very passionate about vaccinating their patients in a timely manner. That's because we have all seen, at one point or another, what some of these horrible diseases can actually do.

If you are thinking about delaying or skipping any vaccines, set up a consultation to get advice and come up with a plan together.

Q. Why do we have so many shots now?

Simple answer: We've been successful inventing vaccines to fight more diseases. It's one of the important advances in modern medicine—vaccines prevent disease, injury, and death. More vaccines are a good thing!

An important point: Many of the vaccine-preventable diseases are viruses. These viral infections cannot be treated with medicine once an infection occurs (for example, hepatitis B, the vaccination for which protects against liver infection and liver cancer).

Vaccines that protect against bacterial diseases are often serious ones, and resistant to many antibiotics (for example, Prevnar, which protects against bacterial pneumonia, bloodstream infection, and meningitis).

And even though the number of shots has gone up, the total load on the immune system has gone down. Today's vaccines are smarter and better engineered than the shots from a few decades ago. In fact, the total number of immunologic agents in the entire childhood vaccination series today is less than what was in just two vaccines forty-five years ago! Our children are getting smarter, safer vaccines today and better protection than we ever got as kids. We are preventing what is preventable.

Q. Do vaccines cause autism?

No.

How can we be so certain, you ask? First, consider the valid scientific research disproving a link (and yes, there is plenty of it).

There have been anti-vaccine groups since the smallpox vaccine was created in 1798. Modern day anti-vaccine folk have teamed up with wellness influencers, and together, they are making lots of noise and spooking new parents.

Medicine has not ignored these concerns. Vaccines have received intense scrutiny over the past twenty-five years in the search for the cause of autism. Numerous studies have been done, and no link has been found. And the 1998 case report that started the modern era of vaccine hesitancy was shown to be a fraud.

Alison Singer, executive director of the Autism Science Foundation and mother of a child with autism spectrum disorder, has said it best: "The question has been asked and answered and it's time to move on . . . we need to be able to say, 'Yes, we are now satisfied that the earth is round.'"

NEW PARENT-TO-BE 411:

Five Vaccine Myths

1. **Too many vaccines, too soon.** Thank goodness we have so many vaccines! Nine of the shots in the routine vaccination series today protect against three different forms of bacterial meningitis (Hib, Strep, and Neisseria). No, you didn't get those shots as a child. But these are not diseases you want your child to get naturally. We are lucky to live in today's world where far fewer kids suffer or die from infectious diseases. And we give vaccines as soon as it is safe and effective to do so to protect those who are the most vulnerable—our babies.
2. **We need to green our vaccines.** While it's clever to play the environmental green card, vaccines are cleaner than the air our kids breathe, the water/breast milk/formula they drink, and the food they eat. Mercury-based preservatives are no longer in routine childhood vaccines, and breast milk contains more aluminum salt than what is in vaccines.
3. **Vaccines cause autism.** While anti-vaccinationists love to make this argument, the research and clinical evidence simply does not support it. Autism has a strong genetic basis, and kids with autism are born with autism—long before they get any shots. There are readers who will tune us out at this point, we know, but science is science and facts are facts. Period.
4. **You can't trust doctors—they make money on vaccines.** Pediatricians would make a heck of a lot more money if our patients weren't vaccinated. We would be busier than we are now, caring for extremely sick children. *Pediatricians find this argument comical (and ridiculously untrue, by the way).* The truth: Docs go into pediatrics to help kids grow up healthy.
5. **It's all a government conspiracy with Big Pharma.** This would be the largest worldwide conspiracy in history. Just ask your pediatrician if they vaccinated their own kids.

Q. When is the first vaccine given?

The hepatitis B vaccine is recommended for all newborns shortly after birth. It has been a part of the American Academy of Pediatrics' recommended immunization schedule in the United States since 1991. Mother-to-child transmission is the most common way a child becomes infected with hepatitis B. Without vaccination and medical intervention, many of these children go on to have a chronic, lifelong hepatitis B infection, which can lead to liver failure and liver cancer.[20]

Pregnant women are tested for hepatitis B virus (HBV) during each pregnancy. If the mother is acutely infected or is a chronic carrier of hepatitis B and the HBV test is positive, it's essential that their newborn receive hepatitis B vaccine and a dose of immunoglobulin within twelve hours of life to prevent the spread of infection.

If the mother tests negative for HBV, a newborn may receive the first of a series of three doses of hepatitis B vaccine between birth and two months of age.

Q. Can we delay giving the hepatitis B shot?

Yes, but there are very rational reasons to give it to all newborns after birth.

You might think that babies whose moms have hepatitis B are the only ones who really need that birth dose. Here's why that's not the case.

- **The blood test isn't perfect.** Women who receive prenatal care get tested for evidence of hepatitis B infection. However, not all birthing parents receive prenatal care and others acquire hepatitis B after the test has been done and before delivery. Hepatitis B infection can be silent and symptom-free initially. Since time is of the essence to prevent hepatitis B transmission to a newborn, it is currently impractical to screen mothers for hepatitis B during labor to determine which newborns should get the vaccine right after delivery.
- **It's easy to slip through the cracks.** We know you are the ideal patient who shows up to all their prenatal visits and has their prenatal lab work in a file on their smartphone! However, some pregnant women (believe it or not) get no prenatal care or claim they did not know they were pregnant when they arrive in the ER in labor. No one knows if that person has hepatitis B or not. Again, it would be exceedingly difficult to get the lab results back in time, even if all birthing parents were tested on the spot to find out. Picking and choosing which baby absolutely needs that hepatitis B shot based on the mother's lab work allows some of those at-risk babies to slip through the cracks of a busy labor and delivery floor. So there is less of a chance of this happening if all babies get this shot.
- **Early exposure of newborns is the worst kind of exposure.** Newborns who are infected between birth and one month of age have the greatest risk of having chronic, lifelong hepatitis B. They have a 90 percent chance of having this disease for life.
- **Babies develop the best immunity.** You may view your newborn as a fragile little thing, but their immune system works extremely well! Babies mount a better response to the hepatitis B vaccine than their parents do, with about 95 percent lifelong protection from the disease. They have about 85 percent protection after just the first dose.

- **You don't have to have sex to get it.** Hepatitis B spreads through blood, saliva, and sexual contact. It's true there are some people at higher risk of acquiring hepatitis B, such as IV drug users, prostitutes, and healthcare providers. But 50 percent of kids under age ten who become infected with hepatitis B don't get it from their moms, sexual contact, IV drugs, or tattoos. Someone can acquire hepatitis B from sharing a toothbrush, being in contact with a child with a bloody nose on the playground, or contact with a childcare provider with an open cut on their hand. Since you cannot check the hepatitis B status of all humans your baby is exposed to on a daily basis, it is safer to protect your baby before they spend time out in the world.

BOTTOM LINE: An at-risk baby must receive hepatitis B vaccine within a twelve-hour window to prevent the spread of the disease.

DR. B'S OPINION:

Hep B Vaccine

If a birthing parent has hepatitis B, there is no choice. Her newborn needs hepatitis B preventive treatment (the vaccine and immunoglobulin) within twelve hours of life. If a birthing parent doesn't have hepatitis B, it is still smart to give that shot before your baby enters the real world.

CHAPTER 12

Feeding Your Newborn

"My opinion is that anybody offended by breastfeeding is staring too hard."

—David Allen

What's in This Chapter

- **Feeding options**
- **Breastfeeding basics**
- **Getting ready**
- **The first few days**
- **Troubleshooting tips**
- **Formula feeding**

It's one of the key decisions you must make for your baby right away: How will you feed them?

Right now, they are getting all their nutrition through the umbilical cord lifeline to you. Once that cord is cut at delivery, your little one is going to be looking around for something to eat!

For your baby's first year of life, there are three food options: breast milk, infant formula, or a combination of both, called combo feeding. Solid food gets added to the menu around six months of age.

What you decide to feed your baby is your choice. But believe us, the forces of human nature (albeit, well meaning) will try to influence that decision. Between family, friends, and crowdsourcing online, you will find the whole world seems to have an opinion about what you should do.

This chapter helps you make an informed decision. But we will also be very honest. We—like every major medical organization in the world—recommend that all babies be breastfed. Why? Human breast milk is the ideal nutrition for human babies. Breast milk has living ingredients, including all those antibodies nursing moms have been making their entire life. So we will encourage you to give it a try, if it's an option for you. We just hope you will give it your best effort, because *any* breast milk you feed your baby is a gift. And we'll give you tons of practical tips to support you and navigate the early, common challenges that people encounter!

However, unlike some experts, authors, or so-called friends, we won't make you feel guilty if you decide on formula or can't make a go of breastfeeding. While nothing is an exact match to human milk, modern infant formula is about as close as it gets. You should feel confident that you are feeding your baby a perfectly acceptable product that fulfills their nutrition needs. Babies thrive on infant formula or combo-feeding with breast milk and infant formula. If there are reasons, you cannot breastfeed or exclusively breastfeed or do not desire to breastfeed, don't beat yourself up about it!

Breastfeeding Basics

The best advice we can give you is to think about (and prepare for) breastfeeding now. Remember when you took driver's ed? Breastfeeding education is similar in that you won't really know how to do it until you get behind the wheel. But if you have the general concepts down, you'll feel much better about your first test drive.

We'd like to give a shout-out to a special expert here at *Expecting 411*: Linda Hill, a registered nurse and a certified lactation consultant (IBCLC). Linda and Dr. B have worked together for twenty-five years. We appreciate her sharing her thoughts and advice. Look for Linda's tips throughout this chapter.

Q. What are the options for feeding my newborn?

Your newborn has three food options: breast milk, infant formula, or a combination of both (known as combo feeding). These will continue to be the three items on your baby's menu for the first year of life. You'll add solid food around six months of age.

Q. Is it true that breast milk is better for my baby than formula?

Yes. There isn't really anything to debate here. Human milk is more suitable for a human baby than any artificially prepared product. It also has health advantages for the nursing parent. We include the entire list of advantages for both parent and baby in this chapter. We'll also help you prepare to breastfeed and troubleshoot the early challenges that new parents frequently face.

DR. B'S OPINION

While I recommend breastfeeding for all the numerous health benefits, your baby will be just fine if they are formula-fed or combo-fed.

Q. What are the real advantages of breastfeeding?

There are advantages for both baby and mom. Let's take a look at each:

Breastfeeding Advantages for Baby

1. **Breast milk has the ideal ingredients for a human body.** Breast milk is living food. It's dynamic, meaning its composition changes over time to meet the needs of a growing baby.
2. **It carries the mother's antibodies to protect baby** from various infections.

3. **It reduces the severity of certain infections,** like stomach viruses and the common cold. It contains a protein called lactoferrin that fends off bacterial infections and supports other important tasks (such as iron absorption).
4. **It is hypoallergenic.** It is rare to be allergic to human milk.
5. **It is a gut builder.** Breast milk naturally contains good germs called probiotics (bifidobacteria) and nutrients (such as human milk oligosaccharides, or HMOs, and IgA) that encourage those microbes to grow called prebiotics. Prebiotics promote healthy digestion and immunity. In short: Breast milk builds the baby biome.[1]
6. **It reduces risk of obesity, diabetes, inflammatory bowel disease, asthma, and some forms of cancer later in life.**
7. **It reduces a baby's risk of sudden infant death syndrome (SIDS).**[2]

Breastfeeding Advantages for Mom

1. **It is always ready to serve, at the perfect temperature.**
2. **It's free, sort of. It does take time to breastfeed and/or pump every day.** Yale researchers estimate the opportunity cost for a nursing parent is about four hours a day.
3. **It reduces a woman's risk of breast, ovarian, and endometrial cancer and other disorders, such as osteoporosis, diabetes, high blood pressure, heart disease, and rheumatoid arthritis.** Any amount or duration of breastfeeding lowers your risk of developing breast cancer before menopause. Currently, one in eight women will get breast cancer.[3] You can lower your risk of many of the listed disorders by nursing for at least a year of your life (not necessarily with just one baby). Nursing for at least one month can lower your risk of having a heart attack or stroke after menopause.
4. **It can be a form of birth control, but don't rely on it exclusively** (unless you want a toddler and a newborn in the house!).

BOTTOM LINE: Breastfeeding is worth the effort it takes to learn how to do it.

Q. How long should I breastfeed?

The American Academy of Pediatrics recommends exclusively breastfeeding for the first six months of life, adding complementary solid foods at that point, and continuing to nurse until two years of age (and beyond, if desired). The latest statistics show that 83 percent of American babies go home from the hospital breastfed. But only 56 percent are still receiving any breast milk at six months of life. The numbers are even lower for babies who are breastfed until one year of age.[4]

Q. If breast milk is recommended for the first two years of life, why do most American families stop before then?

Great question, but more important, how can you help change those statistics?

No matter how many breastfeeding books you read or classes you take, you have to learn how to do it as you go along.

NEW PARENT-TO-BE 411:

Breastfeeding Lingo

Breastfeeding has a language all its own. Here is a quick overview:

- **Colostrum.** The first milk that your breasts produce. Some women start making (and leaking) it before the baby is even born. It is a high-protein drink, filled with mom's antibodies that boost the immunity of a newborn. It has fewer calories than mature milk because of a lower fat content.
- **Mature milk.** The milk that arrives on the third or fourth day after birth. It is about 50 percent fat.
- **Foremilk.** The milk that comes out in the first several minutes of feeding. In general, it contains slightly less fat. Babies who "snack" end up getting mostly foremilk, leading to more frequent feedings (and possibly fussiness).
- **Hindmilk.** The milk that comes out in the later part of a feeding. It is slightly higher in fat than foremilk. Babies who drain a whole breast in a feeding tend to be more satisfied, for good reason.
- **Let-down.** When your milk rushes into the milk ducts as your baby suckles or as you pump. Most women feel this let-down.
- **Engorgement.** In the first days when you make mature milk, your breasts may feel full, tender, lumpy, and hard.
- **Plugged ducts.** An area of the breast has obstructed milk flow, creating a hard, tender, lumpy area. These areas are at risk of getting infected (mastitis—ouch!).
- **Inverted nipples.** Your nipples have an indentation in the center. It can make it more difficult for your baby to latch on.
- **Flat nipples.** Your nipples are flush against your breast tissue. Like inverted nipples, flat nipples can make it difficult for baby to latch.
- **Breast shells.** Plastic devices that pull out inverted nipples. They can also be worn to protect sore nipples from rubbing against your bra.
- **Nipple shields.** Plastic devices that protect sore or cracked nipples. These are also used for moms with flat or inverted nipples. Unfortunately, they can sometimes limit the amount of milk that flows to the baby's mouth.
- **Lanolin.** A thick emollient that helps heal cracked nipples. Brand-name products include Lansinoh and Purelan. They are available at breastfeeding boutiques and big-box stores.
- **Compression.** The squeezing of breast tissue during nursing to improve milk flow and encourage baby to drink. It can also be done while pumping to express more milk.
- **Paced bottle feeding.** Holding a baby upright and holding a bottle of expressed breast milk/formula horizontally to simulate a feeding session at the breast. This technique makes baby less frustrated when they resume nursing.

In truth, breastfeeding is like running a race with the hardest hurdles up front. Most nursing moms don't make it past those hurdles to realize it's a straight shot to the finish line. And if you don't think you can make it over those hurdles . . . ask for help!

Here are the five key reasons why nursing moms struggle, along with our solutions:

1. **Breastfeeding has a learning curve.** Breastfeeding is a learned process. It's not as natural as you might think, and it can be a real pain (literally and figuratively) for the first couple of weeks. Babies know how to suck, and your body knows how to make milk. But the technique of getting the baby latched on correctly requires a great deal of patience and sometimes four hands. Throw in a hormonal roller coaster after delivery, and you'll understand why many people give up. Then comes ***engorgement***. This is what happens when the milk actually comes in. You will wish that it was a bad dream and hope that your old breasts will be back when you wake up—engorgement often means tenderness, pain, sore nipples, and more. Breast infections caused by bacteria (mastitis) and yeast are also common in the early days and weeks of nursing. These are treatable, but they are unpleasant and reduce the desire to continue breastfeeding.

   The solution: Get professional help to learn how to get the baby latched on appropriately.

   DR. B'S OPINION

   If you can survive the first couple of weeks, breastfeeding is as easy and natural as you think it should be!

2. **You're exhausted and lack support.** You are the only one who can feed your baby for the first few weeks while you establish your milk supply to meet your baby's demands. That means you never get a stretch of sleep longer than three hours at a time—at the same time you are recovering from childbirth.

   The solution: Sleep when your baby sleeps (don't try to do laundry or catch up on social media). After a few weeks, you can start pumping (expressing) your breast milk. Then your partner (and anyone else who is willing) can take a turn feeding your baby with a bottle of expressed breast milk. Put any other friends and family to work cooking dinner, changing diapers, and soothing your baby. This will give you the freedom to concentrate on breastfeeding your baby.

3. **You don't have enough milk.** It doesn't happen that often, but some people cannot produce enough milk to meet the demands of their baby. Trying to rev up the milk supply takes a lot of effort, medication, and persistence. And even then, the milk might not come in for some people. The reasons: ***advanced maternal age*** (over thirty-five), some types of breast surgery, or hormonal issues (such as metabolic syndrome and thyroid disease). Watching a hungry baby scream at the breast 24/7 can make any parent want to throw in the towel.

   The solution: You may be able to increase your milk supply by nursing often, pumping between nursing sessions, and taking medication to increase milk production. And remember, every ounce of breast milk counts—even if you don't breastfeed exclusively. Your baby still reaps the benefits from breast milk.

4. **You return to work.** Working parents, in general, have trouble finding time to pump. To completely keep up with your baby's demands, you need to pump

every three hours (nearly impossible, right?). But remember, pumping some breast milk is better than none at all. This is not an "all or nothing" situation.

The solution: Figure out what works for you. Some nursing moms can only pump once while at work and continue to nurse while at home. Your body can adjust to many different feeding patterns . . . which means you can continue some level of breastfeeding even after you head back to work.

5. **Your baby has a problem that makes breastfeeding difficult.** If your baby was born prematurely (before thirty-seven weeks), has acid reflux (***GERD***), or a significant food allergy, it may be even more challenging to breastfeed successfully.

   The solution: Get professional help from a lactation consultant and your baby's doctor regarding pumping, supplementing, or eliminating foods in your own diet to accommodate for your baby's dietary issues.

Q. If I have trouble breastfeeding, whom should I turn to for help?

You already have relationships with healthcare providers who can help—your obstetrician, family OB provider, midwife, doula, and pediatrician. All of us have some experience handling common breastfeeding issues.

However, if you feel like you are a dog paddling in the middle of the ocean, your best bet is to call in another expert. Enter the lactation consultant.

Certified lactation consultants (IBCLCs) are individuals who are specifically trained and certified to handle breastfeeding challenges and can be the difference between breastfeeding failure and success. There are other professionals who are breastfeeding educators, but we prefer certified IBCLCs because they go through a formal training and certification process. Ask your OB provider for a recommendation.

Helpful Hint

Insurance companies are required to cover breastfeeding support services. As always, the devil is in the details—different insurance providers will offer varying benefits. As soon as possible, contact your insurer or company's HR department to determine your policy's benefits.

Partner Tips

Here are our top three suggestions for helping your nursing partner:

1. **Be supportive of breastfeeding.** Breastfeeding can be an emotionally charged experience, especially if your nursing partner encounters problems. You need to be there to support the decision to breastfeed. And you should both participate in a breastfeeding class.
2. **Become an honorary lactation consultant.** Breastfeeding takes a lot of patience and often four hands. (To let you in on a little secret, your expert author, Dr. M, needed three people and twelve towels rolled into various shapes to properly position her and her first baby for breastfeeding!)

You will become the honorary lactation consultant since you will have a bird's eye view of the way your baby latches on to your nursing partner. Watch how the lactation consultant does it and take notes.

Until the nursing parent and baby get the hang of it, you may need to place your baby open-mouthed onto the breast as your nursing partner holds their breast upward. So don't think you are off the hook because your partner is the one actually nursing!

3. **Pick up the slack.** It's also helpful if you take charge of all other baby needs (soothing, diaper changes, etc.) as well as household needs (laundry, meal preparation, etc.) so your exhausted nursing partner can catch some much-needed shut-eye between feedings.

Q. If I am not able to exclusively breastfeed or I stop nursing, what do I feed my baby?

Commercially made infant formula is the acceptable substitute for breast milk in the first year of life. We'll give you a brief overview later in this chapter, but check out our companion book *Baby 411* to help you navigate the formula aisle at the grocery store.

Note: Whole milk, soymilk, goat's milk, and rice milk are not substitutes for breast milk in the first year of life.

Q. If I decide not to breastfeed, will my body still make milk? Do I need to take a medication to stop it?

Yes, your body will naturally make milk. And no, you don't need medication to stop it.

After delivery, your hormones will tell your body to produce milk for your newborn. But your body will only continue to make milk if it is regularly encouraged to do so. That encouragement comes either naturally, with a baby nursing at the breast or artificially, using a breast pump.

If neither of those things happen, your body will quickly stop producing milk in a week or so. You can wear a tight sports bra and apply ice packs for ten minutes once every hour to accelerate this process. You also might want to wear some nursing pads for a few days to conceal any leakage.

Decades ago, people would take medication to dry up breast milk. The risks outweigh the benefits; therefore it is no longer recommended.

Getting Ready

Q. Should I take a breastfeeding class?

Yes, if you have never nursed before. And your partner should go with you. As we mentioned earlier, it really is like taking driver's ed. You will get the big picture idea in a class, but you will learn the finer nuances once you really do it. Nursing is also a team sport. And you are taking the class without your key player (your baby). You will have to teach them the game plan as you go along.

Certified lactation specialists (IBCLCs) usually teach these classes.

Q. My breasts started leaking already. Is this a good sign?

Yes.

While it's no guarantee that you will have enough milk, it does mean that your body is getting ready to go.

Q. I have flat/inverted nipples. Will this be a problem with nursing?

It might be. Babies need an easy target to transfer milk out of the breast and into their mouths. A newborn may get frustrated at the breast because they have difficulty latching on and subsequently eating. Many people do just fine, though. But it's good to take a peek at your nipples right now, so you can prepare yourself for this potential issue.

When people get physically cold, it's normal for nipples to harden and stick out. If this doesn't happen to you, you might have flat or inverted nipples.

- **Flat nipples.** Is your breast perfectly smooth? Try pinching the pigmented area (***areola***) just beneath the nipple to help your baby find it. Avoid baby bottles and pacifiers in the beginning, as your baby will prefer them since they are easier to latch on to.
- **Inverted nipples.** Do you see an indentation in the center of your nipple? Try pinching your nipple. Does it stick out or go in? If it goes in, pull your nipple out before offering it to your baby. If it "hides," then you may want to wear *breast shells* during your pregnancy. You can also use a breast pump after you deliver to help bring out your nipple. *Nipple shields* are useful if the baby can pull the nipple into the shield.

Q. I have small breasts. Will I make enough milk?

Probably. Size doesn't matter. It's what's inside that counts.

You should have enough milk if you have normal breast anatomy (milk ducts, nipples), make hormones that trigger milk production, and have the right amount of stimulation from your baby naturally suckling or using a breast pump.

Fact Check

Women who have small breasts can't breastfeed well.

The truth: While there are some women who do not make enough milk to exclusively nurse their babies, it is not because they have small breasts.

Q. I have very large breasts/nipples. Is this good for nursing?

Sometimes yes, sometimes no.

If you have large, pendulous breasts, you may have more difficulty getting your baby correctly latched. You may want to try the football hold or lying on your side while nursing so you don't have to hold up the weight of your breast.

INSIDER SECRET:
No Two Breasts Are Created Equal

One of your breasts may produce more than the other. In fact, it's quite common. And your baby will figure that out and may develop a preference for the better-producing breast. Some babies will even refuse the breast that has slower flow or less volume.

If your baby doesn't get too frustrated, offer the slower flow breast first because they will nurse more aggressively at the beginning, and that helps increase your supply. And try pumping the lower-producing breast after nursing to improve production.

Does your baby completely refuse one breast? No worries. It's possible to make enough from one breast to completely satisfy your baby. So nutrition isn't a problem. You'll just start to look rather lopsided if you only nurse on one side!

You can also try a nursing pillow (or a rolled-up receiving blanket or burp cloth under your breast) that supports both your breast and your baby.

If your nipples are too large for your baby, you may need to pump and bottle feed until their mouth gets bigger. Real talk: all nursing moms think their nipples are too big for their tiny babies. It is rarely a problem.

Q. I've had a breast reduction. Will this be a problem?

Possibly.

Certain types of breast reduction surgery disrupt the milk duct superhighway. This may mean you do not have enough milk to breastfeed exclusively. You may not even make more than a drop or two at each nursing session. In this scenario, formula-feeding is the most reasonable choice for your baby.

However, no one can predict whether you will be able to nurse or not before you try. And even if you cannot nurse for the long haul, it's great to offer your first milk (colostrum) to your newborn. Work with a lactation consultant to get help with your situation.

Q. I've had a mastectomy. Can I nurse with only one breast?

Yes, in fact I (Dr. B) had a patient whose mother successfully breastfed with one breast for a whole year. It can be done! Each breast is capable of providing enough milk to meet a baby's nutritional needs.

Q. I have implants. Can I still nurse?

Yes.

However, certain types of reconstructive surgery may interfere with your ability to breastfeed exclusively. Also important is whether you experience breast growth during pregnancy. Growth indicates that there is sufficient glandular tissue (which is responsible for milk production) within the breast tissue. If there hasn't been any growth, size A breasts will still be size A breasts, even if you are a size D with implants. Make sense? If you have concerns, consider professional help from a lactation consultant.

The First Days

Right from the start, we want you to have good nursing technique. That prevents those raw, bleeding nipples you've been warned about! It all boils down to good positioning and a good latch.

There are a few basic positions to hold your baby while you nurse. These include a cradle hold, cross-cradle hold, football hold, side-lying, and the koala hold. You'll learn about these positions if you take a breastfeeding class or work with a lactation consultant. But here are some pointers from Linda, no matter which position you choose.

Positioning

- Mom should be comfortable with arms and back supported.
- Mom should not lean over the baby. Instead, use a breastfeeding pillow—a firm pillow that wraps around mom's waist and allows baby to rest supported. Linda's favorite brand is called (don't laugh at the name) My Brest Friend because it provides more support than the competing brands on the market.
- Baby should directly face the breast without having to turn their head.
- Baby's stomach should be pulled in close to mom, tummy to tummy. Using a footstool may be helpful to bring baby closer to mom.
- Baby's ear, shoulder, and hip should be in a straight line.

The other critical issue is making sure your baby's bottom lip latches onto the pigmented area (areola) and not at the base of the nipple. Otherwise, the baby will not be able to transfer milk as effectively and mom will endure some painful nipple trauma.

Comfortable Latch

- Position your baby at the breast so that their nose is directly across from your nipple.
- Aim your nipple up with your thumb so that it is pointing to the roof of their mouth when opened.
- Touch their lips with your breast and they will look up to the nipple as your baby opens their mouth.
- Have their bottom lip latch onto the pigmented tissue (areola) beneath the nipple. Push your nipple into their mouth as you pull your baby into you.
- If it hurts more than ten to twenty seconds beyond the initial latch, break the suction seal, reposition, and try again. *Do not nurse if it hurts beyond the initial latch.* It's normal to feel a tugging sensation. It's not normal to feel pinching, burning, or stinging. You are not doing yourself or your baby a favor by suffering. Pain means you don't have a good latch—or you are paying for previous damage you've already done.

- You should hear gulping ("cuh") noises. Take your baby off if you hear a clicking sound.
- Signs of a bad latch are if your nipple looks like a tube of lipstick or you see a white line across the nipple that eventually leads to cracks, bleeding, and scabs.

Q. When is the first time I should nurse my baby?

Shortly after delivery.

As long as there are no emergency medical issues for you or your baby, you will have a chance to nurse your baby in their first hour of life. They will be awake, alert, and interested in suckling. Take advantage of this moment to bond and start breastfeeding.

After that golden wakeful hour, your baby will want to sleep for the next few hours and will want nothing to do with eating.

Q. Is it okay to supplement with formula until my mature milk comes in?

Yes, it's okay, but it's usually not necessary.

Mother Nature has an elaborate plan for babies and breast milk. Newborns arrive with some extra nutritional baggage to carry them through the first few days of life. That's good because they'd rather sleep than eat. It's also good because your body is making early milk (colostrum) that is antibody-rich but calorie-poor. (It has fewer calories than mature milk, which shows up around day three or four.)

In fact, we pediatricians expect most newborns to lose about 10 percent of their birth weight by the third or fourth day. That's supposed to happen.

At about forty-eight hours of life (at precisely the moment most of you are heading home from the hospital), your baby suddenly says, "Hey, I'm starving, what have you got to eat around here?!"

They'll act completely differently than the first two days and want to nurse nonstop. That demand drives your milk supply up. Although that can be pretty nerve-wracking for about twenty-four hours or so, it's what gets your milk production going.

BOTTOM LINE: You don't need to tinker with Mother Nature's grand scheme by offering formula. Unless there is a medical reason to give formula, let nature take its course.

Q. Can my baby use a pacifier if I am nursing?

Yes. Babies are soothed by sucking. In the first two months of life, sucking on a pacifier may be the only thing that reliably settles your baby. Despite what you may hear, binkies and breastfeeding can mix.

Experts used to believe that pacifiers shortened the length of time that moms continued to nurse. It was almost taboo to offer a binky to a breastfed baby. Research suggests otherwise. Pacifiers don't make a baby or mom stop breastfeeding. Parents who use a binky choose to discontinue nursing for a variety of other reasons.[5]

INSIDER SECRET:

Encouraging Breastfeeding

How can both doctors and parents ensure that breastfeeding is successful? Here are the AAP's guidelines:

- Encourage rooming-in with your newborn at the hospital to learn baby's cues.
- Trained caregivers should formally evaluate breastfeeding (latch, position, etc.) at least twice daily while newborns are at the hospital. (If that doesn't happen, speak up!)
- Supplements (water, sugar water, formula) should not be given to a breastfed newborn unless ordered by the baby's doctor for a medical reason.
- Pacifiers are discouraged until breastfeeding is going well.
- Breastfed babies should see their healthcare provider at three to five days of life and again at two weeks of age to assess breastfeeding.
- Complementary foods (solid food) should be introduced between four and six months of life.
- Babies should sleep in close proximity to their moms to encourage breastfeeding. (Note the word choices here—the AAP is not recommending a family bed.)
- In your early days of breastfeeding, the following four facts of nursing your baby will be especially helpful:

    1. Breast milk production is a supply-and-demand phenomenon. Most women have no trouble making enough milk if the demand is there. Nursing at least eight times in twenty-four hours promotes a good supply.
    2. Colostrum, the first milk, is all your baby needs for the first few days of life. Mature milk, the high-fat stuff, arrives when your baby needs it—around the fourth day of life.
    3. *All* babies are exhausted by the birth process and are not very interested in eating for the first forty-eight hours. They latch on, get cozy . . . and fall asleep after five minutes. This behavior will change (at almost the same moment you leave the hospital!).
    4. Babies are born with 10 percent extra baggage to carry them through the first few days of life. They will lose 5 to 10 percent of their birth weight—expect that. Do not think you are failing at breastfeeding because your baby is losing weight.

In my opinion, breastfeeding and pacifiers are not mutually exclusive—pacifiers are not evil. But it is wise to wait on introducing a pacifier until your baby is a confident breastfeeder (between one and four weeks old) because babies suck pacifiers differently than the breast. Plus, frequent suckling at the breast helps establish mom's milk supply in the early weeks.

I like the Philips Avent Soothie brand of pacifier (which are green with a long nipple), as it is more like the human nipple than other brands. A reasonable alternative to the pacifier is a parent's finger.

Fact Check

Pacifiers interfere with breastfeeding.

The truth: Babies who use pacifiers tend to breastfeed for a shorter period of time than those who don't. But it's not *because* of the binky. Moms who opt to use binkies are the same ones who opt out of breastfeeding. It's just a coincidence—one doesn't cause the other.[6]

Q. What do I need to know about my baby's first few days of breastfeeding?

Let's break this down, day by day . . .

First Day of Life (Zero to Twenty-four Hours Old)

1. Nurse your baby for the first time within an hour or so of birth. They will be awake, alert, and interested.
2. At two hours of life, they will be exhausted and hard to arouse for several (three to four) hours. Don't get too worked up about trying to nurse right now. Take a nap yourself. Or place your newborn skin to skin with you and relax together.
3. Your frequency goal is six to eight feedings in the first twenty-four hours of life.
4. Your baby will probably fall asleep at the breast after a few minutes of nursing. An acceptable feeding session for today is five to ten minutes per breast.

Second Day of Life (Twenty-four to Forty-eight Hours Old)

1. Today's goal is working on your technique. It may take a second set of hands to position the baby while you hold your breast. You will fly solo eventually.
2. Your frequency goal is eight feedings in twenty-four hours. Do not let your baby sleep more than three hours during the day or four hours at night or you will have trouble meeting this goal.
3. Aim for your feedings to last at least five to ten minutes per breast. Do not take baby off the breast at ten minutes if they are still actively sucking.
4. If your nipples are cracked and bleeding, you need help with your technique.

Third Day of Life (Forty-eight to Seventy-two Hours Old)

1. Your baby is suddenly awake and sometimes insatiable. You will likely have a very long night. As long as your baby has lost less than 10 percent of their birth

weight (and has no other risk factors—see below), keep your chin up and resist the temptation to supplement with formula. Your baby's demand is precisely what your body needs to create the supply of milk.

2. Make sure your technique is okay and you are comfortable when your baby latches on.
3. Your frequency goal is eight feedings in twenty-four hours (it should be an easy goal to reach today!).
4. The length of feedings goal should be at least ten minutes per breast.
5. You may feel that your baby is on your breast nonstop. If that is the case and your nipples are sore, take a break if you have nursed for more than forty-five minutes. Let someone else have a chance to soothe your baby. (Letting baby suck on someone's finger may be helpful.)

Fourth Day of Life (Seventy-two to Ninety-six Hours Old)

1. Hello, milk! There is usually little question of whether your milk has arrived. How will you know? Your breasts will be much larger, heavier, and tender. You should feel full before you nurse, and softer after you nurse. You should also see milk when you burp your baby (and sometimes when you shower). The change in your baby's poop will also tell you the milkman has arrived.
2. If your breasts are rock hard and your ***areolae*** (the darker colored ring around your nipple) are flattened against them, you are officially engorged. This lasts for a day or two. See troubleshooting tips on page 288.
3. Your frequency goal is eight feedings in twenty-four hours. Do not let your baby sleep for more than 3.5 hours during the day or a four-hour stretch at night.
4. Aim for your feedings to last at least ten to fifteen minutes per breast. Once your milk supply is well established (around four weeks of life), some women prefer to nurse with one breast per feeding. For now, use both at each feeding, as it stimulates your milk production.

You should be on your way now. Your baby should be gaining about an ounce a day.

Helpful Hint

When you are told that babies feed every two to three hours, time is measured from the beginning of one feeding until the beginning of the next. If the feeding session itself lasts forty-five minutes or an hour, that may leave less than an hour before it's time to nurse again. Your goal is to nurse at least eight times a day. This may be every two to three hours or it may be a series of cluster feedings every ninety minutes, followed by a four-hour stretch. As long as the number of feedings add up to at least eight in a twenty-four-hour period, it is fine.

Troubleshooting for the First Days

As we have already alluded to, the early days of breastfeeding can be challenging. While you are in this stage of your pregnancy journey, you don't need a comprehensive review of all the potential problems and solutions. We don't want to completely bore you (or spook you). Just know that we can help you, when that time comes.

Q. My plan is to exclusively breastfeed, but my healthcare providers are telling me I need to supplement my newborn. Is this really necessary?

Yes, there are a few medical situations where it is necessary. Parents who are certain they want to breastfeed are often devastated if they need to temporarily supplement with donor breast milk or formula.

The key point to remember: You are not a failure. It isn't the end of the world. And offering donor breast milk or formula for a short time won't sabotage breastfeeding success.

1. **Premature newborn.** If your baby is born at less than thirty-five weeks gestation, they probably won't be able to directly breastfeed initially. Depending on how premature your baby is, they might not even eat by mouth at first. You can pump to stimulate your milk production and provide your expressed breast milk.
2. **Late preterm newborn.** Babies born between 34 and 36 6/7 weeks gestation tend to be very sleepy, lazy, and inept at efficient suckling at the breast. So until your baby gets the hang of it, you may need to offer the breast and then some pumped breast milk in a bottle after each nursing session to fulfill their nutritional needs. If you don't have enough milk, formula will work. You can nurse exclusively once your baby's skill and energy level improves, they are gaining weight appropriately, and you are making at least three ounces of milk combined from both breasts for each feeding. This usually takes a week or two, or until your baby reaches the day they were *supposed* to be delivered.
3. **Low blood sugar (hypoglycemia).** Some newborns have trouble maintaining an adequate blood sugar level. Low blood sugar can become a vicious cycle. Babies with low blood sugar lack the energy to eat, which leads to persistently low blood sugar. Besides its negative impact on feeding, sustained low blood sugar can lead to brain injury and seizures. Hence, the temporary solution is to offer sugar gel in addition to nursing until your baby maintains normal blood sugar levels. For a full-term baby, born between thirty-seven and forty weeks, this may be for a feeding or two, or a day or two at most.
4. **Excessive weight loss.** A newborn that loses more than 10 percent of their birth weight usually needs both breast milk and formula until they start to gain weight. As we mentioned earlier, it is normal and expected for your baby to lose 10 percent of their weight from birth. But more than 10 percent means that your baby is dehydrated. Dehydrated babies are not happy babies. They lack energy to eat (another vicious cycle) and so they lose more weight, end up with low blood sugar, and develop jaundice (more on this next). Don't let your baby become a martyr in the name of breastfeeding. If they are dehydrated and your

mature milk hasn't arrived yet, supplement with formula. It prevents them from having other medical issues. Remember, this is temporary until your baby gains weight and your mature milk is plentiful enough.

5. **Significant jaundice.** Let's talk about poop for a minute. Humans clear out a waste product (called ***bilirubin***) in their poop. Bilirubin has a yellow pigment to it. In the first few days of life, a newborn doesn't clear out much bilirubin because their liver (which breaks it down) doesn't function at 100 percent and they aren't pooping very much (since they aren't eating much). As a result, all newborns temporarily collect some bilirubin in their skin, leaving it with a yellowish tint (called physiologic jaundice). This resolves on its own around three to five days of life once they eat a lot, poop a lot, and have fully functioning livers.

   For a variety of reasons, some newborns get significantly jaundiced. If there is more bilirubin than the skin can handle, it collects in the brain and can cause permanent brain damage (called bilirubin-induced neurologic dysfunction, or BIND). It goes without saying that everyone wants to avoid this! There are several ways to prevent BIND, but the first and simplest thing to do is to get a newborn to eat and poop more. The more baby eats, the more baby poops, the more they get rid of their bilirubin load. For a breastfed baby, that means supplementing with formula for a few days.

   Once you see the poop turn from black to dark green to yellow (that yellow-pigmented bilirubin makes it change color) and your mature breast milk is in, the bilirubin levels will drop and you'll be able to resume nursing exclusively.

6. **Maternal reason.** Sometimes, medical problems arise after delivery that prevent the birthing parent to nurse at first. Those problems include postpartum bleeding, high blood pressure, etc. If this happens to you, don't let it get you down. Nurse as much as your OB provider allows and let your baby have some donor breast milk or formula until you have recuperated. You need to be healthy to be able to make milk. If you can, pump to protect your milk supply.

INSIDER SECRET:

Paced Bottle Feeding

If you are bottle feeding (formula or expressed breast milk), hold the bottle as horizontally as possible without allowing air into the nipple. This is called paced bottle feeding. It makes the baby work a little bit to eat, simulating what it is like to nurse at the breast, and slows down the feeding. Slowing down the pace of the meal also helps the baby recognize their satiety and feeling of fullness.

If you hold the bottle upright with a slight angle as most people instinctively do, the baby will guzzle the milk like they are drinking from the tap and may take more than they really need to because it is pouring into their mouth. It also makes them less enthusiastic about the work required to suckle and transfer milk when they are at the breast.

Q. I'm worried my newborn isn't eating enough and my mature milk isn't in yet. How will I be able to tell?

We'll give you the red flags here. The good news: Your first visit at the pediatrician's office is typically a day or two after you go home from the hospital, when your baby is three or four days old. It's an important visit to see how feedings are going and assess your baby's weight. But here are some warning signs. Notify your baby's doctor if:

- You don't have a dramatic change in your breasts by the fifth day of life.
- You don't hear your baby swallowing ("cuh" or "ca-ca" sound) when they are at the breast.
- Your baby's poops have not changed from black tar (meconium) to a greenish-yellowish color by the fourth day.
- Your baby does not have at least four wet diapers on the fourth day.
- Your baby is sleepy and hard to arouse for feedings.
- Your baby is nursing nonstop.

Fact Check

Your boobs will sag if you breastfeed.

The truth: Technically this is true, but your boobs will also sag even if you don't breastfeed. It's one of the joys of going through pregnancy and motherhood. If you are really bothered by your new appearance, we can suggest some nice plastic surgeons in LA and Austin who will be happy to help you regain your perky, pre-motherhood breasts!

You need to avoid gassy foods like beans because it will make the baby gassy.

The truth: Your baby will be gassy no matter what you eat. All newborns are gassy in the first six to eight weeks of life. You don't need to restrict your diet unless you see a real correlation between what you ate and your baby's level of discomfort (it takes four to twenty-four hours to see a problem).[7]

Formula Feeding

Q. Is it okay to feed formula to my newborn?

Yes. Your baby will be fine if they are formula-fed. Infant formula is an acceptable substitute for human breast milk for a baby's first year of life. We are fortunate to live in modern times and have safe, nutritious options to feed our babies. All commercially made infant formulas are highly regulated, resemble human milk as much as possible, and contain thirty essential nutrients to meet Food and Drug Administration requirements in the United States. The number of infant formula options can feel overwhelming. There are some differences in the macronutrients (proteins, fats, and carbohydrates) and added ingredients that may be beneficial in digestion and the developing immune system.

Here are the key advantages to formula:

- **It's about as close as it gets to human milk.** Formulas are specially prepared to contain the appropriate amount of fat, protein, carbohydrates, and other nutrients that growing babies need.
- **It's convenient.** You can take a formula bottle anywhere you go. And yes, there are portable bottle warmers for picky babies. (It's somewhat less convenient at two a.m. when your baby is screaming while you frantically have to warm up a bottle.)
- **It isn't dependent on the nursing parent.** Yes, any willing and able-bodied person can feed a baby a bottle of formula anytime during the day or night.
- **There are options.** While not all babies can tolerate cow, soy, or goat's milk-based formula, there are several alternatives for babies with food allergies.

BOTTOM LINE: Do not feel guilty if you choose to formula-feed or combo-feed your baby or cannot breastfeed. There are plenty of great options!

Q. I have chosen to feed my baby formula. What formula do you recommend?

The American Academy of Pediatrics (AAP) advises using a cow or goat's milk protein-based formula with iron for healthy babies from zero to twelve months of age. That's it. Easy, right? But with ninety infant formulas on the market, it may feel like a very difficult decision!

Here's the thing—the FDA requires all US-made infant formulas to resemble human milk, with thirty essential nutrients. So your baby will get their nutritional needs met regardless of which product you select. But we do encourage you to be a label reader and decide what is most important to you. See https://bit.ly/AAPFormulaAdvice for the AAP guidelines for choosing a baby formula.

Like human milk, all infant formulas contain macronutrients (protein, fat, sugar) and micronutrients (vitamins and minerals). While not FDA required, some formulas also contain probiotics, prebiotics, and omega-3 fatty acids (***DHA***) and omega-6 fatty acids (ARA) in an effort to be more similar to human milk. And a few infant formulas are certified organic and/or use non-GMO products for families who desire it.

The most important differences between formulas are the protein base and the ratio between whey and casein.

Q. How much and how often do I feed my baby?

For the first few days of life, a newborn might take up to an ounce (30 ml) every few hours. After the first few days, offer your full-term baby three ounces in a bottle and see what they do with it. From day three to two weeks old, babies usually eat about two to three ounces every three to four hours. They gradually want more to eat over the next several weeks. But as you might guess by the standard bottle size, babies eventually max out at six to eight ounces per feeding.

How will you know when your baby wants more to drink than what you have offered? Easy. They will finish off what you gave them and look for more! And the beauty of babies is that most of them just eat what they need to and then stop when they are full. Look at the baby. They do not need to finish every bottle. So if you follow your baby's lead, they will probably eat just the right amount.

We recommend paced bottle feeding (see the Insider Secret box on page 302). This slows down the pace of the feeding and allows the baby to sense a feeling of fullness. Don't let them chug it!

Q. Do I need to bring my own formula to the hospital?

Yes, if you plan to formula feed your newborn and you have a specific formula you want to use. Hospitals typically stock a couple of major brands in ready-to-feed (no mixing required) single-use bottles. These are easy to use, since no preparation is needed. But there is no need to stick with ready-to-feed formula, or even the brand you are given at the hospital, once you get home.

CHAPTER 13

Home Stretch

"Can I just spray a little PAM down there right before the baby comes out?"

—Baby Mama

What's in This Chapter

- **Childbirth classes**
- **Inductions**
- **C-sections**
- **Vaginal births after cesareans (VBACs)**
- **True labor versus false labor**
- **Top labor fears**
- **What to pack for delivery**
- **What to have at home**

Most pregnant people spend their entire pregnancy preparing for the big day. As you get closer to this becoming an actuality, we know you have many questions about the nuts and bolts of the whole experience.

This chapter will cover common concerns at the end of your pregnancy and all the things you should think about *before* you go into labor. View this chapter as the dress rehearsal. The next chapter (Labor Day) walks you through what really happens at the big show. We recommend you read both of these chapters before those first contractions start.

Labor Lingo

Bookmark the next two pages. We'll refer to these terms in both this chapter and the next one.

- **Dilation:** The ***cervix*** begins to open to let the baby out. Your OB provider measures it with their fingertips on an internal pelvic exam. We all measure the diameter of the opening of the cervix in centimeters. It ranges from zero to ten. When a cervix is not open at all, it is "closed" or "zero centimeters dilated." When the cervix is completely dilated it is called "complete" or "ten centimeters dilated." See the following diagram.

Dilation **Cervix widens or opens**

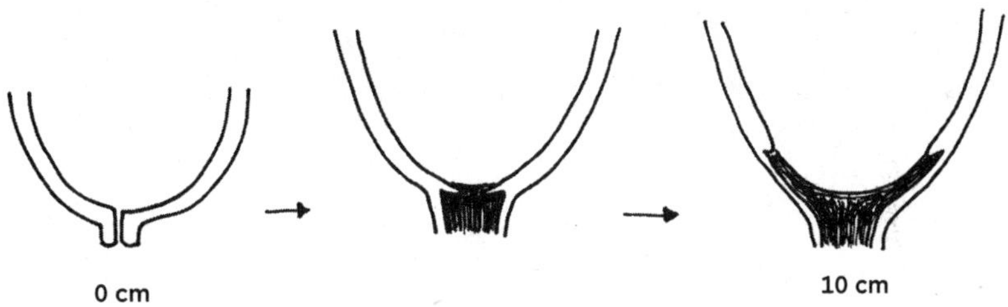

- **Engaged:** This term refers to the process of the baby's presenting body part (usually the head) moving down and settling into the pelvic cavity. This often occurs in the last month of pregnancy, but it may happen earlier if this is your second or third baby. People refer to it as "dropping" or "***lightening***," and you may see that your belly changes shape and you can breathe easier. But if you didn't have to pee enough already, you will now feel like you should set up shop on the potty.
- **Station:** This measurement compares where your baby's head is in relation to the location of specific bones in your pelvis (the ischial spines). It tracks your baby's descent into the birth canal. See graphic below.

  The most commonly used system (yes, there's more than one) ranges from -5 to +5, where -5 means the baby's head is 5 cm above the narrowest portion of your pelvic bones (ischial spines) and +5 means the baby's head is at the opening of your vagina. Your OB provider determines the station by an internal pelvic exam. See the following diagram.

Station **Baby's head descends through mom's pelvis**

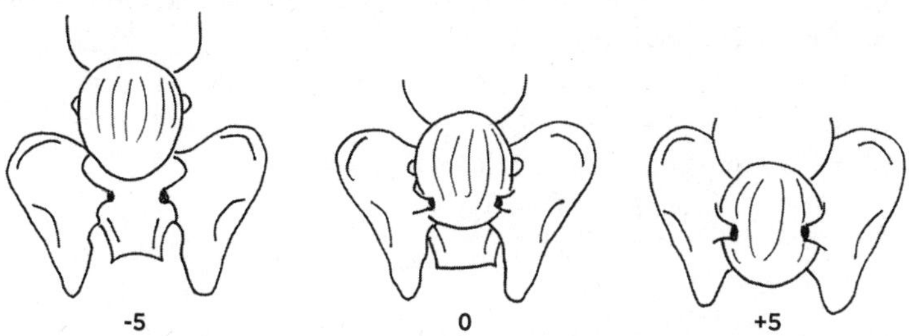

- **Bloody show:** We know, this is a terrible name. It translates to a blood-tinged mucus discharge from the vagina, which often signals the onset of labor.
- **Effacement:** The cervix also starts to thin out as it prepares for birth. Again, your OB provider can determine this from an internal pelvic exam. Docs measure effacement in percentages. So, for example, you will be "0 percent effaced" when the cervix is at its longest and hasn't started to thin yet (most of your pregnancy). And you will be 100 percent effaced when you begin pushing. See the following diagram.

Effacement **Cervix softens or thins out**

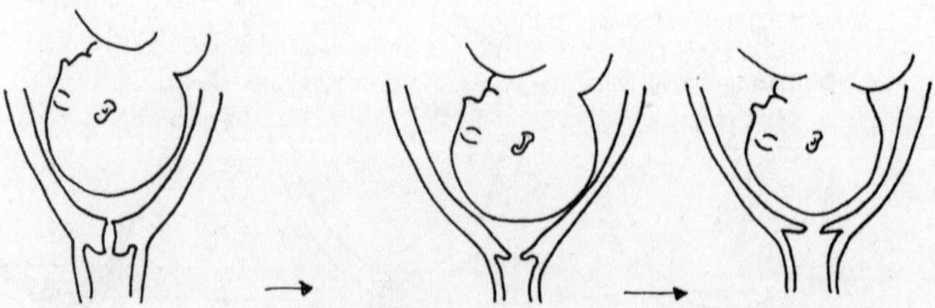

- **Ripe cervix:** The term used to describe your cervix as it thins and softens in preparation for delivery.
- **Mucus plug:** A yellowish, pinkish thick substance that acts as a plug (hence the name) by blocking the cervix during pregnancy. You may lose your mucus plug as the cervix starts to open up. This is often a sign that labor will begin soon. Some women actually see a big blob of mucus. But most don't notice anything until they are in the heat of labor and bloody show begins. And sometimes, a mucus plug comes out well in advance of labor.
- **Presentation:** As the end of your pregnancy nears, your OB provider will check to see if your baby plans to exit the birth canal going head-first (called ***cephalic*** or ***vertex***)—the safest and least complicated way. The head, in this case, is the presenting part, which means it is the first body part to emerge. Ninety-five percent of babies are vertex.

  Occasionally, babies make their exit a bit more challenging by sitting in a ***breech*** position. That means that the baby's butt (or foot in some cases) is the presenting part. And a few indecisive babies lie sideways (***transverse lie***) or diagonally (***oblique lie***).

  It's helpful to know what your baby's plans are, so your OB provider can make plans of their own for your delivery. OBs get that information by doing a physical exam and using an ultrasound if needed.

Childbirth Classes and Birth Requests

Q. There are a variety of childbirth classes available in our community. Which one should I take, and when should I take it?

If this is your first baby, it's a good idea to take a childbirth education class. Most hospitals that have maternity services offer classes in childbirth, parenting, breast-feeding, and infant CPR. Some even offer ***C-section*** classes for people who know in advance that they will have this procedure as well as classes on epidural and spinal ***anesthesia***.

But do not feel like you are wedded to take a class at the hospital at which you will deliver. Your OB provider may be able to recommend a particular class or a childbirth educator who does private home classes for one, two, or more expecting couples. And if you are using a doula, they will likely be doing some classes with you and your partner.

Helpful Hint

If you go on bed rest or simply cannot find a course that works for your schedule, there are plenty of online childbirth courses you can take.

Q. Are there different approaches to childbirth? Which ones should I know about?

Yes, you'll find classes that teach the Bradley method or the Lamaze method.

The *Bradley method* of childbirth is named after Dr. Robert Bradley (an American obstetrician) who developed this technique in the 1940s. The goal: natural, drug-free childbirth.

It is now taught as a twelve-week course that educates a couple on how to cope with the pain of childbirth by using deep breathing and relaxation techniques. The Bradley method was one of the first to involve fathers in the birthing process (instead of keeping them pacing in the waiting room, which was typical at that time).

The woman's partner takes the role of coach, helps to keep the person giving birth focused on the delivery, aids with breathing exercises, and gives constant reassurance. They also provide different forms of massage to help ease the discomfort. (Our tip: Don't buy a whistle, even if you are playing the coach.) Bradley classes prepare patients for possible unexpected outcomes but argue against the use of pain medication and C-section unless absolutely necessary.

The *Lamaze method* of childbirth is named after Dr. Fernand Lamaze (a French obstetrician) who also debuted this method in the 1940s. Lamaze gained acceptance in the United States and is now the most popular of all childbirth techniques.

The Lamaze technique also teaches breathing exercises during labor (this is the one most of us know as "hee-hee-hoooo"—that is, taking a short, quick inhalation before uttering each "hee" and a longer inhalation before each "hoooo").

Unlike the Bradley method, Lamaze teaches various distraction techniques to help cope with the pain of labor, such as concentrating on a pleasant memory like a vacation or an older child. Lamaze techniques also include using a "birthing ball," hot and cold packs, and changing positions to help ease the pain of labor. The Lamaze method is not as strict or regimented as Bradley and holds a neutral position on pain medication, as well as other forms of intervention during labor (such as Pitocin to stimulate labor, vacuum/forceps delivery, and C-section).

If you are unsure on what is best for you, do some research to learn about these two techniques. Many women choose to use a little from each method to help cope with labor. For example, you could use the Lamaze method of breathing during a painful contraction, then try the Bradley method of long, deep, relaxing breaths in between contractions.

BOTTOM LINE: The Bradley method teaches women to focus on their pain in order to help control it, whereas the Lamaze method teaches distraction from pain. For more information, check out Bradleybirth.com and Lamaze.org.

DR. M'S OPINION:

Birthing Classes

If you plan to attempt labor without an epidural or any type of pain medication, I absolutely recommend two things: 1) take a birthing class (see above on Bradley and Lamaze) and 2) seriously consider having a doula at your side. Among their many roles, doulas are a great resource for childbirth education, and many offer prenatal classes as part of their global fee/package.

If you plan to have an epidural, taking a general childbirth class should be just right for you. You do not necessarily need to take a Lamaze and Bradley class. Here are the things you should find out:

1. Does the class teach a particular birthing philosophy or method? Or is it broad-based, offering several suggestions? (Think about what is best for you.)
2. What is the class size? (Small groups of five or fewer couples make it more individualized.)
3. Is the instructor certified? (You want to know what credentials the person has to teach the class.)

Whatever you plan to do, what I've learned over the last two and a half decades of helping women have babies is that the more flexible you are with respect to how your labor will go, the more likely you are to have a great labor. We can guess but never know for sure how someone's labor will go. Being flexible and trusting the person taking care of you is paramount to your birth story.

Q. What is hypnobirthing?

Hypnobirthing is having a baby while you are under hypnosis.

Classes on this technique teach expectant mothers and birth companions how to deal with anxiety, fear, and pain while in labor. The concept: Create harmony between the mind and the body, remove bad thoughts (fear or anxiety), and let the body function as nature intended.

Obstetrician Dr. Grantly Dick-Read came up with this concept in the 1930s, but several techniques have popped up since the 1980s. Hypnotherapist Marie Mongan developed the most popular one used today.

Hypnotherapists who specialize in childbirth hypnosis can offer an approach tailored toward individual women. If you have other phobias about childbirth—like being in a hospital or being poked with needles—this may be especially helpful for you.

FEEDBACK FROM THE REAL WORLD:

Dr. B's Eight-Hour Birthing Class

There are a variety of scheduling options for birthing classes: hour-long classes offered over several weeks, a full-day class, and even some weekend retreats held at swanky resorts so you can combine a babymoon and education.

Before you pay your course fee, I highly recommend you get an endorsement from your OB provider or even a friend. And take a class that fits both your schedule and your philosophy.

Because of our schedules, my husband and I chose an eight-hour marathon course at our delivery hospital. The course was almost more agonizing than my labor! We got up and left after a couple of hours. I figured I would just follow directions when I was told to push, which I did.

INSIDER SECRET:

Childbirth Prep for Everyone

Many hospitals offer sibling classes and tours for the expectant big brother or sister. This may be useful so your toddler or preschooler isn't completely freaked out by the birth.

If this is your first baby, now is a good time to take an infant CPR class. You'll have very little spare time for classes once the baby is actually born.

Q. Do you recommend that I have a birth plan?

Do you need to have a written birth plan (now often referred to as a "birth request" or "birth preference")? No, but it can be helpful. Should you talk to your doctor about your vision for labor and delivery? Absolutely. If you are lucky enough to see one or two providers for your entire pregnancy and one of the two of them will deliver you, talking verbally about your requests can suffice. But having a written copy is a good idea for the hospital so hospital staff, the nurses taking care of you, and your OB provider know exactly what you would like. If you are part of a larger group practice and you aren't sure who will be there on your delivery day, writing it all down is very important.

Your preferences don't need to be extremely detailed, but should cover basic points about your request for pain medication, who you want in the room (so your well-meaning mother-in-law can't sneak in if you don't want her to!), how you want to labor, how you want to deliver, and how you want to spend your initial hour after delivery.

In reality, you don't need a notarized document to use a birthing ball, dimmed lights, or play your Spotify playlist. Nor is a written request required to avoid using pain medication. No one is going to sneak an epidural into your back! OB providers want you to have the most amazing experience possible, with a healthy mom and baby as the end result.

That said, you should talk to your OB provider about your wishes so they have an idea of how you see your labor and delivery. Do you want a natural childbirth? Do you want an epidural as soon as it is humanly possible? Discuss this with your doctor.

If you want to bring in a five-foot plastic ficus tree to decorate your delivery suite (Dr. B had a patient do this), it may be best to check with your OB provider first.

At the same time, it's important to remain flexible. Let's put that into bold caps: **REMAIN FLEXIBLE.** No one knows what lies ahead during labor and sometimes in-the-moment medical decisions must be made if unforeseen circumstances arise. Everyone's goal is to have you and your baby make it safely through delivery.

NEW PARENT-TO-BE 411:

Seven Things You Can Control During Labor

1. **Music.** You can pick any genre you like or decide you want complete silence!
2. **Support.** You can decide who is by your side and who sits in the waiting room (or flies out to see you ***after*** you get home).
3. **Mobility.** You choose whether you prefer to move around or remain in one place during labor. (The type of pain medication you receive may affect this decision.)
4. **Lighting.** During labor, you can do whatever you like. Your OB provider will need good lighting after delivery, however.
5. **Use of pain medication.** It's your call. It's also possible to change your mind during the experience (most, but not all, of the time).
6. **IV fluid.** Depending on your individual situation, you may be able to decide if you want a capped IV ("Hep locked") or if you don't mind an IV that runs fluid and keeps you hydrated during childbirth.
7. **Birthing position.** If you opt out of an epidural for pain control, you can squat, use a birthing bar, or select a variety of other positions to get through your contractions as labor progresses.

Fact Check

You'll get an enema when you go into labor.

The truth: Some people note in their birth requests that they want to avoid getting an enema when they are in labor. Truth is, enemas are not part of routine delivery protocol anymore—this went out of style about the same time as leisure suits.

It's true, though, that most people will have some sort of a bowel movement during the pushing phase of labor. It is almost inevitable: You use the same muscles to push the baby out as you do to poop.

The pressure of the baby's head pushes down on your rectum as the baby descends through the vagina. We know, it's embarrassing, but you can't control this and from the OB provider's end, this is as natural as breathing. The only one who has to know is your OB provider (and trust me, we don't care). We will quickly move it out of sight. We are so quick, in fact, that one of my patients even dubbed me "Poo-dini" for the speed at which I cleaned her up and magically "hid" her poop from her hubby.

Q. What are my options for where I can deliver? How do I decide what is the best fit for me?

The three main options are a hospital, birthing center, or at home.

Other options such as the car, back of an ambulance, or in a wheelchair in the elevator coming up from the ER happen on occasion, but obviously no one plans this!

Let's look at the different options and why the type of delivery you want will influence this decision:

Hospitals. If you are strongly considering an epidural, then you should deliver at a hospital. And if you are a high-risk pregnancy, it is safest to deliver at a hospital.

If you want to have a physician deliver your baby, you will most likely need to deliver at a hospital as well. If your OB delivers at more than one hospital, you may consider choosing the one that is closest to you or take a tour to see which you like best. Here are some things to consider when you assess potential delivery hospitals:

- How many delivery rooms are there?
- Is there a neonatal intensive care unit (NICU)?
- Is there a specialist in the care of premature or sick newborns (***neonatologist***) in the hospital 24/7? What happens if you need one and there isn't one on staff?
- Are there residents (doctors in specialty training) working in the hospital?
- Is there an ***anesthesiologist*** (the doc who performs the epidural/spinal anesthesia) in the hospital at all times? What happens if there isn't one?
- How far is the hospital from your home?

Birthing centers or home. If you have a low-risk pregnancy and plan to have a natural childbirth, then you have several options (birthing center, home, etc.). Of course, you may still choose to have a natural childbirth in a hospital, too.

If you plan to have a midwife deliver your baby, find out whether she delivers at a hospital, birthing center, or at home. If you have your heart set on a home birth, don't just assume your midwife will be able to accommodate your request. It pays to ask!

And remember, if you choose a birthing center or home birth, find out what the backup plan is should an emergency arise. You'll want to know how a facility and OB provider outside of a hospital handle medical emergencies. This may help you decide where you feel the most comfortable.

Talk to your friends, explore your options, and talk to your provider to discuss what option is best for you.

Helpful Hint

Many hospitals offer maternity tours—both in person and virtual. It's a great idea for you and your partner to get the lay of the land. First of all, hospitals can be scary to some people and seeing where you will be is comforting to most women. Second, if you are driving in while in labor (or more than likely being driven by your partner), emotions are running high and knowing where to park ahead of time is paramount! You can find out if and when the hospital you plan to deliver at offers tours on their web page.

NEW PARENT-TO-BE 411:

Where to Deliver

According to a recent survey, 98.4 percent of American babies today are born in a hospital. Of the other 1.6 percent, 67 percent are born at home, 28 percent deliver at a birthing center, and 5 percent deliver elsewhere (presumably in a car on the way to the delivery destination!).[1]

DR. M'S OPINION:

Birth Is Birth

If there is one message that I would love for every pregnant woman to read and remember, it's this: No matter how you have a baby, with pain medication or without, vaginally or via a C-section, planned or unplanned, it is one of the most empowering events you will ever go through. There is no single "right" way to have a baby. Some women are able to choose how they want their birth story to unfold, and others aren't. Some have complications, and the clinical picture changes your OB provider's recommendations. Some women go into labor thinking one thing and change their mind. Some opt to push a baby out, and others opt for a C-section. The bottom line here is, no matter how you have your baby, your birth story is uniquely yours. Birth is not defined by how, but by courage, strength, transformation, and love.

Inductions

Q. My doctor has offered to do an induction. What is it? Is this a good idea?

An induction is the use of medication or other methods intended to bring on labor. Whether or not it is a good idea depends on the reason for the induction.

There are many medical and obstetrical reasons for recommending an induction, such as ***preeclampsia***, spontaneous rupture of membranes without labor, and going considerably past your due date (***postdates***), to name a few. If your doctor recommends an induction for a medical reason, it's probably the safest plan for you and your baby. In the United States, up to 18 percent of all labors are induced.

If you are contemplating an *elective* induction or one for non-medical reasons—like your doctor will be out of town on your due date, you want your child to be a Virgo with Pisces as a rising sign, or you really want your baby to be born on a date other than your mother-in-law's birthday—you should carefully weigh the pros and cons. Medically speaking, it isn't always the best idea. And, according to ACOG, elective inductions should not be done before thirty-nine weeks.

Although inducing a woman's labor is a safe procedure when done in a hospital, there are still inherent risks in using induction medication (such as Cervidil, misoprostol, and/or Pitocin). That being said, inducing someone on their second or third child is much quicker and easier than inducing a patient pregnant with their first child.

OB providers rate your cervix prior to induction to see how ready or favorable it is. This is expressed as a ***Bishop score***, an equation that takes many variables into account—where the baby's head is in relation to certain bones in your pelvis, the dilation and effacement of your cervix, etc. (See more details on the Bishop score in the

FEEDBACK FROM THE REAL WORLD:

Elective Inductions

To give you some perspective, here is a good example of when an elective induction just makes sense. I had a patient who was pregnant with her third child. She had fast labors with her other babies, and her second child came after only three hours of labor.

She was from another country, didn't speak much English, and lived a good sixty minutes from the hospital where I perform my deliveries. Setting a date for an induction gave her time to set up a sitter for her two older children and the security of knowing she would deliver in the hospital . . . instead of in a car in the middle of a freeway during rush hour.

It also gave me time to line up a labor and delivery nurse who spoke fluent Russian to help translate and make her more comfortable.

New Parent-to-Be box below.) The greater the number on the Bishop score, the more likely you will have a successful vaginal delivery.

BOTTOM LINE: Discuss your concerns with your OB. If you want an elective induction, you should decide together with your OB that this is the right thing for you and your baby.

NEW PARENT-TO-BE 411:

Your Bishop Score

Want to know if you have a "favorable cervix" for being induced? Here's how the pros do it. Docs use a scoring system created in 1964 by Dr. Edward Bishop—hence, the Bishop score. It's extremely good at predicting if a woman is likely to have a successful vaginal delivery should she be induced.

A doctor examines a woman's cervix for the following measurements:

- Cervical consistency. (Is the cervix soft, medium, or firm?)
- Position of the cervix as it relates to the vagina. (Is it way the heck in the back, or can it be easily reached?)
- Amount of cervical dilation and effacement. (How thin is it?)
- Station of the presenting part. (Where is the baby's head in relation to specific bones in your pelvis?)

Here's how the scoring works:

Score	Dilatation	Effacement	Station	Position	Consistency
0	Closed	0–30%	-3	Posterior	Firm
1	1–2 cm	40–50%	-2	Mid-position	Moderately firm
2	3–4 cm	60–70%	-1 to 0	Anterior	Soft
3	5 cm or greater	80% or greater	+1 or +2	Anterior	Soft

A point is added to your score for:

- Preeclampsia
- Each prior vaginal delivery

A point is subtracted from the score for:

- Postdate pregnancy
- Nulliparity (never having had a baby before)
- Premature or prolonged rupture of membranes

That is probably more than you ever wanted or needed to know about the Bishop score. But here's the key part: Below is the percentage of pregnant people who end up with a C-section, given a certain Bishop score:

C-Section Frequency Rate, based on Bishop score

Bishop Score	First-Time Delivery	Previous Vaginal Deliveries
0–3	45%	7.7%
4–6	10%	4%
7–10	1.4%	1%

Unless there is an emergency, OB providers generally only attempt induction when a pregnant person has a favorable Bishop score. What is favorable versus unfavorable?

Unfavorable (a score of 5 or less): If you have this score and you need an induction, you would qualify for medication to ripen your cervix (a prostaglandin-based product, such as Cervidil or misoprostol). This helps improve the Bishop score and decreases your risk of having a really long labor and, at some point, needing a C-section.

Favorable (a score of 7 or more): Your cervix is very ripe or "favorable" and there is a high likelihood of having a successful vaginal delivery.[2]

Q. When would an induction take place?

Unless there is a good medical reason, your labor shouldn't be induced before thirty-nine weeks. Why? Sometimes due dates aren't exact and your 38 $3/7$ week baby might really be a thirty-seven week baby who is technically a premature or ***late preterm*** infant. These babies still have risks of having immature lungs, poor sucking technique, low blood sugar, and jaundice. This is not the way to start life if you can avoid it. In fact, ACOG is so serious about this that most hospitals won't allow these "elective" deliveries, even with an ***amniocentesis*** proving that the baby's lungs are mature. The reason? An amnio may prove the lungs are mature, but it doesn't prove that the baby's brain, intestines, and other organs will be ready for prime time.

Q. What are the reasons that I might get induced?

There is a long list of both medical and obstetrical reasons for induction. For some pregnant people, having the baby is safer than continuing the pregnancy. You may be induced if you haven't gone into labor on your own before forty-one or forty-two weeks (***postdates***). You may also be induced if you have a certain medical problem that puts you or your baby at risk if the pregnancy continues.

Here is a list of possible reasons to induce labor. While we haven't included every last possibility, here are the big ones:

Medical Reasons

- Lupus
- Preexisting diabetes
- Preexisting maternal kidney disease
- Preexisting maternal high blood pressure

- Preexisting chronic lung disease
- Severe depression, anxiety, or other psychiatric conditions

Obstetrical Reasons

- Too little ***amniotic fluid (oligohydramnios)***
- High blood pressure of pregnancy (***preeclampsia*** and ***eclampsia***)
- Syndrome of high blood pressure, blood cell and liver abnormalities (***HELLP syndrome***)
- Certain types of gestational diabetes
- Pregnancy goes beyond forty-one weeks (***postdates*** or ***post-term pregnancy***)
- Water bag breaks prematurely (***premature rupture of membranes***)
- Some cases where the placenta has begun to separate from the wall of the uterus (***placental abruption***)
- Certain maternal infections (for example, ***chorioamnionitis***)
- Severe fetal growth restriction
- Complications due to Rh blood type incompatibility (***Rh incompatibility***)
- Non-reassuring non-stress test (docs are concerned about abnormalities of the baby's heart rate detected on a monitor)
- Placental dysfunction
- Pregnancy-related liver problems (***cholestasis of pregnancy*** and ***acute fatty liver***)
- Severe pregnancy-related skin problem (such as ***PUPPS***)

Other Reasons

- You live a far distance from the hospital.
- You have had rapid labors with prior pregnancies.

Remember to check the glossary in the back of the book for an explanation of all these technical terms.

Q. What does it mean when someone gets induced?

It means you put someone into labor who previously was not in labor.

If you and your OB provider decide that it is time to schedule an induction, you set up an appointment at the hospital.

Yep, it's just like scheduling a haircut, except that the times may not be quite so ideal.

Occasionally, your OB provider detects something at an office visit that requires immediate induction (like severe high blood pressure or too little amniotic fluid). You might have to head straight over to the hospital or you may get the green light to run home quickly to grab your stuff first. Unlike your hairdresser, the hospital *will* take you if there is an emergency!

You will get admitted to the hospital and be evaluated in the same manner as if you went into labor on your own. Then, if your cervix is not ready or ripe (see the New

Parent-to-Be 411 box on the Bishop Score on page 316), you will get medication to ripen it.

Next, you get another medication, called Pitocin (see the following Q&A), through an IV to get labor started. We'll cover the details on how this all works in Chapter 14, "Labor Day."

> FEEDBACK FROM THE REAL WORLD:
>
> **Induction Times**
>
> At the hospital where I practice, induction times are as follows: eight a.m., ten a.m., eight p.m., ten p.m., midnight, two a.m., and four a.m. You can imagine how the woman getting induced at two or four a.m. feels! As awful as it is, inductions are scheduled at most busy hospitals during very odd hours. The reason is that the day is filled with other scheduled surgeries and procedures, like C-sections and external cephalic versions, as well as everyone who walks in the door in labor. To avoid staffing issues and to make sure that inductions aren't constantly delayed and canceled, they are often done at night.

Q. What medications are used to induce labor?

Doctors use two different types of medications:

1. **Prostaglandins.** Prostaglandin is a natural agent your body makes that softens the cervix during labor. (If you recall from Chapter 9, "Lifestyles," men also secrete prostaglandins with their sperm in their ejaculate.) For an induction, doctors will sometimes use prostaglandin medication placed directly near the cervix to achieve the same results for pregnant people with an unfavorable or unripe cervix.
    - Cytotec (misoprostol) is a prostaglandin made into a pill. It is placed near the cervix via a vaginal exam and dissolves over time.
    - Cervidil is a prostaglandin in a mesh-like preparation that is placed near the cervix (also with a vaginal exam—let the good times roll!) and removed after twelve hours.
2. **Oxytocin.** Oxytocin is a naturally occurring hormone made in the pituitary gland of your brain that causes uterine contractions and starts labor. Pitocin is the brand name of the synthetically made form of oxytocin used to stimulate contractions if your cervix is ripe. You get this medication through an IV. Your OB provider controls the amount of medication you get because the IV is connected to a pump. You usually start off with a small dose, then your OB provider increases the amount gradually until you reach a desired contraction pattern (usually that means until you are having contractions two to three and a half minutes apart). The amount you will need and for how long you will need it depends on how responsive your uterus is to the drug, what your Bishop score is prior to needing it, and how well your baby is tolerating labor. Some

people need very little, and others need a lot. The goal here is to give you just enough so that you have a contraction pattern that allows your cervix to dilate and your baby's head to descend. Likewise, doctors want to avoid giving you too much, to avoid contractions that are too frequent or last too long. While you are on oxytocin, you are continuously monitored so that your OB provider can keep tabs on both your contraction pattern and the well-being of your little one.

We'll give you more info on Pitocin in Chapter 14, "Labor Day."

Q. Will my doctor break my water bag during an induction?

Probably.

In addition to medication, your OB provider may also decide to perform an ***amniotomy*** (that's a fancy word for breaking your water bag).

Doctors use a nifty little instrument that looks a lot like a crochet hook. We sneak it up along our fingers, which are sitting in the cervix, hook the amniotic sac, and rupture it. It doesn't hurt you any more than the discomfort of having your cervix examined. And it doesn't hurt the baby at all.

This will release prostaglandins that help ripen the cervix. Most people notice a dramatic change in the intensity of their contractions after their water bag breaks.

Q. I've heard about a balloon that can be used. Do I really need that?

It depends. It's called an intracervical balloon, and it's basically the same balloon attached to a catheter that can be used to drain urine from your bladder.

The tip of the catheter (with the balloon deflated at this point) is placed into the cervix that is dilated at least ½ cm. It is held there while the balloon is inflated with saline. It is then taped to your leg to help hold it in place. Once this balloon falls out, your cervix is usually already 2–3 cm dilated.

The balloon is used to help decrease the time that a woman is in the latent or early phase of labor, and it really does work.

A few things to know:

1. It can be painful for some people, so some patients opt to get an epidural or have pain medication prior to the balloon insertion.
2. It isn't used in everyone. If you are more than 2 cm dilated, a balloon is usually not needed.
3. Talk to your doc about this if you have any concerns. I often find that many patients have gotten conflicting information from friends and family members, and many rumors can be dispelled with a simple conversation with your OB provider.

Q. My doctor said he could "sweep my membranes" to help get me into labor. I'm not sure what this means or if it will hurt. What will they do?

That term is just awful, isn't it? It is also sometimes referred to as "stripping the membranes," but that doesn't sound much better.

Despite the inelegant word choice, it definitely describes what doctors can do. Yes, it's uncomfortable. And yes, it might jump-start your labor.

Sweeping or stripping the membranes is done in term or post-term pregnancies, usually in your OB provider's office. To sweep your membranes, your OB provider checks your cervix with a gloved finger. Next, they will place their finger through your cervix and sweep it between your amniotic sac (water bag) and the wall of your uterus. You may feel some intense cramping like period cramps.

This causes your body to release prostaglandins, which help to soften the cervix and may cause contractions. There is no guarantee, though, that stripping your membranes will lead to labor. It's common to have spotting for up to a day or two afterward. If bleeding becomes heavier than this, call your doctor.

Q. I've heard inductions hurt a lot more. Is that true?

Yes and no.

The main difference between an induction and going into labor on your own is how rapidly your contractions start.

If you go into labor on your own, your body may start having irregular contractions over a period of days that slowly get stronger and closer together. You have some time to get used to the pain of the contractions as they slowly increase in intensity.

With an induction, those same contractions occur, but your doc or midwife is making them come on more quickly. The strength of each contraction is not necessarily stronger with Pitocin versus the natural oxytocin that your body makes, but you will experience the contractions in a much more condensed time frame.

Q. What are the risks involved with inducing labor?

The most common problem (which is rare) is that the medication used for an induction overstimulates the uterus, causing it to contract too frequently.

Overall, the risk of anything happening from the use of Pitocin is very low. But overstimulation of the uterus means that too many contractions occur at intervals that are too close together. The uterine muscle has no time to relax between contractions. This can decrease the amount of blood flow to baby, causing a drop in baby's heart rate. If this happens, your OB provider can lower the dose or stop the Pitocin, and the effects wear off very quickly. If the baby recovers well, your OB provider will restart the Pitocin at a lower dose.

If the baby cannot tolerate the stress of the contractions and their heart rate pattern becomes concerning, a ***cesarean section*** is in order. Note: Your OB provider should be knowledgeable about Pitocin and should be monitoring you closely during the induction to modify the dosing, if necessary.

Like any other medication, misuse of Pitocin can cause some pretty nasty complications—which is why you want a skilled OB provider using it. But diligent and judicious use of Pitocin is a safe and effective way of inducing and augmenting labor.

INSIDER SECRET:

Self-Induced Labor?

You've probably heard it all by now, those wacky off-the-wall ideas to induce labor. Eating Thai food, taking an invigorating walk, having a salad drenched in balsamic vinegar. Or standing on your head while chewing the root of a rare lemongrass found only in the Himalayas (okay, kidding on the last one).

Can anything actually make you go into labor besides Mother Nature? Answer: Nothing is a sure thing, but you can certainly try.

If you are a heterosexual couple, you have a source of natural prostaglandin—in your partner's semen. Prostaglandin is the ingredient in many of our induction agents, and when it comes in contact with a cervix that's ready, it may induce labor. (That's the reason that "pelvic rest" is recommended for pregnant people who are at risk for preterm labor.)

Nipple stimulation is another technique that almost always causes uterine contractions. It releases oxytocin, the body's natural Pitocin and stimulant of uterine contractions. In fact, prior to the widespread use of Pitocin, doctors used nipple stimulation to induce labor and evaluate a baby's heart rate pattern during these contractions. Today, however, nipple stimulation is never recommended as a way to put yourself into labor.

As uncomfortable as you are (and we've been there, trust us), you should wait for your labor to begin naturally or talk to your OB provider about an induction.

Fact Check

More deliveries happen during a full moon or changes in barometric pressure.

The truth: Does a full moon's gravitational pull affect amniotic fluid in much the same way it affects ocean tides? There have never been any studies on whether this is true or not, but it's hard to believe that the moon affects the small amount of water surrounding the baby in the same way as tides in the Atlantic Ocean.

There certainly are more visits to labor and delivery units during a full moon—but it's unclear why this happens. And these visits do not translate into more babies being born under a full moon. Many people are sent home after their contractions subside without any dilation of the cervix.

C-Sections

Q. I'd love to have a C-section and get this all over with. How do you feel about elective C-sections?

The official name for this is *primary elective cesarean section*. It means this will be your first C-section, and you are requesting one without a real medical or obstetric reason.

DR. M'S OPINION:

Elective C-Sections

I think that primary elective C-sections can and should be performed for patients upon request in certain circumstances. I say that with a caveat: They should *only* be performed if the patient is well informed. What is well-informed? This means that the OB provider has discussed the potential risks, benefits, and alternatives with the patient and their partner; there was ample opportunity for questions to be asked and answered; and the patient still desires to proceed.

Elective C-sections have been trendy in the United States for the past five to ten years. The C-section rate in the United States increased dramatically from 5 percent in 1970 to 32.3 percent in 2023.[3] In fact, 2 to 4 percent of all US deliveries are primary elective C-sections.[4] Some countries, like Brazil, deliver between 50 and 85 percent of their babies by elective C-section for "perineal preservation" (keeping the vagina and surrounding tissues intact).[5]

Why would you want one? Some people are afraid of labor and a vaginal delivery. There is fear of pain, or that your genital area will never be the same, or that you'll be incontinent as a result and won't ever be able to run or jump on the trampoline with your kids again. Others just fear being in labor for hours and then needing a C-section anyway.

And elective C-sections are certainly convenient. They can be scheduled on a specific date, and you can have everything taken care of at home. It's also true that there is no risk of vaginal or anal tearing.

However, let's be clear here—it is *major* surgery and there are risks. As with any surgery, you face a risk of infection. Additionally, you're at risk for excessive bleeding after delivery (postpartum hemorrhage) and possible injury to surrounding body organs like the bladder, ureters, and intestines during surgery.

On top of that, your baby faces the small risk of having difficulty breathing at birth, which sometimes requires admission to the neonatal intensive care unit (NICU). When a baby is delivered by C-section and does not squeeze through the birth canal, they may have some residual amniotic fluid in their lungs at birth that has to be cleared out (***transient tachypnea of the newborn*** or ***TTN***).

We don't point these things out to scare you, but the truth is C-sections are not risk-free, and the decision to perform one shouldn't be taken lightly.

Here are some things to keep in mind if you are considering an elective C-section:

- Sit down with your partner and your doctor and make a list of all the potential risks and benefits so that you can make the best decision for you.
- Your doctor will consider your age, ***body mass index***, accuracy of estimated gestational age, future reproductive plans, personal values, and cultural context before advising you.
- If you understand all the risks and benefits of each mode of delivery, and there are no absolute reasons not to have a C-section, most American doctors will perform elective C-sections.

Your baby should not be delivered electively prior to thirty-nine weeks, period. And most US doctors as well as hospitals won't allow this.

Q. My doctor said they will do an elective C-section. How will this affect any future pregnancies I may have?

If you decide to have an elective C-section this time around, odds are any future babies you have will also be delivered by C-section.

Each c-section that you have increases the risk of having a ***placenta previa***, ***placenta accreta/increta/percreta***, and ***uterine rupture*** (see Chapter 17, "The Complicated Pregnancy," Complications #37 and #39). It also increases the possibility of a postpartum hysterectomy. Because of this, no one recommends elective C-sections for people who plan to have many children ("many" is hard to quantify, but certainly more than three).[6]

INSIDER SECRET:

Risks and Benefits of Primary Elective C-Sections

Interestingly, a panel of medical experts recently compared the risks and benefits of primary elective C-sections and normal vaginal deliveries and concluded that the information to date "does not provide the basis for a recommendation for either mode of delivery."[7]

And surprisingly, there was *no difference* in complication rates between the two types of delivery.

As OB-GYNs, we recognize that more research needs to be done. But what do we know about primary elective C-sections from the limited studies that we have? Here are the risks and benefits to both mom and baby:

Maternal Risks

- Longer hospital stay
- Higher risk of anesthetic complications
- Greater complications in future deliveries
- Increased risk of inadvertent injury to adjacent organs, such as the bladder and intestines
- Increased need for hysterectomy to stop excessive bleeding (surgical removal of the uterus)
- Increased risk of significant blood accumulation in the wound
- Increased risk of blood clots that can lead to death[8]
- Increased risk of heart attack after delivery

Q. I'd really like to deliver vaginally and not have a C-section. Is there anything I can do to prevent this from happening?

This is how most people feel. Although a few people would prefer to have an elective C-section, most would rather avoid it if possible.

There are a few cases where a C-section is planned for a medical or obstetric reason. For instance, you need a C-section if your baby is positioned to exit butt or foot first (***breech***) or your placenta is lying directly over your cervix (***placenta previa***).

Of course, even if you don't *plan* for a C-section, one might be recommended during delivery. Hence, you go into labor expecting to have a vaginal delivery and some situation arises where your doctor recommends a C-section (see box on next page). These are most often unpreventable.

Occasionally, a baby is too big to fit through a woman's pelvis—this happens sometimes because baby's head is too big or the pelvis is too small. The size of a baby can be hereditary (if you were a large baby, you will likely have a large baby), but it can also be due to excessive weight gain during pregnancy or uncontrolled dia-

Maternal Benefits

- Decreased risk of significant bleeding after delivery (***postpartum hemorrhage***) that might require a blood transfusion
- Fewer wetting accidents (***urinary incontinence***) during the first year after surgery

Fetal Risks

- Longer hospital stay if your baby has breathing problems at birth
- Increased risk of breathing difficulties at birth if delivery is earlier than thirty-nine weeks of gestation
- For infants delivered before thirty-nine weeks of gestation: increased rate of prematurity complications such as breathing difficulties, low blood sugar, and difficulty maintaining body temperature that require admission to the neonatal ICU (NICU)
- Risk of accidentally cutting the baby (fetal laceration). Although it only happens 0.8 percent of the time, yes, it's possible to accidentally superficially cut part of the baby when making the incision in the uterus.

Fetal Benefits

- Lower risk of fetal death
- Lower newborn infection rate
- Reduced risk of bleeding inside the skull
- Reduced risk of lack of oxygen at birth and brain damage
- Fewer birth injuries, such as injury to the nerves supplying the shoulder, arm, and hand (***brachial plexus injuries***)

betes. Keeping your weight gain in the appropriate range and your blood sugar under control, if you are diabetic, can lower your chances of having a C-section.

Your doctor doesn't want to do a C-section, either, if they can avoid it. But docs cannot always predict what happens during labor. If your doctor says the baby won't fit or is concerned about the baby's heart rate (and therefore is concerned about the amount of oxygen reaching the baby's brain) then a cesarean delivery is the best thing for you and your baby.

BOTTOM LINE: Be an informed patient and trust your OB provider. Ask questions and make sure you understand your OB provider's recommendations, including current and future implications.

Q. What's the difference between a planned or scheduled C-section versus an unplanned or emergency C-section?

A scheduled C-section occurs when you know in advance that you or your baby has an issue requiring a C-section or you are deciding to have an elective C-section. In

NEW PARENT-TO-BE 411:

Reasons You Might Need a C-Section

1. Baby is in a position that is dangerous to deliver vaginally (***breech*** or ***transverse***)
2. Some types of twins (if one or both twins are in breech or transverse position)
3. Triplets or anything greater
4. Certain fetal abnormalities/birth defects
5. Placenta lies over the cervix (***placenta previa***)
6. Abnormal placenta (***placenta accreta, placenta increta, placenta percreta***)
7. Abnormal uterus (***bicornuate uterus***, ***uterine didelphys***)
8. Previous C-section with a vertical uterine incision (often done when delivering preterm babies)
9. Previous surgery performed to remove ***uterine fibroids*** (some but not all require future C-sections)
10. Estimated baby weight over ten pounds
11. Significant tear in the genital area (fourth-degree laceration) during previous delivery
12. History of a baby's shoulder getting severely stuck (***shoulder dystocia***) during a previous delivery
13. Mother has a medical condition that makes vaginal delivery too risky

most cases, you will have adequate time to talk with your doctor about everything it entails and to go over the risks, benefits, and alternatives.

Unplanned or emergency C-sections happen when a vaginal delivery was otherwise planned for or was already in progress. Some condition then arises (see list below) requiring a C-section for a safe delivery. These are often heat-of-the-moment decisions and depending on the condition may involve quick movement into the operating room (like what you see in the movies).

Q. When would a scheduled C-section take place?

As with an induction, the magic number for having a scheduled C-section is thirty-nine weeks. At any point before thirty-nine weeks, your doctor must have a medical or obstetric indication to justify delivery.

A baby born between thirty-seven and thirty-eight weeks has between a ten and twenty-six times greater risk of having immature lungs at birth compared to babies born between thirty-nine and forty-one weeks.[9]

We should point out here that you do not need to have an amniocentesis to deliver prior to thirty-nine weeks if you are being delivered for a serious medical or obstetri-

Unplanned/Emergency Section

1. Baby is too big to get through the birth canal (***cephalopelvic disproportion***)
2. Fetal distress/non-reassuring fetal heart rate. If your baby is at risk and you are not close to delivering, a C-section is needed
3. Labor stops. Either you stop dilating or your baby's head stops descending through the birth canal (***failure to progress***).
4. Severely elevated blood pressure with or without seizures or blood cell/liver abnormalities (***preeclampsia, eclampsia, HELLP syndrome***) and delivery is not imminent
5. Failed attempt at a vaginal delivery using a vacuum or forceps
6. Placenta starts to tear away from the wall of the uterus before delivery (***placental abruption***)
7. Umbilical cord slips out of the vagina after the water breaks and before delivery (***umbilical cord prolapse***)
8. ***Uterine rupture***
9. Umbilical cord vessels or placental blood vessels lie over the cervix (***vasa previa***)
10. Baby is breech, but it was not diagnosed before labor. Yes, it happens.

See Chapter 17, "The Complicated Pregnancy," for details on all of these situations.

INSIDER SECRET:

A Look into Emergency C-Sections

An emergency C-section can often be very scary for both the person in labor and their partner. While this is a rare event, we want you to be prepared. That's why you are reading it here before you go into labor.

Here is an emergency C-section scenario: Monitors detect that the fetal heart rate is dropping. Many nurses and doctors and other hospital personnel enter the delivery room, attempting to help increase the fetal heart rate. This may include changing your position, turning off your Pitocin (if you are receiving some), placing an oxygen mask over your face (it will smell like plastic), giving you intravenous medication (if indicated), and performing a vaginal exam.

If they are unsuccessful, all of these people (and about twenty more!) rush you into the operating room. Many monitors are placed on your arms and chest, people are moving around at lightning speed, and yelling orders left and right—there's a lot of commotion! I warn my patients that it will be a zoo, and it will be scary. I ask them to try to keep calm, trust us, and let us do what we need to do to get their baby out as quickly as possible. If a baby's heart rate is low enough to cause concern, we know there is less oxygen getting to their brain. We know that baby's life and health depends on a rapid delivery. That's why everyone is moving so quickly to help get your baby out.

Remember, no one can predict what will happen in labor. In fact, it's a common saying among obstetricians and midwives that the most predictable thing about labor is that it's unpredictable! Although this situation rarely arises, it is important to trust the decisions made by your delivery team to ensure the delivery of a healthy baby.

cal reason, such as severe preeclampsia at thirty-five weeks. The risk to the mom and baby are greater if the baby stays in versus coming out a little premature.

Q. My doctor and I have decided that it's best for me to have a repeat C-section for my second delivery. Is there anything I should think about?

Yes, there are a few things to keep in mind. First, there is likely some scar tissue that formed as you healed from your first C-section. Scar tissue forms in everyone in varying degrees after any surgery. As doctors, we never know how much until we go back in a subsequent time. So, if you have a lot of scar tissue, the surgery may take a little longer. When scar tissue replaces normal tissue planes, and anatomic structures aren't in their normal positions, docs have to be very careful and operate more slowly to make sure we are in the right area.

The good news regarding scar tissue is that it does not have nerve endings, and what that usually means is that your postoperative pain tends to be less the second, third, and fourth time around.

Something else to think about is that you already have a child at home and you will now have a newborn. Moving around for the first two weeks is slow. Make sure you have help—your partner, a parent or two, siblings, friends, or a postpartum doula or nurse.

Vaginal Birth After Cesarean (VBAC)

Q. I had a C-section with my first pregnancy. Will I be able to deliver vaginally this time?

The answer is not straightforward. It depends on whether your doctor performs ***VBACs*** (vaginal births after cesarean sections), whether the hospital where they deliver allows them, and what type of uterine scar you have.

There are two main types of C-section incisions: *low-transverse* and *vertical* (also known as *classical*). The names describe the type of incision that is made on the uterus (not the outer cut on your skin, but the one on the *inside*, on your uterus).

Most C-sections (over 95 percent) are of the low-transverse type. Classical or vertical incisions are rare and are mostly done to deliver a very premature infant.

If you used a different OB provider with your previous delivery, and particularly if your delivery was in another country or wasn't straightforward, you'll need your medical records since the doctor's operative notes describe which type of incision you had.

If you had a vertical incision, you cannot have a subsequent vaginal birth. That's because you have a 4 to 9 percent risk of ***uterine rupture*** (where the scar bursts open during labor). This is a risk that obstetricians and ACOG are not willing to take, as it can be catastrophic.

If you had a low-transverse incision, it may be possible for you to have a VBAC. The risk of uterine rupture after only *one* previous low-transverse C-section is much lower—between 0.7 and 0.8 percent.

Reality Check

Many hospitals and physicians stopped allowing VBACs in 2002. VBAC rates started to decline in the mid-1990s and continued sharply into the 2000s, mainly secondary to the new ACOG guidelines at the time and growing concern with liability. Specifically in 1999, ACOG altered its guidelines to be more restrictive. It aimed to manage the risks associated with VBACs and required immediate availability of medical personnel and facilities for emergency C-sections. It also required that any given hospital performing VBACs have an OB-GYN on hand, which disallowed many ***community hospitals*** from doing them.

Q. I'm worried that even if I decide to have a VBAC the second time, I will end up with a C-section again anyway. What are my chances of having the baby vaginally?

If you look at the studies, you have a 60 to 80 percent chance of success.

The problem is that we cannot reliably predict how any one individual patient will do, but we are able to give you a reasonable guess when we look at all factors unique to you, including ethnicity, age, BMI, history of vaginal delivery, indication for your prior C-section, and whether you have a history of a VBAC.[10]

In general, if you had your first C-section for a specific reason that tends not to reoccur with a subsequent pregnancy (such as a breech baby or a non-reassuring fetal heart pattern), you're more likely to have a successful vaginal delivery (between 75 to 86 percent).

If you had your first C-section because you stopped dilating or your baby's head was too big to fit through your pelvis, your success rate is lower (50 to 80 percent).[11,12] Talk to your doctor about your wishes and to get their recommendation.

NEW PARENT-TO-BE 411:

No VBACs allowed

There are certain women who should absolutely not have a vaginal delivery because of the high risk for uterine rupture.

You are a high-risk person if you have a previous classical or T-shaped uterine scar, previous uterine rupture, or two or more previous uterine scars.

Also, you can only have a VBAC delivery at a hospital—no home births, birthing centers, etc. That's because if you run into any complications, you need immediate access to an operating room and personnel capable of performing an emergency C-section. That's why home births are a no-go in this scenario.

VBACs are also off the table if a complication arises that requires a C-section—like a placenta previa or a breech baby.

General Concerns

Q. Should my partner come to my appointments in the final weeks?

Your partner can join you at any and all office visits. Ask your OB provider if they feel there are any "not-to-be-missed" appointments on the horizon.

Q. I am delivering at a teaching hospital, and I don't want an intern examining me while twenty other folks look on. Is there a way to ensure crowd control?

Every teaching hospital is different.

If this is an important issue, you should discuss your concerns with your OB early on in your pregnancy. And remember that this is *your* birth experience. If you absolutely do not want medical students or residents in the room, it is your right to say so.

You can decide how many people are in there (you won't care at a certain point—trust us)—whether it's just one additional intern or enough to require stadium seating.

DR. M'S OPINION:

Preparing for Delivery!

In my practice, I strongly recommend that partners are present for the thirty-four- to thirty-six-week visit because after the routine exam, I take couples into my office and go over what they need to know about labor and delivery.

This includes when to call, where to call, what labor feels like, when to go to the hospital (and where to park!), when I show up, my philosophies on fetal monitoring, augmenting labor with Pitocin, epidural/pain control, vacuum/forceps delivery, and C-sections. We also discuss episiotomies and our overall attempt to avoid them. You should be with an OB provider who wants you to have the day ***you*** desire. I tell my patients that I had my labors the way I chose, and my goal is for them to have the same. So we discuss "birth preferences" and why we would change course if need be as labor begins and progresses.

This visit also gives my patients a chance to ask other questions about what they may or may not want in labor, what to pack in their bag, how many family members/friends can be in the room, etc. And it's my chance to remind them about choosing a pediatrician, cord blood banking if they choose to do so, making a decision on circumcision, and having a properly installed car seat ready to go.

Talk to your doctor about the kind of hospital they practice in, teaching or non-teaching, and discuss your concerns.

Q. When does the baby "drop" in preparation for delivery?

The fetus is basically swimming around until about thirty-three weeks, when they move to a head-down position (***vertex***).

But even once they move into this position, their head may still be "floating" in the pelvis, meaning that it has not dropped. Your friends (who are intensely watching your belly) may tell you that once the baby drops, your labor is imminent. That's not necessarily true.

Some babies may not drop until actual labor begins, especially with second and third pregnancies. Other babies may start heading into the pelvis as early as thirty-five weeks.

Q. I had a very large baby with my first pregnancy. What are the odds that I'll have another big kid with this pregnancy?

You and your OB provider are visiting on a weekly basis now. Since they are measuring you every week, you both are probably taking bets on how big your baby will be.

If you had a large baby the first time, the odds are pretty darn good that you will have another big baby. Specifically, if you had a baby that was over 4,000 grams (eight and a half pounds) the first time, you are five to ten times more likely to deliver a baby greater than 4,500 grams (almost ten pounds) the second time around. This is compared to women who have had smaller babies.[13]

Second and third babies tend to be larger than first babies, and boys tend to be larger than girls.

Finally, your own birth weight is a predictor of your newborn's birth weight. If you were a big baby, there's not a whole lot you can do to change your baby's fate.

Q. I've heard that massaging my genital area (perineum) once a week in the last month of my pregnancy will help prevent tearing or the need for an episiotomy. Is this true?

Although the theory on this topic used to be that it wasn't helpful, we now believe that starting perineal massage (or massaging the tissue at the opening of the vagina and in between the vagina and rectum) between thirty-four and thirty-five weeks can help quite a bit during delivery. First, it can increase the pliability of the tissue (stretchiness) which can then minimize tearing. Most OB providers don't cut episiotomies anymore except on rare occasion, so having tissue that stretches better allows the fetal head to do less damage on its way out and this minimizes tearing. Most pelvic floor physical therapists recommend doing this and can be great resources for learning how.

Q. This is my second baby, I'm at thirty-seven weeks and already dilated 3 cm. Will I go into labor before forty weeks?

It's pretty common for women who have already had a baby before to be sitting around with a dilated cervix. Your body knows what to do, and that is one of the reasons that second and third labors are so much quicker, on average.

You do not need to race home, pack a bag, and head over to the hospital if your OB provider tells you that you are three or four centimeters. In fact, many pregnant people with prior deliveries, and even a few who haven't had a baby before, walk around for weeks at three to four centimeters without having regular contractions and don't even know it.

Q. How will I know I am really in labor versus having false contractions?

Braxton-Hicks (BH) refer to "practice contractions," and they occur at various times during pregnancy, but can increase in intensity during your last month, especially if this isn't your first baby.

They happen at random, often in the middle of the night, and are associated with a hardening or tightening of your belly. Some women do experience mild menstrual-like cramping associated with Braxton-Hicks, but typically, they are not very painful.

The most important difference between ***Braxton-Hicks contractions*** and real labor contractions is that BH contractions do not dilate the cervix and real contractions do.

Real labor contractions are *painful*. They often have a pattern to them, so, for example, they will begin at intervals of twenty minutes apart and gradually shorten—becoming ten, seven, and then five minutes apart. They are often, but not always, accompanied by an increase in mucous discharge and sometimes, bloody show. And they only last for about a minute or a minute and a half. Braxton-Hicks contractions can last for much longer, sometimes even up to thirty minutes.

Reality Check

People who have given birth before start having contractions earlier in their subsequent pregnancies and have them more often than those who've never given birth. By the time you are on your third or fourth pregnancy (if you are one of the brave), you are having so many Braxton-Hicks that you feel like you will be delivering in your kitchen!

DR. M'S OPINION:

How to Tell the Difference

Real contractions hurt. I have only had one patient in fourteen years who felt like she was having some mild stomach discomfort and was actually nine centimeters dilated! We all want to be that woman (believe me, I prayed for it every night starting at about twenty-six weeks in my own pregnancies), but in reality, 99.9 percent of us will feel labor when it happens.

NEW PARENT-TO-BE 411:

True Labor Versus False Labor

True Labor

- Contractions occur at regular intervals
- Contraction intensity and discomfort gradually increases
- Intervals between contractions gradually decrease
- Discomfort occurs in the lower back and abdomen
- May be accompanied by increased vaginal discharge or bloody show
- Contractions cause cervical dilation
- Contractions do not stop with rest, hydration, or medication

False Labor

- Contractions occur at irregular intervals
- Contraction intensity and discomfort remain unchanged
- Intervals between contractions remain long
- Discomfort is mainly in the lower abdomen, or no discomfort other than tightening
- No accompanying bloody show
- The cervix does not dilate
- Discomfort from contractions is relieved by rest and medication

Q. When do I call my doctor?

All physicians do things a little differently. Find out what *your* doctor wants you to do and when they want to be called. As an OB, here is what I tell my patients:

- **If you are beyond thirty-five weeks:** Call when contractions are consistently five minutes apart for two hours.
- **If you are less than thirty-five weeks:** Call if you have more than four to six contractions in an hour and they do not resolve with rest and drinking lots of water.
- **If your water breaks:** This is not usually the first sign of labor. Your water bag most often breaks after you have been contracting for a while. Alternatively, your doctor might break it for you at the hospital. If it does break, it's not always like the movies, where you are mulling over peas in the frozen foods aisle, and suddenly you are standing in Niagara Falls. Often it's just a leak that doesn't stop or a constant sense of wetness. Call your OB provider for this one, no matter how far along you are in your pregnancy.
- **If you have vaginal bleeding:** A little bit of spotting (pinkish or brownish discharge) is okay as your pregnancy comes to an end, especially if you have had recent intercourse or your OB provider has recently checked your cervix. Anything more than spotting and anything bright red deserves a phone call to your doc. And any bleeding at all during a high-risk pregnancy (preterm labor or placenta previa, for example) should be discussed with your OB provider as well.
- **Decreased fetal movement:** Monitor your baby's daily movements. In the final weeks of pregnancy, your baby's movements will be smoother and less noticeable than those jolting kicks in the second trimester (because your baby has less space to move around). But you still need to feel them. Call your OB provider if you detect fewer movements.

Partner Tip

When you call the OB (you are likely making the call because your partner is so uncomfortable she wants to die), keep your cool, and stick to the facts. We know you haven't been sleeping, and you're nervous/excited/full of adrenaline about what's to come.

I'll be very honest here. When docs get that phone call in the middle of the night, it often wakes us out of a deep sleep. It takes us a few moments to get focused. It's hard to follow someone talking at an auctioneer's pace and going into excruciating detail about how the new chair is ruined because of the bloody show all over it.

My personal favorite example is a patient's husband (who I love dearly after going through two pregnancies with him). He gave me an in-depth rundown on the contraction pattern like a football game commentary. I listened patiently (at four a.m.) for over four minutes as he told me about the timing and length of each contraction from start to finish, the intensity of each, what his wife was doing during each contraction, what she ate for dinner, and finally what she threw up! I still give him a hard time about this, and we always have a good laugh.

BOTTOM LINE: Keep it simple. Here's an example: "Hi, Dr. M. It's Paul Smith, Sarah's husband. She has been contracting every five minutes for about three hours, is having some bloody discharge, and is really uncomfortable. We'd like to go to the hospital now." That's perfect. It's easy for us to understand, sticks to the facts, and allows our sleepy brains to get a handle on the situation.

Q. My mother had very quick deliveries. I don't want to deliver on the highway. Are my chances any greater with my mom's history?

Let's start with a definition of "very quick deliveries" or in technical terms, a ***precipitous labor***. That's a labor that lasts less than three hours from start to finish.

While there aren't any firm stats on this, it happens in about 2 of every 100 births.

It's more likely to naturally happen if you have delivered a baby before because your first baby paves the way for the next one. Or you've had a prior precipitous delivery. Or you have a large pelvis. Or you have a well-positioned and smaller than average baby. It can also happen artificially if you receive too much Pitocin or use cocaine.

I hate to disappoint you, but it's a myth that labor patterns run in families. (Especially if your mom told you she had quick, easy deliveries!) It's true, though, that you may inherit the shape of your pelvis (aka "good birthing hips") from your mom, which can be a positive.

But you have to factor several other variables that affect the ease or difficulty of labor and delivery. For instance, you might want to see if your hubby has a big head (literally)—and then pray, for delivery sake, your baby doesn't inherit that trait!

Partner Tip

If you aren't taking a childbirth class at the hospital where you are delivering, be sure to know where to go when your partner begins labor. Arrange to take a tour or do a practice run, so you know where to park and where to go at two a.m.

Q. Do tall people have easier deliveries than short people?

Yes. People less than five feet tall (especially those who have never given birth before) have twice the risk of having a C-section. Why? That's often due to the baby's head being too big to fit through the woman's pelvic bones (***cephalopelvic disproportion***).

The C-section rate *increases* as the pregnant person's height *decreases*—maxing out at 30 percent of people who are under four feet, six inches tall.

If you have normal stature or are just slightly smaller than average, you don't have any higher risk of a complicated delivery. And if you were teased in high school for being head and shoulders above your classmates, you can now thank (instead of curse) your parents' genes. They may just make your labor easier.[14]

INSIDER SECRET:

The Top Thirteen Fears About Labor—And How to Defeat Them

From the home office in Beverly Hills, California, we present the top thirteen fears about labor:

13. I want a natural childbirth, and I'll end up with a C-section.
12. I'll be in pain, and it will be too late to get pain medication.
11. Something bad will happen to the baby.
10. Something bad will happen to me.
9. There will be horrible traffic on the highway, and I'll deliver in my car.
8. I won't know what contractions will feel like or when I'm really in labor.
7. I'll never deliver, and I'll be pregnant forever.
6. My body will never be the same after this.
5. I'll never want to have another baby after I deliver this one.
4. My doctor will be in Jamaica when I go into labor.
3. If my partner sees anything down below, they will never want to be intimate with me again.
2. My epidural won't work; I will have chronic back pain or be paralyzed after receiving one.
1. I will poop during my delivery.

How can you ease your fears? Educate yourself! Read books, watch videos, take a childbirth class, and talk to your doctor/midwife/doula.

You have to feel comfortable asking your OB provider about your concerns and anxieties. This is the whole reason for choosing an OB provider that you love and trust.

Of course, it's normal to have these thoughts run through your head in the middle of the night when you get up to pee, keeping you from going back to sleep. Your brain will rest easier if you get these questions answered. (Of course, the disrupted sleep patterns are still out of our control.)

Wondering about your pain medication options? We discuss all pain medications in Chapter 14, "Labor Day." It will help you know what your options are.

Q. When should I pack a bag for the hospital, and what should go in it?

Pack it up at between thirty-three and thirty-four weeks.

And keep it light—it's not like you're going to summer camp for a month. Your partner (or whomever is staying with you at the hospital) should pack a bag, too.

Yes, this seems early, but if you pack now, you won't have to panic if you break your water bag at two a.m. when you are thirty-five weeks.

Keep items you will need during labor separate from things you'll need while you recover. Here's a packing list:

- **Your own toiletries.** Bring toothbrush, toothpaste, shampoo, conditioner, face soap, face lotion, and lip balm (this is a lifesaver during labor!).
- **A robe.** You can also bring your own PJs to sleep in after delivery is over. You'll wear a hospital gown during labor and occasionally the first day or two postpartum.
- **Hair ties.** A vaginal delivery is often long, and there can be vomiting, sweating, and crying. Having hair in your face during any of these situations is less than ideal. During a C-section, your hair will be under a surgical cap (like we all wear in the OR), and it's easier to keep it tucked in when it's first pulled back with a hair tie.
- **Socks for labor and slippers or flip-flops for afterward.** Socks are cozy and help people feel warmer in the often chilly rooms. Many women get more swollen after delivery, and flip-flops may be the only shoes that fit! You are also getting up and down quite a bit from your bed to lift, feed, and change your baby, and flip-flops are the easiest thing to get on and off quickly.
- **An outfit to go home in.** Select a comfy maternity outfit because your baby bump won't disappear for several months.
- **An outfit for the baby to go home in.** A two-piece outfit is better since the baby will have their umbilical stump for a couple of weeks or so. One-piece outfits or "onesies" can rub on the stump.
- **Food and drink**. Check with your doc regarding hospital policy on eating/drinking during labor. If allowed, you may want to bring things to sip on or hard candy to suck on.
- **Pillows.** Some people like to bring their own pillows. If you do, be forewarned that they may go home a little bloody as deliveries can be a messy sport.
- **Camera/video camera.** Yes, you will want to capture these very special moments with photos and video. But you probably shouldn't stream the birth live unless your partner is deployed in the military. And some doctors/hospitals don't allow recording of the birth, so ask beforehand.
- **Cord blood collection kit if you are using one.** Some patients opt to bank (store) their child's cord blood, which is the leftover blood in the umbilical cord and placenta after the cord has been clamped and cut. If you are planning to do this, you'll need to bring your kit to the hospital with you. For a full discussion on cord blood banking, check out Chapter 11, "Parenthood Prep."

- **List of relatives/friends to be notified once baby is born.** Everyone will be waiting on pins and needles for the text or call, and you don't want to leave anyone out!
- **Insurance card and driver's license or another form of picture ID.** These two are absolute requirements for admission to a hospital, so make sure they are in your go bag.
- **A copy of your birth requests.** Your birth requests aren't formally documented in your medical chart, so it's helpful to have a copy (or two) of your requests on hand so that you can share them with the people who will be taking care of you.
- **A phone charger.** Your stay at the hospital will likely outlast your phone's battery, especially if it's not already fully charged when you are admitted.
- **If you are a second- or third-time parent, pictures of your older child/ren to put in the room when they come to visit.** It's nice for older kids to see that although there is a new baby in the family, mom and dad haven't forgotten about them. Having a picture of them near your hospital bed is a sweet reminder of this.
- **Make a playlist on your phone so you can listen to hours of uninterrupted music if you want.** For most people, the right kind of music is extremely during labor or a C-section. Think of music that soothes you, calms you, and then if planning to push a baby out, music that encourages you to do that, too!
- **If allowed, whatever else you need that provides comfort to you or you feel will aid you in the labor/delivery experience.** I've had patients bring anything from an old sweater knitted by her grandmother to a baby blanket that was hers when she was a baby.
- **The baby's car seat, properly installed.** The hospital will only release the baby home in a vehicle that contains an infant car seat. And no, the hospital staff won't give you a car seat demonstration at checkout. You are responsible for doing this before you use it for the first time. (See the Helpful Hint below.)

Helpful Hint

Installing an infant car seat isn't as easy as it should be—and this vexes many first-time parents. Yet correct installation is crucial to protect your newborn.

To get help with choosing the right car seat for your baby and installation, the National Highway Transportation Safety Administration is the government entity that regulates car seat restraints. Check out their extremely helpful website at NHTSA .gov. There, you can determine which car seat your baby needs, watch videos on proper installation, and find a car seat inspector nearest your home. There are even some certified safety technicians that can do a virtual inspection for you.

Partner Tip

Yes, you need to pack a bag, too! Staying with your partner overnight in the hospital both during labor and afterward is paramount. It helps more than you will know to have someone there when you are vulnerable, tired, nervous, and overwhelmed. Here are a few must-haves for your bag:

- Two sets of clean clothes
- Toiletries
- A phone charger
- A separate camera if you plan to use one
- A copy of your partner's medical power of attorney
- A good pillow (you may be sleeping in a recliner chair or cot)
- Comfy shoes
- A list of good take-out places near the hospital
- Anything that won't fit into her bag

Q. I'm trying not to freak myself out, but I keep seeing on social media that bad things can happen during labor and delivery. Do I need to be legally prepared for that?

Although rare, yes, sometimes there are unforeseen complications during childbirth. And rarely, a pregnant or postpartum woman needs to be on a ventilator or is unable to make decisions regarding her healthcare and the healthcare of her fetus or newborn. For this reason, we think it's always a good idea to create a medical power of

INSIDER SECRET:

Other People's War Stories

You may not know this, but there's a sorority for people who've given birth before. And like all sororities, the initiation ceremony is a secret ritual that's only known to those in the club.

Most of us in the club won't tell you the fine details of our labor and delivery experience (aka the initiation ritual). We only share it with other members who are already in the sorority.

This unwritten rule is usually followed. We abide by it because we don't want to scare the living daylights out of you. And Mother Nature has a way afterward of replacing those memories with the amazing joy of holding a newborn.

If it's your mother we're talking about, they won't tell you because they were either completely knocked out with laughing gas when they gave birth to you . . . or they want more grandchildren.

However, there are a few sorority girls who break the rules. A few Chatty Cathys want to relive their labor experience with you, even if you don't ask them to share these personal details.

We suggest finding a good exit strategy if you encounter one of these people at the summer office party or in line at Costco. Hearing these stories is not helpful to your mental state, nor terribly useful to your prenatal education.

After you deliver, welcome to the club. And remember, mum's the word.

attorney (also known as an advance healthcare directive) prior to your delivery date. This allows you to designate a trusted person (an "agent") to make medical decisions for you in the event you lose capacity to do so yourself.

This must be a written document, created by you when you are of sound mind, witnessed by two people (neither one can be your "agent") or a notary public. You can either download the form online yourself or ask an attorney to create one for you. Each state has its own requirements, so be sure to check laws in the state you live and will be delivering in.

Nesting

In the final weeks before delivery, your nesting instinct will kick in. Just like a momma bird, you too will have an overwhelming urge to prepare your nest for your little one. If you want to use all that energy in a productive way (instead of rearranging your kitchen cabinets, which is what Dr. M did), here are our suggestions:

Have these items for YOU when you return home:

- **Lots of big sanitary pads.** I mean the big ones, like you used in high school before you discovered the beauty of tampons.
- **Nursing bras.** These are much easier for all the taking on and taking off that will be happening if you are planning to breastfeed or pump.
- **Nursing pads.** Think of these as pantyliners for your bra! They will help keep leaks from happening before, after, and in between feeds.
- **Peri wash bottles.** Most hospitals will give you the one you will be using in the hospital, but if not, it's great to have at home to keep.
- **Lanolin ointment.** If you are nursing, this is a lifesaver for cracked nipples. It also works well for your baby's diaper rash!
- **Ibuprofen.** Brand names: Advil or Motrin.
- **Stool softener.** Most women won't have a bowel movement for one to two days after a vaginal delivery and sometimes up to four days after a C-section. Taking a provider-approved stool softener like Colace or Miralax can definitely help make the first time pooping after birth easier.
- **Comfortable sleepwear.** Not that you will actually be sleeping!
- **Breast pump and all of its paraphernalia if you plan to use one.** You can also research renting a hospital-grade breast pump from a local hospital, nursing supply store, or lactation consultant.
- **Nursing pillow.** Dr. B's favorite is My Brest Friend for comfort and best positioning.
- **Soothies.** Gel pads for soothing nipples.

Have these items for BABY when you return home:

- **Diapers.** If you are doing disposable diapers, you won't need the newborn size for too long, so don't buy a box full of them. Babies quickly go to "Stage 1."
- **Diaper rash cream.** Anything that's zinc oxide or petroleum based will do. Aquaphor is a personal favorite.

- **Baby wipes.** Yes, they are safe to use.
- **A bassinet or crib for baby to sleep in.** While a newborn can sleep in a crib starting at birth, many parents prefer to use a small bassinet or co-sleeper for the first few months of a baby's life. Newborns like the cozy space. And bassinets make it easy to keep your baby nearby in your bedroom for those night feedings. It's best to buy a new bassinet or crib, if possible, as safety standards change over time.
- **Baby clothes.** If you didn't get an entire wardrobe at your baby shower, steer clear of buying expensive newborn outfits that are outgrown in a matter of weeks. No-name onesies are more practical, cheaper, and easier to clean after spit-up happens!
- **Sleeper pajamas.** Pick the right fabric for the season your baby is born. Light cotton works for summer, and fleece is fine for winter.
- **Swaddle blankets.** Learn how to do the baby burrito wrap from the nurses at the hospital. You may also want to check out the miracleblanket, which is very popular for newborns.
- **Burp cloths.** You'll need lots of those. Cloth diapers make great burp cloths.
- **Pacifiers if you plan to use them.** If you are breastfeeding, I suggest the Soothie brand, which is more similar in shape to a human nipple.
- **Bottles if you plan to use them.** You never know what might happen so get at least one for emergency use.
- **Formula if you plan to use it.** Pediatricians usually recommend a cow- or goat-milk-based formula, but ask your baby's healthcare provider for advice if you have specific health concerns.
- **Digital rectal thermometer.** Yes, this is how you need to take your baby's temperature. Fancy ear thermometers, pacifier thermometers, etc., are not accurate enough for a newborn.
- **Perfume- and dye-free bathing soap.** Brand names: Aveeno, Cetaphil, Dove.
- **Perfume- and dye-free laundry detergent.** Brand names: Tide Free and Gentle, All Free and Clear.
- **Distilled bottled water** to prepare formula.
- **2 x 2 or 3 x 3 gauze pads** if your son has a circumcision in his future.
- **Big tub of petroleum jelly.** Brand name: Vaseline. Good for when you need to use the rectal thermometer, circumcision care, and as diaper rash cream.
- **Emory board/nail file.** Newborns are too young for nail clippers.
- **Saline nose drops.** Good for stuffy noses.
- **Vitamin D drops.** Brand name: D-vi-sol. Your baby will need a vitamin D supplement.

Partner Tip

Want to score bonus points? Line up a babysitter and/or petsitter now for the big day. You may be out of your home for twenty-four hours or more, and Fido can't cross his legs for that long! Your partner will be relieved to not have to worry about this item.

PART FOUR

The Big Event

Showtime! We cover your labor day with a detailed look at vaginal deliveries, C-sections, and VBACs (vaginal births after cesarean). What to expect at the hospital, birthing center, or if having a baby at home. Then it's everything you wanted to know about epidurals but were afraid to ask. After the baby is born, we look at your baby's first few minutes, days, and weeks. We also discuss other key postpartum issues, such as care for mom after delivery, weight loss, baby blues, and more.

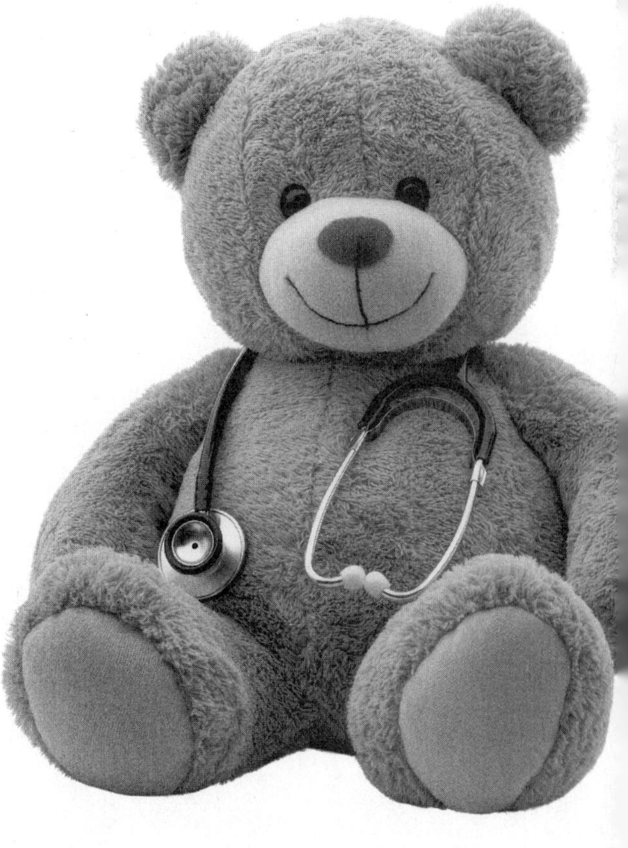

CHAPTER 14

Labor Day

"I like trying [to get pregnant]. I'm not so sure about childbirth."

—Mary Ann Evans

What's in This Chapter

- **The three stages of labor**
- **Hospital births**
- **Labor positions**
- **C-sections**
- **Medications**
- **Epidurals**
- **Home births**
- **Birthing centers**
- **Complications**
- **Once the baby is born**

Let's pretend that you, indeed, are in labor, and there is no turning back. Of course, you'll want to read this chapter before this day actually happens (you won't want to read it in between contractions).

First, we'll discuss giving birth at a hospital—what to expect, who will be helping with the birth, and so on. We'll then discuss the labor process at a birthing center and at home. No matter where you go, this chapter will give you all the details you will need to prepare for the big day (or night!).

Labor: An Overview

Q. What is labor anyway?

Labor means you have regular uterine contractions that make your ***cervix*** open (dilate) and thin out (efface). It is what allows the baby to descend from inside your uterus, through the birth canal (vagina), to the outside. There are three stages of labor, defined by the changes that occur in your uterus and cervix.

First Stage

- Begins with the onset of labor and ends when your cervix is ten centimeters dilated and 100 percent effaced (completely thinned out).

- The average length of this stage for first-time moms is between ten and fourteen hours.
- The length is shorter for women who've delivered babies before.

Second Stage (Pushing and Delivery)

- Begins when the cervix is completely dilated and ends with the birth of the baby (this is the pushing phase of labor).
- The average length for first-time parents is between one and two hours.
- The length of this stage is shorter for people who've done this before, averaging less than an hour.

Third Stage (Afterbirth)

- Begins with the birth of the baby and ends with delivery of the placenta.
- The average length for this stage for all vaginal deliveries, whether this is your first or your fourth, is between five and fifteen minutes.

BOTTOM LINE: Labor takes longer if you've never done it before. For women who haven't had a child before, the average length of labor is anywhere from ten to eighteen hours. This is broken down into eight to sixteen hours for the first stage (see above) and one to two hours for the second stage.

For women who have had at least one baby, labor is usually much quicker. Typically, the more babies you have had, the quicker the labor. The average is four to six hours for the first stage and less than one hour for the second stage.

These ranges are slightly longer if you get regional anesthesia (epidural or spinal anesthesia).

Reality Check

Most people go into spontaneous labor (inductions don't count!) at night or in the wee hours of the morning. And they usually deliver in the afternoon or early evening.

Q. How does it all work?

Delivering a baby is a fascinating, well-orchestrated process.

Labor involves a few key players: your cervix, your uterus, two hormones (oxytocin and prostaglandin), and, of course, your baby. The production and release of oxytocin from your brain tells your uterus (which is really just a big, specialized muscle) to contract.

The contractions are doing important work. They help to open the cervix, which has been tightly closed since the start of pregnancy. They also push the baby's head against the cervix—this helps to open and efface the cervix further.

The cervix must be fully thinned out (effaced) and fully opened (dilated) to allow the baby's head to pass through the vagina. Contractions also help (along with your efforts) to push the baby through the vagina. They will become more intense, last longer, and come closer together until the birth of the baby.

During active labor, the fluid-filled amniotic sac where your baby has lived for the past nine-ish months may rupture (your water may break) or your OB provider may rupture it for you. Once your water has broken, more prostaglandins are released and your contractions become more intense.

Q. What causes labor?

No one knows.

Yep, we've been able to map the human genome and invent vaccines to stop cancer . . . but we still don't know what actually causes a person to go into labor.

One theory: The baby triggers labor. At some late stage of pregnancy, your baby sends a signal (whether it is hormonal, from the baby's adrenal gland, or the release of a certain fetal protein) that enters into your bloodstream. This substance is thought to signal your body to start labor, probably through the release of maternal oxytocin. Oxytocin is the hormone that stimulates contractions. (Pitocin is a synthetic form of oxytocin that is routinely used to induce labor.)

That's why all those tricks to induce labor (balsamic vinegar salad dressing, anyone?) don't work, until your baby tells your body to do its thing.

Q. Once my labor starts, how long does it usually take to deliver?

Everyone asks this question, but there is no easy answer.

Families often like to make bets and create large pools with spreadsheets that rival March Madness brackets. But even for someone like me who does this a few times a week, it's tough to predict. Here are the variables that are involved:

- How many babies you've had in the past
- Duration of previous labors
- Baby's estimated weight
- The reason for the induction (if you are induced)
- Your ***Bishop score*** (see Chapter 13, "Home Stretch") at the start of labor (or your induction)

Your OB provider can give you a ballpark estimate of how long you will be in labor. Just don't ask them to bet on it!

A Walk-Through of the Hospital Experience

Q. How do I know when I should go to my birthing center/hospital?

Most of the time its best to call your OB provider to discuss your symptoms and have them help you decide if it's time—that's what we're here for! But here is some basic knowledge so you'll be a bit educated on when it's time to call or go:

1. If you see bright red blood, whether a small or large amount.
2. If your bag of water breaks. We don't always have women rush to the hospital if this happens because the decision for when to go is nuanced and depends on

a few things. Is this your first baby or not? Is the ***amniotic fluid*** clear? Green? Brown? Bloody? Are you group B strep positive? Do you live far from the place you will be delivering? Are you at term (past thirty-seven weeks) or preterm (before thirty-seven weeks)? Call your provider to discuss.

3. Contractions that are regular in timing and painful, occurring every five minutes, lasting at least a minute, for at least an hour.

Q. Where am I supposed to go at the hospital?

Know where you are going *before* the big day. If you take a tour of the hospital's labor and delivery floor, this is the perfect time to inquire. You can also just ask your OB provider.

Some hospitals want you to go through the emergency room and others prefer that you come straight to labor and delivery. Figure out which entrance is best (hospitals usually have several) and on which floor labor and delivery is located.

FEEDBACK FROM THE REAL WORLD:

Don't Park in the Red Zone!

It's also important to know where to park! One patient's husband was so flustered by his wife's labor that he parked in a red zone outside the ER. When he went back down to get his wife's things, he found that his car had been towed!

Q. Will I automatically get admitted to the hospital?

No. You only get to stay if you prove you are actually in labor. So don't just show up at the hospital on the day you'd *like* to deliver and hope they will let you in.

Most labor and delivery units have a triage system to help decide who stays and who goes. Usually, a labor and delivery nurse will do your initial assessment and check your vital signs. You get to pee in a tiny container (yeah, we know, again, and it's nearly impossible at this point) and change into a hospital gown. Heads up—it is open in the back, so if your whole family has come with you in the hope that today is the big day, turn with caution!

Then you'll have to answer a million questions, some of which are irritating if you are actually in labor, since you are trying to think and breathe at the same time. (You won't feel like discussing your dietary preferences or the last time you had a bowel movement!)

Next comes the monitor hookup. You will wear two small plastic devices that are fastened to your belly by Velcro straps. One is an external fetal monitor (a monitor used to pick up the baby's heart rate and pattern) and the other is a pressure-sensing device (Tocometer or TOCO; a monitor used to pick up uterine contractions).

If you are leaking, you will get a special examination to determine whether you've broken your water bag. Depending on the delivery hospital, it will be a nurse, midwife, resident (doctor in specialty training), or obstetrician who does the exam. That person inserts a sterile speculum into your vagina to collect a specimen of fluid and determine if it's really amniotic fluid (or just pee or vaginal discharge).

If you aren't complaining of leaking, the healthcare provider will examine your cervix with their fingers. This isn't very comfortable, but it's quick and necessary.

The hospital staff gives all of this information to your obstetrician. And if your water bag has broken or you are officially in labor, you will be admitted.

Q. What happens after I am admitted?

Once you get the green light for admission, one of the friendly hospital staff escorts you to the labor room. You'll either walk or catch a ride in a wheelchair.

All hospitals are different when it comes to labor rooms. You might spend some time in a smaller room in early labor, and then move to a larger room when you become more active and delivery is imminent. Or you'll labor in one room and deliver in an operating/delivery room. Or you may have one deluxe suite for the entire time.

After you get into bed and you're in that attractive hospital gown, if you do have a birth plan/request, now is a great time to hand it over to your nurse, and they should review your preferences with you. After that, the usual protocol is to hook you back up to the fetal monitors and give you an IV. (It involves a tiny tube going into a vein in your arm or hand, but your contractions are more painful than that so you really won't care.)

IV stands for intravenous line—a small tube (known as a catheter) that allows access into one of your veins so that you can receive fluids and medication. The healthcare provider who starts the IV will collect some of your blood at the same time. That's used to check your blood type, do a complete blood count (looking for signs of infection, ***anemia***, or a low platelet count), and obtain a specimen for a cord blood collection kit if you are doing one. Some hospitals also have requirements to check hepatitis, syphilis, and HIV status when someone is admitted. It is standard to get IV fluid to keep you well hydrated, unless your doctor specifies differently. Dehydration can be a risk factor for a labor that fails to progress (and leads to a C-section).

Note: You only get pain medication through that IV if you request it. Contrary to what you might hear in childbirth class, no one can give you anything without your consent.

Once you are settled in and the procedures are over with, you might as well get cozy (as much as possible). You'll be hanging out with your partner for the next ten to fourteen hours as you go through the first stage of labor.

Q. I thought I was in labor but the nurses told me I was still in early labor and sent me home. How will I know when it's time to go back?

Good question. This happens frequently with first-time moms, so don't feel bad! If your water bag has broken or you are bleeding, you are not often sent home. If your contractions aren't close enough or your cervix isn't that dilated and isn't changing on repeated exams, you may be sent home and asked to return when you are further along in your labor. So be on the lookout for more painful contractions, contractions that are closer together than when you left the hospital, ***bloody show***, or your water bag breaking. All of these changes would warrant either a phone call to your provider or a second visit to labor and delivery.

Q. I tested positive for Group B strep during pregnancy. Is there anything special that needs to happen?

Yes.

If you tested positive for Group B strep (GBS) during your pregnancy, you will get IV antibiotics during labor to protect your baby. We discuss why this is so important in Chapter 6, "Tests."

Penicillin (or ampicillin) is the antibiotic specifically used for GBS. If you are allergic to penicillin or one of its relatives, there are other antibiotic options. Your prenatal records (which should be at the hospital) document medication allergies, but it's always a good idea to tell your nurse if you have any drug allergies.

Reality Check

If you go into labor before thirty-seven weeks and haven't been tested for Group B strep, you will be treated as if you are positive and you'll get IV antibiotics during labor. This is extremely important since your GBS status is unknown and premature babies are at much higher risk of getting infected with GBS.

Q. Can I eat or drink anything before I head to the hospital?

It depends. If you're heading for an induction, eating is a great idea, but most women don't want to eat if they are already in labor because they likely aren't hungry and are often nauseated or vomiting. And if you're heading in for a scheduled or unscheduled C-section, there is no eating or drinking at all since you need to have an empty stomach before surgery.

Q. Can I eat or drink anything while I am in labor?

Docs used to tell people in labor that they could have nothing but ice chips once the labor process began. There are two reasons for that:

Labor makes some people queasy, and that often leads to vomiting. It's easier to clean up water than a chicken burrito with extra hot sauce.

And if you end up needing an emergency C-section, it's best to have an empty stomach during surgery. (If you need general anesthesia, that food could end up in your lungs and potentially cause pneumonia. More than you wanted to know, right?)

But those rules have changed a little bit. Ask your OB to find out the specific guidelines you should follow. Once you get to the hospital, you probably won't be allowed to eat, but most hospitals have relaxed their guidelines in recent years. At the very least, you can sip on liquids throughout labor. You might also be able to eat ice pops or suck on hard candy. Find out the answer to this question at your pre-labor hospital visit.

Partner Tip

If you decide to get a burger on the way into the hospital, leave off the onions. Your laboring partner will smell your breath constantly for the next several hours . . . and we probably don't have to warn you about how moody they'll be during labor.

Vaginal Deliveries

NEW PARENT-TO-BE 411:

A Hospital Vaginal Delivery in Thirteen Easy-ish Steps

Step 1: You go into labor and get admitted to your hospital or birthing center. Or you arrive for your induction.

Step 2: You move to your delivery or birthing suite.

Step 3: You get hooked up to monitors.

Step 4: You get an IV placed and blood drawn (it's only one needle stick!).

Step 5: You and your partner hang out while your contractions become more frequent and more uncomfortable during the first stage of labor.

Step 6: Your nurse checks on you often and your OB provider (or another healthcare provider) examines you to check your progress every couple of hours.

Step 7: You notify your medical team if/when you would like to receive any pain medication.

Step 8: If you desire pain medication by epidural, an ***anesthesiologist*** arrives to place it.

Step 9: You reach ten centimeters dilation, and it's time to push.

Step 10: Find a position that works for you, and go for it. Your partner, support people, and medical team keep you focused and pushing.

Step 11: Your baby arrives! Piece-o-cake, right?

Step 12: Umbilical cord is cut.

Step 13: The placenta is delivered.

Q. Who will examine me?

This is going to depend on the hospital (see below) and where your OB provider is at the moment.

- **Public hospital:** A nurse or the obstetrician on call will examine you.
- **Community hospital:** A nurse, your OB provider, or the person on call for your OB provider will examine you.

- **Teaching hospital:** A nurse, midwife, resident, or attending physician will examine you. However, even in a teaching hospital, it's possible that your own doctor is the one doing most or all of the internal exams.

While you are in the first stage of labor (remember, that's ten to fourteen hours on average), your OB provider may need to check on other patients who are in labor, or they may need to run back to their office to see patients.

If there is a problem or your doctor needs to know how far along you are after three or four hours (and they are at the office seeing patients), they may ask the nurse to examine you and relay the information to them.

If there is an absolute emergency requiring a procedure or intervention and they are not at the hospital, a resident or fellow (doctor in specialty training) in a teaching hospital or a colleague in a community hospital might evaluate you.

BOTTOM LINE: Your job: trust that you will be in very capable hands.

Vaginal Delivery in a Nutshell

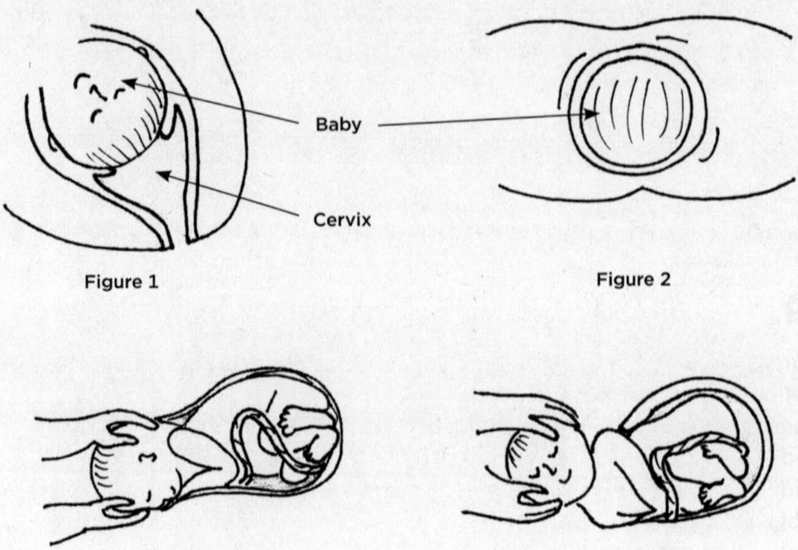

Figure 1 Figure 2 Figure 3 Figure 4

Baby remains in the uterus until the cervix is dilated 10 cm (Figure 1), then makes their way down the birth canal until the head emerges (Figure 2). Your practitioner delivers your baby's head first, followed by the shoulders (Figure 3). Then the rest of the baby is delivered (Figure 4).

INSIDER SECRET:

The Three Types of Hospitals

Public. These hospitals primarily (but not exclusively) care for under-resourced populations in cities. Some of them are also teaching hospitals.

Community. These are smaller hospitals that provide standard care. The doctors on the hospital staff usually have private practices near the facility.

Teaching. These hospitals are affiliated with medical institutions that train medical students, physicians in specialty training (interns, residents, fellows), and other healthcare professionals. Senior physicians (attending physicians) supervise those in training and see clinic patients or have their own private practices. Teaching hospitals are often regional referral centers for complex medical cases.

Q. How many internal exams will I have?

It depends. Ideally, exams should be minimized, particularly after your bag of water has broken. In general, you may get one about every two to six hours during labor.

These exams help your OB provider figure out how your labor is progressing. If your labor is going slowly, expect more exams.

You get *more* if you are being induced and you start with a low Bishop Score (see Chapter 13, "Home Stretch").

You get *fewer* if your water bag is broken right off the bat, particularly if you are known to be Group B strep positive. Every internal exam introduces some bacteria into the cervix and uterus, even if your OB provider uses sterile gloves. That's why your doctor will try to limit the number of internal exams once your amniotic sac is ruptured.

Q. Will I be able to use the bathroom during early labor?

During the early stages of labor, if you need to go to the bathroom, there are a few options assuming you don't have an epidural (see page 363). You can get up and walk to the bathroom and use the potty, or you can have the nurse place a bedpan beneath you if you are too uncomfortable to move around.

Q. Will I be able to walk around, take a shower, or use a bouncy ball during labor?

It depends on if you have an epidural or not.

If you *don't* have an epidural (or until you get one placed) and your baby's heart rate tracing looks good on the monitor, most OB providers will let you walk around, get into a bathtub, or use a birthing ball (see the Insider Secret box below).

DR. M'S OPINION

You can bring anything you want to help you labor, but here's the bottom line: Be flexible about how your labor will go. A successful delivery ends with a healthy mom and baby. It doesn't matter how you accomplish that goal. And you don't get graded on style points!

Most of the time, you just need to check in periodically. You get hooked up to the fetal heart rate monitor for twenty minutes to be sure all is well and then you get another forty minutes of freedom.

If you really want to roam around during labor, see if your delivery hospital offers *ambulatory monitoring.* That's a portable monitor that connects to a computer and allows staff to track your baby's heart rate while you pace the hallway and move into different positions.

If you *do* have a typical epidural, you won't be able to walk around because the nerves that are used to help your muscles move are being blocked by the pain medication. Some hospitals now offer *walking epidurals* that do allow for more movement. Talk to your OB provider about what is available to you.

Helpful Hint

Don't assume that your hospital's labor room will have a bathtub or shower. There may only be a few select rooms that offer those amenities. If you want one of those rooms, request it in advance or when you get admitted.

INSIDER SECRET:

Birthing Balls

Some women prefer to be sitting up and leaning forward during a contraction. A birthing ball may help you do this. Some updated birthing centers and maternity wards come complete with beds that have a trapeze bar above the bed and side rails that moms can hold on to while laboring.

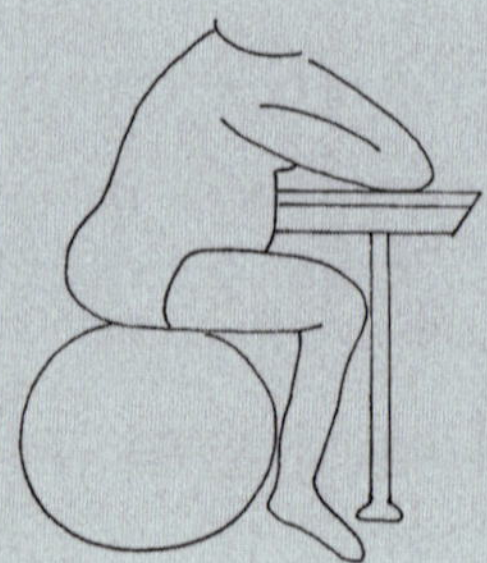

Q. How is the baby monitored while I am in labor?

In a hospital setting, an external fetal monitor (EFM) is used. It's a plastic monitor that is placed on your belly with a little bit of cold lubricant. Once a nurse finds the baby's heartbeat, it is secured with a large Velcro strap to hold it in place. It's the same monitor used for non-stress tests (NSTs) in your OB's office.

This monitor gives a visual picture of your baby's heart rate and pattern, similar to an electrocardiogram (EKG). Unless you are up walking around or going to the bathroom, you are hooked up to the monitor, and there is a continuous reading of your baby's heartbeat.

The American College of Obstetricians and Gynecologists recommends that your healthcare provider check these monitor tracings every thirty minutes during your first stage of labor and every fifteen minutes in your second stage of labor. For high-risk pregnancies, the provider should check the monitor tracings every fifteen minutes during the first stage and every five minutes in the second stage.

If you deliver at home, your midwife will probably use a stethoscope to listen to the baby's heartbeat (fetoscope) or a handheld Doppler device, like the one used to check the baby's heartbeat during your prenatal visits. Birthing centers also use Doppler devices to listen to the baby's heart rate.

Q. I've heard about a monitor that attaches to the baby's scalp. Is that necessary?

Occasionally, an *internal* monitor called a fetal scalp electrode (FSE) is necessary. This monitor attaches to the baby's head via a tiny little wire. Yes, the wire actually screws into the skin of the scalp. We know it sounds dreadful, but they should only be used when we really need to get more information about your baby. These situations include:

- concern about the fetal heart rate or pattern.
- inability to use an external fetal monitor because mom is obese.
- position of the baby makes external monitoring difficult.

We know the thought of a tiny wire being put into your baby's scalp is the last thing that anyone would want (us included). But it's necessary sometimes. No, it can't do any permanent damage. And no, it can't go into your baby's brain. Most babies will have a little superficial mark on the scalp that ends up scabbing up and falling off, without any reminder that something was ever there.

BOTTOM LINE: Monitors should only be used for good reason, and your OB provider should explain to you in detail why you need one.

Q. My friend's doctor put something inside of them to measure their contractions. What was that? Will I need that, too?

This is called an intrauterine pressure catheter (IUPC).

The IUPC is a thin little sterile plastic catheter that slides up along the inner wall of your uterus (next to the baby) and measures the pressure of your contractions from inside your uterus. It is more accurate than the monitor placed on the outside of your belly.

An IUPC may be used in many situations such as when it is difficult to pick up contractions with an external monitor (often in obese patients), when it is unclear whether more or less Pitocin is needed, and to help predict uterine rupture in trial of labor after cesarean (TOLAC) patients. Your OB provider will tell you if one is necessary.

Internal monitors are rarely needed in labor.

Q. I'm worried the umbilical cord will be wrapped around the baby's neck. Can we do an ultrasound when I go into labor to check for that?

Yes, it might happen. But, no, you shouldn't worry.

One in every four babies is born with the cord around their neck (***nuchal cord***). But doing an ultrasound to find out is not going to change the way your OB provider manages your labor or delivery.

The cord usually gets wrapped around some part of the baby (neck, shoulder, leg) during the first or second trimesters as they swim around in the amniotic fluid with a leash (the umbilical cord) attaching them to the placenta.

At delivery, your OB provider will sweep their fingers behind your baby's neck after the head comes out to feel for the umbilical cord. If it is present, it's usually loose enough for us to gently slip it over your baby's head.

BOTTOM LINE: While you might think doing an ultrasound during labor to check for a cord wrapped around the baby's neck is a good idea, it won't really change what happens during delivery. Knowing that a cord is there would just scare most people during labor—which is not a good thing!

Q. Will my OB provider know if the cord is wrapped around my baby's neck before delivery?

Sometimes yes, sometimes no.

If the cord is *loosely* wrapped around the baby's neck, shoulder, body, or limbs, docs often have no idea until the baby is born.

Rarely, the cord is *tightly* wrapped around any one of the above-mentioned body parts—this can be "seen" by looking at the baby's heart monitor. If the umbilical cord is getting compressed when you are having contractions, it shows up on the fetal heart monitors as a very specific, recognizable pattern. If the pattern persists, it could mean the baby is not tolerating labor very well.

Sometimes changing your position helps the situation. If the baby's heart rate drops too low or too often, your OB provider may suggest doing an ***amnioinfusion***. Using a small catheter (called an intrauterine pressure catheter, or IUPC), your OB provider puts sterile water back into the uterus.

The increased water helps the umbilical cord "float" in the hope of lessening compression of the cord during each contraction. If that doesn't help and you are nowhere close to delivering and the fetal heart rate keeps dropping, your OB provider will probably recommend a C-section.

Q. Will my doctor hold my hand the entire time?

The answer is most likely no, but varies, depending on your doctor (or the doctor on call who manages your delivery) or midwife. And it's a question you should ask at some point during your prenatal care so you feel comfortable with the plan.

Here are the different possible scenarios:

- **Scenario #1:** Your delivery doctor checks on you at the beginning of labor, a nurse checks on you throughout labor, and then your doctor shows up as the baby's head is coming out.
- **Scenario #2:** Your delivery doctor checks on you a few times throughout the day or night, arrives when you are completely dilated or have started pushing, and stays with you until delivery.
- **Scenario #3:** Your delivery doctor checks on you frequently throughout your labor and stays with you the entire time you are pushing until you deliver.

Note: There is no right or wrong approach here—the key is you should be informed regarding what to expect and comfortable with that plan.

How do doctors know how your labor is going if they aren't in the room with you? Thanks to modern technology, many doctors can see their patients' heart rate tracing and contraction patterns on their home or office computers. Yes, there is even an iPhone App for that—AirStrip OB that provides mobile monitoring for docs on the go.

As a result, your doctor can keep an eye on the whole process while a labor and delivery nurse is physically present at your side. Alternatively, your nurse can and should give periodic phone updates to your OB provider.

Q. Will my nurse hold my hand the entire time?

No. But you will see quite a bit of them, and they'll be very helpful.

When you get admitted to the hospital, a labor and delivery nurse is assigned to you. They will help to get you settled in and comfortable. They'll check on you often, answer many of your questions, occasionally perform cervical exams, assess the baby's heart rate tracing, and support you during delivery.

However, your nurse will probably be assigned to more than one patient, and they won't be in the room with you the entire time. It's also possible you will end up with one nurse during labor and another one for delivery if your labor goes beyond your first nurse's eight- or twelve-hour shift (but we'll be optimistic you won't be in labor that long!).

The positive here is that you and your partner will go through labor together without a third party constantly in the room with you. You can really let your hair down and swear like a sailor if you like.

Your nurse will be around if any problems arise during labor and with you (and only you) when it's time to push.

Helpful Hint

Occasionally, a laboring person and the nurse assigned to them just don't see eye to eye. If this is the case, talk to your OB provider to see if you can have a new nurse assigned to your care. You want to have a good birth experience, so speak up for yourself if you feel uncomfortable (or make your partner do it!).

Q. If I have a doula, will they be there the entire time?

Yes. You hire them to be your personal labor coach/instructor/companion for the entire duration of labor and delivery.

Most doulas join you at your home when labor begins, and then transition with you to a birthing center or hospital.

Doulas are especially helpful if you choose to go through labor naturally without pain medication. This is a hard but not impossible feat that's easier with a doula by your side.

Q. Can my partner hold my hand the entire time?

Yes! Gone are the days of making husbands or significant others cool their heels in the waiting room while their sons and daughters are being born down the hall.

Today, we encourage your partner to be with you the entire time. Your significant other's physical, mental, and emotional support is critical and can help you have a smoother delivery.

Q. My doctor wants to use Pitocin to "augment" my labor? What does that mean?

Doctors commonly use a medication called Pitocin (a synthetic form of oxytocin) to induce labor. Pitocin is also used to help move along (augment) your labor.

Sometimes, labor slows or contractions aren't strong enough or close enough together to dilate a pregnant person's cervix and move the baby down the birth canal. Or their water bag may have broken and they aren't having any contractions at all. Helping labor along may prevent the need for a C-section.

You'll get Pitocin through your IV. Usually the dose of Pitocin for augmenting labor is lower than what's needed for inducing labor. If you're at a birthing center and your OB provider decides that you need Pitocin, you need to be transferred to a hospital.

Before deciding to augment your labor, your OB provider will carefully assess your

NEW PARENT-TO-BE 411:

Pitocin and Autism?

One of the internet myths you may hear about is that children have an increased risk of developing autism when the woman's labor is induced or augmented with Pitocin. Let's unpack the facts here, so you can rest assured that this is a safe medication for you and your baby.

Over a decade ago, some autism researchers explored alterations in the levels of the neuropeptide oxytocin in children with autism spectrum disorder. At the time, this was a hotbed of research, and some healthcare providers even prescribed oxytocin nasal spray to their autistic patients. Ultimately, a large-scale meta-analysis of data failed to prove any link, and no significant benefit was found in treating these children.[1,2]

Because Pitocin is a synthetic form of oxytocin, researchers at the time were also curious to see if there was an association between Pitocin use during labor and autism rates.[3] One published study in 2013 showed an association, but it did not prove that this medication causes autism. And there is a big difference between association and causation. A major study conducted by Harvard and published in *JAMA Pediatrics* put this issue to rest. The study reviewed an entire population of more than 1 million babies, some of whom included siblings, over thirteen years, and compared children delivered with or without the use of Pitocin. They found no evidence of a link to autism.[4] ACOG guidance agrees: There is no conclusive evidence that Pitocin causes autism.

contraction pattern, how much your cervix is dilated, and how far your baby has descended into the birth canal. They'll also pay close attention to your baby's heart rate in response to your contractions, to make sure your baby will be able to tolerate the stronger contractions that will occur with Pitocin.

This is one of those medical scenarios where your doctor needs to make the call, based on the situation. Some doctors are more liberal about using it than others. But starting Pitocin should include a thorough conversation with your doctor explaining their reasons behind the recommendation.

BOTTOM LINE: Talk to your OB provider about any questions or concerns you may have. Keep the lines of communication open when any change in management occurs (a new nurse arrives, a decision to use Pitocin is made, etc.). You need to know what your OB provider is thinking and vice versa.

Q. Will my water break on its own? If it doesn't, what happens?

Your water usually breaks on its own, either at the beginning of labor (which is why you arrive at the hospital in the first place) or at some point before delivery.

If it doesn't happen spontaneously, your OB provider will probably break your water bag because it releases natural prostaglandins that move your labor along.

There are a few situations where your OB provider would want your bag to be left intact for as long as possible (or want it to happen naturally). Those include women with HIV, hepatitis B and C, or those who are Group B strep (GBS) positive who have *not* received antibiotics. It's best for GBS-positive women to get at least one dose of antibiotics before their water bag breaks.

It is rare for a baby to be born with a water bag intact.

INSIDER SECRET:

All About Cauls

A baby who is born with its amniotic sac completely intact is called "en caul." This occurs in 0.1 percent of all deliveries. In medieval times, being born "en caul" was a sign of good luck. The family often kept the amniotic sac as an heirloom or sold it to others as a good luck charm to fend off witches and protect one from death by drowning. Since very few people today are familiar with this tradition, you won't get much for it on eBay. If this happens to you, just brag to your friends.

Q. My doctor says there is an arrest of dilation. What does that mean?

As we discussed above, there is a typical pattern for labor. However, everyone is different, and there is a range of what is considered normal.

Sometimes, the process of labor slows down too much or stops altogether. This is called either ***arrest of dilation*** (where your cervix stops dilating normally) or ***arrest of***

descent (where the baby's head stops descending through the pelvis and birth canal). There are very specific criteria that OB providers use to determine if your labor is officially not progressing normally. And those criteria differ depending on if you have delivered a baby vaginally before and if you have an epidural.

Labor varies between individuals, and it's important that whoever is taking care of you recognizes that. Of course, there are cases where a laboring person really isn't progressing and this can happen at any point during labor—even if you're dilated at ten centimeters.

Arrest of dilation and arrest of descent can happen for the following reasons:

Problem with the Uterus

- Cervix dilates very slowly.
- Cervix stops dilating.

Disproportion of Baby's Head Size to Woman's Pelvic Size or Shape

- Baby's head is too large to fit through your pelvis.
- Your pelvis is too small or of a particular shape that doesn't allow the baby's head to fit through.

Abnormal Presentation

- Baby's head is in a position that makes descent into the birth canal difficult or impossible.

If you have weak or infrequent contractions, your OB provider will probably start Pitocin to kick-start contractions.

Reality Check

We realize there is a lot of pressure these days to have a natural childbirth—no drugs, no interventions, etc. But there are situations where using a drug like Pitocin or breaking your water bag (or both) makes your labor progress more effectively. For a person who has never gone through childbirth before, this may be just the ticket to avoid a C-section—the ultimate intervention. Here are the common scenarios where you might need help:

- Broken water bag without contractions.
- Contractions too far apart and thus the cervix stops dilating.
- Contractions are not strong enough to move baby's position.

Q. What are my delivery options if I am not dilating properly or my baby's head isn't descending?

The baby needs to come out eventually (as staying inside your uterus until kindergarten is not an option). Your OB provider keeps a close eye on your progress during labor, and if they think your labor has either dramatically slowed or stopped progressing altogether (and you are already on IV Pitocin and your water bag has broken), there are two options:

- **Option #1: Operative vaginal delivery.** This involves using forceps (rarely used today) or a vacuum extractor to help deliver the baby. This can only happen if you are already ten centimeters dilated (fully dilated), your baby's head is low enough in your pelvis to safely help them out and you are delivering with an obstetrician who has an operating room immediately available in case an emergency C-section needs to be done.
- **Option #2: C-section.** Sometimes a patient will choose to have a C-section instead of an operative vaginal delivery, and sometimes an operative vaginal delivery doesn't actually work and the only other option is a C-section. Talk to your OB provider before you go into labor about these alternatives so you will feel comfortable about Option #2 if Option #1 (an operative vaginal delivery) is not possible.

Q. Is it common to have an episiotomy?

Twenty years ago, it seemed like every person delivering a baby vaginally had an episiotomy. That's because doctors thought that making a clean, surgical cut (***episiotomy***) to the area between the vagina and rectum (perineum) reduced the trauma to that area. And if that was the case, women after birth would have fewer bladder and bowel accidents (incontinence), problems having sex (sexual dysfunction), and body parts, such as the bladder, uterus, or rectum, sagging into the vagina (pelvic organ prolapse). It was also thought that a surgical incision was easier to sew up than the multiple tears that some people get during delivery.

However, here's what we know now, after many years of scientific research: Doing routine episiotomies can lead to more third- and fourth-degree tears (see box below), ultimately leading to chronic vaginal pain, pain during intercourse, and an anal sphincter muscle that doesn't function properly.

Episiotomies are also linked to an increase in bleeding (***postpartum hemorrhage***) and infection at the surgical site. And the procedure does not protect a woman from incontinence or pelvic organ prolapse in the future, as previously thought.

So episiotomies are no longer routine. There are about 4 million babies born every year. In 1992, 1.6 million episiotomies were performed in the United States. Compare this to a 3.4 percent rate nationally in 2024. This marks a 73 percent reduction in episiotomy rates in the past fifteen years.[5]

However, there are still a few rare situations where you might need one. Your OB provider often has to make this difficult judgment call at the very end of delivery. For

DR. M'S OPINION:

Episiotomies

I very rarely perform episiotomies. I might do one if I need more room in the case of a vacuum-assisted vaginal delivery or a shoulder dystocia. It's a last-minute judgment call after all the pros and cons have been weighed and there has been verbal consent with my patient.

example, if your baby's shoulder gets stuck behind your pubic bone (***shoulder dystocia***), your OB provider will perform certain maneuvers to free the baby's shoulder. An episiotomy may provide the extra room for the baby to deliver safely.

BOTTOM LINE: Episiotomies are no longer routine. You need a good reason to have one.

Q. So how can I avoid tearing during delivery?

It's common to tear during delivery, especially if this is your first baby—your vagina isn't the size of the Grand Canyon! And people who have a shorter perineum (the tissue between the vaginal opening and anus) or more fragile tissue may tear more. That's genetic, and you can't control it. But here are three strategies that can help.

1. **Don't have an episiotomy unless it's medically necessary.** Talk to your OB provider about it.
2. **Pelvic floor physical therapy and/or perineal massage.** Your OB provider can refer you to a therapist for pelvic floor physical therapy and to teach you how to do perineal massage at home, starting at about thirty-three to thirty-four weeks. Massaging the tissue makes it more pliable and able to tolerate trauma during delivery.
3. **Have your OB provider massage mineral oil or another lubricant into your perineum while you are pushing.** This along with warm compresses and the pressure of the baby's head helps gently stretch the tissues out to minimize tearing. Having a trained OB provider help guide your baby's head and shoulders out also helps minimize tearing.

NEW PARENT-TO-BE 411:
Vaginal Lacerations

Here is how vaginal lacerations are graded. Warning: Read this box only if you have a strong stomach and enjoy horror flicks. We're not kidding.

1st Degree: The cut/tear involves only the vaginal tissue.

2nd Degree: The cut/tear extends from the vagina into the tissue between the vagina and anus (the perineum).

3rd Degree: The cut/tear extends from the vagina, through the perineum, and into part or all of the muscle of the anus (the anal sphincter).

4th Degree: The cut/tear extends from the vagina through the perineum and anal sphincter and extends into the lining of the rectum.

Q. I've heard about using different birthing positions. Must I be lying down to deliver?

Nope. There are a variety of positions you can use. There are only two rules:

Rule #1: You can't deliver standing up (because your OB provider cannot stoop beneath you to catch your baby)—although some people find squatting comfortable.

Rule #2: Birthing positions are limited if you have an epidural (but finding a comfortable position should be a non-issue if your epidural is effective). With an epidural, your options are lying down, lying on your side, lying in a reclined position, or using a bar to help support you in a more upright position.

Here are a few birthing positions if you don't have an epidural:

- Sitting
- Lying on your side
- Squatting
- Sitting on all fours
- Reclining on a bed or in a tub of water

There is no perfect position for labor, and frequent changes of position can help you relax and get a little more comfortable with your contractions. As your labor progresses, try various positions until you find one that works for you.

Q. I've heard horror stories about "back labor," where all of the pain associated with contractions is in your back. Is there a way to prevent or avoid this pain?

Some laboring people feel most of the discomfort in their lower back during a contraction (back labor). Some people don't have any back pain with contractions, and a few feel pain both in the back and the lower abdomen.

People who have back labor usually have a baby whose head is in the "sunny-side up" position (***occiput posterior*** or ***OP***). That means the baby is looking up instead of down (***occiput anterior*** or ***OA***). Up to 20 percent of babies are in the OP position during labor. But many of them rotate into a more favorable position during the later stages of labor . . . so only 5 to 10 percent are born OP or "sunny-side up."

There is no way to prevent having your baby end up in the OP position, but there are some positions that you can be placed in during labor to help turn your baby. Your nurse, midwife, or doula can help with this as most are very knowledgeable about how to help turn these babies during labor. Some women have a certain shape to their pelvis that makes it hard for a fetus to be in a position other than OP. So, unfortunately, doctors can't prevent back labor, either.

But here are some tips to help relieve the discomfort of back labor:

- Massage
- Warm compresses
- Positioning yourself on all fours or on your side
- Lying all the way on your side, almost on your stomach (which might help the baby turn), while hugging a pillow

Q. What happens if I need to pee or poop during labor?

Yes, you will probably pee and poop when you are pushing. Now, take a deep breath and mentally prepare yourself and your partner for it. It's completely normal and happens often.

Q. What if I have an epidural? Will I know if I need to pee or poop?

If you have epidural or spinal anesthesia, you won't be able to feel your bladder fill up with urine and you won't have the urge to urinate. So your nurse will insert a thin tube that goes through your urethra and into your bladder (a catheter) that will collect the urine. No worries—this procedure happens after the medication coming through the epidural has already kicked in. You will be numb and won't feel a thing. The catheter comes out right before you start pushing.

Pooping is another matter. Despite having an epidural, you will still be able to feel pressure, specifically rectal pressure. That pressure sensation is usually the baby's head as it descends into the birth canal, pushing down on the rectum below. It is the head pushing on the rectum that makes you feel like you need to have a bowel movement. So any time a person in labor says, "I feel like I have to poop," they get a cervical exam first before they are allowed to try to poop. It's poor form to deliver a baby into a bedpan or the toilet!

Partner Tip

You may witness your labor partner poop. That's only one of the visuals that partners can find disturbing. Try to erase those visions from your mind. Just remember how much you love this person and how much of a sacrifice they are making to bring your baby into this world.

And try not to faint. The labor and delivery staff has more than enough to do without you becoming a patient, too. Stand with your knees partially bent, and if you feel lightheaded, sit down and put your head between your knees. Also, make sure you are eating and drinking even though your partner in labor is not.

Fact Check

It's standard protocol for your OB provider to shave your pubic hair before delivery.

The truth: This is true and false. Doctors do not shave women prior to a vaginal delivery. But some of your pubic hair will get shaved if you are going to have a C-section. And in fact, it is better and safer for us to do it at the hospital immediately before surgery for two reasons: 1) Shaving or waxing the day or two prior to surgery allows bacteria to colonize in the hair follicles and increases your risk of an infection; 2) It's really hard for you to see down there! If you have had laser hair removal prior to becoming pregnant, that's fine. But there's no need to schedule a Brazilian wax session before you go into labor.

Q. When will I know it is time to push?

This answer depends on whether you have an epidural or not.

*If you are laboring **without** an epidural*: You'll probably feel the need to push when your cervix is dilated to eight or nine centimeters. While it's okay to bear down lightly, it's best to avoid pushing until the cervix has completely dilated to ten centimeters. Resist the temptation to push, and just breathe.

Why? You can cause tears in your cervix if you push at less than ten centimeters. These tears can be really difficult to repair and can make you bleed excessively (***post-partum hemorrhage***). Not good. Your labor and delivery nurse or doula will help you breathe through your contractions and bear down lightly until you have reached ten cm and can really start pushing.

If you are laboring ***with*** *an epidural*: There are two scenarios.

- **Scenario #1:** You may start to feel rectal pressure (like you have to poop). At that point, your OB provider or a nurse or midwife will check your cervix to see how dilated you are and where the baby is situated in the birth canal. If you are ten cm and the baby's head has descended low enough in the birth canal, you get the green light to start pushing.
- **Scenario #2:** If the baby's head is still pretty high in the birth canal, your OB provider may decide to let you "labor down." That means your contractions can do a little more work on their own before you start pushing. Why? Pushing when the baby's head is still high in the birth canal (a "very high station") will tire you out. Once the head descends a little farther, you can begin pushing.

Note: Sometimes with an epidural you won't feel anything and won't have a clue when it's time to push. Your OB provider will have to tell you that you are at ten centimeters, the baby's head is low enough, and you need to start pushing. If your epidural is that good, give your anesthesiologist a tip to pay for their next greens fees or spa day (or at least say thank you when they check on you after delivery).

BOTTOM LINE: With first-time deliveries, most people push between thirty minutes and two hours.

Q. What's the best way to push?

Everyone finds their own best way to do it, and we trust that you will, too. Push in the position that feels best to you and one where the OB provider helping to deliver your baby says you are making progress. If you do not have an epidural, you will be more mobile and thus have more options. Here are some of them:

- Lie on your back, slightly reclined. (This is the most effective way if you have an epidural.)
- Pull your legs back by reaching under your thighs, curl your chin to your chest, and push.
- Hold bedside rails or handles on each side and someone else holds your legs back.
- Sit more upright and hold on to a birthing bar above your head.

If you feel like you aren't being effective in one position, try another until it feels right.

In any position, you'll be told to start pushing at the beginning of each contraction. And this is how pushing usually goes:

1. Take a deep breath in through your mouth and then let it out. (That's your cleansing breath to help open up your lungs and get your mind and body ready for what they need to do next.)

2. Your next breath is another deep breath in, which you hold (do not exhale) as you bear down in your lower abdomen and vaginal/rectal area. This is similar to how you push if you are constipated—bad analogy, but it's exactly the same.
3. After pushing for approximately ten seconds (if you can only do it effectively for seven or eight, that's okay), you can exhale.
4. Take another deep breath in to do this all over again two more times.
5. Aim for three pushes in each contraction.
6. Some people want their "team" (partner, nurse, OB provider) to count for them and others do not. Tell your team what your preference is. Counting faster is not an option.

FEEDBACK FROM THE REAL WORLD:

Pushing

If you begin to push while exhaling, all of your power leaves with the air you are exhaling. Just try doing a practice one right now. You'll see that things are more effective if you hold your air in and push, compared to if you let your air out while pushing.

Push like you are really constipated and you're trying to get the poop out (again, awful analogy, we know).

Yelling and screaming makes your pushing less effective and thus makes your delivery even longer—the opposite of what you want. (But we do understand why you feel like doing this, as we've both been there.)

Q. Can I have a mirror to see the delivery?

Yes. Of course, you are welcome to watch the baby being delivered. Some people are motivated by seeing that their pushing is effective. Others, however, have no desire to see the show. It's your choice.

Q. What happens after the baby's head comes out?

At least 90 percent of the time, the head is the toughest thing to get out. So the hardest part is usually over! Once the head comes out, your OB provider will likely ask you to rest for a second (that means don't push) so that they can quickly check to see if the umbilical cord is wrapped around the baby's head (don't panic, just read the question about that earlier in this chapter). Slowing down the delivery also reduces the trauma to you and your baby.

Once your doctor knows the umbilical cord is safely away from your baby, they will help guide the baby's anterior (top) shoulder out and then tell you to push again to deliver the baby's posterior (bottom) shoulder and then the rest of the body.

Reality Check

You may say some pretty *#&%$! things while you are pushing. And there may also be some X-rated shots in there as well. So, if you are recording the event, you may not want to share video footage of your child's birth with anyone else. It's always best to preview the video by yourself before sitting down in a home theater to view it with a twenty-person audience.

Q. My sister has three children, and they were all born "sunny-side up." What does that mean?

Let's first explain what all the positions are and what they mean. Your OB provider will know what position your baby is in by doing a cervical exam and feeling the bones that make up the baby's skull.

Doctors locate the back part of the baby's head (the occiput) in relation to the woman's body to figure out the position. Envision that person is lying down on their back. Here are the baby's possible delivery positions:

- **OA (occiput anterior):** Baby looks straight down as they come through the birth canal (pictured at right).
- **LOA (left occiput anterior):** Baby looks down and the back of their head points toward woman's left side.
- **ROA (right occiput anterior):** Baby looks down and the back of their head points toward woman's right side.
- **OP (occiput posterior):** Baby looks straight up as they come through the birth canal (aka "sunny-side up"; pictured at right).
- **ROT (right occiput transverse) and LOT (left occiput transverse)**: Babies who look up and are pointing left or right (LOP or ROP) are also called sunny-side up (see illustrations below).

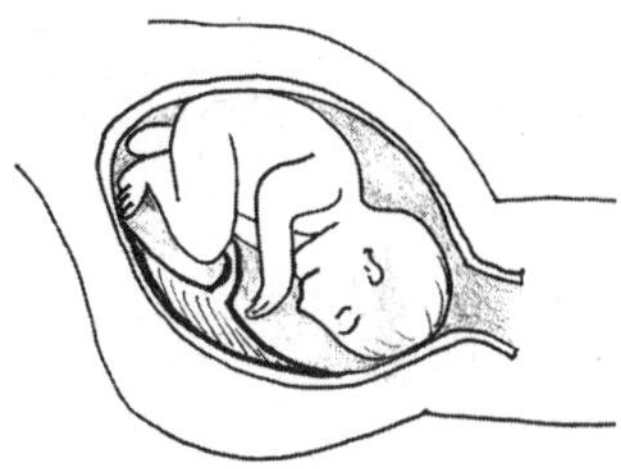

Occiput anterior

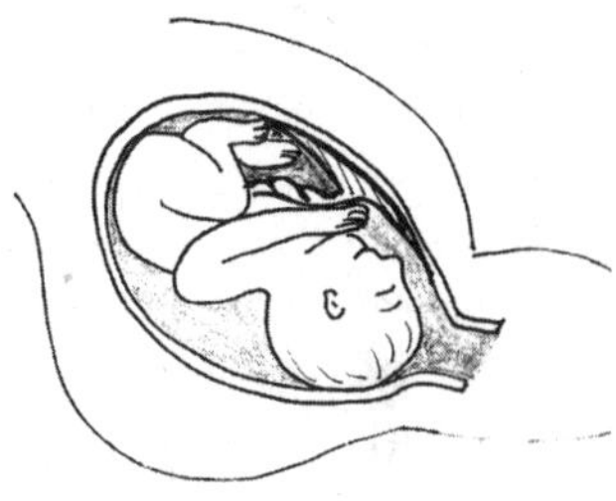

Occiput posterior

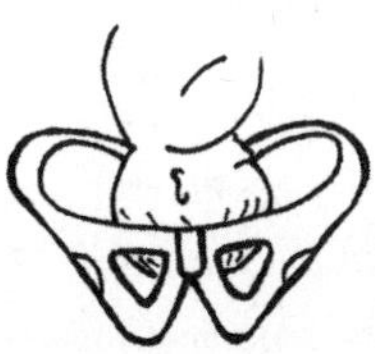

Right occiput transverse

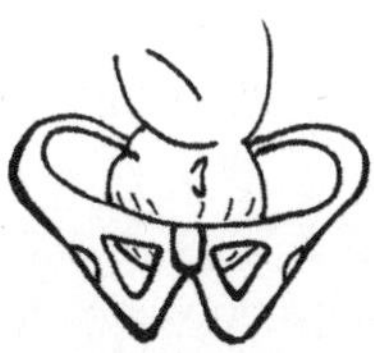

Left occiput transverse

NEW PARENT-TO-BE 411:

The Newborn Skull

How does the baby's skull manage to fit through the birth canal during delivery? A newborn's skull is not like an adult's. Instead of a solid mass of bone, a newborn's skull is made up of several separate bones. These fuse together during the first year of life—but at birth, these bones are separated, and that allows the skull to mold and squeeze through the pelvis.

Q. Can the baby be delivered vaginally if they are in an odd position?

Usually, the answer is yes.

Babies in the ROA, OA, or LOA positions (see above for discussion) are the easiest to deliver because it's easiest for the baby to maneuver through the pelvis when their head is looking down.

Babies can get where they need to go in other positions, but the delivery may take longer or require assistance (vacuum extractor or forceps).

Occasionally, babies don't fit because of how they are presenting in the birth canal or because of the shape of the woman's pelvis. Babies whose heads are rotated sideways (***occiput transverse positions***, referred to as ROT or LOT) are the ones most notorious for this problem. Women with babies in these positions often require a C-section.

Refer back to Chapter 13, "Home Stretch," for more details on the position of baby (lie, station, presentation, etc.).

Q. Can my partner cut the umbilical cord? Is it okay if they don't want to cut the cord?

It is completely up to you and your partner.

Some partners are dying to do it, and others don't even want to talk about it.

If your partner does want to cut the baby's cord, they will do it after the baby has come out and after your OB provider has placed two clamps (about one inch apart) on the cord. (Don't worry, your doctor will tell them when it's their turn to go to work.)

Your partner will cut the cord with a pair of scissors (provided by your OB provider) between the two clamps. The umbilical cord is a little rubbery (or "al dente," as one patient's husband who is a chef referred to it!), so it often takes a few snips to complete the job. This never hurts mother or baby.

DR. M'S OPINION

I always ask my patients and their significant others in advance, and then I ask again on D-day. Sometimes people change their mind. If your partner doesn't want to cut the cord, that is perfectly okay.

Partner Tip

Sometimes there is quite a bit of blood still left in the vessels between the clamps. Cutting the cord can cause a little bit of a "spray effect" (which is why I always turn my head away when the cord is being cut). Be prepared to get a teensy bit messy!

Q. I've been told that we should wait to cut the umbilical cord until after it stops pulsating. Why?

ACOG advises waiting, based on research showing that delayed cord cutting has health benefits for newborns.

It turns out that waiting sixty seconds after delivery to cut the cord gives babies extra blood from the placenta, lowering the risk of anemia, improving iron stores in baby (particularly important for preterm babies*) as well as decreasing the risk of brain hemorrhage and supporting brain health and neurodevelopment in the first year of life.[6] A decade ago, doctors would routinely cut a newborn's umbilical cord pretty quickly.

However, here are some key considerations with these guidelines:

- If your baby is in distress and there is an immediate concern for their health, your doctor will cut the cord right away and hand the baby over to the pediatric team ASAP.[7]
- If you are considering cord blood storage, there may be less blood to save. The baby gets the remaining blood from the placenta, leaving little if any left to collect.

So should you cut the cord sooner or later? We think you have to weigh your options, but we ultimately support delayed cord clamping. If you have a family history of certain disorders that may benefit from cord blood banking, cutting the cord and collecting and storing that extra blood may be a better option. If you don't, give your newborn a little mini-transfusion boost.

Reality Check

A new fad among natural childbirth enthusiasts is the "lotus birth" or "umbilical nonseverance." The concept: The baby hangs out with their dead, rotting placenta (which is attached to them) until the umbilical cord eventually separates from the belly button (that's two to four weeks on average). To state the obvious, there is absolutely no health benefit to this practice—only risk. A bloody, decaying placenta is a wonderful breeding ground for germs, which can subsequently infect the baby. We would be much more impressed with lotus birthing if it meant giving birth in a really cool sports car.

Q. When will I be able to hold the baby for the first time?

If the delivery goes smoothly and the baby is doing well, you can hold your baby as soon as they come out. The majority of moms request this to begin bonding with their baby. And in fact, this special time, often referred to as the "Golden Hour," is an extremely important time for both mom and baby. Having skin-to-skin contact with a newborn (often by laying the baby on mom's chest) helps them regulate their breathing, temperature, and acclimate to mom's smell. For you, it not only helps with bonding and oxytocin release, but it also decreases the shaking that can happen after delivery.

However, if the baby has an immediate problem (such as trouble breathing), they may get whisked over to the warming table in your delivery suite or even off to the neonatal intensive care unit.

This is very unsettling to new parents who have a perfect vision planned of those

*Pregnant people share a significant amount of iron with their growing baby in the third trimester, particularly in final thirty-two to forty weeks. Babies who are born prematurely are at risk of developing anemia because they miss out on that last bit of iron transfer. This is why preterm babies benefit the most from delayed cord clamping. They are also at greater risk of needing immediate support after delivery, so your doctor and the newborn care team will help determine which is the greater priority in the moment.

first moments together with their newborn. If this should happen to you, remember that your baby's health is the utmost priority. Even if you don't get to bond in those precious minutes right after delivery, you still have time later—and we promise it won't impact your long-term relationship with your child.

Reality Check

Your newborn will be bloody, often covered in cheesy white stuff (***vernix***) and sometimes poop (***meconium***). If the thought of this happens to turn your stomach, you have the option of having the baby dried and warmed right next to you at the warming table, and then handed over to you. They won't have their first real bath for a couple of hours after delivery, so they won't be totally clean, however.

Q. When does the OB collect blood for cord blood banking?

Very shortly after delivery. Here is how the scenario usually goes:

The baby comes out, and your OB provider (usually) puts them right up on your chest. If a couple wants to bank their baby's cord blood, your OB provider places two clamps on the cord right after delivery and the cord is cut (either by your partner or by your OB provider).

Once the cord is cut, your OB provider places a needle into the largest vessel in the umbilical cord to drain as much blood as possible into a bag or syringe. The goal is to get as much blood as possible before the vessels spasm and the placenta begins to separate from the wall of the uterus. Once that happens, no more blood flows through the umbilical cord.

Q. When do I get to feed the baby for the first time?

Assuming all is well after the vaginal delivery and your baby doesn't need to go to the nursery for any reason, you can start feeding them right away.

Some babies want to eat immediately. It is easy to tell because they start moving their lips and sticking out their tongues.

Other babies are rather sleepy—or coughing and sneezing to try to get all the fluid out of their lungs. Don't worry if your baby doesn't want to eat right away. Breathing is a higher priority than eating, so they will need to get the hang of it first (remember, they just learned how to do this the moment they came out).

Whether you are nursing or formula feeding, those first feeding moments can be awkward since you probably have no idea what you are doing. None of us do. Don't be embarrassed to ask for help. Your baby is very forgiving.

Q. How/when does the placenta come out?

The placenta is typically delivered within five to fifteen minutes after the birth of the baby. Trust us, it's a lot easier to deliver the placenta than the baby!

Most OB providers actively manage this stage of labor by gently pulling down on the umbilical cord, helping it separate from the wall of the uterus. You may also get a dose of Pitocin (through an IV) to help with delivery of the placenta and prevent excessive bleeding after delivery.

After you deliver your placenta, doctors do a few things to help your uterus contract and reduce blood loss. Your uterus is massaged from the outside of your abdomen, and you may get a dose of Pitocin (particularly if one was not given just prior to delivery of your placenta). The Pitocin helps your uterus contract even after you have delivered. The goal is to get your uterus to rapidly contract after delivery of the placenta—this helps slow bleeding. Your uterine contractions close off the arteries that previously supplied the placenta, which reduces blood loss.

Q. What if my placenta doesn't come out?

Occasionally, the placenta doesn't separate well and deliver.

Your OB provider can give a dose of Pitocin to help the uterus contract and expel the placenta. If that doesn't work, your doc may need to reach into your uterus with a gloved hand and separate the placenta from the wall of the uterus. This pleasant procedure is called a "manual extraction of the placenta." This is often very difficult, especially if the uterus has already started to shrink or if the placenta is really stuck to the uterine wall.

Very rarely, a woman has to go to the operating room to have the placenta removed with a surgical procedure.

BOTTOM LINE: The placenta needs to come out. In most cases (thank goodness!), it does so on its own.

Q. Does all the tissue from pregnancy come out by itself?

Your OB provider inspects the placenta once it is delivered to confirm that it is intact. A close inspection of the placenta, umbilical cord, and associated membranes (amniotic sac) is made to ensure that there aren't any pieces missing. Every once in a while, part of the placenta or fetal membranes doesn't come out and remains in the uterus (***retained products of conception***).

Very rarely, a person has to go to the operating room to have any remaining tissue removed with a surgical instrument (***postpartum D&C***).

Helpful Hint

"Products of conception" refers to all of the tissue that forms as a result of the sperm meeting the egg. That includes the fetus, placenta, umbilical cord, and amniotic sac.

Q. Is someone going to clean me up after all this?

Yes!

Either your OB provider or nurse will take care of that. It varies.

They'll use warm water with clean towels to clean up all the ***vernix***, blood, and sometimes ***meconium*** that will be all over your thighs and genital area. You are cleaned up immediately afterward because it is much easier to get everything off when it is wet.

After delivery of the placenta, the entire introitus (opening of the vagina), vaginal canal, and vulva are assessed for any lacerations. Those requiring stitches are cleaned, numbed with an injection of a local anesthetic like lidocaine (if you did not have an epidural), and sutured. Aftercare for the perineum consists of witch hazel pads with ice for everyone, laceration or no laceration.

C-Sections

NEW PARENT-TO-BE 411:

A C-Section in Fourteen Easy Steps

Here's the basic rundown, whether you have an elective or an emergency C-section. Some things vary between individual doctors and hospitals. And unless it's a major emergency, you are awake for the whole experience.

Step 1: Your doctor explains why they feel it is necessary that you have a C-section. They explain the risks, benefits, and alternatives, and you ask all of your questions.

Step 2: You read and sign a consent form stating that you understand and accept the risks, benefits, and alternatives.

Step 3: You drink a very sour-tasting antacid (think Warheads candy) to help neutralize stomach acid in the event you throw up. (Part of you wants to drink it because you are beyond thirsty. The other part of you wants to puke just smelling it. Take it down like a tequila shot. You'll be sorry if you sip it.)

Step 4: You get wheeled or walked into an operating room (OR), and your partner waits outside while everything gets set up. Don't let the sterile environs of the OR scare you. The OR is a white room with big lights hanging from the ceiling. It looks just like a set from *Grey's Anatomy*. You'll see a big anesthesia cart, a bed where you will be lying, and a big table to the right with all of the surgical instruments, needles, and towels on it (usually covered with a drape until just before surgery). There is also an incubator where the baby goes immediately after delivery.

Step 5: The anesthesiologist (your new best friend) inserts a small needle into your back and injects numbing medicine. You will probably have ***spinal anesthesia*** (discussed later in this chapter) unless you have been in labor and already have an ***epidural*** in place. If your epidural is already in place from being in labor, you will be given more medication through the catheter that is already in your back (no more needle sticks!).

Step 6: You lie down on the OR bed with your head on a pillow and your arms out to the side. I know you'd rather fold your arms on your chest or place them down at your side . . . but you might inadvertently move them into the surgical field where docs are operating (thus contaminating it), hit your doctor's hand while they are holding a sharp instrument (I don't need to explain why that might be bad), or accidentally grab your doctor's tush (which actually happened to me once!). You'll have an IV in one arm and a blood pressure cuff on the other, which both do better with outstretched arms. And your hands will stay out of trouble.

Step 7: A member of the OR team places monitors on your chest and one on your finger (see question on next page for details). FYI: All of this is really cold. The room, the air, the monitors. Many hospitals use a disposable paper gown called a "Bair Hugger" that is attached to a machine that blows warm air into it. This warms you up pretty quickly. You can also ask for warm blankets if you are still cold.

Step 8: The anesthesiologist will test you (using a cold alcohol wipe or a sharp object) to make sure you are numb. Once that's certain, you have a catheter tube placed through your urethra into your bladder (I know it sounds bad, but remember, you're numb!).

Step 9: You get prepped for surgery. Your pubic hair is shaved in the spot where the incision will be, and you are painted with an antibacterial soap to sterilize the area.

Step 10: You get draped for surgery. The OR team arranges a sterile drape over you, leaving only a small area over your lower abdomen open for your doctor to work. The drapes (yes, like curtains) are hung from to poles on either side so that your chest and head are visible, but you can't see what is going on below.

Step 11: Now your partner arrives to be by your side, wearing disposable, sterile, yet fashionable scrub attire. (If you've ever had fantasies of being with Dr. McDreamy, enjoy that visual now.)

Step 12: The OR team counts instruments and sponges and then has a "time out." (No one's in trouble—this helps avoid medical errors.) Your surgeon states a few obvious things out loud (like your name, any allergies you have, and what surgery you are having) to make sure that everyone is in agreement.

Step 13: Your doctor tests once more to make sure that you are indeed numb and begins the C-section.

Step 14: Your doctor begins surgery by making an incision (a cut) on the skin and works their way down to the uterus. Once they get into the uterus, they will rupture the amniotic sac (if not already ruptured) and lift the baby out. (You will feel pressure on your chest just before delivery as the OB pushes the baby out—this is a weird tugging sensation.) Next, your placenta is removed. Then, everything that was cut to get the baby out is sewn back together while you meet your baby. Voilà!

Q. Why would I need a C-section?

We can think of about twenty-three reasons. Check out Chapter 13, "Home Stretch," in the box entitled "Reasons You Might Need a C-Section" on page 326.

Q. Do I need an IV?

Yes, absolutely.

There must be immediate access to a vein for any type of surgery. Through the IV, you can get fluids, antibiotics, and medication.

Q. What if I need to pee?

You won't feel the sensation that your bladder is filling up if you have spinal or epidural anesthesia. That's dangerous because the bladder can stretch out and not correctly function later on—or may rupture. That's why doctors put a tube (Foley catheter) into your bladder through your urethra to constantly collect your urine. The procedure is done after your numbing medicine has kicked in. And it is removed about twelve hours after surgery when you can again pee on your own.

Q. Why is my blood being drawn?

When your IV is placed, some blood is drawn at the same time to check your blood type, Rh type, and get a complete blood count (CBC). Yes, you had those same labs checked in your doctor's office, but the hospital needs it to match donor blood in the remote chance you need a blood transfusion.

The CBC reveals if you are anemic prior to starting surgery and if you have an adequate number of platelets to clot your blood.

Q. What are all the monitors for?

You are hooked up to several monitors when you have surgery (thankfully, none of them hurt). We'll go over them so you won't feel like an alien. They help your doctors make sure your body is tolerating surgery.

- **Blood pressure cuff.** The cuff wraps around the upper part of your arm and stays for the duration of the surgery. It periodically fills with air (and gets pretty darn tight), reads your blood pressure, and then deflates.
- **Heart monitor.** You'll have three sticky patches on your chest with wires that go to a heart monitor. (Warning: They are *cold* when they go on.) The anesthesiologist uses this monitor to check your heart rate and pattern.
- **Pulse oximeter.** A small clip or sticker goes on your finger. This little thing, believe it or not, tells us how much oxygen is in your blood.

Q. What kind of anesthesia will be used?

Spinal anesthesia is the most popular choice for a C-section.

You'll feel a little poke and burn when the anesthesiologist injects local anesthesia to numb up your skin. Then they use another very thin needle to find the right space in your spinal canal and injects numbing medication.

The main difference between a spinal and an epidural is that with a spinal you get one shot and you're done. With an epidural, a tiny tube (catheter) remains in your back to be able to periodically inject more medication.

Spinal anesthesia is used for C-sections because the operation is pretty quick. Epidural anesthesia is used for vaginal deliveries since a person might be in labor for eighteen hours and need more medication. Often, the anesthesiologist will administer a pain medication called Duramorph (a longer-acting opioid medication) when they are doing spinal anesthesia for a C-section or an epidural. This provides very good pain relief for the first twenty-four hours after you deliver.

However, if your C-section is a non-elective one and you already have an epidural, your anesthesiologist will keep this going. Doctors also use an epidural if you are having additional surgery at the same time as the C-section (like removing a large ovarian cyst or doing a planned hysterectomy) or your doctor projects that your surgery may go longer or be harder than usual (example: this is your third C-section).

It's rare to need general anesthesia (where you are asleep) except with some emergency C-sections. It's only used when there is an immediate concern about the well-being of a fetus, there is no time to put in regional anesthesia (a spinal or epidural), or there is a reason you cannot have regional anesthesia.

For details, see the "Medications During Labor and Delivery" section later in this chapter.

Reality Check

A C-section puts you at a slightly higher risk of getting a postpartum infection than delivering vaginally. That's because making a cut in the skin can lead to a wound infection. To prevent this, doctors routinely give a dose of antibiotics through your IV before the start of surgery.

Q. Will I be cleaned up like I am having surgery?

Yes, because you are having surgery.

An antibacterial soap-like substance (usually clearish-pink and sticky, but there are many varieties) is used remove as much of the bacteria living on your skin as possible. We know you are clean, but no matter how clean you are, we all have bacteria living on the surface of our skin, and these are the same bacteria that can cause wound infections after surgery.

Q. Is my partner allowed to be in the operating room?

Yes!

Your OB provider wants your partner or support person to be there with you. However, if they are the queasy type, tell them not to look over the sterile blue sheet! Even with a routine C-section, it looks like a war zone on the other side. The only time this is not true is if there is an absolute emergency and you have to be put to sleep. In this scenario, as hard as it is, your partner will have to wait in the hallway outside the operating room.

Q. Can anyone else be in the OR?

Usually not.

But all hospitals have different policies. Some will allow two people to be with you. Just ask.

Q. Can we video the delivery?

This varies depending on the hospital and physician.

Here's a typical scenario: You can usually video the part of the delivery when the baby is actually coming out. Then you can video the baby in the warmer and getting cleaned up. Often, you cannot video the surgery itself, leading up to delivery or afterward. And really, unless you are a pre-med student, why would you want to?

Q. Can I view the delivery with a mirror?

It depends on your hospital's policies (and whether or not you have a strong stomach).

If this is important to you, ask in advance. It's common to be queasy during the surgery anyway, then consider whether you actually want to see someone cutting you open, touching your internal organs, covered in your blood.

It may be better to have someone videotape the delivery and then decide later whether or not you want to see it.

FEEDBACK FROM THE REAL WORLD:

Fainting Dad

I once had a dad look over the curtain just as I was taking his wife's uterus out of her abdomen to start sewing it up. He politely asked what the purple thing was that I was holding in my hand. When I replied, "Oh, it's just your wife's uterus," he turned bluish-white, started getting wobbly in the knees, and almost passed out. A word to the wise: Don't look if you have a weak stomach. We have two patients to take care of already (mom and baby); we don't need three!

Q. How long will it take?

A routine C-section takes about twenty-five to thirty minutes.

But if you've had a previous C-section or prior abdominal surgery, scar tissue could increase the time needed to perform your surgery. Your anatomy is now different, so doctors have to avoid damaging tissue that may not be in its usual place.

Emergency C-sections done for fetal distress are much quicker. If your baby is in severe distress, your OB provider can deliver them in a minute or two.

Q. Will my partner be able to cut the cord?

Yes, but it's not quite the same as in a vaginal delivery.

Because everything must be sterile in the operating room on the doctor's side of the blue curtain, your partner cannot come over to make the cut.

The delivering doctor initially cuts the cord. After the nurse or pediatrician takes the baby, another clamp (a small plastic one) is placed on the umbilical cord very close to the baby's skin. If desired, your partner can use a pair of scissors to trim the remaining cord hanging above that clamp.

Q. Is it still possible to collect the cord blood for cord blood banking?

Yes.

It is just as easy to collect cord blood during a C-section as with a vaginal delivery. Just remember to bring your kit to the hospital and hand it to your nurse when you are admitted. Many hospitals carry cord blood collection kits in case you forget yours at home.

Q. Where will the scar be?

Usually, your doctor will make the cut horizontally (a ***Pfannenstiel incision***) across the lower part of your abdomen just above your pubic bone. These days, most doctors try to make the cut as low as possible (in the upper part of your pubic hair) to avoid having a visible scar.

Some doctors make vertical skin incisions (from your belly button to your pubic bone)—but those are usually only done in emergencies or under special circumstances, like when a post-delivery hysterectomy is planned.

Q. Will I have stitches or staples?

It depends on your doctor.

Historically, most doctors used stitches on all the layers underneath the skin and staples to close the skin. Right before the woman went home (three to four days after surgery), the doctor would remove the staples and place Steri-Strips (little sterile pieces of surgical tape) over the healing skin. Staples were popular because they are quick and easy to do, with presumably the same wound healing results.

In the past few years, however, some good studies have compared the outcomes in patients receiving staples versus stitches during a C-section closure. The verdict: Stitches are better than staples. While there is no difference in the discomfort or cosmetic outcome, the wound separates (and reopens, yikes!) less often when stitches are used. And it only takes about ten minutes longer to stitch up the belly. Well worth the wait![8]

Q. What will happen to the stitches on the uterus?

The stitches (sutures) on the inside of your body are self-absorbable so they don't need to be taken out. Your doctor will close your skin with either stitches or staples.

If staples are used to close your skin, those will be taken out right before you go home from the hospital.

Q. When do I get to see the baby?

You will see the baby right after delivery. But where your baby goes next as you move from the operating room to a recovery room depends on the hospital.

Many delivery hospitals try to keep mother and baby together. If the baby does not have any medical issues requiring attention in the newborn nursery, mom and baby go to the recovery room together. A labor and delivery nurse looks after mom, and a nursery nurse comes to evaluate the baby.

If the baby needs to be observed more closely, they go to either the newborn nursery or the neonatal ICU (NICU). We know it's hard to be separated, but your baby's health is the first priority.

If you are in a hospital where it isn't possible to keep mom and baby together, you head to the recovery room and your baby goes to the newborn nursery for a while. You reunite about three to four hours later when you settle into your postpartum room. Truthfully, you will fall asleep, so that time will pass quickly!

Q. When do I get to nurse the baby?

If you are delivering at a hospital where mom and baby stay together, you can nurse in the recovery room.

If you can't nurse immediately, don't fret about it. There will be plenty of opportunities to bond!

If you are delivering at a hospital where you need to recover first, you can nurse your baby when you are brought to your postpartum room a few hours later.

Reality Check

The operating room may feel chaotic to you—but it's really a highly organized place. Don't feel overwhelmed by it all. If you deliver twins or other multiples, expect two or more pediatric or NICU teams and warmers in the delivery room.

Q. Who will be sure the baby is okay after delivery?

In the operating room, there is a team for you and a team for your baby. Every hospital has its own policies, but there is (at least) one specially trained pediatric nursery nurse at even the most routine, low-risk C-sections. At the other end of the spectrum, there may be a neonatologist, NICU nurse, and a respiratory therapist in the OR—all awaiting the delivery of a newborn in a high-risk situation.

The pediatric team takes the baby from the sterile surgical field over to a warming table or "warmer" and dries off/warms up and stimulates your baby to take some nice big breaths. This clears out the fluid from their lungs.

Meanwhile, the team does an initial survey of your baby, including vital signs,

Apgar scores and measurements (head, chest, length, and weight). For details, see the "Once the Baby Is Born" section at the end of this chapter.

If all is well, the nurse wraps your baby up like a little burrito and hands them to you and your partner.

Reality Check

Unless you live in a rural community, your own pediatrician will probably not be in attendance at your C-section. It will be a pediatrician or pediatric specialist on the hospital staff or a nurse. Your personal pediatrician will be notified by the hospital. Depending on the pediatric practice, you may see your own pediatrician or the pediatric hospitalist while you and your baby remain at the hospital.

Q. What will the first few days after my C-section be like? When will I be able to walk? What can I eat?

You'll see more about this in Chapter 15, "Postpartum: What's Next?," but here is a brief rundown:

People recover surprisingly quickly after a C-section despite the fact that it's major surgery. Every doctor has their own set of post-operative rules (and so do hospitals), but most of us are on the same page. Here's how we do it at my hospital just so you have a general idea of how things will go.

Assuming you aren't feeling queasy, you will be allowed to drink water four hours after surgery. Take my advice here . . . drink *slowly*. Yes, you are dying of thirst. But if you take down too much, too quickly, it will all come back up again. You will probably be able to sit up and even start to walk within six to twelve hours after surgery. Once the lovely catheter that is in your bladder is removed (about twelve hours after surgery), you will need to get up to walk to the bathroom when you have to go. Most hospitals encourage new moms to start walking pretty quickly after delivery. Walking gets your intestines moving again (they can slow down after abdominal/pelvic surgery). But most important, walking prevents blood clots from forming in your lower legs. (More on this in Chapter 15, "Postpartum: What's Next?")

You will probably get to eat real food twelve to twenty-four hours after your C-section. Check with your doctor to see if family members or friends can bring in outside food for you to eat, as most hospitals are not known for their amazing cuisine.

Fun fact: You may not have a bowel movement for three to five days after having a C-section. This is normal, but it's a good idea to let your doc know if you haven't gone number two in four to five days.

Medications During Labor and Delivery

NEW PARENT-TO-BE 411:

Anesthesia and Analgesia

There are special medications used to keep a person comfortable, relaxed, and pain-free during medical procedures. Doctors categorize them based on how the medications work.

The two basic terms to remember are ***analgesia*** (pain relief only) and ***anesthesia*** (the absence of pain, along with immobilization, usually achieved with sedation).

Medications are taken by mouth, inhaled, or given through an IV or shot. While some medications act locally at one site, others act regionally (over a larger area of the body). And general anesthesia acts on the whole body.

This list covers the types of medication used in labor, delivery, and postpartum care:

- **Sedatives:** Drugs that calm you down, ease your agitation, and let you sleep.
- **Narcotics:** Potent pain relievers derived from opium or an opium-like compound. They can also affect mood and behavior. People can become dependent on them if used long-term.
- **Epidural anesthesia:** Pain relief medication that numbs the nerves from the waist down. A small needle goes into the epidural space of the spine, and then a thin catheter tube remains to give continuous flow of pain medication for the duration of labor. It takes about ten to twenty minutes to kick in. The epidural provides excellent pain relief. You will have some leg weakness, but you should still be able to push effectively. Once the epidural is discontinued, you will regain full sensation and muscle strength.

Epidural

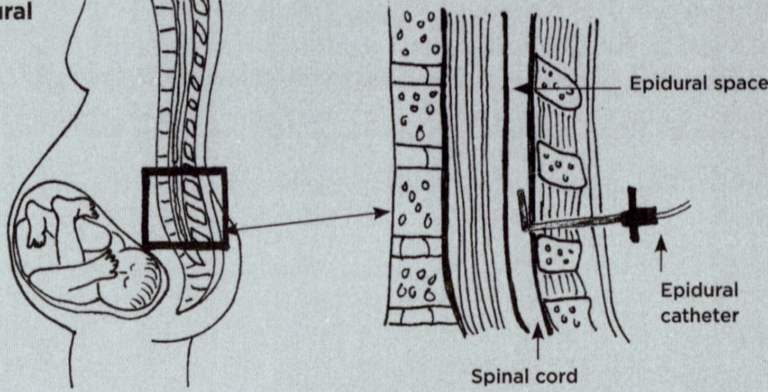

- **Spinal anesthesia:** Pain relief and numbing medication that affects nerves from the chest down. A small needle goes into the spinal canal for a single injection of medication. The medication begins to work immediately. You will be pain free and numb in the lower half of your body. It wears off after a couple of hours.

- **Pudendal block:** Local pain relief medication that is injected in the pudendal nerve (vaginal) area to quickly numb the vagina and vulva (perineum). It is used during the second stage of labor or after a delivery to do a repair.
- **Saddle block:** This is spinal analgesia that only numbs the buttocks, thighs, and genital area (perineum). It used to be popular, but it is rarely used today.
- **General anesthesia:** This is only used in true emergencies, when a baby needs to be delivered immediately, if you refuse regional anesthesia, or you are unable to receive regional anesthesia. You get medication to fall asleep, then a muscle relaxant, and finally pain relief. If you are asleep and all your muscles are relaxed, you also need a ventilator to breathe for you while you are under anesthesia. Once you are asleep, a breathing tube is placed through your mouth into your windpipe (trachea) to attach to the ventilator. After the procedure is over, the medication is turned off, you begin to awaken, and the breathing tube is removed.

Q. I want pain medication! When can I get my epidural?

There are really just two circumstances where you can't get an epidural:

1. It's too early because you aren't in labor.
2. It's too late because the baby's head is coming out.

It takes about five minutes for the anesthesiologist to set up and fifteen minutes until pain relief is on board. Our advice: Don't wait until pain is excruciating to request an epidural. Why? Because your friendly anesthesiologist may be busy helping another person in labor and won't be able to get to you right away. So if you know you want an epidural, speak up.

Here are the official guidelines on epidurals from ACOG: "Maternal request is sufficient medical indication for pain relief during labor." They also note that epidural anesthesia does not increase the risk of having a C-section.[9]

Helpful Hint

Once you get your epidural, you may want to read the paper or get out the backgammon board until it's time to push.

Fact Check

Epidurals cause autism.

The truth: Epidurals are not a cause of autism. Neither are Tylenol, cell phones, or vaccines!

Epidurals lead to chronic back pain.

The truth: You may be tender at the injection site for up to a week or two after delivery. If you have chronic back pain, it is more likely to be from the very awkward positions you are in while breastfeeding, holding your newborn, and sleeping.[10]

Q. I've heard that epidurals slow labor down. I don't want to be in labor any longer than I have to. What should I do?

Don't worry that the epidural will slow things down. In fact, some studies have shown that getting an epidural early may *decrease* the time to full dilation. This research is still up for debate, but the most recent data supports this theory.[11,12]

However, your doctor should look at each patient individually. You'll have to ask your OB provider if they have any concerns.

Q. What is a spinal headache? How likely is it that I would get one?

A spinal headache (***postdural puncture headache***) occurs in 1 to 3 percent of women who receive epidural anesthesia.

The needle used in the procedure can puncture the membrane that surrounds the spinal cord. This causes a leakage of spinal fluid, leading to a severe headache and upper back/neck pain for a day or two.

The difference between a spinal headache and a regular headache is that a spinal headache goes away or improves when lying flat. Bright lights may also bother you.

Most anesthesiologists recommend simple treatment for the first twenty-four hours—bed rest, hydration, and pain medication. About one-third of patients have pain severe enough to need additional help.

If you fall into that group, you may need something called an epidural blood patch. This involves injecting a small amount of your own blood into the epidural space. The blood forms a clot and seals the hole like a patch on a tire. This will cure the headache almost instantly. Occasionally, the blood patch needs to be repeated, but this is not very common.

Q. What are the risks of having spinal or epidural anesthesia?

The risks are very low of having a problem if you have a well-trained anesthesiologist taking care of you. But you should be aware of potential side effects and complications before you sign off:

- Low blood pressure
- Itching
- Fever
- Large bruise (hematoma)
- Infection (abscess)
- Allergic reaction to medication
- Nerve damage

- Inadequate pain relief
- Spinal headache (postdural puncture headache)
- Transient drops in fetal heart rate
- Painful sensations in the buttocks and legs
- "High spinal" where nerves to the neck and brainstem are numbed
- Death (very rare but possible)

Q. The hospital that I am delivering at only provides laboring people with spinal anesthesia, not epidurals. Should I get one?

Spinal anesthesia only lasts for an hour or two. Once it wears off, you can't get any more. That's why it's better for C-sections than for vaginal deliveries. But it can be used for the second stage of labor (the pushing stage).

Remarkably, there are still some hospitals that don't offer epidurals to laboring people. If that is your only option, talk with your provider about when it might be right for you.

Q. Can everyone get an epidural?

Pretty much, yes. There are a few conditions that might make an anesthesiologist reluctant to place one. Doctors are very cautious about these things for safety reasons. Here are those situations:

- You are taking blood thinner medications.
- You have an extremely low platelet count.
- You have a bleeding disorder.
- You have a serious heart condition.
- Your blood pressure is unstable.
- You have had corrective spine surgery.

Anesthesiologist Dr. Steve Rutman has this advice: Do a pre-labor visit with your anesthesiologist. "If you have a medical condition that you feel might complicate getting an epidural, have your OB call the anesthesia department at your delivery hospital and arrange a prenatal visit with an anesthesiologist. This allows the doctor to suggest additional tests before you go into labor to see if an epidural is safe. You can also make a plan for forms of pain relief so everyone knows what to expect when you arrive to have your baby."

Reality Check

Anesthesiologists do not like surprises!

Q. I've heard of people taking fentanyl or another opioid for pain relief before an epidural. What do you think?

If you are so uncomfortable that you are contemplating narcotics, just get an epidural instead.

Morphine, butorphanol, and fentanyl are IV narcotic medications used early in labor to dull the pain of contractions. They are also offered to some people when labor induction involves using an intracervical balloon. The drug goes into your bloodstream, and although it helps to dull your pain, it also goes through the placenta, to your baby. If you have a long labor (that means you, first-time moms), it can be taken early on because it usually wears off before delivery.

But if your labor is quick, your baby might be born with narcotics on board. In higher doses, it can make a baby's breathing rate dangerously slow and cause them to be very lethargic. That's never a good way to start out life. Those babies need another drug after birth to reverse the narcotic's effects.

Q. I don't want any pain medication. What are my options to reduce the discomfort of labor and delivery?

If you want to attempt labor and delivery without pain medication, we'd highly recommend having a doula. It is so important to have an experienced person to coach, massage, and encourage you through this very tough and painful process.

A doula will help you to relieve and cope with the pain by changing positions, breathing, sitting on a birthing ball, taking a bath, being massaged, and using different focusing techniques. Ask your friends, OB provider, or local hospital for references.

Home Births

For this section, we recruited an experienced midwife to discuss the home birth experience. Heather Milovina, a certified nurse midwife (CNM), WHNP-BC (Women's Health Nurse OB provider), and certified pre- and postnatal massage therapist, has practiced in California and Hawaii. Heather is also Dr. M's sister, so the price was right.

Here's the take-home message: Birthing at home with a skilled attendant can be a joyful and safe experience for low-risk people. Midwives provide both medical and emotional support during your prenatal care and labor.

When you go into labor, your midwife will likely come to your home during early labor and remain there through delivery. You may also have an assistant midwife, doula, or other healthcare OB providers present. Your partner and any other family members you desire to have with you can be your support team. The birth attendant will bring most of their own supplies but will request you have some items on hand in advance.

The midwife monitors your progress by assessing your vital signs, doing periodic vaginal exams, and checking fetal heart tones using a fetoscope or Doppler. Home birth attendants try to avoid internal fetal monitoring, IVs, episiotomies, and artificial rupturing of the fetal membranes, unless absolutely necessary.

You can give birth on your bed, in a birthing tub, bathtub, or even on your living room floor if you like. You can decide where you feel the most comfortable.

Once you give birth, your baby is placed into your arms to begin bonding and breastfeeding. The midwife will examine your baby thoroughly, weigh and measure them, and administer vitamin K and eye ointment if agreed upon beforehand.

After you deliver the placenta, the midwife will perform any necessary suturing and clean you and the birthing area. As Heather points out, "The only evidence that a birth just occurred is your new baby!"

The midwife stays for a couple of hours after your delivery to make sure both mother and baby are stable, to answer questions, provide care instructions, and ensure you have eaten a meal.

If a complication arises, midwives are trained in neonatal resuscitation and CPR. They will also have oxygen with them and medications to stop bleeding. But if you need advanced medical care, you are transferred to the nearest hospital or medical facility.

"When you choose to birth at home, you are free to wear what you want, labor and birth in any position, eat and drink freely, and have any friends and family present if you desire," Heather told us.

To help you cope with contractions, your midwife may suggest using herbal medicine, homeopathy, hydrotherapy, massage, acupuncture, and various breathing techniques. They'll also give continuous hands-on assistance.

If your birth is proceeding normally (which over 90 percent do), a midwife does little more than monitor the health and progress of you and your baby. They provide positive, loving support. Although every midwife brings their own style, there are standards of care that are universally followed.

Reality Check

ACOG has a policy statement that respects families' rights to make informed decisions about childbirth. They also want people planning a home birth to be aware of the potential risks. The American Academy of Pediatrics does not recommend home births because there is a two- to three-fold increased risk of infant mortality, which is about 1 in 1,000 births.[13] The AAP supports hospitals and accredited birthing centers as the safest place to deliver. If a family chooses to deliver at home, they recommend the following precautions:

Rapid transport should be available, if necessary, to a nearby hospital. There should also be at least one medical provider attending the delivery whose only job is to care for the newborn. It's rare, but situations arise where both mother and newborn need immediate care.

BOTTOM LINE: Think twice about delivering at home, especially if a hospital isn't nearby. And have at least two skilled providers in attendance at a planned home birth.

Reality Check

Even though you deliver at home, your baby still needs close monitoring on a daily basis for weight loss and jaundice. Be sure your care attendants follow up at twenty-four and forty-eight hours of life in case your baby needs additional care. Your baby should also have a newborn follow-up appointment with your pediatrician at four to five days of life.

Birthing Centers

If you have a low-risk pregnancy and want a natural birth experience (but don't want to deliver at home), a birthing center might be right for you.

Most birthing centers *do not* do inductions, use Pitocin or continuous external monitoring, offer epidurals or spinals, or perform operative deliveries (involving the use of a vacuum or forceps) or C-sections.

Birthing centers *do* provide a relaxed, comfortable setting with less intervention than hospitals and allow you to return home shortly after the birth if you so desire. Midwives or licensed nurses perform deliveries at birthing centers. Obstetricians typically do not.

The ideal birthing center experience closely follows the New Parent-to-Be 411 box "A Hospital Vaginal Delivery in Thirteen Easy-ish Steps," on page 351.

Reality Check

If there is a complication during your labor that requires immediate medical care, you will be transferred to the nearest delivery hospital. Even though this is not your ideal vision, remember the goal is a healthy baby and mom.

This Wasn't in the Birth Plan!

While one hopes for that picture perfect delivery, sometimes things don't go by the book. This section discusses items that weren't what you outlined in your birth preferences.

Freak-out warning: Most of these complications are uncommon. This section is for those of you who want the complete picture. For everyone else, who might find this material disturbing, you may want to skip to the next section, "Once the Baby Is Born."

NEW PARENT-TO-BE 411:

Ten Things That Can Go Wrong During Labor and Delivery

Now, for those who choose to read on, here are the top ten things that can go wrong with labor and delivery. If you end up in one of these scenarios, take a deep breath and let your healthcare team do what they are trained to do: Get you and your baby through delivery safely.

1. **Non-reassuring fetal heart pattern.** If the monitors show that a baby is continually stressed during labor, your OB provider is going to move things along to get your baby out safely. That may mean doing an operative or assisted vaginal delivery (that is, using forceps or a vacuum extractor—more on this below) or a C-section.
2. **Malpresentation.** Your baby may have their own idea of how they would like to make their entrance into the world. But sometimes their choice is unrealistic. If we know ahead of time that your baby is breech, you need a version or a C-section. But some malpresentations are discovered during labor. That makes for either a complicated vaginal delivery or an emergency C-section.
3. **Arrest of dilation or arrest of descent.** If you are exhausted AND your doc has already given you Pitocin AND broken your water bag AND your baby is still high in the pelvis and not moving down the birth canal, or you have stopped dilating over many hours, yes, you will need a C-section.
4. **Chorioamnionitis**. About 1 to 5 percent of people get an infection in the placenta, amniotic sac, and surrounding fluid. It's more common if your water has been broken for more than twenty-four hours before delivery. Once your water breaks, the clock is ticking.
5. **Meconium**. Babies who are stressed prior to or at delivery may pass their first poop before they leave the womb. That poop can be seen in the amniotic fluid. If the meconium enters the baby's lungs, it can cause inflammation and problems breathing. So it's important to clear the baby's airway. If your water breaks and your OB sees the meconium, a neonatal team is called to attend the delivery. Yes, even more people get to see you naked: You won't care at that point.
6. **Shoulder dystocia**. After the baby's head comes out, the shoulder that is on top gets stuck behind the woman's pubic bone. This is one of the few situations that will make your OB provider sweat (literally and figuratively). Your baby needs to be delivered pronto and the doctor is going to do what it takes to make that happen. There are many maneuvers to try, but if they are not working to deliver the baby, doctors and midwives actually purposely break the baby's collar bone (***clavicular fracture***) or upper arm (***humerus fracture***) to deliver them. Severe shoulder dystocias can cause a

(continued)

temporary (90 to 95 percent of the time) injury to the nerves of the baby's shoulder, arm, and hand (***brachial plexus injury***).

7. **Neonatal resuscitation**. When your baby is born, the healthcare providers in the room make sure your baby is vigorous, breathing, moving, and turning nice and pink (see Apgar discussion below). If they are not doing what the team expects them to do, they may need to be warmed up, receive oxygen, have their nose and mouth suctioned, or even receive CPR. Your first reaction is, "Is my baby going to be okay?" The answer is almost always yes, but give your team time to help baby make the big transition to the real world. And yes, some babies need more medical support in the intensive care nursery (NICU) until they prove they can manage life on their own.
8. **Labored breathing**. Babies who are delivered by C-section don't get the amniotic fluid squeezed out of their lungs like those who get pushed through the birth canal (unless your doc makes an incision as small as I do and babies are still squeezed out though a tiny incision!). As a result, some babies may have temporary labored breathing for the first few hours after delivery (called ***transient tachypnea of the newborn*** or ***TTN***). Occasionally, babies delivered vaginally will have this, too. If your baby has TTN, they are monitored for a little while in the nursery before getting their first snuggles with you.
9. **Operative vaginal delivery**. An uncomplicated vaginal delivery is the goal, but sometimes that just isn't in the cards. If having a forceps or vacuum extraction will help get your baby out safely, it is the right answer.
10. **Minor birth injuries**. If you have a vacuum extraction, your baby could have a very large goose egg on their head (a collection of blood called a ***cephalohematoma***). It's temporary, and you can cover it up with those cute little hats for their first baby pictures. Other babies may have bruised faces and little broken blood vessels from delivery. Medically, the only concern here is a slightly greater risk of your baby becoming jaundiced in the first few days of life.

Q. My doctor just broke my water bag and said that there was meconium (the fluid was greenish-brownish). That shouldn't happen before the baby is born, right?

First of all, let's define "***meconium***." "Meconium" is a Latin word that means "poppy juice." It is a dark green sticky substance consisting of mucous and fecal material that forms in the fetal intestine (which is apparently the same color as poppy juice).

Meconium is released as the baby's first bowel movement at or near the time of birth. Typically, this does *not* occur prior to delivery.

Sometimes a fetus under stress will release meconium into the amniotic fluid prior to delivery. How do we know? There are two possible clues: once your amniotic sac is ruptured, the fluid is greenish/brownish. Or, in some cases, if there is no fluid leaking out at all after rupture of membranes, doctors may suspect meconium.

What causes this stress? Lack of sufficient blood supply and lack of oxygen. This may be caused by many things, including ***placental abruption***, ***preeclampsia***, ***fetal growth restriction***, ***oligohydramnios***, placental insufficiency, and fetal infection.

Q. Is there anything to do now that my baby has passed meconium and I am still in labor?

No, not really.

If the amniotic fluid is only slightly tinged with what is called "light meconium" and your baby looks like they are doing well based on their heart-rate pattern, there is nothing to do but observe.

If, on the other hand, the amniotic fluid is more like split pea soup in appearance or "thick meconium," and there is concern about the fetal heart rate, an ***amnioinfusion*** may be done, although not routinely recommended by ACOG.

An amnioinfusion is a procedure where a very thin sterile catheter is placed through the vagina up into the uterus, next to the baby. This does not hurt nor bother your baby. Through this catheter, doctors can infuse sterile water into the uterus to help wash out some of the thicker meconium. This is also done if a baby is showing signs of fetal distress based on a compressed umbilical cord.

Once your baby is delivered, their nose and mouth will be suctioned (as well as the upper part of their throat) to remove any meconium prior to them taking their first breath. This prevents the meconium from getting beyond the baby's vocal cords and potentially into their lungs. As you might guess, this is a situation where your baby isn't immediately placed on your chest.

Q. My friend had a baby that got stuck after the head came out. Why does this happen, and how do I know that won't happen to me?

This is called ***shoulder dystocia***, when baby's shoulder gets stuck behind mom's pubic bone (after the head comes out).

Here's what you need to know: Shoulder dystocia is rare, occurring in just 0.6 to 1.4 percent of all vaginal deliveries. It often happens without warning and is one of those unpredictable obstetric emergencies. So while there is no guarantee it won't happen during your delivery, you can rest somewhat easier by realizing it does not occur frequently.

There are some risk factors for shoulder dystocia (see below), but most cases just happen out of the blue.

And if it does happen, your OB provider will perform some special maneuvers to help free the little one's shoulder and deliver the rest of the baby.

Q. What are risk factors for having a shoulder dystocia?

A big baby (***macrosomia***) is the number one risk factor. You are most likely to have a big baby if you have diabetes (either preexisting or gestational, with poor sugar control), obesity, or a pregnancy that goes beyond its due date. Other risk factors include having a previous baby who was delivered with shoulder dystocia or who was large or needed a vacuum or forceps to help with delivery.

This is why OB providers recommend C-sections when the estimated fetal weight is 5,000 grams or more (11 pounds) in non-diabetic patients and 4,500 grams or more (10 pounds) in diabetic patients.

That said, most cases of shoulder dystocia occur in patients with none of the above risk factors.

Q. Is it true that sometimes instruments are used to pull the baby out?

Yes.

This is called an *operative vaginal delivery*; it occurs in 10 percent to 15 percent of US deliveries. Operative deliveries use either forceps or a vacuum extractor.

The decision to do an operative vaginal delivery is often made in the heat of the moment—when it is clear there is either a risk to the woman or baby. Operative deliveries are also needed in cases of extreme maternal exhaustion where the woman is just beat and can't push anymore. Additionally, they are used if woman suffers from a medical condition that requires them not to push during the second stage of labor. This might be severe maternal heart disease or certain rare conditions that increase the pressure in a person's brain, such as having too much spinal fluid and vascular aneurysms.

Talk to your OB provider about the hypothetical need for an operative vaginal delivery during one of your prenatal visits. You won't have time to have a relaxed discussion about it in the delivery room.

Here's an overview of each method:

Forceps: These puppies look like salad tongs on steroids. The OB provider places them on either side of the baby's head. Older physicians who are very experienced in this vanishing art occasionally choose this method of delivery.

Vacuum extractor: This is the instrument of choice for most OBs. The typical vacuum extractor is a flexible plastic suction cup (although a metal or inflexible cup is also occasionally used) placed over a specific area on the baby's head to help ease them out.

An OB provider can only perform an operative vaginal delivery in certain situations. To be successful, the cervix must be fully dilated (10 cm), and the baby's head must be low enough in the birth canal.

Here are three good reasons to use forceps/vacuum extractor:

- **Lack of oxygen to the baby's brain.** If your doc sees the fetal heart rate dropping and not recovering, the baby must come out.
- **Mother's health at risk.** To shorten the pushing stage of labor if mom has severe heart disease or brain conditions that makes pushing risky.
- **Exhaustion.** If the woman no longer has the energy to push.

And, by contrast, here are reasons *not* to use forceps/vacuum extractors:

- **Your labor is long.** You should not have an operative vaginal delivery just because your OB is tired of watching you push and really wants to get home to catch the last few minutes of a basketball game.
- **An immediate C-section isn't an option.** You should not have an operative vaginal delivery just because having an immediate C-section is not an option where

you are laboring (such as a home birth or birthing center). You should be transported emergently to a hospital for a C-section. If a doctor can't deliver a baby after trying with either a vacuum or forceps, a C-section is the only option, so these procedures can only be done in a hospital with immediate access to an operating room.

- **You haven't consented.** You should never have an operative vaginal delivery without your consent.

If you have a well-trained OB provider, it is relatively rare to have a complication from a vacuum extractor or forceps delivery (there is a 3 to 5 percent risk). But you need to be an informed patient, so that's why we list possible complications (see the box below). If reading this will give you nightmares, just skip right over it!

NEW PARENT-TO-BE 411:

Possible Operative Vaginal Delivery Complications

Possible complications of vacuum extraction:

- Big bruise (collection of blood) under the baby's scalp and above the skull (***cephalohematoma***)
- Cut on the baby's scalp
- ***Jaundice***
- Bleeding in the space between thin membrane that lines the bones of the skull and the thin membrane that covers the baby's brain (***subgaleal hemorrhage***)
- Bleeding in the back of the baby's eye (***retinal hemorrhage***)
- Bleeding in the baby's brain (***intracranial hemorrhage***)
- ***Shoulder dystocia***
- Soft tissue injury to the woman if vaginal or cervical tissue gets trapped under the suction cup

Possible complications of forceps:

- Facial and head bruises on the baby
- Facial nerve injury to the baby
- Scratch on the outer part of the baby's eye (corneal abrasion)
- Skull fracture of the baby
- Bleeding in the baby's brain (***intracranial hemorrhage***)
- ***Shoulder dystocia***
- Soft tissue injury to the mother
- Maternal bleeding

Q. I know the way your labor goes can't be predicted, but mine seems to be going off track, and I don't feel like my nurses or provider are communicating with me. What can I do?

Unfortunately, sometimes during the labor and delivery process, patients don't feel heard. This is the reason that earlier in this book we stressed finding an OB provider whom you feel comfortable with and whom you trust. But there are many situations where even if you trust your provider, they aren't the one delivering your baby or you haven't even seen the doc or midwife who will be delivering you (some will only come at the end for the actual delivery), and you don't feel comfortable with your nurse or other team members caring for you. Ultimately, you need to trust your instincts and stand up for yourself. If you feel like you aren't getting the communication you need to better understand things, ask to speak with your provider on the phone. If you feel like you and your nurse just don't mesh, you can ask to speak to the charge nurse to have a different nurse assigned to you. If you feel uncomfortable speaking out yourself, you can ask your partner or friend/family member with you to talk with them.

Once the Baby Is Born

Now let's pretend your baby was just born. Congratulations! What happens next? Ideally, your OB provider puts your baby on your chest and you are able to do skin-to-skin contact for the next hour (often referred to as the "Golden Hour"). This is important for you and your little one. It's not always possible, but if you have a chance to request this, please do!

The following list can be done on the chest of the woman, or in the warmer. The order of things may vary a bit, but here's the general idea:

1. **Drying and stimulation**. Your baby will be covered in blood and vernix. In other words, your baby is all wet. And that means they are going to get cold pretty fast. So the staff will vigorously dry them off with towels and either place them skin-to-skin on your chest or put them on a small exam table that has a heater (warming table). The vigorous rubdown stimulates your baby to breathe and gets their circulation going.
2. **Suctioning**. Their mouth and nose get suctioned to remove thick secretions.
3. **Apgar scores**. Your baby gets graded on how they are adjusting to life outside the womb. They get a score of zero to ten at one minute of life and again at five minutes (see more on Apgar scores in question below).
4. **Measurements**. Your baby has their weight, length, and head circumference measured and recorded.
5. **Assistance as needed**. If your baby has a significant problem (limp, blue, not breathing, low heart rate), the staff provides any support necessary while they are on the warming table in the delivery room. If your baby needs ongoing support, they go to the nursery or NICU. If your delivery or birthing center does not have a NICU, and your baby is very ill, they may need to be transported to another facility.

6. **First meal.** If your baby is doing well, they should nurse or take a bottle of formula within the first hour of life. (They'll only be interested in sleep for the next few hours after that.) After baby and parents have time to bond, they have a few more things on their to-do list.
7. **Eye ointment.** It is recommended that all newborns get antibiotic eye ointment to protect them from a serious eye infection.
8. **Vitamin K injection.** It is recommended that all newborns get one dose of vitamin K, as most babies are born with low levels of vitamin K. Low vitamin K levels can lead to vitamin K deficiency bleeding (VKDB), which can lead to significant bleeding into vital organs, like the brain. It is given as an injection (shot) to give optimal protection quickly. In case you are wondering, it would take several weeks to months of taking an oral Vitamin K supplement to treat a vitamin K deficiency—leaving susceptible babies at risk for severe bleeding.
9. **Hepatitis B vaccine.** The United States, as well as many countries worldwide, recommends universal protection for all newborns against a serious viral infection called hepatitis B. The top three ways this infection is spread is by blood, body fluids, and birth. It is often a silent infection, and an infected person can be symptom-free initially. While women receiving appropriate prenatal care are routinely screened for hepatitis B, not everyone receives optimal prenatal care and it is also possible to acquire hepatitis B during pregnancy. So a mother can unknowingly pass it to her newborn during the birth process. For a more detailed discussion, see Chapter 11, "Parenthood Prep."
10. **ID band and security clip.** Your baby is official now. They'll wear an ankle band bracelet (usually two—one on each ankle) that matches yours (so no one swaps babies in the nursery). Many facilities also attach security clips to newborns for additional peace of mind. We call them "Baby LoJacks."
11. **Observation time.** Your baby needs to be watched closely for the first couple of hours. The nursery nurses will do a complete head-to-toe exam, and monitor their heart rate, respiratory rate, body temperature, and oxygen level. That's the time your baby also gets any blood drawn for lab tests should any be necessary (blood sugar, blood count, blood culture). The nurses also notify your baby's doctor about the birth if your pediatrician makes hospital visits. If not, a hospital-based pediatrician will be responsible for caring for your baby while they are there.
12. **First bath, first checkup.** Your baby can get cleaned up after they prove they can maintain their body temperature. This is optional in most hospitals, and some parents choose to forgo the bath for a few more days. After all those hurdles, your baby is ready to just hang out with you in your postpartum room. Your pediatrician or a hospital-based pediatrician will examine your baby within twenty-four hours of birth.

We could write a book on the details of your baby's first exam and what you're supposed to do next. Oh wait, we already did! Check out *Baby 411* for the sequel to this story.

Q. What Apgar score do you need to get into Harvard?

This is actually a trick question—they only accept standardized test scores. But the medical staff cares very much about your baby's Apgar scores because it tells them how your baby is transitioning to life outside the womb. Here's how we do the grading:

Appearance (color)

Pulse (heart rate)

Grimace (reaction to stimulation)

Activity (tone)

Respiratory rate

Each category is scored zero, one, or two, with a maximum of ten points, but it's rare to get a perfect score, even for babies born to moms who are doctors (believe us, we tried to sway the hospital staff when we both delivered our kids, but the highest was a 9!). OB providers do an assessment at one minute of life, again at five minutes, and occasionally at ten minutes. Babies who go through difficult deliveries often have a low (less than five) Apgar at one minute, and then perk up (greater than seven) at five minutes. Babies that don't improve their scores may need observation and assistance by the medical staff.

Q. What happens to the placenta?

The placenta is an amazing conduit of food and oxygen, a disposal system for fetal waste, and a manufacturer of hormones and amniotic fluid. But once the baby is born, the placenta's job is done. So it gets delivered, too.

The fate of your placenta depends on whether there were any problems during your pregnancy or labor. If so, your OB provider may ask a pathologist to take a look at it to help identify a placental abruption or infection.

Otherwise, your placenta ends up in a red biohazard bag and gets discarded with all other medical waste products.

If you want to keep your placenta and you are delivering at home, you can do whatever you wish. If you are delivering at a hospital or a birthing center, you will need to get clearance from your medical provider and the birth facility. Discuss this with your OB provider in advance.

Believe it or not, some folks are adopting the ancient Chinese practice of "placental encapsulation." The placenta is steamed with lemon, ginger, and chili, then dehydrated for several hours. It is then prepared into a powder form and placed in a capsule to ingest. You can find a local "certified independent placental encapsulation specialist" in some hipster cities (yes, Austin, Texas, and Beverly Hills, California, we are talking about you), or you can take the DIY approach (yes, it's on Pinterest; not kidding). Fans tout the health benefits of ingesting the hormone-rich tissue, but medical organizations say there is no evidence to support this practice.

Alternatively, you might decide to bury your placenta in the ground and plant a tree over it (like Matthew McConaughey did. Let's hope Matthew's dog isn't a digger!).

Partner Tip

You will think of your beloved in a whole new light now after witnessing the miracle of birth together. Next time they yell at you for leaving the toilet seat up, remember this moment and how much you love them.

Whew, that was tough—no matter how you had your baby! But you did it and you now have a newborn in your arms. Enjoy!

CHAPTER 15

Postpartum: What's Next?

"Giving birth is like taking your lower lip and forcing it over your head!"

—Carol Burnett

What's in This Chapter

- **Tips for vaginal deliveries**
- **Tips for C-sections**
- **Seven reasons to call your doc**
- **When can I drive?**
- **When can I hold my toddler?**
- **Birth control**
- **Stretch marks**
- **Nutrition tips**
- **Baby blues**
- **Postpartum depression**

Let's pop into a time machine and read the recommendations for women who just gave birth back in 1949. Yes, this is from an actual handout given to women who just gave birth:

"If you smoke, try to limit your cigarettes to five a day, particularly if you are breastfeeding."

"If you drink, try to limit your drinking to one highball a day." (We love that term, highball!)

And our personal favorite: *"If you are having trouble breastfeeding, you may consider stopping and switching your baby to the bottle, as this will allow you to have more time to sew, cook, tend to your flowers and look well-maintained when your husband comes home from work."*

My, my . . . we've come a *long* way, ladies!

This chapter will prepare you for the changes your body will go through after delivery, both immediately and a few weeks down the line. We are talking about physical, hormonal, and emotional changes—and there are plenty of them! Learn about them now so you'll know what is normal and what isn't. And you will be more prepared to deal with it all.

Care After Vaginal Delivery

Q. Why is the nurse massaging my belly?

Your uterus needs to shrink down after delivery. A soft uterus whose muscles aren't contracting (***uterine atony***) can lead to excessive bleeding (***postpartum hemorrhage***). This, as you might guess, is not good.

Your OB provider will massage your belly just after the placenta is delivered, then your nurses will do it periodically over the next forty-eight hours. In fact, you'll be sick of everyone touching your belly to see if your uterus is hard.

Q. How do I care for my tear or episiotomy?

Most women suffer some kind of trauma down there after a delivery. If you tore or had an ***episiotomy***, healing can be pretty uncomfortable and may take a few weeks (particularly if this is your first). Here are some things that may help:

- Put an ice pack over your genital area (vulva/perineum) for the first twenty-four hours after delivery.
- Use warm water (easiest if you put it in a squirt bottle) to cleanse the area after urinating or having a bowel movement. This helps ease discomfort and prevent infection.
- Use a topical analgesic such as Dermoplast spray (contains benzocaine, menthol, aloe vera, and lanolin).
- Use witch hazel (pads or spray).
- Use ibuprofen around the clock (every six hours) for the first forty-eight hours after delivery. This helps with pain as well as swelling and inflammation.
- Avoid lifting too much or being too active.
- Avoid using soap directly on the outside of the vagina for a few days, as it will sting like the dickens if you do.
- Take a stool softener like docusate (Colace) or polyethylene glycol 3350 (MiraLAX) to help with your first few bowel movements. Drink lots of water and eat prunes and have more fiber (cereals, flax seeds, chia seeds, raspberries, blackberries).

If you are recovering from a third- or fourth-degree tear/episiotomy, here are some additional tips:

- Use a donut (soft ring-shaped cushion) when you are sitting down.
- Take sitz baths (your pelvic area sits in a few inches of warm water) two to four times a day to help with some of the discomfort.
- Change your sanitary pads frequently.

INSIDER SECRET:

Five Amazing Things Your Body Does Just After Delivery

1. Your uterus shrinks from a size large enough to hold your baby to the size of a large grapefruit.
2. The lining of your uterus (the ***endometrium***) begins to regenerate just sixteen days later.
3. You lose more blood than would fill a pint-size container of ice cream . . . and live to tell about it.
4. Your body's hormonal changes (after the placenta is delivered) trigger your breast milk production.
5. You lose ten to fifteen pounds in a matter of minutes.

Q. My vaginal area is bruised. How long will that last?

A bruise (or in medical lingo, a *hematoma*) can result from the veins in your genital area being torn during delivery. The blood gets trapped under your skin and your skin turns dark red, purple, or black (sounds fun, right?).

Sometimes this can look dramatic and can extend up above your pubic hair line on your lower abdomen or down either thigh. Or this bruise can cause part of your vulva (the labia in particular) to swell.

Although it looks as if it will never go away, it will. But this takes time. A small vulvar hematoma may take only a week to disappear, just as a small bruise on your leg would. A large hematoma (particularly if your vulvar area is swollen) may take weeks or months to completely resolve. Using ice for the first twenty-four to forty-eight hours will help.

Q. I pushed for three hours, and the outer part of my vagina is pretty swollen. What should I do?

Ice, ice, ice.

This is the best thing to do for the first twenty-four hours after delivery if you have a lot of swelling (***edema***). If your swelling is pretty severe, keep the ice on for forty-eight hours. Most of the swelling is improved after forty-eight hours and your body will take care of the rest in the next week or so.

Q. I have a few tears on my vagina—how long will they take to heal?

It depends on how many and how deep.

Some women get tiny cuts and abrasions on either side of the urethra and into the vagina. Those usually heal up in three to four weeks.

But it may take six weeks or more to heal if you have deep tears along the sides of the vagina (***sulcal tears***), lacerations of the ***cervix***, or a third- or fourth-degree tear.

Partner Tip

Time heals all wounds. But tread lightly about lovemaking right now! Your partner won't get the green light for at least six weeks after delivery.

Q. I'm scared to use the bathroom after delivery!

We promise, it's usually not that bad! Here are a few things that can help: After peeing, use a peri wash bottle filled with warm water, then pat dry with toilet paper. You can follow with lidocaine spray, witch hazel pads, or ice for comfort. For bowel movements, we recommend staying hydrated, using stool softeners or a magnesium supplement, and taking Sitz baths (soaking in warm water).

Care After a C-Section

Q. When will I be allowed to drink something?

Usually, you can have a few sips of water two to four hours after surgery. But if you feel nauseated or you're puking, you don't get anything to drink until that subsides.

When they do hand you a drink, start with small sips even though you'd love to gulp it down (you'll feel like you just walked through the desert). Chugging it will only make you feel nauseated. Our advice: Nurse your drink.

Q. When can I eat something other than chicken broth?

You get a yummy liquid diet for the first twelve to twenty-four hours after a ***C-section***. It's a very appetizing assortment of Jell-O (you can select the color!), broth, juice, and teas. Yes, it feels like torture, but your doctor wants to be sure your stomach and intestines are ready to handle liquids before moving up to solids.

If you are drinking like a champ and aren't nauseated or vomiting, you get to eat real food (if you call hospital food "real food") sooner. Many hospitals allow your friends and family to bring food in for you, so you can skip the hospital fare.

POSTPARTUM

Reality Check

Although the tradition used to be that you needed to pass gas prior to eating after surgery, things have changed. Today, you can eat after showing that you can keep down liquids.

Passing gas usually happens within a day or two after surgery. Be prepared to answer the question "Have you passed any gas?" about twelve times a day as everyone coming into your room (the nurse's aide, the nurse, your doctor, and maybe even your mother-in-law) will certainly ask.

Partner Tip

As long as you get approval from the doctor, bring in a nice meal from the real world for your recovering partner. Whether it's their favorite pasta dish or the sushi they've been craving for nine and a half months, it will be very much appreciated. No matter where you deliver in this country, we guarantee that hospital food isn't like home cooking!

Q. My OB provider wants me to take a few laps up and down the hall. Why?

There are several reasons. Mainly, it prevents blood clots and constipation!

First of all, you are still at risk for blood clots even though you aren't pregnant. Up to 30 percent of all blood clots (***DVTs***) associated with pregnancy occur after delivery. Following World War II, doctors started recommending that people walk the day after having a baby. Prior to this, people stayed in bed for about a week.

Moving around makes your veins work to move blood around and prevents stagnation, which is a risk factor in developing a blood clot.

Second, many people experience gas pain and constipation after a C-section. Walking helps to pass gas (bet you didn't know that!). So put your little one in their mobile bassinet and hit the hallways. You don't have to go very far, but walking two to three times a day is the goal.

NEW PARENT-TO-BE 411:

Blood Clot Prevention

All hospitals should use precautionary measures to prevent blood clots in the legs with surgery patients. Blood clots can easily dislodge from the legs and travel up to the lungs, causing a life-threatening condition called a pulmonary embolism. There is a real risk of getting a blood clot after surgery, and there is a real risk of getting a blood clot after having a baby. Put the two together in the form of a C-section and the risk is even more significant. In fact, there is a five- to ten-fold increased risk. (This is not meant to freak you out. It's meant to explain to you why all the medical staff takes this so seriously.) Here are the possible methods your hospital will use to prevent clots:

How to Prevent a Blood Clot

The last thing you want after surgery is a blood clot in your leg (***deep vein thrombosis*** or ***DVT***). There are two things you need to do to prevent this:

1. **Get out of bed.** Start pacing the halls (feel free to count all the different colors of Jell-O you see in food trays).
2. **Wear your compression stockings or SCDs (sequential compression devices).** These are not-so-attractive devices that wrap around your lower legs to help prevent blood clots. Compression stockings are tight from the toes to the upper thigh. They increase circulation and prevent blood from pooling. SCDs are soft plastic inflatable devices that are placed around each leg and hooked up to a machine that alternates inflating and deflating. It feels like a mini leg massage and helps prevent blood from stagnat-

ing and pooling. They can be somewhat annoying, especially in the middle of the night when you are trying to sleep.

If you have additional factors putting you at risk for developing a blood clot, your doctor may prescribe a blood-thinning medication for additional prevention. Heparin or enoxaparin (Lovenox) injections may be given until a patient is walking. This is used most often in people who are obese or those who are not able to walk after a few hours.

Who is at risk? Here are the factors:

- Obesity
- Advanced maternal age (over thirty-five)
- Family or personal history of blood clots
- Antiphospholipid antibody syndrome
- Other inherited blood clotting disorders
- C-section
- Immobilized
- Twins or other multiples

Remember, every postpartum person is at increased risk for blood clots. So your doctors and nurses are watching you closely!

Q. How do I care for my healing body? How do I care for the wound until it heals? Can I take a shower or a bath?

Every doctor has their own recommendations, so find out from yours what they suggest.

Most doctors remove your bandages before you leave the hospital. If you had staples closing a skin incision, they will be removed as well. These are replaced with small little pieces of surgical tape. Ask your doctor when you can put ointment, salves, or scar treatments on your incision.

Your doctor will probably tell you that it is okay to take a shower, but make sure to dry your wound area with a clean towel (bacteria grows when things are moist). Some doctors say taking a bath is okay; others disagree.

Taking good care of your body is the best way to help your incision heal. Avoid heavy lifting, avoid being on your feet for too long, and avoid constipation. Drink lots of liquids, eat well, and sleep when you can.

We know this is tough because between Dr. M and Dr. B, we have four children—so we know that the advice "sleep when you can" may seem like a cruel joke!

Q. My wound seems to be opening up and draining. This is bad, right?

Right!

There shouldn't be *any* liquid draining from your incision once you get home—not clear, not bloody, not yellow.

You need to call your doctor right away—it doesn't matter how minor this seems.

Q. Do my stitches/staples need to be removed?

The stitches that are on the inside of your body dissolve on their own. And if you've got stitches on your skin, those usually dissolve as well.

If your doctor used staples on your skin, they will be removed three to five days after your surgery if you had a low horizontal incision in or just above your pubic hair (***Pfannenstiel incision***). This is done at the hospital before you go home. It sounds painful, but most people feel nothing more than a little pinch and it takes only a few minutes. Then, the incision is covered with pieces of sterile paper.

If you had a vertical skin incision (from your pubic bone to your belly button), your doctor will take the staples out after seven to ten days at their office.

Care for Both Vaginal and Cesarean Deliveries

Q. I've got the shakes. Is something wrong with me?

Nothing is wrong with you—and you are not cold (although that won't stop well-intended family members from covering you with blankets).

No surprise here, but you've got some major hormonal shifts happening. That's what makes you shake.

You may shake as you transition in labor from the first stage to the second stage, after you get a spinal or epidural block, and after delivery. Some people shake so severely that their teeth chatter and it's difficult for them to hold their baby.

Yes, it's annoying, but it's normal and it goes away within 30 to 120 minutes after delivery.

Q. I'm having lots of bleeding. Is this normal?

Yes.

Don't be concerned if you have some gushing in the first day or two after delivery. It will be worse when you nurse your baby and when you stand up. Occasionally, you'll even pass small clots. You'll wear the equivalent of Depends for the first few days. (How nice, you and your baby can both wear diapers!)

Expect to bleed for about four to six weeks after delivery. It should slow down in volume and become darker until it is brownish-yellowish. So what is and isn't normal?

Red Flags: Postpartum Bleeding

- Bleeding that is continuously dripping or pouring out of you (like an open faucet).
- Continuously passing large clots (the size of a golf ball or larger).
- Bleeding that starts getting heavy again a week or two after delivery.
- Feeling lightheaded or dizzy.
- Loss of consciousness.

- Feeling your heart beating rapidly.

If you have any of the above symptoms and are still in the hospital, call your nurse immediately. If you are at home, call your OB provider immediately.

Q. What happens if there is too much bleeding?

It's normal to lose a lot of blood during delivery. So what's *abnormal*?

A ***postpartum hemorrhage*** is defined as losing more than 500 milliliters (half a liter) of blood following a vaginal delivery, or 1,000 milliliters of blood after a C-section.

Your body usually does just fine losing up to 1,000 milliliters of blood because your blood volume increased during the last nine months that you were pregnant. Losing *more* than that can be dangerous.

Here's what happens if you lose too much blood:

- You will get more fluid running in through your IV.
- Your OB provider will do pretty aggressive uterine massage to help the uterus firm up and stop bleeding. They'll also order some medication, usually methylergonovine (Methergine) or a synthetic prostaglandin called carboprost tromethamine (Hemabate) while they investigate the reason behind the bleeding.
- You may have blood drawn to check your blood count and to determine the levels of certain proteins and blood clotting factors.

The next step depends on why you are bleeding. If you have an undiagnosed laceration on the cervix or vagina, your doctor will repair it. If there are some pieces of placenta or membranes still stuck in the uterus (***retained products of conception***), your doctor will check your uterus to remove any remaining tissue. If you had a previous C-section or other uterine surgery, your OB provider needs to check to see if your old scar has opened up.

If your bleeding does not slow down despite intervention, you may need to have surgery. Depending on the reason, surgery can range from a dilation and curettage (***D&C*** aka cleaning the inside of the uterus with a surgical instrument) to major abdominal surgery to stitch the uterus in order to help it contract or tie off certain arteries supplying blood to the uterus.

A blood transfusion is necessary if your heart rate, blood pressure, or oxygen saturation is unstable and your OB provider is concerned you have lost too much blood. In some emergencies, women may need blood products other than red blood cells. Some people get platelet transfusions and blood clotting substances. This is more often necessary for women having a postpartum hemorrhage compared to almost any other kind of hemorrhage occurring in non-pregnant patients.

Very rarely, if nothing else works, a hysterectomy has to be performed in order to save your life. Don't panic. Did we mention this is extremely rare?

Reality Check

If you had a postpartum hemorrhage with your first pregnancy, you have a 10 to 15 percent chance of having it again with your second delivery. If you have had it in two previous deliveries, the risk rises to 20 percent with your third.

INSIDER SECRET: Blood Transfusions

No one gets a blood transfusion unless it is absolutely medically necessary. It is recommended only when your health is seriously at risk. Your doctor may decide that you need a blood transfusion because you have lost at least 30 percent of your total blood volume or your heart rate, blood pressure, or oxygen saturation is unstable.

But you still have to sign the consent form to authorize it. Our advice: Sign off if your doctor recommends it. But do so only after all of your questions have been answered and you understand their reasoning for recommending it.

If you end up in this situation, you won't have time to use donor blood from a friend or family member (designated donor). Even if your spouse or mother has the same blood type, there isn't time to have their blood checked and matched to yours (that can take days, and you need that blood within a matter of minutes to hours).

You will receive a blood transfusion from the blood bank. Blood donations are thoroughly screened to minimize any spread of infection, including HIV.

What are the risks? Although donor blood is extensively screened, the risk of contracting hepatitis B from a transfusion is 1 in 200,000 if you haven't already been vaccinated. The risk of getting hepatitis C is 1 in almost 2,000,000 and the HIV risk is less than 1 in 2,100,000.[1]

It's also possible to have a mild immune reaction with fever, chills, or hives. That's why patients sometimes get a dose of acetaminophen (Tylenol) and diphenhydramine (Benadryl) prior to getting a blood transfusion to prevent these symptoms. Rarely, a person has a more severe immune reaction where antibodies are made against the blood being transfused. [2]

Q. Why do the nurses have to keep checking me all night long? I just want to get a little sleep!

We know and agree with you.

You were up all night in labor, pushed for an hour, finally got the hang of breastfeeding, kicked out all the visitors, and dozed off for a few minutes.

Next thing you know, a nurse or nurse's assistant waltzes into your room to chat (and they are all so dang perky at two a.m.!), pushes on your belly, listens to your chest, checks your pad (your diaper equivalent), and takes your vital signs.

It's true—the hospital is the worst place to get some rest.

However, the first twenty-four hours after delivery are important. There are rare but serious complications that can occur after having a baby. The hospital needs to keep a close eye on you because a change in your vital signs can be an early sign of infection, bleeding, or a blood clot.

So how's a girl supposed to get some sleep? Here are two tips:

1. Ask your nurse to put a note on your door to request that all hospital personnel visit you during a certain window of time. That way you won't have someone

waking you up every time you've just fallen asleep. It works great at night, but you can also request this during the day. (Murphy's Law says that the birth records person, the food tray delivery, cleaning person, and staff photographer will all pop by when it's nap time.)

2. See if your doctor can write an order to let your nurse skip one set of vital signs at night. Assuming all is well, this is usually possible.

Q. I'm having some trouble peeing. Is this common?

Many people have trouble urinating after delivery (especially the first few times).

If you had an epidural or spinal, you also probably had a catheter draining urine from your bladder during labor. Occasionally, those catheters cause some temporary bladder irritation. And very rarely, a person gets a ***bladder infection***.

Catheter or not, you may have some trouble. You might not have the same sensation of your bladder filling up, or have trouble stopping your urine stream, or have a few accidents (leak a little) for several weeks after delivery. Fun, we know.

Rarely, people sustain a temporary nerve injury that leads to difficulty urinating. If you can't pee within six hours after delivery, you'll probably need to have a catheter placed to drain the urine from your bladder. (You don't want a stretched-out bladder that doesn't function well later on.) Once that catheter goes in, your OB provider might decide to leave it in overnight and let your bladder rest. It then comes out and you can try again.

Q. I'm feeling a bit short of breath. Is this okay?

No.

This can be normal, but it can also be one of the first signs of a problem. Tell your nurse or OB provider, especially if you are also having chest pain.

Here's a scary list of possible reasons for shortness of breath after delivery. We realize that this may give you an anxiety attack . . . which also causes shortness of breath! The possible causes for shortness of breath:

- Anxiety attack
- Asthma flare-up
- A temporary condition where a portion of the lungs does not expand completely (***atelectasis***)—more common with C-sections and prolonged Pitocin use
- Congestive heart failure (an overworked heart)
- Infection in the lungs (***pneumonia***)
- Fluid buildup in the lungs, seen occasionally after C-sections and with preeclampsia (pulmonary edema)
- Blood clot that gets stuck in the lung's blood vessel (***pulmonary embolism***)
- Amniotic contents enter a woman's bloodstream (***amniotic fluid embolism***)

BOTTOM LINE: Hit that nurse call button if you have shortness of breath, just to make sure things are okay.

Q. I'm having some yucky vaginal discharge with an odor. Is this normal?

No, usually not.

The concern here is an infection in the lining of the uterus (***endometritis***). Besides foul-smelling discharge, you can have a fever, chills, lower abdominal pain, abnormal vaginal bleeding, and exquisite uterine tenderness (severe pain when the top portion of your uterus is pushed upon).

So who's most likely to get endometritis? People who have had a:

- C-section—especially if it is done before twenty-eight weeks or you had a prolonged labor before having an emergency C-section
- Prolonged rupture of membranes (your water bag was broken for twelve to twenty-four hours prior to delivering)
- Long labor with multiple vaginal exams

Postpartum endometritis is pretty rare in vaginal deliveries (less than 3 percent) and scheduled C-sections (5 to 15 percent). It's most common in emergency C-sections done after labor starts (up to 20 percent of the time).

Reality Check

Your vaginal discharge may have an unpleasant odor as your bleeding decreases in the weeks after having a baby. Old blood is kind of stinky.

Q. My legs and feet are swelling. Is this a bad sign?

Not necessarily.

Many people get more swollen *after* having a baby than beforehand. Your body has a lot of extra fluid circulating around (remember your blood volume is double that of a non-pregnant person). Until your kidneys can filter out all that extra fluid, you may be a little puffy, particularly in your legs and feet. Waking up on postpartum day number two and having cankles is usually nothing to panic about.

So when does swelling need immediate attention? A ***deep venous thrombosis*** (***DVT***) is a blood clot that usually forms in the lower legs. Watch for pain and swelling in one leg significantly more than the other. A clot can dislodge from the legs and travel through the heart to the lungs, where it gets lodged in an artery. This is called a ***pulmonary embolism*** (PE).

The other potentially serious issue is called ***preeclampsia***. Only pregnant and postpartum women get this disorder. It involves high blood pressure and leaky kidneys, which allows protein to seep from your bloodstream into the urine. It usually occurs in the later stages of pregnancy (after thirty-two weeks), during labor and delivery, or up to six weeks after delivery.

Surprisingly, one-fourth of all cases of preeclampsia happen *after* delivery. Not every woman with preeclampsia has swelling. But tell your doctor if you notice rapid onset and severe swelling of the legs, hands, or face.

Q. I am not going to breastfeed. Do I need to take something to make my milk dry up?

In the past, doctors used to prescribe a medication to stop milk production. But the FDA no longer approves this drug because of safety concerns.

If you do not desire to breastfeed or have decided to stop breastfeeding, here are a few helpful steps in making it as easy as possible:

- Talk with your OB provider and/or pediatrician first.
- If you started nursing, drop one session every two to three days.
- Wean your feedings to once or twice a day before stopping altogether.
- After you nurse or pump for the last time or if you don't plan to breastfeed at all from the start, bind your breasts tightly with a bandage wrap followed by a tight sports bra. Intermittent ice packs can help as well.
- If you are full of milk (***engorgement***), use ice packs to help with the swelling. Avoid taking a hot shower (turn your back so that the hot water doesn't hit your breasts directly, just your back) or stimulating your breasts since this will cause more milk production. Then you'll have to start the process all over again!
- Use ibuprofen every six hours as directed to help with pain.

It can take up to two weeks for breast milk to dry up. It does not happen overnight. If you have concerns, asking for help from a lactation consultant can be very helpful.

Q. My best friend told me to use a belly band right after I deliver to help my stomach shrink back faster, but I had a C-section. Can I still do that?

A belly band or belly binder is a piece of fabric that wraps around your entire belly, from just above your pubic bone to well above your belly button, and helps hold everything in a bit tighter when moving around after a delivery. Once the baby is out, it takes time (and some work) for your uterus and all the layers of your abdomen to go back to the way they were (or close). Although many companies tout quicker shrinkage with their products, nothing does that other than time and exercise (when you are cleared). But most OB providers agree that belly binders help support women in the postpartum period and make it easier when walking and moving around. And you can use them whether you had a C-section or a vaginal delivery, with one caveat. If you had a C-section, you may opt for one with legs to step into versus one that is purely a wrap. The lower edge of the wrap can rub along your incision and cause irritation and swelling.

Q. How long will I stay at the hospital/birthing center?

If you have a vaginal delivery at a hospital, you will usually stay there for twenty-four to forty-eight hours. If there are complications, you may have to stay longer.

If you deliver at a birthing center (all deliveries there are vaginal deliveries), you will usually go home after six hours. Most women do not stay past twenty-four hours.

If you had a cesarean delivery, the typical stay is three to four days.

Reality Check

If you deliver at a birthing center or at home with a midwife, most OB providers will do a home visit the day after you deliver to check on you and your baby.

DR. B'S OPINION:

Hospital Stay Length

If this is your first baby, stay at the hospital as long as you can. Most insurance companies cover the cost (forty-eight hours for a vaginal delivery and ninety-six hours for a C-section) and the clock begins the moment you deliver (not when you are admitted in labor). Your real labor begins once you take your newborn home—take advantage of all the "free" help.

Heck, even if it's your fifth baby, you may want to stay as long as someone is lined up to care for your other children!

Q. Can my partner sleep with me at the hospital?

Usually, yes.

We won't guarantee that your partner's foldaway cot will feel like your memory foam mattress at home, but it sure is nice to have a support person there day and night. Even if it's not your partner, a willing relative or close friend there with you is a welcome presence.

Ask your OB provider, hospital, or birthing center to get specifics.

Q. Can my baby stay in the same room with me at the hospital?

Yes, it's called "rooming-in."

This is encouraged because rooming-in promotes breastfeeding and bonding with your newborn. The only time this is not possible is if your baby needs to be observed or treated in the nursery or the NICU for a medical problem. If that situation arises, you can visit, cuddle, and feed your baby in a comfy recliner in the nursery. Not ideal, we know, but it's all about your baby's health.

By the way, you are also allowed to ask the nursery to babysit for an hour or two if you really need to get some shut-eye. Yes, the nurses will bring your baby back if they need to eat. No one tries to sneak formula into a breastfed baby while they are camping out in the nursery!

Q. What are my pain medication options? Are they safe for breastfeeding?

You have a few options, and all of them are safe to take while you are breastfeeding.

Vaginal delivery. People vary in how they deal with pain, and some have more pain than others due to their own histories as well as circumstances surrounding delivery. Some nursing parents have extraordinary pain with breastfeeding. Others have pain as their uterus starts to shrink back down to its normal size.

Most people need some type of pain medication, at least for the first few days. Overall, the number one pain medication of choice for postpartum discomfort is ibuprofen (brand names: Motrin, Advil). It is both a pain reliever and an anti-inflammatory agent (that is, it reduces swelling). That makes it superior to acetaminophen (brand name: Tylenol), which is only a pain reliever. As an OB, I recommend taking ibuprofen every six hours around the clock for the first two days and then as needed. Just be sure to take it with a little bit of food in your stomach since it can cause some stomach irritation.

Cesarean delivery. Virtually everyone needs pain medication after having a C-section. Remember, it *is* major surgery. You will have pain at the incision (wound) site, as well as from all the layers of stitches that were put in underneath the skin and on the uterus. You may also have discomfort as your uterus contracts to shrink back down to normal size.

Sometimes in the early stages of recovery when you aren't yet eating (or you've just puked for the fourth time), you are given something called ketorolac (Toradol), which is an intravenous form of ibuprofen. You may also need to take narcotic medication by mouth in addition to ibuprofen for the first week or two. Most people who have had an uncomplicated C-section do not need to take pain medication regularly after two weeks.

How do you know you need more than ibuprofen? If you cry every time you think about nursing or pooping or you can't walk around upright due to pain, you need more than ibuprofen.

Your options include acetaminophen with codeine (Tylenol 3), acetaminophen with hydrocodone (Vicodin), or acetaminophen with oxycodone (Percocet). These are narcotic pain medications that are safe when used in prescribed dosages for short periods of time. They are a problem for nursing parents only if you take them in large doses (above and beyond what is prescribed) or if you take them for a long period of time. Using them for a short time after delivery is okay.

Helpful Hint

Narcotic/opioid medications can make you constipated. Take a stool softener, increase your fiber intake, and stay hydrated if you are taking these medications.

Q. I'm worried about how my three-year-old will react when they come to visit me for the first time after having the baby. Is there anything I can do to help make things easier?

Yes.

Most siblings do just fine. Usually they are very nice to their new brother or sister (and *not* so nice to their parents who have the gall to shake up their little self-centered world).

DR. B'S OPINION:

Helping Older Siblings Adjust

Older siblings take about six to eight weeks to adjust to the "new normal." They are going through a grieving process of sorts. Expect some acting out. To a toddler or preschooler, any attention—good or bad—is attention. Give your child attention so they don't have to resort to acting out.

DR. M'S OPINION:

Alone Time and Older Children

It's nice to set aside some "alone time" with your older child or children. Let them pick somewhere they want to go or something fun they want to do and have a little "date" with them. Even if you sneak away from the baby for an hour, it's a very special thing for your older child.

What can you do to make that first meet and greet a good one?

- Greet your older child ***without*** the new baby in your arms.
- Let your older child climb in your arms, give you a big hug, and chat.
- Ask your child if they want to hold their new sibling while sitting on your lap. If they don't, that is okay.
- Have a large picture of your older child prominently displayed in your hospital room. (Thanks to Bess, my children's pediatrician, for this recommendation as well as many others!)
- Have the new baby give a gift to the older sibling. And yes, your older child can also select a gift to bring to the new baby. (You may have to remind your child that newborns have no use for Thomas trains or Barbie dolls just yet!)
- Have a "birthday party" for the new baby. What toddler can resist cupcakes?

Q. What if I want to have my tubes tied? When is this done?

If you are having a C-section, you can have your tubes tied just after the baby is delivered and the uterus is sewn up.

If you are having a vaginal delivery, you have one of two options.

Option #1: *Postpartum tubal ligation, done right after delivery.* If you have an epidural, we'll just continue using it so that you won't need general anesthesia for the surgery. Your doctor makes a small incision just below the belly button and then brings each tube up to the incision, so they can be tied and cut.

Option #2: *Removal of your fallopian tubes (bilateral salpingectomy), done at least six weeks after delivery.* Most doctors nowadays perform these *laparoscopically*. That means your doctor makes two or three tiny incisions in your belly and operates through long instruments placed in those incisions. This is day surgery (outpatient surgery) and requires general anesthesia. We used to just remove a portion of each fallopian tube, rendering them incapable of allowing the egg and sperm to meet. The reason the tubes are now removed completely if you no longer want children is to help protect you from getting ovarian cancer. I know, this sounds strange, but we now believe that some forms of ovarian cancer originate in the fallopian tubes, so if you aren't going to use them anymore, it's safer to just remove them.

Once You Go Home

Q. When do I follow up with my OB in the office?

Vaginal delivery. Your OB will probably want to see you in two weeks unless there is a specific concern, although sometimes your OB provider will ask to see you in six weeks.

Your doctor will tell you the plan when you are discharged home from the hospital. You will also get a list of symptoms that deserve an earlier appointment. Those include fever, breast pain/redness, worsening abdominal pain, severe lower leg swelling or pain, or more bleeding instead of less.

Cesarean delivery. Most OBs see C-section patients back in the office in one to two weeks. Check prior to discharge for a recommendation.

No matter when you see your OB provider for the first time in the office, you will most likely be asked to come back a few weeks later for a "final six-week postpartum visit." This visit usually includes a Pap test, a discussion of birth control methods or IUD placement, and advice on returning to pre-pregnancy activities. Then with a touch of separation anxiety (we feel it, too!), you say goodbye to a familiar face for six to twelve months!

Q. I have a fever. My doctor says I need to see them. Why?

Having a fever (temperature greater than 100.4°F) between one to ten days after delivering a baby *always* warrants a call to your OB provider. These are the top seven reasons for a fever:

- **Endometritis.** Look for foul-smelling discharge, abdominal tenderness, chills.
- **C-section incision or vaginal tears/episiotomy infection.** Look for pus or discharge from your abdominal incision or episiotomy/vaginal laceration site and redness/tenderness of the skin surrounding it.
- **Mastitis.** Look for flu-like symptoms (fever, chills, muscle aches) and redness/pain in one breast.
- **Bladder infection (UTI).** Look for pain with urination, lower abdominal pain, urinary frequency.
- **Atelectasis.** Look for shortness of breath, difficulty breathing.
- **Pneumonia.** Look for difficulty breathing, coughing.
- **Pelvic abscess.** Look for abdominal tenderness, bloating, fatigue.
- **Deep venous thrombosis.** Look for leg swelling/pain and possible redness, typically in just one leg.

Red Flags: Fever

Call your OB provider if you experience:

- Fever, defined as greater than 100.4°F and/or chills
- Excessive bleeding
- New or increasing pain in your genital or rectal area
- Pain with urination or inability to urinate
- Leg pain or swelling, particularly on one side
- Breast pain or redness
- Severe abdominal pain not responding to or requiring more pain medication

Q. When can I drive a car?

Whether you had a vaginal delivery or C-section, OBs have one simple rule: Do not operate heavy machinery (car, truck, or large farm equipment, if you are so inclined) while under the influence of narcotics! That includes Tylenol 3, Vicodin, Percocet, or any other narcotic.

Here are some general guidelines. Be sure to check with your OB provider before hopping into the driver's seat.

Vaginal delivery. If you are just taking ibuprofen and had an uncomplicated vaginal delivery, you should be able to drive again within a week. If you had a third- or fourth-degree tear or episiotomy, you may want to check with your doctor first.

Cesarean delivery. Your doctor will probably tell you not to drive for two weeks after surgery. This is frustrating, but there are good reasons.

1. You'll be taking narcotic pain medication longer than your friends who delivered vaginally (probably at least a week or two).
2. You use your abdominal muscles when you drive, especially when you move your foot quickly from the gas pedal to the brake. It may be difficult, if not impossible, to slam on the brakes in the days following major abdominal surgery. So bite the bullet for a mere fourteen days and ask a friend or your mother-in-law to pick you up to take you to your next appointment.

Reality Check

You will be very tired during your first few months as a new parent, so be extra careful on the road. Sleep deprivation can take a real toll on your driving ability.

Q. When can I walk up stairs?

Vaginal delivery. You can walk up stairs right away if you didn't tear or have an episiotomy, or your tear was very small. Just do it very carefully.

If you had a more substantial vaginal tear or episiotomy, it takes more time to heal. Going up and down stairs will hurt. You may want to use one level of your home or apartment for most of your daily activities and limit stair walking during the first week or two.

Cesarean delivery. You should also camp out on the first floor of your house if you have lots of stairs. It's okay if you need to go up or down once or twice a day. Just be careful and take it slowly. Plan to have your baby sleeping nearby at night, so you aren't going up and down the stairs after sundown. The chance of slipping is greater at night because it's dark and you are tired.

Two to three weeks after delivery, you should be able to go up and down stairs without any difficulty.

Q. When can I lift my toddler again?

Yes, your maternal instincts (and guilt) will make you want to pick up your toddler and show them the love. But listen to your OB provider before you act on that instinct.

Vaginal delivery. You can lift your child as long as you had an easy delivery. If you had major complications at delivery or you are healing from a large vaginal tear or episiotomy, you are in the "I have more healing to do" category. For you, wait a week or so before lifting or carrying your toddler. But ask your OB provider for a specific plan. Your toddler can still jump up on you and sit in your lap, just without you assisting them.

Cesarean delivery. Avoid lifting your toddler for four to six weeks. Your toddler can crawl up or be placed on your lap by someone else, but it's not a good idea to carry them around after major surgery. Why? Your wound (incision) is weaker than the surrounding tissue while it is healing. It is much easier to have an incision open up during the first few weeks after surgery than at any other time. You won't want to deal with the consequences of that! This includes cleaning the wound and packing it with sterile gauze every day. If it doesn't heal on its own, you will have to go back to the operating room to have it closed surgically, weeks or months down the line. This is not a fun experience, trust us!

DR. M'S OPINION

I hate to see the look on my patients' faces when I advise them not to lift their older kiddos for at least four to six weeks after a c-section. I know you are dying to pick your toddler up (I was, too), but it's just not worth the risk.

Q. When can I start exercising again?

Check with your provider before you start doing any kind of exercise after delivery. OBs usually give the green light after six weeks (occasionally longer with C-sections), but your personal history determines when it is safe for you. Ask first.

ACOG says that women can gradually resume exercising when they feel ready. Some people who have had uneventful vaginal deliveries with little genital (perineal) trauma feel well enough to take a light, brief walk a week or so after delivery. But if you had a third- or fourth-degree laceration, you may need to hold off exercising for up to eight weeks.

Once your OB provider gives their official blessing, you can resume all pre-pregnancy activities and exercise regimens. But remember to start slowly. Begin with walking, yoga, mild hiking, and swimming. You can't expect to jump back into the sixty-minute weight and cardio routine that you were doing prior to getting pregnant. Remember that all of your joints and ligaments can be loose for up to five months after delivery.

And let's talk about those abdominal muscles. Most people develop some degree of a gap between their abdominal muscles as their pregnancy progresses. That gap (called the ***diastasis recti***) takes about two months to close. In some people, it never closes, and there's always a gap. It's important to let your body heal and close the muscle separation prior to beginning any intense abdominal workouts. Start easy and save the heavy-duty crunches for eight to ten weeks after delivery.

Here are some postpartum exercise tips:

- Stretch for five to ten minutes before *and* after exercising.
- Wear comfortable clothing.
- Keep well hydrated with water or a sports drink.
- Wear a comfortable and supportive bra.
- Clear your mind of all the other things going on. This is your time to relax, think, meditate, and get back into shape.

Q. Umm, I still look pregnant. When will this baby bump go away?

Yep, none of your friends told you that either, did they?

Why? Remember there are two things that grow during pregnancy: your uterus and the skin over it.

After delivery, your uterus shrinks down to the level of your belly button immediately and stays there for a day or two. By two weeks after delivery, the uterus has gone down to halfway between your belly button and your pubic bone.

In most women, the uterus returns to normal size (about the size of your fist) by six to eight weeks after delivery. As your uterus shrinks down in size, your tummy will, too.

The skin covering your belly is another story. It has been stretched out over the last nine months by your expanding uterus (rivaling Santa Claus's physique). This takes time and then some hard work to put it back the way it was.

Reality Check

In some women, the skin over the abdomen is so stretched during a pregnancy it never really goes back. In these cases, no amount of diet or exercise will return the elasticity of the skin to its pre-pregnancy form. If this bothers you, options include wearing support garments (like Spanx) or having a plastic surgeon surgically remove the excess skin (***abdominoplasty***).

Q. I feel like I am having contractions again. Is this okay?

Just when you thought it was over, right? Actually, you continue to have contractions after delivery because this helps your uterus shrink. That, in turn, decreases postpartum bleeding and gets your uterus back to its normal size.

You'll probably feel contraction pain while nursing—and don't be shocked to see a small gush of blood that follows. Contractions decrease in frequency and intensity with time, and you won't even notice them five to seven days after delivery. Postpartum contractions are more intense (but go away more quickly) with each subsequent delivery.

INSIDER SECRET: Kegel Exercises

You've probably already figured out that you don't quite feel the same below your waistline. Don't be too dismayed. You need to give your body time to heal—and that takes six to eight weeks. Just look at your baby's noggin, and you'll understand why your muscles are so weak right now!

Good news: You can actively help your pelvic floor muscles get back in shape. Kegel (KAY-gull) exercises help tighten up all of the muscles in the vaginal area, including the muscle that keeps you from having accidents (urethral muscle). These exercises not only help reduce incontinence, but they get you back in shape for the day you are ready for sexual intercourse. We promise that desire will return at some point.

Here is a step-by-step guide to all things kegel:

- Start this process while you are urinating.
- After you begin to urinate, try to stop the stream of urine.
- Hold this position for a few seconds.
- Release and resume urinating.
- Do this a few times each time you go to the bathroom.

When you first start, you probably won't be able to stop the entire flow of urine (or any of it if you are like we were!). Don't panic. Keep trying. As your muscles get stronger, you might win the gold medal when kegels become an Olympic sport. Just kidding on that one, but you will be surprised at what you will be able to do.

Besides kegels, your regular exercise regimen will help tone your pelvic floor and abdominal muscles, too.

Q. I am having bloody discharge. How long does that last? Can I use tampons?

The bloody discharge is called ***lochia***. What you see is blood and sloughed-off tissue from the lining of the uterus. That lining was held in check by hormones during your pregnancy, and now it's time to clean house.

It's normal to have lochia for thirty to forty-five days after you've given birth. Here's the 411 on lochia after birth:

- **Days one to seven:** Lochia contains quite a bit of blood, so it will be bright red.
- **Days seven to ten:** Lochia is less bloody and more watery and pinkish in color.
- **Day ten until four to six weeks:** Lochia turns brown, then yellowish in color.

Lochia should progressively decrease in volume and get less bloody in appearance. And, no, tampons are not recommended.

BOTTOM LINE: Most women have lochia for four to six weeks.

There may be some days during this time that you think, "Oh, wow, I've stopped bleeding!" only to be met with more lochia the next day. This is normal, and the flow may wax and wane over a few weeks.

Sorry, but you've got to stick with pads until six weeks have passed from the time of your delivery.

Red Flag

If your bleeding/lochia is becoming heavier and is bright red, contact your OB provider.

Q. When do I get my period again?

It really varies from woman to woman. It also depends on whether or not you are breastfeeding.

Many women who are breastfeeding do not have periods at all. Some have irregular spotting and even fewer have regular menstrual cycles.

If you are not breastfeeding, you will probably see your period (menstrual cycle) return within six to ten weeks after delivery. Sorry, the party's over. It's back to the feminine hygiene products aisle because by twelve weeks, up to 80 percent of non-breastfeeding women have resumed their menstrual cycle.

Reality Check

Here's a little fact you need to know: About 75 percent of women do *not* ovulate prior to their first period. But that means a quarter of all moms *can* get pregnant right after having a baby. And yes, this includes those of you who needed assisted reproductive technology like IVF to get pregnant the first time!

Q. How long after delivery should I wait to have intercourse?

Doctors usually advise waiting six weeks after having either a vaginal delivery or a C-section to resume intercourse.

This will probably be an easy sell for you. Most women do not feel like being intimate right after having a baby. Do not be discouraged! You will eventually get your groove back.

You are going through a lot right now. Here is just a small sampling of reasons why you feel like you do after delivery:

- You are exhausted beyond belief.
- Your hormones are all over the place, making you an emotional wreck.
- You have a few extra pounds to lose and don't feel very sexy.
- Your boobs leak all the time (also not very sexy).

DR. M'S OPINION

Most of the time, we docs don't have to twist your arm when it comes to refraining from sex. In fact, most of my patients are begging me to tell their partners that they can't have intercourse for even longer!

- Your baby is attached to your body 24/7, and you just want a few moments in the day where no one is touching you.
- Your baby needs you all the time. You think your spouse also "needs" you. There is not enough of you to go around.
- You had a big vaginal tear with delivery, and the thought of sex makes you cry.

The best advice we can give you is to talk to your partner about your feelings. The sexual part of your relationship is as important as any other aspect of your relationship.

Make sure your doctor gives you the green light before proceeding. For instance, if you had a big vaginal tear (third- or fourth-degree laceration) or a wound infection, you may need to wait longer than six weeks.

Always, always use lubrication jelly for the first several times you get back in the saddle if you are breastfeeding.

FEEDBACK FROM THE REAL WORLD:

Parenthood Is Not for the Weak-Hearted

As doctors, both authors have endured sleep-depriving residency training programs. Back in our day, this was a rite of passage in medicine that required us to work eighty-plus hours a week (for about four dollars an hour) to somehow prepare for a medical career. After finishing this experience, we both thought having a newborn in the house would be a piece of cake.

WRONG!

By far, new parenthood is the most exhausting job we have ever had. When you are a resident, you get to go home and sleep after being up all night on call. When you are a new parent, you are up every two or three hours for two to four months straight!

Who'd be interested in sex with that kind of sleep schedule?

Partner Tip

Don't feel rejected if your partner doesn't share your desire to be intimate. Just be patient—really patient.

Q. I've heard having sex for the first few times is really painful. Is that true?

We're sorry to say that usually the answer is yes, especially if you are breastfeeding.

The walls of the vagina are thinner than usual after having a baby and continue to be that way while you breastfeed, due to lower levels of estrogen. So even if you didn't have a tear or episiotomy, sex may be uncomfortable or even painful.

Sometimes, women who had episiotomies or natural tears/lacerations have more discomfort with intercourse initially. It depends on the degree or severity of the cut or tear, whether or not there was a subsequent infection, how quickly your body heals, and a few other factors. Check with your OB provider before having intercourse. If you had a fourth-degree laceration or episiotomy, you may need to wait longer than the typical six weeks.

Q. I'm breastfeeding, and I have absolutely no interest in being touched at the end of the day. Is this normal?

Yes, this is normal.

Your estrogen levels are extremely low, and you are exhausted from having a new baby around.

Many breastfeeding women feel like they get plenty of touching by having a baby at their breast all day long. While breastfeeding is not sexually arousing, it's common to feel touched out, like you don't have anything left at the end of the day for another person who wants to touch you.

Some nursing parents may also feel their breasts are for baby now, not for playing around. Your partner may feel frustrated, so talk about your concerns and fears. Your desire will return after your baby gets a little older and you stop breastfeeding.

The AAP recommends exclusively breastfeeding for at least the first six months of life if possible, and they support continued breastfeeding for two years or beyond, if possible, alongside the introduction of solid foods. But we don't want you to wait until then to have intercourse again. So here are a few ways to breastfeed and make love:

- After the first few weeks, you can begin pumping or "expressing" breast milk. Let your partner do a bottle feeding or two of expressed milk in the evening. This gives you a mental and physical break. Hopefully, you'll be more interested in sex if you get a respite from breastfeeding. Added bonus: Some women find it arousing for their partners to have spit-up on their shoulder. (Really! Once you see it, you'll understand.)
- Lubricate, lubricate, lubricate. Always use a lot of lubrication since your body won't lubricate normally for a while. Buy the industrial-size drum of Astroglide—does Costco sell this yet?

Sometimes, if nothing is working, you can ask your doctor to prescribe a topical estrogen cream to help plump and heal your vaginal tissue. The cream doesn't have enough estrogen for it to be absorbed into your bloodstream, so it's very safe to use when breastfeeding.

DR. M'S OPINION:

Back in the Saddle

Many of my patients are so uncomfortable that they swear they will only have one child because there is no way they will ever be able to be intimate again to get pregnant! The good news is that a) once you are done breastfeeding, the symptoms typically go away, and b) there are a plethora of water-soluble lubrication options. Use lubricant every time you have intercourse to help prevent chafing and tearing.

Q. When do I need to use birth control again?

Easy—once you start having intercourse again.

Assuming you are healing well and get the green light from your OB provider, you can resume sexual relations at six weeks. Even though you are breastfeeding, you can still get pregnant. Let's put that in bold caps: **YOU CAN STILL GET PREGNANT.**

And even if you needed assisted reproductive technology to become pregnant last time, YOU CAN STILL GET PREGNANT!

Your OB provider will go over your birth control options at the six-week postpartum visit. If you are breastfeeding, you still have a variety of options. Those include a non-hormonal vaginal ointment that maintains the pH in the vagina, a progesterone-only pill, the Depo-Provera injection, an IUD, the withdrawal method, or condoms.

If you aren't breastfeeding, in addition to the items just mentioned, you have the option of using combination oral contraceptive pills ("the Pill"), a contraceptive patch, or ring.

If you are finished having babies, you might consider permanent sterilization in the form of tubal removal, or even better, a vasectomy for your male partner.

Q. Does breastfeeding work as contraception?

The short answer is no.

Do not use breastfeeding as a form of birth control unless you want to have a toddler and a newborn in your house. I've seen countless utterly shocked moms get a positive pregnancy test before their baby's first birthday.

It's true that most women who are breastfeeding on a regular basis do not menstruate regularly or at all. But this DOES NOT MEAN that you can't get pregnant. You can ovulate at any time, and this is especially true as you begin to wean your baby and breastfeed less. And all it takes is one little sperm making his way down the right tube at the right time.

If you don't want to use other forms of birth control, at least use a condom.

FEEDBACK FROM THE REAL WORLD:

Murphy's Law and Pregnancy

I can't tell you how many patients I have who didn't use contraception after having a baby because "we got pregnant using IVF, so there is no way I can get pregnant again," "we got pregnant using medication and IUI, so there is no way I can get pregnant again," or "it took us ten months to get pregnant the first time so there is no way I can get pregnant right away." These are the same patients who are frantic on the phone (while holding a four-month-old in their arms) because they took a pregnancy test after feeling weird symptoms and it was positive.

Having Another Child

At some point, you will actually have sexual intercourse again. I remember a patient who, after my six-week pep talk, had a horrified look on her face. She literally begged me to tell her husband that the "no sex" rule ends at six months and not six weeks. However, her second child was born when her first was fifteen months old.

Even if you don't think you will feel like having sex again in this lifetime (and most of us don't), at some point you will! That said, you have to consider if/when you want to have another child.

Q. How long should I wait between one pregnancy and the next?

For your own health and your next baby's, a recent study by the US Centers for Disease Control and Prevention concluded that the optimal gap between births is at least eighteen to twenty-three months.[3]

It is especially important to wait to conceive again if you had a C-section so that the uterine muscle can fully heal before expanding again to carry another pregnancy.

We asked Dr. Kaylen Silverberg, Medical Director of Texas Fertility Center in Austin, Texas, for his advice. He recommends having children at least two years apart. Why? It provides quality time with the first baby and time for a woman's body to recover from pregnancy, delivery, and breastfeeding. And he says, "Most importantly—it gives couples time to reconnect!"

Q. How will I know if I am ready to have another baby?

There are many things to think about before getting pregnant again. Everyone is different.

Some people are ready to have another baby with one still in diapers and others don't even want to start trying until second grade is over. But if you are planning another one, you may want to ask yourself a few tough questions first:

- Do you work? If so, do you have time for another baby right now?
- If you have a baby or toddler at home, are you getting enough rest or still waking up repeatedly in the middle of the night?
- Will you be financially ready to have another baby?
- How does your partner feel about having another baby?
- Do you have enough time and energy right now to give attention to a newborn and still continue to care for your other child/ren?
- Do you have help (parents, siblings, other relatives, friends, a nanny)?

BOTTOM LINE: There is no perfect time to have another baby. And it often happens without much planning.

Partner Tip

Your vote is equally important when it comes to your family planning. It takes two to tango. Speak up!

General Appearance

Q. I have an outie belly button right now. Will it go back to being an innie?

Most of the time your belly button goes back to what it was, albeit a little bigger. If you had an innie, you'll have an innie again, and the same goes if you started with an outie. This process may take some time, though.

The only time this isn't true is if you developed an umbilical hernia (a break in the fascial layer beneath your skin, allowing your intestines to pop through every once in a while). If you developed a hernia during pregnancy, you will likely continue to have an "outie," and this won't change unless you have your hernia surgically repaired.

Q. I feel like I have a "bowl full of jelly" in front of me. My stomach is so stretched out, and it jiggles every time I walk around. Will I be like this forever?

I know it's strange. Before you deliver, your belly is hard and tight. Now there's a crazy amount of skin that seems to move with your every move!

Your growing baby and uterus stretched out your skin and the underlying tissue and muscle over the past nine months. Now that your uterus is empty and the baby is out, that same skin has nothing big to cover.

You will notice a big decrease in size over the first fourteen to twenty-one days after having your baby. Then, just as it took nine months to stretch out, it often takes a long time for everything to go back down.

Wearing an abdominal binder or Spanx-like support garments can really help make you feel better when you walk around for the first two to four weeks. And there is actually a garment called the "c-panty" that can be extremely helpful after C-sections.

Q. My aunt told me that she wore her pre-pregnancy jeans home from the hospital after she had her baby. Is that possible?

No, she is lying. Really. We know she swears she did, but believe us, she didn't. Either that or her doctor kept her in the hospital for three to six months after having her baby.

Your uterus will be at about the level of your belly button, and your hips are wider from the normal expansion that occurs prior to delivery. Don't even attempt to try on pre-pregnancy jeans until it's been at least six months. Otherwise, you will find yourself sweating and cursing on the floor as you try to inch them up your thighs (yes, I was dumb enough to try that!).

Endocrine Issues

Q. I'm sweating all the time. Has my body thermostat changed or is this just hormonal?

It is very normal to find yourself waking up in a puddle in the middle of the night, to the point where you need to change your shirt. These "hot flashes" can also happen in the middle of the day.

Experts believe this is due to the drastic change in hormones that has just occurred in your body. You delivered a baby, and with that event, a huge cascade of hormonal changes happened in your body. Your estrogen levels have plummeted, and you are in a temporary state of "menopause."

Don't panic, we said *temporary*. The constant feeling of being hot and bothered usually doesn't last more than a month or two. However, let your OB provider know if you are experiencing these symptoms. Rarely, a thyroid problem can develop after pregnancy and mimic these symptoms.

Q. I'm sweating all the time. Has my body thermostat changed, or is this just hormonal? I've been feeling really off since having the baby, and I just had labs done. My OB told me I have postpartum thyroiditis. What does that mean? I've never had thyroid problems before so I'm scared.

Postpartum thyroiditis is thyroid dysfunction that occurs within twelve months of delivery and can include an overactive thyroid (hyperthyroidism), an underactive thyroid (hypothyroidism), or both. This happens in 5 to 10 percent of all women after childbirth, but it is not diagnosed commonly, as it often occurs months after delivery (when someone is no longer seeing their OB provider regularly) and causes very vague symptoms. If the thyroid is overactive, symptoms include fatigue, irritability, weight loss, palpitations, and/or heat intolerance. If underactive, fatigue, constipation, depression, inability to lose weight. And as you can see, all of those symptoms are found to varying degrees in postpartum women!

Don't worry! In most, this condition resolves spontaneously; however, in 30 percent, classic hypothyroidism will develop (regardless of whether someone originally had hyper- or hypothyroidism).

Once diagnosed with a blood test, you will likely be kept under surveillance by an internal medicine doctor, family doctor, or endocrinologist (hormone doctor).

Q. I had gestational diabetes. What happens now that I'm not pregnant anymore?

The beauty of gestational diabetes is that it goes away after delivery. Human placental lactogen (a hormone made by the placenta) is what usually causes gestational diabetes. Since the placenta is gone now, so is the culprit, uh, we mean, the hormone.

You are no longer classified as a diabetic and can eat normally. Yay!

But you still have a few things to be aware of:

1. You are at risk for having gestational diabetes with your next pregnancy.
2. You are at risk for developing type II (adult onset) diabetes later in life.
3. You need to do another glucose challenge test (very similar to the one you took during pregnancy when you drank that really sweet, flat syrupy drink) at your six-week postpartum visit (if not then, within twelve weeks of delivery).
4. If you pass the test, tell your primary care provider that you were diabetic during your pregnancy. They need to follow you more closely to watch for diabetes in the future.
5. If you don't pass the test, you get referred to your primary care provider for an evaluation.

Cardiovascular Health

Q. I had preeclampsia. What happens after I deliver?

Preeclampsia is a disease that is specific to pregnancy (we discuss this in detail in Chapter 17, "The Complicated Pregnancy," see Complication #20). Most cases occur after thirty-two weeks of gestation or during delivery. Occasionally, it develops earlier than thirty-two weeks or after pregnancy in the postpartum period.

If you had preeclampsia during your pregnancy or delivery, your doctor will monitor your blood pressure closely in the postpartum period. If you were placed on magnesium sulfate to prevent seizures, you will likely continue it for twenty-four hours after delivery. Your doctor will check your lungs regularly to make sure there isn't any fluid buildup (pulmonary edema).

The good news: Your blood pressure should return to normal shortly after the birth.

The bad news: You have a greater risk of preeclampsia with future pregnancies. You also have a higher risk of developing high blood pressure in the future. Many hospitals now have programs in place to continue monitoring women with preeclampsia in the weeks and months after they leave the hospital. This includes regular blood pressure monitoring and visits with a cardiologist.

Skin and Hair

Q. My hair texture is changing again, and I am starting to lose my hair. What can I do?

Wasn't it fantastic to have massive hair growth and shiny, radiant hair during your pregnancy? You can thank your high estrogen levels for that.

But now that your pregnancy is over (and those pesky little hormonal shifts continue to happen), many women begin to notice something new: hair loss.

We aren't just talking about a little more hair on the brush. Nope, we are referring to chunks of hair falling out in the shower, while brushing or styling, and even while just resting your head on a pillow or your loved one's shoulder.

You'll only appreciate this hair loss if you were one of the unlucky ones who suffered from facial and body hair during your pregnancy. That will start to fall out, too.

It's a long time to wait, but most women get their pre-pregnancy hair back six to eighteen months after delivery.

Staying on a prenatal vitamin or switching to a postnatal vitamin can help, but nothing will stop this.

FEEDBACK FROM THE REAL WORLD:

Alarming Hair Loss!

I used to wonder why my office got so many frantic phone calls from women who were one, two, three . . . or six months postpartum, stating that a lot of hair was falling out. I would tell my nurse to reassure them; I didn't really know why they were so upset. After having my first child and seeing the equivalent of a full wig plastered across the shower floor, I finally understood how this process could be so alarming!

Q. Ugh, those stretch marks—will they ever go away?

Unfortunately, once ***stretch marks*** appear, they are there to stay. If you want to feel a little better, their initial reddish, purplish color does fade over time to a silver-gray color.

If you don't want to wait or are done having kids and can't take the lines anymore, consult a dermatologist or plastic surgeon about using laser therapy. Just make sure to lose all of your baby weight first.

Q. I have splotches on my skin now (melasma/chloasma). Will they go away?

The splotches may fade, but they typically do not go away completely on their own. Stay out of the sun, because that will only make it worse.

If it doesn't fade and still bothers you, consult with a dermatologist. They may offer certain prescription creams or laser treatment. Neither treatment may work completely, but it might help severe cases.

Q. When can I start using all of my retinol-based creams that I had to stop during pregnancy?

When you are done breastfeeding.

Q. When can I get Botox again?

When you are done breastfeeding. Hang in there, mama, you've made it this far.

Blood

Q. I am Rh-negative. I got RhoGAM during my pregnancy. Is there anything else I need to do?

It depends on whether your baby is Rh-negative or Rh-positive.

All babies that are born to Rh-negative women get their blood type checked in the first twenty-four to forty-eight hours of life. If your baby is Rh-*positive,* you should receive another dose of RhoGAM. You need to receive your dose of RhoGAM within the first seventy-two hours after delivery to be fully protected.

Q. My OB provider said I lost a lot of blood during my delivery and that I was anemic (based on a blood test done after delivery). What should I do?

Most of the time, taking an iron supplement and eating foods that are rich in iron will correct the ***anemia***.

The typical advice is to take the iron supplement once, twice, or three times a day (your OB provider will get more specific on frequency and dose). Yes, iron supplements cause constipation. Ask for a slow-release iron supplement, which is less constipating, or take it with a stool softener. (See Appendix A, "Medications," for details.) Occasionally, we will recommend an IV iron infusion if levels are so low that it would take forever to replace all of it with oral supplementation.

Iron-rich foods are always important as your body absorbs iron from a food source much better than from a vitamin. This includes chickpeas, lentils, chicken, turkey, red meat, liver, spinach, dried apricots, prunes, raisins, egg yolks, iron-enriched cereals and grains (read the label), artichokes, and mollusks (oysters, clams, and scallops).

DR. M'S OPINION:

Vitamin C

Vitamin C helps your body absorb iron better. So have a vitamin C–rich food or drink along with your iron supplement. Foods containing higher amounts of vitamin C include guavas, strawberries, citrus fruit (lemons, oranges, grapefruit), kiwi fruit, rose hip extracts, raspberries, nectarines, mangoes, peaches, peppers, broccoli, curly kale, tomatoes, cauliflower, and brussels sprouts.

Immune System

Q. I wasn't immune to rubella when I had my prenatal blood work done. What do I do now?

Because we don't give the MMR (measles, mumps, rubella vaccine) during pregnancy, you should receive a rubella vaccine after you deliver. This is routinely given before you leave the hospital if you are not immune. It is safe to receive while breastfeeding.

Q. I wasn't sure if I had chickenpox when I was little, and when my OB provider checked at the beginning of pregnancy, it showed that I hadn't. What should I do now?

You should receive a varicella vaccine. It is a two-part vaccine, with the second dose given four to eight weeks after the first dose. Although we don't give it during pregnancy, this vaccine is safe to receive while breastfeeding.

Q. Do I need a whooping cough vaccine?

Yes, if you did not get it during pregnancy.

The guidance from ACOG is that pregnant women should receive a Tdap vaccine with each pregnancy, ideally between twenty-seven and thirty-six weeks. This allows the mom's antibodies to be transferred to the baby. If you did not receive Tdap during pregnancy, you should definitely get it now. It is safe to get it even if you are breastfeeding.

If the last tetanus shot you remember getting was at your own pediatrician's office, you need to get the Tdap—T stands for tetanus, d stands for diphtheria, and "ap" stands for acellular pertussis (you might know it better as whooping cough).

Before 2005, adults used to get Td for their tetanus booster shots (recommended every ten years)—there was no "ap."

We know that our immunity to whooping cough wanes over time, but there was never a booster vaccination available for pertussis before now. Because of that, adults would be the ones to get whooping cough and go undiagnosed (thinking it was a cough they just couldn't shake or bronchitis). Sick adults would then spread it to those who were the most vulnerable: infants too young to be vaccinated. Yes, that includes your newborn.

Today, all parents, grandparents, and adult caretakers should get the Tdap vaccine if they spend time around a newborn baby.

BOTTOM LINE: Tell your newborn's adoring fans (grandparents, aunts, uncles, etc.) to get their Tdap shots if they want to hold your new baby.

Partner Tip

If you don't have a primary care doctor, now is the time to get one. You should get your Tdap shot as well as the seasonal flu vaccine to protect your precious cargo at home.

Tummy Issues and Nutrition

Q. Are there any special vitamins or nutrients I need more of?

You should continue taking your prenatal vitamins (preferably with ***DHA***) or switch to a postnatal vitamin for as long as you breastfeed.

Breastfeeding women also need 1,300 mg calcium and 800 IU of vitamin D. Your prenatal vitamin probably won't have enough calcium in it, so take a calcium supplement to make up the difference. It's also important to get calcium from your diet. Your body absorbs the calcium from food better than the calcium found in a supplement.

One eight-ounce glass of milk contains about 300 mg of calcium. Other ways to get about 300 mg of calcium include one cup (eight ounces) of yogurt, two cups of cottage cheese, one cup of orange juice fortified with calcium, one cup of soy milk fortified with calcium, six oranges, or two slices of calcium-fortified bread.

Helpful Hint

Take your prenatal vitamin and your calcium supplement at different times of the day. All that calcium cannot be absorbed into your system at the same time.

Q. I managed to escape pregnancy without developing hemorrhoids, but boy, do I have them now after pushing. What can I do?

Hemorrhoids are just varicose veins that develop around the anus due to the pressure of the baby during pregnancy and the pushing forces that occur during a delivery.

They can get pretty big (like the size of a large grape or even bigger) and sometimes they hurt more than your genital area after delivery!

You can use ice packs, witch hazel pads, and a topical steroid cream or suppository (like 1 percent hydrocortisone) to help shrink them back down to normal. Being constipated doesn't help matters. So take a stool softener and eat anything that is high in fiber (fruits, vegetables, whole grains, prunes, bran).

Red Flag: Hemorrhoids

If you are having excruciating pain from hemorrhoids, contact your provider right way. That's because a clot can form in the vein, called a thrombosed hemorrhoid—although this is rare.

Q. I had my baby three days ago and still haven't had a bowel movement. Is that normal?

Yes.

Many women will not poop for a few days after delivery. The good news is that it gives some time for your girl parts to heal before having to bear down while pooping and stretch out some tender, healing tissue.

However, you will do yourself a big favor if you go when you feel the urge to go. We know you are scared to go, but holding it in will only make things worse a few days down the line. And load up on fiber, water, and a stool softener shortly after delivery so you aren't in misery when nature calls. If you had a third- or fourth-degree tear, ask your OB provider about taking something more than a run-of-the-mill stool softener. You may benefit from something a little stronger, at least until you have a few softer bowel movements.

Reality Check

As we discussed, narcotic pain medication can cause constipation as a side effect. So, if you have taken any, either take a stool softener and increase your fiber to combat the effects of the medication, or you can try switching over to ibuprofen for pain relief instead.

Q. How much weight will I lose now that I have delivered?

The good news: You will lose quite a bit of weight right after delivery. Specifically, you lose seven to eight pounds of baby, one to two pounds of placenta, and at least two pounds of amniotic fluid and blood.

That's a ten- to twelve-pound weight loss at the time of birth!

Then, you get rid of your extra fluid in the week or so after delivery just by peeing and sweating it out. That's another two to four pounds without even heading to the gym.

The bad news: It takes some time to get back to your pre-pregnancy weight. So be realistic, patient, and optimistic!

Q. Can I go on a diet if I am breastfeeding?

We know you don't want to hear this, but the answer is no.

While breastfeeding, you actually need about 300 to 500 calories more than what you normally eat. If you aren't getting enough to eat or drink, you and your breast milk will suffer.

Your baby is still very needy, taking what they need at your body's expense. For instance, if you don't get enough calcium in your diet to provide an adequate amount in your breast milk, your body conveniently takes it out of your own bones. And if you are truly starving yourself to lose weight, your milk quality and quantity will suffer. As a result, you aren't doing your baby any favors.

The goal: Be healthy, make wise food choices, and exercise—but save the dieting until after you are done breastfeeding.

Urinary Tract

Q. I pee a bit every time I laugh—and that's not very funny. What do I do?

It is very normal to leak a little urine after having a baby. This may last for a few days or up to a few months.

Many women also report not having great bladder control until after they are done breastfeeding, their estrogen levels rise again, and the vaginal/vulvar/urethral tissue gets plumped up. The very first step to addressing incontinence is doing kegel exercises. (See the box on page 415 for kegel how-tos).

If you feel kegels haven't cured the problem, there are some other options:

- **Topical estrogen cream.** If you apply this cream religiously once or twice a day, it may help revitalize the tissues down there. It's available by prescription only, so you will need to ask your doctor for it.
- **Timed voiding.** This means that you go into the bathroom, sit down, and try to urinate every two hours whether you feel like you have to go or not. Many of us tend to hold our urine, thinking, "Oh, I will just do one more thing before I go." Try to train yourself to empty your bladder regularly.
- **Pelvic floor physical therapy.** A pelvic floor physical therapist can be instrumental in helping to strengthen the pelvic floor after delivery, which in turn can help with not only urinary incontinence, but also pelvic floor weakness and pressure, fecal incontinence, and painful intercourse. You can ask your OB provider for referrals.
- **The Emsella device.** This is a chair that some providers have in their offices that does 12,000 kegels in twenty-eight minutes. Yep, you heard that right—12,000 kegels in a single session. Most women couldn't even do that many in a month! The Emsella uses high-intensity focused electromagnetic energy to contract and strengthen the muscles of the pelvic floor while you sit there fully clothed. If your provider doesn't have one, check to see if others do in your area.
- **Surgery.** Bladder reconstructive surgery is a last resort and reserved for severe cases. A woman must have completed childbearing and be unsuccessful with all other treatments.

Most of the time, your symptoms will resolve by six months after delivery.

Emotional/Mental Health

Q. How long am I going to feel exhausted?

Let's see here. You just worked really hard to grow and then deliver a baby. Regardless of whether you had a vaginal delivery or a C-section, your body has been through a great deal and is expending a lot of energy toward healing.

You also lost quite a bit of blood during delivery and you are likely a little (or a lot) anemic.

And now for the biggie, you have a newborn and are likely not sleeping well through the night. Newborns sleep a lot, but not all at the same time. You'll probably be awakened every two to three hours at night for the next eight weeks.

No one can really prepare you for the sheer exhaustion you will experience. But it is a rite of passage for all new parents. You will survive, even though some days you might wonder!

It's critical to take care of yourself, for your baby's sake. Eat well. Nap when your baby naps. Do not be tempted to clean up, get baby announcements out, or do laundry during naptime. And believe it or not, regular exercise actually helps lessen fatigue.

While some parents report that they are exhausted until their kids go off to college, expect to start feeling better after three months (assuming your baby starts sleeping longer at night).

Q. I just had my baby a week ago and I find myself crying for no apparent reason. I'm also really irritated with my husband. Is this normal?

Yes.

In fact, it's so normal that up to 80 percent of women feel this way. It's called ***postpartum*** or ***"baby blues"***. This is different than postpartum *depression*.

Postpartum blues typically occur in the first four to five days after delivery and can last for up to two weeks. You might feel moody, anxious, impatient, irritable, or weepy. It's kind of like PMS.

The blues occur for a number of reasons: major hormonal shifts, lack of sleep, and anxiety over caring for a new baby. You may not always feel sad when you are crying. In fact, you may sob as you say out loud, "I have no idea why I am crying!"

When you have the baby blues:

- You are eating normally.
- You have no difficulty sleeping (when you get a chance to!)

Remember these key points when we compare the blues to postpartum *depression*.

Q. I just had my baby ten weeks ago, and I am still crying every day. I'm having a hard time getting out of bed to take care of my baby. Is this something I should be concerned about?

While this doesn't happen to everyone, there is an explanation. It's called ***postpartum depression*** (***PPD***) and it happens to as many as 10 percent of all new mothers.

Symptoms may occur a few days after delivery or not until months afterward. Symptoms can be mild or severe, and often alternate, so that some days seem okay but other days are really tough to get through.

The difference between postpartum blues and postpartum depression is that PPD does not go away.

Symptoms include severe fatigue, overwhelming feelings of sadness and guilt, and trouble sleeping and eating.

It is vitally important that you speak to your provider about your feelings, and if possible, include your partner or other loved ones in the visit. The more help you can get, the quicker you can begin to feel better.

Helpful Hint

A psychiatrist specializing in women's reproductive mental health, Dr. Lucy Puryear, shares her insider tip on deciphering postpartum depression: "In my experience, the single best question to ask a new mother who I suspect is suffering postpartum depression is, 'Are you able to sleep when the baby is sleeping?'" If the answer is no, seek professional help.

DR. M'S OPINION:

Postpartum Blues

No one really tells you about postpartum blues. I sure didn't learn about it in medical school, residency, or from any of my girlfriends. It wasn't until I went through it myself that I learned about it.

I now make it a point to tell my patients before sending them home so that they know what to expect and that they aren't the only one in the world experiencing these feelings.

Partner Tip

As you may know, partners sometimes gain sympathy weight. Well, partners are also at risk for having postpartum depression. Seek help if you have some of the warning symptoms we've discussed.

POSTPARTUM

Q. I know this sounds strange, but I'm having thoughts of harming my baby. Is this normal?

No, this is not normal.

This may be a symptom of severe postpartum depression or postpartum psychosis. Postpartum psychosis occurs after one out of every 1,000 pregnancies. The onset is sudden and usually occurs two to three weeks after giving birth (but it can happen as quickly as a few days after delivery).

Symptoms include bizarre behavior, hallucinations (hearing or seeing things that are not really there and can't be heard or seen by others), delusions, suicidal thoughts, and thoughts of harming others, including your newborn.

Postpartum psychosis is a medical emergency because it is extremely dangerous for you and your baby. You should contact your OB provider immediately and have another adult with you and your baby at all times.

Partner Tip

Oftentimes, the support person is the one to identify a problem. Keep your eyes open and get help for your partner if you have concerns. Trust your instincts—you know your partner best, and if she seems depressed or you are concerned about other behavior, call her OB provider. Check out the Red Flags for postpartum depression below.

Q. Who is at risk for postpartum depression?

According to Dr. Lucy Puryear, certain women are at greater risk of developing postpartum depression. These are women who are more vulnerable to hormonal changes than others. For them, those major hormone shifts cause depression. Here are the top six risk factors:

- History of depression at any point in life.
- Symptoms of depression during the third trimester of pregnancy.
- Previous history of postpartum depression.
- Family member with bipolar disorder.
- Severe premenstrual syndrome (called PMDD, premenstrual dysphoric disorder).
- Poor marital support.

Q. I keep having these horrible thoughts that something terrible will happen to my baby and it will be my fault. Is it normal to feel this way?

Every once in a while, a mom might come up with a worst-case scenario in her mind, such as, "If I fall asleep while I am nursing in this rocking chair, I might drop my baby." That's normal (and probably wise to consider!).

But occasionally moms find themselves having these thoughts all the time. They have no desire to intentionally harm their babies, and they are very scared of these crazy thoughts. These symptoms can be seen with postpartum anxiety disorder or postpartum obsessive-compulsive disorder.

If you feel this way, do not be afraid to ask for help!

Red Flags: Postpartum Depression[4]

- Lots of crying
- Sad mood
- Short temper
- Feeling hopeless or worthless
- Lack of desire to be around family and friends
- Lack of caring for yourself
- Change in appetite or eating pattern
- Difficulty sleeping, even when the baby is sleeping
- No desire to get out of bed
- Not wanting to hold or touch the baby (not enjoying the baby)

- Difficulty thinking clearly
- Thoughts about your own death, or death of the baby

Reality Check

Although not as common, partners can get postpartum depression, too. If you are experiencing any of the symptoms mentioned above, please reach out to your partner's provider for help.

Red Flags: Postpartum Anxiety

- Overwhelming fear that the baby will become sick or get injured
- Inability to leave the house due to consuming thoughts about the baby's well-being
- Decreased appetite
- Rapid weight loss
- Physical symptoms like a racing heartbeat and shortness of breath
- Panic attacks
- Persistent debilitating anxiety that interferes with normal life and baby bonding

Q. Where do I turn if I need help?

The first place to start is with the person who delivered your baby. They can help you immediately and then refer you to local mental health professionals and support groups in your community. There is nothing to be embarrassed about. And believe us, you are definitely not alone!

Q. My birth didn't go at all like we had planned. In fact, it was pretty traumatic, and I feel like I may still be in shock. What should I do?

It's always so hard when complications arise, and a planned birth doesn't go the way it was imagined. Whether there was an emergency that required more interventions than desired, a planned vaginal delivery that ended in a C-section, or even a baby needing to go to the NICU for more specialized care right after delivery, having a traumatic birth can have long-lasting impacts on your mental health. The first thing to know is that you are not alone. (A Birth Trauma Awareness Week is held in July due to how often this occurs.) Start talking about it and ask questions. Ask your OB provider to go over the details of what happened so you can have a clearer understanding. When you have all of your medical questions answered, many women feel better. If not, you can seek out a therapist or psychiatrist that specializes in birth trauma. There are many options in most areas in the United States, and you can find one by just searching online or asking your OB provider for a referral.

PART FIVE

Special Concerns and Problems

Let's hope you don't have to read this section. But if you need it, you can find info on the top twelve emergencies during pregnancy plus the fifty-one most common pregnancy complications. Sickness happens—so we cover the most common infections and ailments.

Are you over age thirty-five? We also look at the special issues with "advanced maternal age" pregnancies, plus provide a detailed view of preterm labor and babies. Multiples have their own special challenges . . . We cover this in-depth with info on twins, additional testing, and more.

Finally, the last chapter, "When It Doesn't Work," covers miscarriage and stillbirth. Plus, we have a detailed glossary, index, and info on our other books.

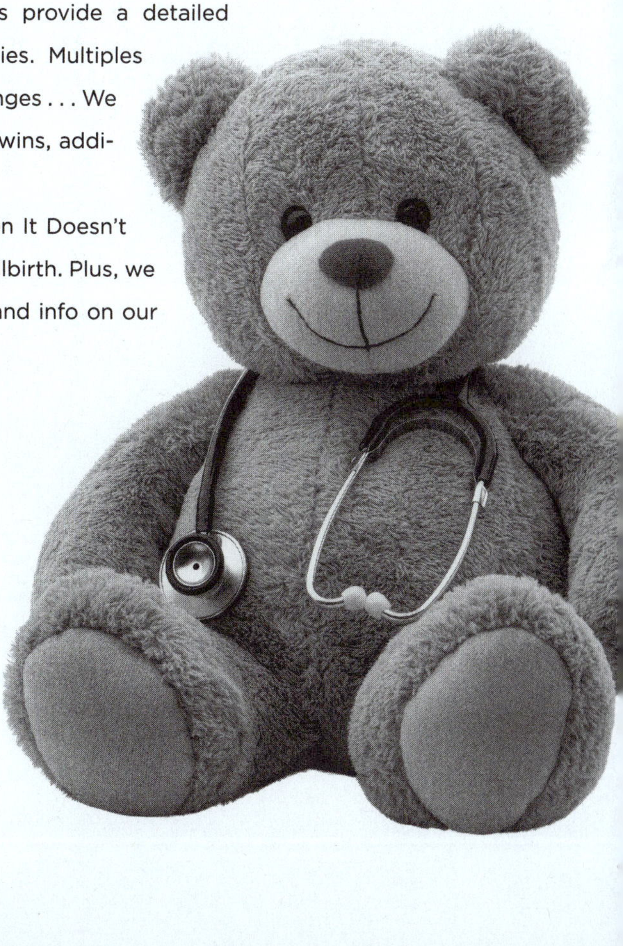

CHAPTER 16

Pregnancy 911

"Don't worry, I've never lost a patient.
I never lose anything. Have you seen my stethoscope?"

—Hawkeye, *M*A*S*H*

What's in This Chapter

- **On-call etiquette**
- **Headache**
- **Vomiting**
- **Fever**
- **Abdominal pain**
- **Contractions**
- **Vaginal bleeding**
- **Decreased fetal movement**
- **Leaking fluid**
- **Trauma and accidental injury**
- **Swelling legs/feet**
- **Seizures**
- **Shortness of breath/chest pain**

Let's face it. We all pause for a moment before calling our doctor about a concern. We don't want to seem like we are obsessing over something that is probably nothing. We don't want to wake our overworked providers up at three a.m. over something that could wait until the morning.

This chapter should help you troubleshoot the most common and the most urgent medical problems during your pregnancy. It will help you determine when you really do need to call your provider (even at three a.m.) and when it's probably okay to wait until the office opens. It also prepares you for what your doc will ask you when you call.

A key point: This chapter does not, in any way, replace the need to check with your OB provider. If you are worried, pick up the phone! Your OB provider will not get upset with you. But having this information on your nightstand may help you worry less and trust your instincts more.

The goal of this chapter is to help you troubleshoot, and to do it quickly. If you want to read up on the topics we refer to here, head over to Chapter 17, "The Complicated Pregnancy," for all the ugly details.

On-Call Etiquette

Q. What's the best way to communicate with my OB provider?

Before we get into specifics on emergencies, let's go over a few tips:

1. **Who you gonna call?** Before the need arises, find out how your OB provider handles phone calls during the day and after hours. Who answers the phone? And what number do you call?
2. **Volunteer information.** If your OB provider shares on-call responsibilities with other doctors (which is likely), don't expect the on-call doc to know your medical history or have it accessible. Tell the on-call doctor how far along you are and if you've had any complications, as well as the problem you are calling about.
3. **Skip the snack.** If you have to head to the hospital, do *not* eat before you go. It's better to do certain tests and procedures on an empty stomach. Since you don't know what lies ahead, hold off on the food. Do grab a toothbrush and some reading material.
4. **Call before running anywhere.** If you think there is a problem, you should always call your doctor or midwife before rushing to the emergency room (unless you are calling 911). Your doctor may be able to manage things over the phone, and if not, your doctor can notify the hospital that you are coming in (and be ready to meet you there).
5. **Take your temperature.** If you think you have a fever, take your temperature with a thermometer *before* calling. The OB provider will ask, so you might as well be ready to tell them exactly what your temperature is instead of saying, "I think I feel warm."
6. **You make the call.** While it's nice for your partner to speak with your OB provider, it's best if you call yourself. Your OB provider will ask a number of questions that will be tough for your partner to answer, such as "How many days ago did your green vaginal discharge begin?" or "When was the last time you had a bowel movement?"
7. **Make sure your phone accepts anonymous calls.** Most docs call from blocked phone lines—make sure your cell phone is not blocking such calls.

Helpful Hint

Just a heads-up—if you encounter one of the problems in this chapter during office hours, your OB provider may manage it differently than in the middle of the night or on a weekend. During normal business hours, your doctor will be able to see you in their office and have full access to a lab or imaging facility. If you need urgent attention at other times, the only way to accomplish an evaluation is through an urgent care facility, emergency room, or admission to the hospital.

Q. How do I decide what is a medical emergency?

Much of this is just common sense.

Unless your life or the life of your fetus is in imminent danger, it's best not to call 911. But there are situations when you need paramedics and a rapid trip to the emergency room.

Let's go over a little medical lingo before we discuss specific emergencies. If you've ever watched *Grey's Anatomy* or *The Pitt*, you know that doctors will "triage" or prioritize patients to be treated based on the severity of their problem.

For the purposes of this chapter, this is how we will triage (that is, categorize) pregnancy emergencies:

- **911:** Call 911. (This is a life-threatening emergency and requires emergency medical assistance right away.)
- **Priority 1:** Needs medical attention TODAY! (You need same-day medical attention, but someone can drive you to your doctor or the emergency room or an urgent care center.)
- **Priority 2:** Needs appointment in the next day or two.
- **Priority 3:** Watch and wait. Needs appointment if there is no improvement or worsening of symptoms.

Red Flags: When Do I Need an Ambulance?

Here are the top pregnancy emergencies that require immediate attention by a trained medical provider and immediate transport to the nearest hospital. Call 911 if you experience:

- **Severe vaginal bleeding.** Extremely heavy vaginal bleeding that does not stop or gets worse needs medical attention. Blood is continuously dripping or pouring out of you (like an open faucet) or you are passing multiple blood clots. Bleeding along with abdominal pain or dizziness/faintness is also a red flag.
- **Severe chest pain.** Make the call especially if you are also short of breath.
- **Labor and rectal pressure.** If your labor has progressed at home and you are planning to deliver in a hospital, contractions that are coming every two to three minutes, especially with rectal pressure, warrant quick transport to a hospital. You most likely don't have to poop—it's the baby's head!
- **Blood when water bag breaks.** If you break your water bag and there is a large amount of blood.
- **Your water bag breaks, and you feel something in your vagina.** It could be the umbilical cord or a fetal part (head, hand, or foot).
- **Severe abdominal pain.** A sudden onset of severe, constant abdominal pain, especially if you also have vaginal bleeding.
- **Sharp abdominal trauma.** Yes, this can happen. If it does, have someone call 911 immediately if you have been stabbed or take a gunshot wound to the belly.
- **Severe blunt abdominal trauma.** If you have a bad fall or motor vehicle accident that results in direct abdominal contact.

Red Flags: When to Head to Urgent Care Yourself

There are times you need urgent care, even if you don't need an ambulance. For example, if your emergency happens after office hours (at night, early in the morning, or on a weekend), it's often best to go straight to the ER. Let someone else drive you and call your doctor on your cell phone while you are en route. The ER doctor who sees you will likely give your OB provider a call to discuss your case and make a follow-up plan.

Here are a few of the top reasons to head to the nearest ER without waiting for the on-call doctor to call you back:

- Abrupt onset of a severe headache that is not responding to pain medication such as acetaminophen (brand name: Tylenol)
- Extreme, unrelenting vomiting
- Excruciating abdominal pain, especially when associated with nausea, vomiting, diarrhea, and/or fever
- Moderate or heavy vaginal bleeding

If you have an emergency when your doctor's office is open, it's best to call there first. Your doctor will either want you to come to the office for an immediate evaluation or go to the ER.

Q. How do I take my vital signs?

For certain problems, it's helpful to report your vital signs to the doctor on call. If it's not an extreme emergency, take your temperature, pulse (heart rate), and breaths per minute (respiratory rate) before picking up the phone.

How to check your pulse: The easiest places to find your pulse are your neck (just under your jawbone on either side) or the inner part of your wrist. Count how many times you feel a beat in fifteen seconds and then multiply that by four. That equals your pulse (how many times your heart beats in a minute). The average heart rate for an adult is 60 to 100 beats per minute.

How to check your breaths per minute: Watch your chest as it moves in and out. Count one breath for each time you breathe in for fifteen seconds and then multiply that by four. This is your respiratory rate. The average respiratory rate for an adult is twelve to twenty breaths per minute.

We assume you know how to use a thermometer, so we won't go through an explanation of checking your temperature. We just have one bit of advice, however: Report the actual reading on the thermometer (by mouth or ear or temporal artery scanner) to your OB provider. Do not add a degree, subtract a decimal point, or do a calculus equation on the number!

Partner Tip

If you are there during an emergency, one helpful role is to take your partner's vitals. Stay calm and follow the above procedures to get accurate readings.

The Top Twelve Obstetrical Emergencies

We will triage symptoms that require medical attention and discuss how quickly you need to act in each scenario. While this is not an exhaustive list, it covers the most common and the most serious issues you may encounter.

We are keeping our fingers crossed that you won't ever need this chapter! This is how doctors and midwives handle emergencies when the office is closed.

1. Headache

Being pregnant can give anyone a headache! Don't be surprised if you have one here or there. They are typical in the first and early second trimesters, even in women who don't have a history of frequent headaches. Headaches are rarely a sign of something serious. But on occasion, your body is telling you that something is very wrong.

Common Diagnoses:

- Tension headache from stress or work
- Dehydration
- Lack of sleep
- Discontinuing caffeine from your diet (caffeine withdrawal)
- Elevated hormone levels
- Migraine sufferers sometimes have more migraines during pregnancy

Uncommon Diagnoses:

- High blood pressure (severe ***preeclampsia***)
- Stroke
- Bleeding between the brain and surrounding tissues (subarachnoid hemorrhage)
- Bleeding in the brain (***subdural hematoma***)
- Infection in the tissue around the brain (***meningitis***)
- Trauma

What to Do:

- Drink water.
- Rest in a cool, quiet room.
- Take acetaminophen (brand name: Tylenol) as directed on the bottle. Do *not* take ibuprofen (brand names: Advil, Aleve, Motrin) or aspirin.
- Have a caffeinated drink (coffee or cola . . . no, it won't hurt the baby).
- Ask for a shoulder/neck/head massage if your partner is around.

What the OB Provider Will Ask You:

- Do you have a previous history of frequent headaches or migraine headaches?
- When did it start?
- Did it wake you from sleep?

- How long has it been going on?
- Have you had a recent head injury?
- Have you tried taking acetaminophen (Tylenol), resting, drinking fluids, or having some caffeine?
- Are you having any other symptoms: Fever? Nausea or vomiting? Stiff neck? Blurred vision? Sensitivity to light? Pain in the upper right side of your belly? Abdominal pain or vaginal bleeding? Dizziness? Loss of consciousness? Seizures? Confusion? Slurred speech?

911: Call an Ambulance

- Severe headache and loss of consciousness/confusion/slurring words
- Severe headache and seizure
- Severe headache and uncontrollable vomiting
- Severe headache after head injury (such as from a car accident, fall, violence)
- The worst headache you have ever had, particularly if it wakes you from sleep

Priority 1: Needs Medical Attention TODAY

- Severe headache and onset of blurred vision
- Severe headache and dizziness
- Severe headache and sudden onset of hand/feet swelling
- Severe headache with fever and/or neck stiffness and light sensitivity

Priority 2: Needs an Appointment the Next Day

- Constant headache without other symptoms that comes and goes, despite trying the measures mentioned above.

Priority 3: Watch and Wait. Needs Appointment If There Is No Improvement or Worsening of Symptoms

- Frequent headaches that resolve with the abovementioned measures
- A dull, intermittent headache with no other symptoms

2. Vomiting

Almost every pregnant woman tosses her cookies at some point, particularly in the first trimester. But vomiting can also be a sign of something more serious, especially when it occurs without morning sickness or when morning sickness has already come and gone.

Common Diagnoses:

- Morning sickness
- Food poisoning
- Eating too much, especially in the later stages of pregnancy
- Labor

Uncommon Diagnoses:

- Gallstones/gallbladder inflammation (***cholecystitis***)
- Inflammation or infection of the liver (hepatitis)

- Inflammation of the pancreas (***pancreatitis***)
- Inflammation or infection of the appendix (appendicitis)
- Kidney infection (***pyelonephritis***)
- Twisted ovary (ovarian torsion)
- High blood pressure (***preeclampsia***)
- ***Acute fatty liver***

What to Do:
The priority is to keep liquids down to prevent dehydration. It's less important whether or not you can tolerate solid food right now. Call your OB provider if you are vomiting so often that you cannot keep liquids down for three to four hours.

- Rest.
- After vomiting, wait five to ten minutes and try to take a small sip of liquid. The best liquids to try are those with a little bit of sugar or carbonation (instead of straight water), like ginger ale, 7UP, Sprite, or Gatorade. You can also try clear chicken broth or bone broth.
- Hold off on milk or dairy products while your stomach is unsettled.
- If you can keep the sips down after ten minutes, try a few more sips every five minutes.
- If you are actively vomiting or extremely nauseated, wait one hour before you test the waters with those sips of fluid.
- If you cannot stop vomiting and/or you are not able to keep down those sips of liquids, call your OB provider.
- Remember to take your temperature first and take note of any other symptoms you may have (see below).

What the OB Provider Will Ask You:

- How many times have you vomited?
- What color is it? Green? Yellow? Bloody? Coffee grounds?
- What have you eaten in the last twelve hours?
- Have you been able to keep any liquids down in the last few hours?
- Have you been around anyone who has been sick?
- Do you have a fever?
- Do you have any of these other symptoms: Diarrhea? Abdominal pain? Low back pain? Headache? Pain with urination?

911: Call an Ambulance

- Vomiting a significant amount of blood (red or brownish fluid)
- Vomiting associated with severe, constant abdominal pain

Priority 1: Needs Medical Attention TODAY

- Vomiting a small amount of blood
- Vomiting so much you haven't been able to keep fluids down in four hours

- Vomiting and dizziness
- Vomiting and chills, low back pain, and painful urination
- Vomiting and a fever greater than or equal to 102°F
- Vomiting bile (yellow/bright green fluid)
- Vomiting and head injury
- Unrelenting vomiting that has continued for more than six hours

Priority 2: Needs an Appointment the Next Day

- Vomiting throughout the day, but you're able to keep some liquids down
- Persistent vomiting and diarrhea
- Vomiting associated with a fever greater than 100.4°F but less than 102°F

Priority 3: Watch and Wait. Needs Appointment If There Is No Improvement or Worsening of Symptoms

- Sporadic vomiting associated with morning sickness in the first trimester
- One or two episodes of vomiting with no other symptoms

3. Fever

Fever is an elevation of the body's regular temperature. Contrary to what you probably learned in school, our body temperature is not 98.6°F, twenty-four hours a day. It varies on a daily cycle based on hormone levels. Our body is coolest at four a.m. (as low as 97.6°F) and hottest at seven p.m. (as high at 100°F). So the true definition of a "fever" is a body temperature of 100.4°F or higher.

Fever is your body's way of responding to an infection or inflammation. You should contact your OB provider any time you have a temperature of 100.4°F or greater.

Common Diagnoses:

- Common cold or flu virus
- Stomach virus
- Food poisoning
- You just received a vaccine (seasonal flu shot, etc.)
- Sinus infection

Uncommon Diagnoses:

- Lung infection (***pneumonia***)
- Inflammation of the pancreas (***pancreatitis***)
- Inflammation and infection of the appendix (appendicitis)
- Blood clot
- Inflammation or infection of the liver (hepatitis)
- Gallstones/inflammation of the gallbladder (***cholecystitis***)
- Infection of the placenta and amniotic sac (***chorioamnionitis***)
- Parvovirus infection

- Listeria infection
- Kidney infection (***pyelonephritis***)

What to Do:

- Rule #1: Before you panic, take your temperature . . . Just because you feel hot doesn't mean your core body temperature is over 100.4°F (what we consider to be a fever).
- Take 650 mg of acetaminophen (brand name: Tylenol) by mouth every four to six hours (do not exceed forty-eight hours).
- Drink more fluids.
- Take note of other symptoms (see below).

What the OB Provider Will Ask You:

- What is your temperature?
- How long have you had it?
- Have you taken any medication? Acetaminophen (Tylenol)? How much? When was your last dose?
- Do you have any other symptoms: Headache? Cough? Runny nose? Sore throat? Nausea? Vomiting? Diarrhea? Abdominal pain? Vaginal bleeding or leaking? Painful urination? Back pain? Chills? Body aches?
- Is anyone at home sick, or have you had any sick contacts in the past week?
- Do you have a rash?

Priority 1: Needs Medical Attention TODAY

- Fever at or over 102°F
- Fever and back/flank pain with or without chills
- Fever with body aches and chills
- Fever and intractable vomiting or diarrhea
- Fever and foul-smelling vaginal discharge
- Fever and severe abdominal pain
- Fever and difficulty breathing

Priority 2: Needs an Appointment the Next Day

- Fever and severe sinus pain
- Fever and upper respiratory symptoms (cough, runny nose, ear pain, sore throat)
- Fever without a clear reason why

Priority 3: Watch and Wait. Needs Appointment If There Is No Improvement or Worsening of Symptoms

- Fever less than 102°F that responds to acetaminophen (Tylenol) and resolves
- Fever less than 102°F with no other symptoms

4. Abdominal Pain

Everyone gets some belly discomfort during pregnancy. It's common to have random, short-lived episodes of abdominal pain during any trimester. It happens in the first trimester as your uterus begins to grow . . . and in the second trimester as your round ligaments get pulled. Inevitably, it also happens in your third trimester, either due to the extreme discomfort from having a big baby in your belly or secondary to uterine contractions and labor. The key is to be able to figure out when abdominal pain is normal and when it is not. Doctors worry more about dull, crampy abdominal pain than sharp, knifelike pain.

Common Diagnoses:

- A growing uterus (mild tightening/cramping without vaginal bleeding)
- Round ligament pain
- Muscle strain
- Constipation
- ***Bladder infection***
- Uterine contractions/labor
- Stomach virus (***gastroenteritis***)
- Food poisoning

Uncommon Diagnoses:

- Appendicitis
- Benign tumor in uterus outgrows its blood supply (degenerating ***uterine fibroid***)
- Rupture of an ovarian cyst
- Gallstones/inflammation of the gallbladder (***cholecystitis***)
- Liver inflammation or infection (hepatitis)
- Inflammation of the pancreas (***pancreatitis***)
- Kidney infection (***pyelonephritis***)
- Hernia
- ***Ectopic pregnancy*** (first trimester)
- ***Placental abruption***

What to Do:

- Rest. Sit down or lie down on your left side.
- If your pain persists, gets worse, or you have additional symptoms, call your OB provider.
- Take note of whether you have any additional symptoms (see below).

What the OB Provider Will Ask:

- Where is your pain located? Upper abdomen? Lower abdomen? In the middle? More to one side?
- Does the pain radiate or travel anywhere? Your back? Your leg? Your chest?
- How long have you had the pain?
- Is it constant or does it come and go?

- Does anything you do make it better? Worse?
- Do you have any underlying medical problems (such as high blood pressure or lupus)?
- Are you having any vaginal bleeding or leaking of fluid from the vagina?
- Is your baby moving (if past twenty-six weeks)?
- Are you having any other symptoms? Fever? Chills? Nausea? Vomiting? Diarrhea? Pain with urination? Low back pain?

911: Call an Ambulance

- Severe pain that comes on suddenly and there is no relief for an hour or more
- Severe abdominal pain and heavy vaginal bleeding
- Severe abdominal pain and constant vomiting
- Severe one-sided abdominal pain in the first trimester with vaginal bleeding and/or dizziness before you have had an ultrasound showing that your baby has correctly implanted in your uterus

Priority 1: Needs Medical Attention TODAY

- Abdominal pain and fever, chills, low back pain, or painful urination
- Abdominal pain with nausea and intermittent vomiting
- Abdominal pain and small amounts of vaginal bleeding
- Abdominal pain and watery vaginal discharge
- Severe abdominal pain with known uterine fibroids or an ovarian cyst

Priority 2: Needs an Appointment the Next Day

- Intermittent abdominal pain and no other symptoms
- Mild abdominal pain and a visible bulge in your groin area

Priority 3: Watch and Wait. Needs Appointment If There Is No Improvement or Worsening of Symptoms

- Abdominal pain that gets better and resolves with no other symptoms
- Abdominal pain that improves with rest or use of a maternity belt

5. Contractions

Unless you have a scheduled C-section, you will encounter contractions when you go into labor. It's also natural to have ***Braxton-Hicks contractions*** sporadically toward the end of pregnancy. If this is your second, third, or (wow, we salute you) fourth pregnancy, Braxton-Hicks contractions may be felt as early as twenty to twenty-four weeks.

If you have real contractions in the second or early third trimester, you definitely need to chat with your OB provider!

Common Diagnoses:

- Braxton-Hicks contractions
- Dehydration (leading to contractions)

- A bladder infection (leading to contractions)
- Labor (real contractions in a pregnancy beyond thirty-seven weeks gestation)

Uncommon Diagnoses:

- Preterm contractions (uterine contractions occurring after twenty-two weeks and before thirty-seven weeks that, although uncomfortable, do not cause dilation of the cervix)
- Preterm labor (uterine contractions occurring after twenty-two weeks but before thirty-seven weeks that *do* lead to dilation of the cervix)

What to Do:

These are all things that even my children have learned after listening to me talk with patients on the phone over the last twenty-one years!

- Rest. Sit down or lie down on your left side.
- Hydrate. Drink a lot of water/fluids.
- Time your contractions over the course of an hour. How? Time them from the start of one to the start of the next.
- Take note of other symptoms, such as vaginal bleeding or leaking of water from the vagina, pain with urination, or constant pain.
- **If you are less than thirty-five weeks,** call your OB provider if you are having more than four to six contractions in an hour.
- **If you are more than thirty-five weeks,** call your OB provider if you are having regular uterine contractions every five to seven minutes for an hour.
- **If you are carrying more than one fetus, have bright red vaginal bleeding, have a *cerclage*, or any other type of high-risk pregnancy**, discuss *all* contractions with your OB provider.

What your OB Provider Will Ask:

- How far along are you? What is your due date?
- How often are your contractions occurring?
- How long have you been having contractions?
- Does your pain come and go, or is it constant?
- Are you carrying one fetus or do you have twins? Triplets? More?
- On a scale of one to ten with ten being the most pain you have ever felt, how painful are your contractions?
- Do you have a history of preterm labor in this pregnancy or any previous pregnancies?
- Are you having any vaginal bleeding or leaking of fluid from the vagina?
- What were you doing when your contractions began? Exercising? On your feet all day? Having intercourse?
- Have you been getting enough to drink? Are you well hydrated?
- Do you have any pain with urination? Fever? Frequent urination?

911: Call an Ambulance

- Severe, constant abdominal pain, especially with vaginal bleeding
- Regular, painful contractions occurring every two to three minutes with rectal pressure (particularly in a woman who has already had one or more children)

Priority 1: Needs Medical Attention TODAY

- Painful uterine contractions occurring more frequently than four to six times an hour if you are less than thirty-five weeks gestation
- Painful regular contractions occurring every three to five minutes, for at least an hour or two if you are over thirty-five weeks gestation
- Painful uterine contractions with leaking of fluid/blood from vagina
- Painful, regular uterine contractions with a high-risk pregnancy (***breech presentation***, ***placenta previa***, ***vasa previa***, previous C-section, multiples)

Priority 2: Needs an Appointment the Next Day

- Intermittent contractions that are becoming more regular but are still fifteen to thirty minutes apart
- Uterine contractions and frequent urination

Priority 3: Watch and Wait. Needs Appointment If There Is No Improvement or Worsening of Symptoms

- Intermittent contractions occurring at thirty-five weeks or beyond
- Uterine contractions with dehydration that resolve when you increase your fluid intake
- Uterine contractions occurring with overexertion that resolve when you rest

6. Vaginal Bleeding

About 10 percent of all pregnant women have some vaginal bleeding, with most of these episodes occurring in the first trimester. Typically, a small amount of vaginal bleeding is nothing serious. But it's always a good idea to run it by your OB provider.

Docs are most concerned when the bleeding is bright red, persists, or when it is extremely heavy and accompanied by large clots. OB providers get clues from what color the blood is, how much is coming out, whether or not clots are present, and when in a pregnancy the bleeding occurs.

Common Diagnoses:

- ***Implantation bleeding***
- Vaginal or cervical irritation or injury (from intercourse)
- Vaginal or cervical infection
- Partial placental separation
- Labor (***bloody show***)

Uncommon Diagnoses:

- Ectopic pregnancy

- Threatened miscarriage
- Cervical cancer
- Death of one fetus in a multiples pregnancy (***vanishing twin***)
- ***Cervical insufficiency***
- Premature labor
- ***Placenta previa***
- ***Vasa previa***
- ***Placenta abruption***

What to Do:

- Rest. Lie down if possible.
- Use a pad so that you can quantify how much blood you are losing.
- Note any other symptoms, such as abdominal pain, decreased fetal movement (if you are more than twenty-six weeks), dizziness, and lightheadedness.
- Bring or take a picture of any blood clots/tissue you pass with you to the medical facility.
- Call your OB provider with any amount of bleeding.

Reality Check

At least half the time, your OB provider will not know exactly why you have vaginal bleeding. If there is no obvious diagnosis, doctors assume that it is due to a small degree of placental separation that isn't visible on ultrasound.

What the OB Provider Will Ask You:

- How much blood are you passing? Is it spotting, or are you bleeding as much as a period?
- How far along are you? What is your due date?
- Are you passing any blood clots or any tissue?
- Are you having any abdominal pain or cramping?
- Do you feel faint, dizzy, or lightheaded?
- Is this the first episode of vaginal bleeding you have had during this pregnancy?
- Have you ever lost a pregnancy/had a miscarriage in the past?
- Have you had intercourse recently?
- Have you had any recent abdominal trauma?
- If you are past twenty-six weeks, do you feel your baby moving around?

911: Call an Ambulance

- Severe abdominal pain with moderate to heavy vaginal bleeding
- Moderate to severe bleeding with a known ***placenta previa*** or ***vasa previa***
- Moderate to severe bleeding with a known chronic ***placental abruption***

- Moderate to severe bleeding and dizziness or lightheadedness
- Moderate to severe bleeding after having direct abdominal trauma

Priority 1: Needs Medical Attention TODAY

- Continuous vaginal bleeding
- Spotting with a known ***placenta previa, vasa previa,*** or ***chronic placental abruption***

Priority 2: Needs an Appointment the Next Day

- Minimal red/brown spotting without pain

Priority 3: Watch and Wait. Needs Appointment If There Is No Improvement or Worsening of Symptoms

- Intermittent brownish spotting once you have already confirmed that the fetus is implanted in your uterus (i.e., you've had an ultrasound)

Miscarriage

If you miscarry before six to seven weeks, you can usually manage things at home. You will have bleeding like a very heavy period, and you may pass a few blood clots. You can treat the pain with ibuprofen (Advil, Motrin).

Signs of a potentially more serious condition include severe, unrelenting pain, particularly on one side versus the other, excessive vaginal bleeding (as if a faucet has been opened up), continuous passage of large blood clots, dizziness, or faintness.

See Chapter 22, "When It Doesn't Work," for details.

7. Decreased Fetal Movement

A happy, healthy fetus is one that moves around. Most women cannot feel their baby moving around until eighteen to twenty-two weeks. And even at this point, the movement is sporadic. You may feel movement one day and then not again for two more days. But after about twenty-six weeks, you should begin to notice the baby moving around every day, and this is when we recommend that you start doing ***fetal kick counts***. Be sure your baby is moving during each twelve-hour period.

Common Diagnoses:

- Your baby is sleeping (fetal sleep cycle).
- Your baby is hiding behind the placenta. If the placenta is located between the baby and the side of your uterus closest to the skin on your belly, it will cushion the fetus's movement and make it more difficult to feel.
- You have been moving around all day, and although baby has been moving, you have not been aware of it.

Uncommon Diagnoses:

- Low level of ***amniotic fluid*** (***oligohydramnios***)
- Fetal distress
- Stillbirth

What to Do:

- Many times, a mother suspects that she is not feeling her baby move because she has been moving around all day at home or at work. Stop your activity and see what happens.
- Sit down or lie on your left side.
- Drink something sweet like orange juice or lemonade.
- Eat a snack or meal if it is mealtime.
- Take your hands and lightly move your belly around.
- Count how many times the baby moves over the next hour.
- If you still cannot feel movement over the next hour, call your OB provider.

Most women who have had stillbirths report a decrease or absence of fetal movement for the two to five days prior to diagnosis. If you are uncertain about how much your baby is moving around, and you have tried all the tips above, call your OB provider.

What the OB Provider Will Ask You:

- How far along are you? What is your due date?
- When was the last time you felt the baby move?
- When was the last time you ate or drank anything?
- Are you having contractions?
- Are you leaking any fluid?
- Are you having any vaginal bleeding?

Priority 1: Needs Medical Attention TODAY

- Lack of fetal movement for twenty-four hours, after twenty-six weeks, despite attempting all the efforts listed above.

Priority 2: Needs an Appointment the Next Day

- Baby is still moving around, but there's been less movement in the past day or two.

Priority 3: Watch and Wait. Needs Appointment If There Is No Improvement or Worsening of Symptoms

- Your baby's movements change from quick punches and jabs to larger, rolling body movements, but is still moving. This typically happens after thirty-four to thirty-five weeks.

8. Leaking Fluid from the Vagina

It's normal to have quite a bit of vaginal discharge during pregnancy (***leukorrhea of pregnancy***). Discharge typically is whitish-clear, odorless, and the consistency of mucous. Tell your OB provider if you have leakage of a watery substance from your vagina.

Common Diagnoses:

- Increased vaginal discharge in pregnancy (leukorrhea of pregnancy)
- Vaginal infection
- Semen leaking out after intercourse
- Leaking urine

Uncommon Diagnoses:

- Water bag breaks (rupture of your amniotic sac)

What to Do:

Now, don't get grossed out when we tell you what to do here, but:

- Take a look at the fluid—check the color, texture (watery or mucusy), and odor.
- Try to figure out when the fluid came out. Did you have a full bladder on the way to the toilet? Was it just after urinating? A few hours after having intercourse? Did you just get out of the bath or swimming pool?
- If the fluid is a mystery to you, always call your OB provider. It is better to play it safe and check things out, even if your doc tells you that you peed on yourself. You don't want to have a broken water bag undiagnosed for days.

Reality Check

Most of the time when you break your water bag, you will leak continuously and start having uterine contractions within twenty-four to seventy-two hours. It's pretty rare to be leaking once every few days from a broken water bag.

What Your OB Provider Will Ask:

- How far along are you? What is your due date?
- What color is it?
- How much came out?
- Is the fluid thick, thin, watery, or mucusy?
- Is there an odor?
- Are you having any vaginal symptoms? Itching? Burning?
- Was it one time or is it still happening?
- Was there any bleeding associated with it?
- Are you having contractions?
- Did you just have intercourse? Take a bath? Go swimming?
- Do you have to go to the bathroom? Is your bladder full?

911: Call an Ambulance

- Massive bleeding from the vagina
- Fluid leaking from the vagina with the feeling or sight of something in the vagina—particularly when the baby is in the breech position

Priority 1: Needs Medical Attention TODAY

- Watery fluid continuously leaking from the vagina
- Discolored fluid (dark green, brown, black) leaking from the vagina
- Fluid leaking from the vagina with uterine contractions
- You have leaked once or twice without other symptoms or contractions, and you are less than thirty-seven weeks

Priority 2: Needs an Appointment the Next Day

- You have leaked once or twice without other symptoms or contractions, you are more than thirty-seven weeks pregnant, and it has stopped

Priority 3: Watch and Wait. Needs Appointment If There Is No Improvement or Worsening of Symptoms

- Leaking that occurs only with a full bladder, on the way to the bathroom, or just after you think you are done urinating

Reality Check

Most women will leak urine at some point during their pregnancy. For some, it happens only with coughing, laughing, or sneezing. For others, it's a daily occurrence. It's not pretty, but it's normal.

9. Trauma (Accidental Injury)

Trauma simply means injury to the body. This includes car accidents (minor or major), falls, domestic violence, and assault (burns, gunshot wounds, stabbings, kicks, and punches). Unfortunately, major trauma complicates 3 to 8 percent of all US pregnancies.

Believe it or not, pregnant women suffer trauma more frequently than the average person. Your center of gravity has changed, and you are more likely to suffer a fall by tripping on uneven ground, walking downstairs, or even walking your dog. Your belly sticks out, and it is something you aren't used to. You are more likely to bump into things (the corners of countertops, for example) and get burned at the stove. And an airbag deploying will almost always hit a pregnant belly.

Unfortunately, pregnancy is a time when domestic violence occurs more frequently. As hard as it is to imagine, women do get beaten by partners during pregnancy, including being punched or kicked in the abdomen.

It's possible for the fetus to be harmed any time there is direct trauma to the abdomen. The placenta can be injured and pull off the wall of the uterus (***placental abruption***), interfering with the fetus's blood and oxygen supply. Trauma can also cause first trimester miscarriage, premature rupture of membranes, uterine rupture, and stillbirth.

You need to contact your OB provider if you have *any* abdominal trauma, blunt or sharp—no matter how minor it seems.

Common Diagnoses:

- Falls
- Burns
- Minor car accidents

Uncommon Diagnoses

- Major car accidents
- Domestic violence
- Assault
- Gunshot wounds
- Stabbings

What to Do:
Call your OB provider any time you have had an injury to your belly. Seek medical care as soon as possible if you were in a car accident and had direct abdominal trauma (contact between your belly and the steering wheel, dashboard, airbag, or even tightening of your seat belt). The same goes for any assault injury or fall where you had a direct injury to your abdomen.

WARNING:
Injury Prevention Tips

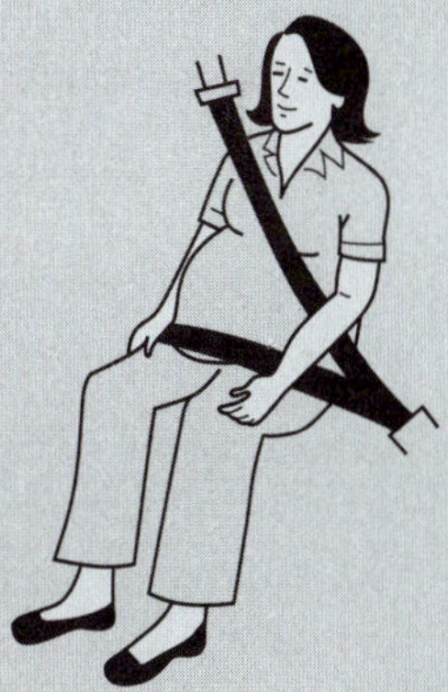

- The bottom portion of the seat belt (the belt) should be placed ***below*** your belly, across your lap (see illustration). Avoid placing it across your belly near your belly button.
- Be careful: Your center of gravity has shifted, and you are more likely to trip and fall when pregnant.
- Avoid activities that will increase your risk of falling: walking dogs, riding horses, wearing high-heeled shoes. (As you already know, I'm a shoe-lover, so this one was tough for me to put in here, but it's the truth.) Or, say, playing in a co-ed rugby tournament.
- If you are in an abusive relationship, seek out help and formulate a plan to leave. You can find resources at National Domestic Abuse Hotline: thehotline.org or 1-800-799-SAFE (7233).

What Your OB Provider Will Ask:

- How far along are you? What is your due date?
- What kind of accident was it?

- Was there any direct abdominal trauma?
- If so, how hard was the impact?
- Do you have any bruising or abrasions on your skin where the trauma occurred?
- Are you having any abdominal pain right now?
- Are you having any vaginal bleeding?
- Are you leaking any fluid from the vagina?
- Is the baby moving (if greater than twenty-six weeks)?
- Do you have any other associated injuries? Sprains? Open wounds? Abrasions? Head injury?
- Was this injury the result of an assault or domestic violence? Are you currently still in danger?
- If you sustained a burn, where is it? How much of your abdomen is involved? Is the skin coming off, or is it just red? What did you get burned with—hot water? Coffee? Something on the stove?

911: Call an Ambulance

- You were in a major car accident.
- You sustained major blunt trauma to your abdomen.
- You were stabbed.
- You were shot.
- You were in a minor car accident but have severe abdominal pain and/or vaginal bleeding.
- You fell and have severe abdominal pain and/or vaginal bleeding.

Priority 1: Needs Medical Attention TODAY

- Direct abdominal trauma (by any method) that doesn't fit into the categories above
- Decreased fetal movement hours or days after direct abdominal trauma
- Severe abdominal pain hours or days after direct abdominal trauma
- Vaginal bleeding hours or days after direct abdominal trauma

Priority 3: Watch and Wait. Needs Appointment If There Is No Improvement or Worsening of Symptoms

- A minor fall. You did not directly hit your belly. You have no vaginal bleeding, abdominal pain, or obvious injury. It's still a good idea to talk to your OB provider, but you probably won't need an office visit.

Reality Check

Up to 40 percent of severe blunt trauma injuries in pregnancy lead to a placental abruption.

But here's a surprise. About 3 to 5 percent of *minor* abdominal trauma also leads to placental abruption.

So even if you think that you are absolutely fine after your little fender bender, it's best to talk with your OB provider and get checked out.[1]

10. Swelling of Your Lower Extremities (Legs/Feet)

Cankles happen.

Nine out of ten pregnant women lose sight of their ankle bones as their pregnancy nears the end. It's frightening, shocking, and often sad when this day happens. And it happens earlier for some women than others.

Although most of the time swelling is a normal phenomenon, sometimes it is a sign that something more serious is happening.

Common Diagnoses:

- Normal swelling (***edema***) that occurs at the end of pregnancy
- Increased salt intake (as a Texan and a Californian, we know how hard it is to say no to chips and salsa)
- Blood vessel changes with pregnancy (venous insufficiency)
- Just got off an airplane
- Forgot to wear your support stockings!

Uncommon Diagnoses:

- High blood pressure (***preeclampsia***)
- Blood clot (***deep venous thrombosis***), particularly if only affecting one leg
- Poorly functioning heart (congestive heart failure) or kidneys

DR. M'S OPINION

T.E.D. hose were a lifesaver for me! They are not sexy, but neither are the cankles you are trying to prevent.

REALITY CHECK:

Swelling Prevention Tips

- Put your feet up whenever possible. Use a stool or low table with pillows stacked on top.
- Decrease your salt intake.
- Exercise.
- Wear comfortable shoes and socks. You may have to get a size bigger than you normally wear to accommodate the swelling that happens as the day progresses.
- Don't cross your legs while sitting down.
- Drink tons of water. This helps your body retain less water. (We know this is counterintuitive since you are swollen, but it's true.)
- Eat a well-balanced diet.
- Ask your OB provider about using support stockings.

What to Do:

- Rest.
- Elevate your legs with a stool or a few pillows.
- Drink more water.
- If one leg is more swollen than the other, call your OB provider.

What Your OB Provider Will Ask:

- How far along are you? What is your due date?
- Did it come on suddenly, or has it been going on for a while?
- Is it symmetrical in both legs, or is there more swelling in one leg/foot?
- Are you having any pain with your swelling?
- Is there any discoloration to the skin of your lower extremities?
- Do you have any chest pain? Shortness of breath? Dizziness? Feelings of anxiety?
- Do you have any medical problems?
- Have you had a lot of salt intake over the last few days?
- Have you been diagnosed with high blood pressure or ***preeclampsia***?
- Are your hands and face swollen, too?
- Are you having headaches, blurry vision, changes in your vision, or right upper abdominal pain?
- Did you just get off an airplane?

911: Call an Ambulance

- One leg dramatically more swollen than the other and chest pain, shortness of breath, dizziness, or a feeling of impending doom

Priority 1: Needs Medical Attention TODAY

- One leg more swollen than the other
- Experiencing pain in one leg in the presence of swelling
- Rapid onset of swelling in legs, feet, hands, and face

Priority 2: Needs an Appointment the Next Day

- Gradual increase in swelling in the lower extremities prior to twenty-eight weeks
- Gradual increase in swelling in the lower extremities and discomfort in both legs

Priority 3: Watch and Wait. Needs Appointment If There Is No Improvement or Worsening of Symptoms

- Gradual onset of swelling in the third trimester, in just the lower legs, ankles, and feet

11. Seizures

A seizure occurs when something (lack of oxygen, lack of nutrients, toxins, drugs, blood, trauma) interrupts the normal electrical circuitry in the cells of the brain (neurons). Seizures are rare during pregnancy, and it is a true medical emergency for both mom and baby.

The key is being able to determine what is really a seizure and what is not. Many people report that they saw a loved one have a "seizure" when in fact that person fainted, lost consciousness, passed out, or had some involuntary body shaking (tremors or chills). While there are a few different types of seizures, here are the key points:

The person having the seizure:

- Loses consciousness or cannot remember a certain period of time.
- Feels a sensation in their skin, muscles, vision, or sensation of taste.

The person witnessing a seizure may see the person:

- Lose consciousness, faint, or appear spaced out.
- Have rigid muscle tone.
- Clench jaws and teeth.
- Have involuntary muscle movements that are jerky and repetitive.
- Pee or poop involuntarily (incontinence).

Common Diagnoses:

- Not enough blood gets up to the head while standing or sitting up too fast (***vasovagal event***)
- Dehydration
- Fainting
- Seizure when someone has a known seizure disorder (epilepsy) prior to pregnancy

Uncommon diagnoses:

- Seizure from severe, uncontrolled ***preeclampsia*** (called ***eclampsia***)
- Seizure from another rare cause, such as drugs or recent head trauma

FEEDBACK FROM THE REAL WORLD:

Don't Wait to Call!

I had a patient, who, bless her heart, called me at nine a.m. on a Saturday morning. She said, "Sorry to bother you, Dr. M, but my husband told me that while we were having breakfast at six-thirty this morning, my eyes rolled back and I started shaking uncontrollably. I don't really remember what happened after that. I knew I should call you, but I didn't want to wake you up."

Moral of the story: For something like this, WAKE UP YOUR DOCTOR!

What to do:

- If you have a seizure, someone should call 911 first and then notify your OB provider immediately!

911: Call an Ambulance

- A true seizure during pregnancy is always considered a medical emergency. Although it is rare to have a seizure caused by ***preeclampsia***, any pregnant woman who has a seizure needs immediate medical attention to rule that out.

12. Shortness of Breath and/or Chest Pain

It's normal for a pregnant person to get short of breath occasionally. Especially near the end of your pregnancy, you may have a brief sensation where you can't take in a big breath of air. This feeling should resolve with rest.

Why do you feel this way? Your growing uterus puts pressure on the diaphragm muscle above your belly and below your lungs. Your lungs have less room to expand. And you weigh more. Last, you need more oxygen not only for yourself, but for your baby as well.

Chest pain is *never* a "normal" symptom of pregnancy and always calls for medical evaluation.

Common Diagnoses:

- Approaching due date
- Overexertion
- Asthma flare-up
- Anxiety/panic attack

Uncommon Diagnoses:

- Blood clot in the blood vessel supplying the lungs (***pulmonary embolism***)
- Severe allergic reaction where your throat begins to swell (anaphylaxis)
- Worsening of a previously known heart condition
- Initial symptoms of a previously undiagnosed heart condition
- Fluid buildup in the lungs from congestive heart failure or severe preeclampsia
- Heart attack

What to Do:

- Rest. Sit down and put your feet up.
- If you are still short of breath after resting, call your OB provider.
- If you have asthma, try using your inhaler (that your doc has previously approved).
- If you have a lung or heart condition, call your OB provider.

What Your OB Provider Will Ask You:

- How long have you been having chest pain?
- How long have you been having shortness of breath?

- Do you have any medical problems? Heart conditions? Asthma? Anxiety?
- Do you have any allergies?
- What were you doing when your symptoms began?
- Does it improve with rest?
- Do you have any abdominal pain? Dizziness? A rash or hives? A severe headache? Blurry vision?
- Does your chest pain travel anywhere? Your back? Your abdomen? Your arm? Your neck?
- Are you having any swelling in your legs and feet? If so, is one leg/foot more swollen than the other?

911: Call an Ambulance

- Severe, unrelenting chest pain
- Unable to catch your breath/severe difficulty breathing
- Total body swelling with or without hives/rash and difficulty swallowing or breathing

Priority 1: Needs Medical Attention TODAY

- Difficulty breathing and you have asthma
- Difficulty breathing, with or without a cough, with known preeclampsia (the development of shortness of breath could signal pulmonary edema or water in your lungs)
- Any type of chest pain other than the 911 emergency kind

Priority 2: Needs an Appointment the Next Day

- Asthma flare-up that is not improving with your rescue inhaler medication

Priority 3: Watch and Wait. Needs Appointment If There Is No Improvement or Worsening of Symptoms

- Intermittent shortness of breath that resolves with rest (particularly in the third trimester)

If you have already delivered your baby and think you have a medical emergency, check out "I'm feeling a bit short of breath. Is this okay?" on page 405, in Chapter 15, "Postpartum: What's Next?" for guidance.

PREGNANCY 911

CHAPTER 17

The Complicated Pregnancy

"Love is all fun and games until someone loses an eye or gets pregnant."

—Jim Cole

What's in This Chapter

- **Top Complications**
- **Medical problems**
- **Maternal issues**
- **Fetal issues**

WARNING: This chapter may induce restless nights full of anxious worrying (as if you already didn't have insomnia).

Yes, there are many things that *can* happen during pregnancy. But most of them *don't* happen. View this chapter as a reference if you have concerns about a condition or if you have been given a specific diagnosis. We haven't listed every possible complication in pregnancy, just the most common ones.

Bottom line: This is a scary chapter. It is full of medical scenarios without any sugarcoating. And some of the discussion here can get rather technical—but we figure if you are dealing with one of these complications, you want a detailed picture of what's happening.

Here's our advice: ***Do NOT read this chapter unless your OB provider is concerned that you actually have one of these issues.*** You have enough to worry about.

This chapter is divided into two major sections:

- Medical complications: Health issues that complicate pregnancy.
- Obstetrical complications: Issues specific to pregnancy itself (either a problem with the mother or the baby).

To make it easier to find what you are looking for, we've grouped these by body system (urinary tract, blood, etc.).

Overview: Medical Complications

A. The Gut (Stomach, Intestines, Liver, Gallbladder, and Pancreas)

1. Hyperemesis gravidarum (excessive vomiting)
2. Cholestasis (liver problem)
3. Acute fatty liver (liver problem)
4. HELLP syndrome (liver problem plus other problems)
5. Cholecystitis (gallbladder problem)
6. Pancreatitis
7. Appendicitis

B. Female Anatomy (Uterus, Ovaries, and Fallopian Tubes)

8. Ovary problem (ruptured ovarian cyst)
9. Ovary/fallopian tubes problem (adnexal torsion)
10. Fibroids (degenerating uterine fibroid)

C. Urinary Tract (Bladder and Kidneys)*

11. Kidney stones
12. Acute urinary retention

D. Blood

13. Anemia
14. Rh incompatibility
15. Sickle cell anemia
16. Thalassemias
17. Low platelet count
18. Blood clot in your leg or lung (deep venous thrombosis, pulmonary embolus)
19. Blood clotting disorders (thrombophilias, factor V leiden, prothrombin gene mutation, protein C or S deficiency, antithrombin III deficiency, antiphospholipid syndrome)

E. Heart and Blood Vessels

20. Preeclampsia and eclampsia
21. Preexisting hypertension and gestational hypertension

*Note: Bladder and kidney infections are covered in Chapter 18, "Infections."

F. Lungs

22. Asthma

G. Hormonal Issues (Endocrine)

23. Hypothyroidism (underfunctioning thyroid gland)
24. Hyperthyroidism (overfunctioning thyroid gland)
25. Preexisting type 1 diabetes
26. Gestational diabetes

H. Systemic Autoimmune Diseases

27. Lupus (systemic lupus erythematosus)

I. Brain and Nervous System

28. Seizure disorder
29. Migraine headaches

J. Mental Health

30. Depression
31. Anxiety disorder
32. Bipolar disorder
33. Schizophrenia

Obstetrical Complications (Mom)

K. Uterus

34. Cervical insufficiency
35. Uterine didelphys or bicornuate uterus (abnormal uterus)
36. Preterm labor

L. Placenta

37. Placenta previa (problem with placental position)
38. Vasa previa (problem with the umbilical cord position)
39. Placenta accreta, increta, percreta (problems with placenta attachment)
40. Placental abruption (placenta separates too early)

M. Amniotic Fluid

41. Polyhydramnios (too much amniotic fluid)
42. Oligohydramnios (too little amniotic fluid)

Obstetrical Complications (Fetus)

N. Position

43. Breech
44. Transverse Lie

O. Size

45. Macrosomia (too big)
46. Fetal growth restriction (too little)

P. Other

47. Genetic/chromosomal defects
48. Post-term pregnancy (past your due date)

INSIDER SECRET:

Rule of Threes

There's a "Rule of Threes" in pregnancy when it comes to many preexisting health conditions. That means one-third of people's symptoms get better, one-third of people's symptoms get worse, and one-third stay the same during pregnancy.

Medical Complications of Pregnancy

A. The Gut (Stomach, Intestines, Liver, Gallbladder, and Pancreas)

1. Hyperemesis Gravidarum

What is it? Supersized morning sickness. Constant nausea and vomiting causes dehydration and weight loss. It occurs in up to 2 percent of all pregnancies.

Usual time of onset: First trimester.

Symptoms: Severe vomiting, weight loss of more than 5 percent of your pre-pregnancy weight, scant/dark urine, headaches, confusion, fainting, occasionally jaundice.

Cause: Unknown. It's thought to be due to elevated hormone levels (especially ***beta-hCG***) during pregnancy.

Treatment:

- Hospitalization.
- Fluid and electrolyte replacement through a vein (IV).
- Anti-nausea medication.
- Vitamin B supplements.
- Once the vomiting is under control and you are rehydrated, start with small, frequent bland meals and take oral anti-nausea medication.
- If you cannot tolerate food over a long period of time, you may need to get your nutrition through an IV.
- Explore complementary therapies: acupuncture, acupressure, and hypnosis.

Issues for Mom: If not treated, hyperemesis can have seriously bad results—malnutrition, jaundice, kidney failure, blood clotting disorders, tears in the esophagus.

Issues for Baby: None immediately. A fetus who endures prolonged stress (which occasionally happens with hyperemesis) could be at risk for medical issues later in life, such as high blood pressure, heart disease, and diabetes.[1]

Helpful Hint

Your doctor will make sure it's not something else causing all your vomiting before chalking it up to hyperemesis. Thyroid disease, gallbladder disease, hepatitis, or even the stomach flu can make you puke excessively.

2. Cholestasis of Pregnancy

What is it? The normal flow of bile in the gallbladder and liver is decreased or stops altogether. Eventually, the excess bile can enter the bloodstream (which makes your skin yellow, or jaundiced, and itchy).

Usual time of onset: Almost always third trimester but occasionally earlier.

Symptoms: Intense itching, particularly on the palms and soles at night, dark-colored urine, light-colored bowel movements, yellowing of the eyes or skin, abdominal pain. These symptoms make it easy to diagnose. But often intense itching is the only symptom.

Cause: Elevated hormone levels in pregnancy cause a dilation and slowing of the bile ducts, slowing the passage of bile through the liver and gallbladder.

Treatment:

- Anti-itch creams and lotions (calamine, aloe, steroid cream) to relieve itching.
- Soaking in cold water or an oatmeal bath to relieve itching.
- Prescription medication (such as ursodeoxycholic acid).

- Immediate delivery may be needed if cholestasis is severe. Even with mild cholestasis, you may still likely deliver early to help prevent possible fetal complications.
- Your doctor will check your liver and bile acid levels with regular blood tests and perform non-stress tests to assess your baby's well-being. Your job is to do daily fetal kick counts and report any abnormality to your OB provider.

Issues for Mom: Using creams and oatmeal baths may do nothing to help relieve the misery. And if cholestasis goes on for a while, you will not absorb fat-soluble vitamins (A, D, E, and K) very well.

Issues for Baby: This complication is more dangerous for the fetus than for the mom. There is a risk of preterm birth (since early delivery is often recommended), passing meconium early (in the womb), and fetal death.

Reality Check

If you have cholestasis with this pregnancy, you have a 70 percent chance of having it again with a future pregnancy. Ugh.

3. Acute Fatty Liver

What is it? A rare, life-threatening condition where the liver is unable to break down fatty acids and they begin to accumulate in a pregnant woman's liver, preventing it from working as it normally does.

Usual time of onset: Third trimester, but occasionally in the second trimester or immediately postpartum.

Symptoms: Nausea, vomiting, lack of appetite, upper abdominal pain (particularly on the right side), fever, and ***jaundice*** (yellowing of the skin and eyes).

Cause: The theory is an enzyme deficiency leads to abnormal metabolism of fatty acids during pregnancy.

Treatment:

- Admission to hospital with an OB, a high-risk obstetrical specialist, liver doctor, and liver transplant surgeon all taking care of you in an intensive care unit (ICU).
- Sugar and fluid replacement through a vein (IV).
- Blood transfusion and transfusion of blood clotting factors if needed.
- Liver transplant (rare).
- Immediate delivery after you are medically stable (usually vaginal but occasionally ***C-section*** is necessary).

Issues for Mom: Liver dysfunction/hepatitis, inability to clot blood, pancreatitis, brain swelling and coma, liver rupture.

Issues for Baby: Prematurity.

4. HELLP Syndrome

What is it? A severe form of preeclampsia (see Complication #20 and "Help, I have HELLP!" on page 482.). HELLP stands for H hemolysis, EL elevated liver enzymes, and LP low platelets. Very rarely, it develops without any high blood pressure or other symptoms of preeclampsia.

Usual time of onset: Third trimester.

Symptoms: See Complication #20 later in this chapter. Bleeding from gums, nose, urethra, rectum. Pain in the upper right side of the belly, yellowing of the skin (***jaundice***).

Cause: Unknown. Theories include a disruption in the balance of hormones that control blood vessels, a decreased amount of blood flow to the uterus, injury to uterine blood vessels, and calcium deficiency.

Treatment:

- Immediate delivery.
- Steroids, platelet transfusion, and plasma exchange if necessary.

Issues for Mom: Very low platelet count, liver dysfunction, severe anemia. It's possible (but rare) to have ***disseminated intravascular coagulation (DIC)*** where your body is unable to clot blood.

Issues for Baby: Prematurity (if you have HELLP before thirty-seven weeks). And since HELLP is essentially a severe variation of preeclampsia (and therefore causes subsequent placenta problems), there is also a risk of growth restriction and fetal death.

5. Cholecystitis

What is it? An inflammation and/or infection of the gallbladder.

Usual time of onset: Late second or third trimesters.

Symptoms: Pain in the middle of or right upper side of the belly that sometimes spreads to the flank area or shoulder blade. Pain is often worse after eating. Sometimes there is also nausea, vomiting, fever, and yellowing of the skin and eyes (***jaundice***).

Cause: Most often, it's because a gallstone forms in the gallbladder. This blocks the passageway that bile uses to travel from the gallbladder to the small intestine. The bile thickens and then becomes infected with bacteria. People with sickle cell disease or similar conditions are at increased risk for ***cholecystitis***.

Treatment:

- Temporary fasting with fluid and electrolyte replacement through an IV.
- Pain medication.
- Antibiotics.
- A tube is temporarily placed from nose to stomach (nasogastric tube) to help drain the stomach, if necessary.
- Surgery to remove gallbladder, if all else fails. The optimal timing of surgery is the second trimester. Minimally invasive (laparoscopic) surgery is safe during pregnancy.

Issues for Mom: Anyone, including pregnant women, can have complications from gallbladder disease, including infection, perforation, or slowing of the intestine. But for pregnant women, these complications can lead to preterm labor. Pregnant moms with cholecystitis are also at risk for pneumonia, ***adult respiratory distress syndrome (ARDS)***, and inflammation of the pancreas (pancreatitis).

Issues for Baby: Preterm labor and delivery.

Reality Check

Any abdominal problem (from appendicitis to gallstones) can lead to preterm labor.

6. Pancreatitis

What is it? An inflammation and/or infection of the pancreas.

Usual time of onset: Late second or third trimesters.

Symptoms: Sudden and severe abdominal pain in the middle to upper abdomen that often spreads to the back, nausea, vomiting, fever, and jaundice.

Cause: Many causes, but in pregnancy it is almost always due to a gallstone blocking the connection from the gallbladder and pancreas to the small intestine. Pancreatic enzymes back up and cause inflammation of the pancreas.

Treatment:

- Temporary fasting with fluid and electrolyte replacement through a vein (IV).
- Treat any electrolyte or blood sugar abnormalities.
- Pain medication.
- Fetal monitoring, if needed.
- A tube is temporarily placed through the nose to the stomach to help drain the stomach, if necessary.
- Total nutrition through IV, if needed.
- Surgery to remove the gallbladder (if all else fails and if the gallbladder is the cause).

Issues for Mom: Pain control—it really hurts. Acute symptoms last for five to eight days. Ninety-five percent of women recover.

Issues for Baby: Preterm labor and delivery. Fetal death is rare (less than 10 percent), but the chance goes up with the severity of the illness.

7. Appendicitis (Assuming You Still Have Your Appendix)

What is it? An inflammation of the appendix.

Usual time of onset: Second trimester.

Symptoms: Pain first, then nausea, vomiting, fever, and sometimes decreased appetite. Although appendicitis pain classically starts around the belly button then moves to the lower right side of the belly, it may not happen that way during pregnancy. The position of your appendix moves as your pregnancy progresses.

- First trimester: Pain is in the lower right side (see "right lower quadrant" in the illustration below).
- Second trimester: Pain is to the right at the level of the belly button.
- Third trimester: Pain is in the middle or on the upper right side (see "right upper quadrant" in the illustration below).

Your Abdomen

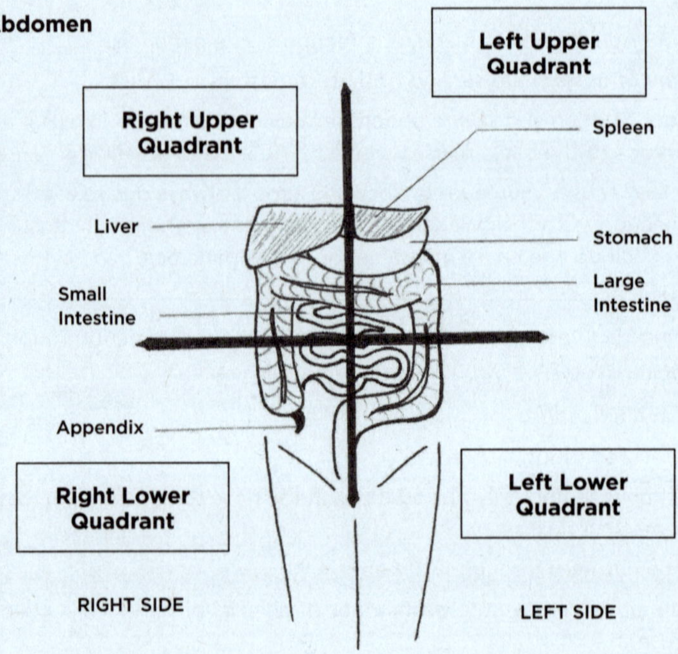

Cause: The appendix gets blocked (often by poop), then swells up and can get infected.

Treatment: Immediate surgery.

Issues for Mom: Pregnancy prolongs recovery from surgery and increases the risk of complications. The worst outcome (which is rare) is widespread infection into the belly and bloodstream.

Issues for Baby: Preterm labor and delivery from the disease or the surgery. Timely diagnosis and treatment significantly reduces risk of death for mother or baby.

B. Female Anatomy (Uterus, Ovaries, and Fallopian Tubes)

8. Ruptured Ovarian Cyst

What is it? It's very common to have a cyst on your ovary during pregnancy. That cyst can go on to rupture and leak fluid into your abdominal cavity—which causes inflammation and pain. Call your doctor.

Usual time of onset: Often late first and second trimesters.

Symptoms: Chronic, mild pain in lower belly that suddenly changes in intensity after a minor fall or intercourse. Or it can just happen out of the blue.

Cause: Most of the time it is the ***corpus luteum***—a cyst on the ovary that initially produces the progesterone needed to sustain a pregnancy until the placenta takes over this job at about ten weeks. Most corpus luteum cysts start leaking and slowly go away on their own. Occasionally, the hormones produced during pregnancy can stimulate these cysts to get very large.

Treatment:

- Take it easy at home.
- Drink lots of fluids.
- Pain medication.
- As long as you do not have a lot of bleeding and the cyst goes away, you can recuperate at home. It's rare to have complications that require hospitalization or surgery.

Issues for Mom: Pain management, bleeding/hemorrhage into the abdomen if the ruptured cyst bleeds. Surgery, if necessary.

Issues for Baby: Possible preterm labor and delivery.

9. Ovarian/Adnexal Torsion

What is it? The ovary and tube twist upon each other, compromising the blood supply to both. The tissues will die if this condition is not resolved.

Usual time of onset: Twelve to twenty weeks.

Symptoms: Acute, severe, one-sided lower pelvic pain, nausea, vomiting, and fever. You may have had similar episodes in the past.

Cause: Often, a mass in the pelvis (such as a dermoid tumor or other cyst of the ovary). The mass makes the tube and ovary heavier than usual, and they are more likely to twist upon themselves.

Treatment:

- Surgery.
- Progesterone supplements if a corpus luteum cyst needs removal before ten weeks gestation.
- If it is caught early enough, your OB will untwist the tube and ovary, and blood flow resumes without tissue damage. And they will remove the mass. If your OB sees that there is tissue death, they will remove the tube/ovary and mass.

Issues for Mom: Pain control, recovery from surgery.

Issues for Baby: Possible preterm labor and delivery.

10. Degenerating Uterine Fibroid

What is it? Fibroids are benign tumors in the muscle of the uterus. If the blood supply to the fibroid is altered, the fibroid tissue dies. It occurs in 5 to 10 percent of pregnant women with fibroids.

Usual time of onset: Twelve to twenty weeks.

Symptoms: You may or may not have had bouts of pain earlier in the pregnancy. But now you have severe abdominal pain in one area (where the fibroid is located on the uterus). Most women can pinpoint the pain with one or two fingers. You may experience nausea, vomiting, and tenderness over the area.

Cause: Rapid growth of uterus during pregnancy decreases the blood flow to the fibroids, which leads to tissue death. When the fibroid breaks down, prostaglandins are produced, which can cause pain and uterine contractions. This condition resolves on its own.

Treatment:

- Supportive care with pain medication (narcotics and anti-inflammatory medication such as indomethacin or ibuprofen if used before thirty-two weeks).
- Prevention of preterm labor.
- Surgery is not an option for this condition during pregnancy.

Issues for Mom: Pain control.

Issues for Baby: Potential adverse effects from indomethacin. Occasionally preterm labor and delivery. See Appendix A, "Medications," for details on this medication.

C. Urinary Tract (Bladder and Kidneys)

11. Kidney Stones

What is it? A kidney stone is made of minerals that have crystallized in the urine. This small mass (which looks like a rock and can sometimes be sharp as hell) gets stuck as it makes its way down from the kidney into the bladder. Kidney stones occur in one of every 1,500 pregnancies.

Usual time of onset: Second and third trimesters.

Symptoms: Flank pain (usually one-sided), pain spreads to the groin or labia, painful urination, and blood in the urine. Less common: nausea, vomiting, lower abdominal pain, fever, and chills.

Cause: Family history or personal history of kidney stones, recurrent ***bladder infections***, increased age, low water intake, hot/dry climate, diet high in calcium/sodium, obesity, and pregnancy. Pregnancy puts women at risk because the tubes (ureters) from the kidney to the bladder function poorly during pregnancy. You also excrete more calcium in your urine when you're pregnant, which is a setup for stones.

Treatment:

- Hospitalization/bed rest.
- Fluid replacement through IV.
- Pain medication.
- Anti-nausea medication.
- Antibiotics, if necessary.
- 60–80 percent of stones pass by themselves; 20 percent need surgical intervention.
- Afterward, drink plenty of water and keep your calcium intake at a normal level (1,200 mg/day). Too much or too little calcium puts you at risk for stones. And it's possible to get these more than once!

Issues for Mom: Severe pain, preterm labor, possible need for surgery, bloodstream infection, pneumonia, ***adult respiratory distress syndrome (ARDS).***

Issues for Baby: Possible preterm labor and delivery.

Reality Check

Passing a kidney stone may be as painful as childbirth—at least that's what men think!

12. Acute Urinary Retention

What is it? You can't pee even though you want to.

Usual time of onset: First and early second trimesters.

Symptoms: Inability to urinate, lower abdominal pain, and occasionally fever.

Cause: Your enlarging uterus blocks the passage of urine from the bladder to the urethra (see graphic to the right). Good news—it's usually no longer a problem when the uterus grows and gets even bigger.

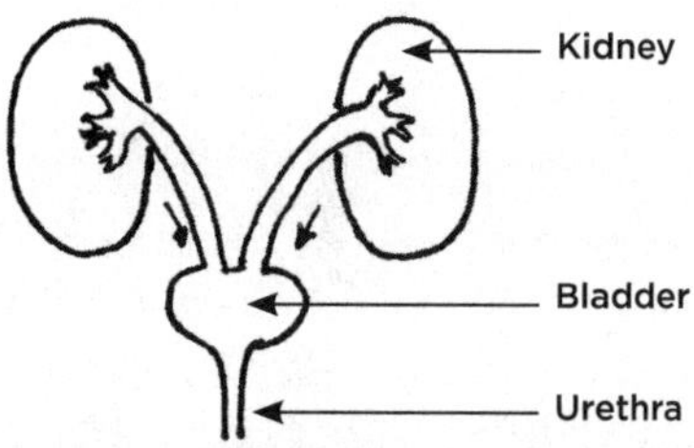

Normal urine flow

Treatment:

- A tube (catheter) is placed into your urethra to release the urine.
- A tube (Foley catheter) remains in place until the issue resolves.
- Move the position of the uterus by manually repositioning the uterus or inserting a device called a pessary.

Issues for Mom: Failure to get emergency care can lead to bladder tears and rupture and occasionally a buildup of waste products in the bloodstream.

Issues for Baby: None.

D. Blood

13. Anemia

What is it? Less than the normal number of healthy red blood cells or hemoglobin that carries oxygen to the body.

Usual time of onset: Second or third trimester.

Symptoms: Fatigue (beyond your usual pregnancy fatigue), a whiter, paler color to the skin, and a whiter color on the insides of the eyes (instead of the usual pinkish or reddish color)

Cause: Numerous! The top reason is your body needs more iron during pregnancy. And your blood volume doubles during pregnancy but the number of red blood cells does not. The increased liquid (blood volume) dilutes the red blood cells (hence, it's called a dilutional anemia). This double whammy is why you need an iron-rich diet and a prenatal vitamin with iron. Other causes: chronic bleeding (such as from hemorrhoids or vaginal bleeding from a chronic placental abruption), inherited anemia (such as thalassemia or sickle cell anemia).

Treatment:

- If you have an inherited anemia, see Complications #15 and #16.
- Iron-rich foods (raisins, dried apricots, clams, shrimp, chicken, liver, red meat, breakfast cereals, dark green vegetables like spinach and kale, as well as lentils).
- An iron supplement, which unfortunately can cause constipation (try Slow Fe if you are already having problems with that).
- Iron replacement through an IV for severe cases.
- Blood transfusion for really severe cases.

Issues for Mom: Common problem: fatigue. Uncommon problem (with persistent, severe anemia): heart failure. Your OB provider checks your hemoglobin level at your first prenatal visit and usually again at twenty-four to twenty-eight weeks. Anemia at the end of pregnancy is risky because you are about to lose 300 to 1,000 ml of blood during your delivery and potentially become severely anemic afterward. The goal is to prevent the need for a blood transfusion.

Issues for Baby: A few studies show a link between maternal iron deficiency anemia, preterm birth, and subsequent low birth weight.[2] Severe anemia (defined as a hemoglobin level less than six) reduces oxygen delivery to the fetus, and that can be serious, as you might imagine.

14. Rh Isoimmunization (Incompatibility) or Rh Disease

What is it? An Rh-negative mom is carrying an Rh-positive fetus. See the New Parent-to-Be 411 box on hemoglobinopathies on page 478.

Usual time of onset: Second trimester, in pregnancies other than a woman's first.

Symptoms: None.

Cause: An Rh-negative mom and an Rh-positive dad conceive a baby. There is at least a 50/50 chance of the fetus being Rh-positive. If there is any crossover of blood from the fetus to the mom (which can occur with minor trauma, vaginal bleeding, ***CVS***, ***amniocentesis***, external ***cephalic*** version procedures, placental abruption, miscarriage, abortion procedures, or at the time of delivery), mom's immune system makes antibodies against the foreign Rh-positive proteins. In any subsequent pregnancies, mom's antibodies can cross the placenta and attack and destroy fetal red blood cells (if the fetus is Rh-positive), causing severe anemia in the baby or even fetal death. This usually occurs in pregnancies other than the first.

Treatment:

- A Rh immune-globulin (RhoGAM) shot is given at twenty-eight weeks of pregnancy.
- A second RhoGAM shot is given within seventy-two hours after delivery if the baby is Rh-positive.
- You also need a RhoGAM shot if you have a miscarriage, abortion, ***ectopic pregnancy***, CVS, amniocentesis, percutaneous umbilical cord blood sampling (PUBS), external cephalic version or any bleeding during your pregnancy. RhoGAM prevents mom's body from producing any potentially harmful antibodies and complicating any future pregnancies. RhoGAM is mercury-free and there is no risk of contracting hepatitis or HIV.

Issues for Mom: No problems.

Issues for Baby: If you have already developed Rh antibodies, your OB provider will closely monitor the fetus for anemia (hemolytic anemia). This anemia is rare (less than 1 percent of the time), but a severely anemic baby needs a special blood transfusion (exchange transfusion) that replaces the damaged red blood cells with healthy ones. A baby with severe Rh disease often needs to be delivered prematurely. Undiagnosed and untreated Rh disease can lead to severe anemia, jaundice, brain damage, heart failure, and death in extreme cases.

Reality Check

The only way to avoid a RhoGAM shot is to test the baby's father. If you can prove he is Rh-negative (and that he's the father), your baby is Rh-negative and RhoGAM isn't needed. You'll need his blood, though, and that requires a needle. This, of course, could lead to an ugly picture of you, your OB provider, and the tow truck guy outside having to tie your beloved down for the blood test! So you can see why it's easier just to get the RhoGAM for you!

15. Sickle Cell Anemia

What is it? An inherited blood disorder that affects red blood cells. The red blood cells carry an abnormal type of hemoglobin (the part of the red blood cell that helps carry oxygen). The abnormal hemoglobin causes the red cells to have a crescent shape as opposed to a spherical shape, and they don't live as long as normal red blood cells. These "crescents" can get stuck in the smaller blood vessels in the body, causing less blood and therefore less oxygen to reach the tissues and organs. Tissue damage eventually occurs.

Usual time of onset: You are born with it. Sickle cell crises, however, are more common during pregnancy, specifically in the second and third trimesters.

Cause: You are born with it. Sickle cell disease is an inherited disease that's more common in people of African, South and Central American, Saudi Arabian, Indian, and Mediterranean (Turkey, Greece, Italy) descent. Sickle cell disease occurs when someone inherits two abnormal hemoglobin genes, one from their mom and one from their dad. Sickle cell trait occurs when someone inherits a normal gene from one parent and an abnormal gene from another parent. People with sickle cell trait are generally healthy, although they can have crises in these situations: dehydration, high altitude, activities that have increased pressure (scuba diving) or lower oxygen (excessive exercising or mountain climbing). Sickle cell crises are more common during pregnancy, specifically in the second and third trimesters.

Treatment:

- Avoid potential triggers (see above).
- Get a flu shot.
- Take 4 milligrams of folic acid a day.
- For a sickle cell crisis, hospitalization, fluid replacement through IV, and pain medication.
- Blood transfusion for severe anemia.

Issues for Mom: Pain (when the abnormal red blood cells get stuck in the blood vessels causing lack of oxygen to the tissues), increased risk for infection (because the disease causes you to have a non-functioning spleen), severe anemia that may require a blood transfusion, increased risk of gallstones and gallbladder inflammation (see the information on ***cholecystitis*** on page 468).

Issues for Baby: If mom has sickle cell disease, it is important to know if the father of the baby has sickle cell disease or trait. See the New Parent-to-Be 411 box on hemoglobinopathies on page 478. Preterm labor and delivery are also a risk.

BOTTOM LINE: Women with sickle cell disease have a higher risk of preterm labor and delivery. And sickle cell crises are more common during pregnancy. Good prenatal care is essential.

Reality Check

All states screen newborns for sickle cell disease with a simple blood test done after twenty-four hours of life. Early detection allows for early treatment. See Chapter 11, "Parenthood Prep," for details on newborn metabolic screening.

16. Beta-thalassemia (Minor)

What is it? An inherited form of anemia more common in people of Middle Eastern or Mediterranean descent.

Usual time of onset: Congenital (you are born with it).

Symptoms: Many patients don't have any symptoms. Some have symptoms of anemia (fatigue, lack of energy).

Cause: Abnormal gene causes abnormal hemoglobin, so red blood cells are less able to carry oxygen to other organs/tissues.

Treatment:

- None, unless you also have iron-deficiency anemia.
- Genetic counseling for parents, particularly if both parents are carriers.
- Take 4 milligrams of folic acid a day.

Issues for Mom: None.

Issues for Baby: It's only an issue if the father of the baby also has a hemoglobin abnormality. For details, see box on hemoglobinopathies on page 478.

17. Thrombocytopenia

What is it? A low platelet count. Platelets are cells that clot blood. Normal ranges are between 150,000 and 400,000 per microliter. It occurs in 7 percent of all pregnancies and can be part of HELLP syndrome.

Usual time of onset: Third trimester.

Symptoms: Bleeding from the nose and gums, easy bruising, and petechiae (pronounced pe-teek-E-eye), which are flat, purplish, pinpoint dots that almost look like freckles. Some people have no symptoms. Good news: It's very rare to just bleed excessively.

Cause: Several. The most common reason is benign gestational thrombocytopenia. Others are lupus, idiopathic thrombocytopenia (ITP), thrombotic thrombocytopenic purpura (TTP), ***HELLP syndrome*** (Complication #4 in this chapter), medications (such as heparin), certain viral infections, and having an enlarged spleen.

Treatment: Treatment depends on the cause.

- For gestational thrombocytopenia: observe and check platelet counts periodically.
- For HELLP syndrome: delivery, magnesium sulfate (see Appendix A, "Medications," for details on this medication).
- For ITP: possible platelet transfusion, steroids, IVIG (see Appendix A, "Medications," for details on this medication).
- Rarely, surgical removal of the spleen when there is no improvement in first/second trimesters. This is only necessary in extremely rare cases of ITP, but never for HELLP Syndrome.

Issues for Mom: Platelet transfusions, like blood transfusions, carry a small risk of acquiring HIV and hepatitis B and C. HELLP syndrome is often associated with ***pre-eclampsia*** (Complication #20).

Issues for Baby: It depends on the cause. For gestational thrombocytopenia, there are no major concerns for baby. In maternal ITP, there is a small risk (12 percent) that the newborn will also have a low platelet count and could be at risk (1 percent) of having bleeding inside the brain. In HELLP syndrome, docs worry about prematurity, growth restriction, and rarely, fetal death (from placental abruption, lack of oxygen, or extreme prematurity).

REALITY CHECK: Hemoglobinopathies

The formal name for a bunch of different diseases that affect hemoglobin (the oxygen-carrying component of our red blood cells) is hemoglobinopathies. They are genetic defects, passed on through your family. You can blame your parents, but it's just your fate—not your fault.

While there are quite a few hemoglobinopathies, the most common are sickle cell anemia, alpha-thalassemia, and beta-thalassemia. State-mandated newborn screening tests can detect these diseases in babies. Since they all cause anemia, they also can be picked up on a routine blood test called a complete blood count (CBC). If the CBC is abnormal, additional testing can determine exactly which hemoglobinopathy you have.

Why is this important? If you have a hemoglobinopathy, your partner should be tested to see if they have one, too, or if they are a carrier. This helps identify couples at risk for having a baby with hemoglobinopathy. It's just a blood test (***hemoglobin electrophoresis***). Considering all the testing you've been through, it's the least your partner can do! Here are a few scenarios:

- If both parents have sickle cell disease, the baby will have sickle cell disease.
- If the mother has sickle cell disease and the father has sickle cell ***trait***, the baby has a 50 percent chance of having the disease.
- If both parents have only the sickle cell ***trait***, there is a 25 percent chance that baby will have the disease.
- If mom has beta-thalassemia, the baby only has a potential issue if the dad is also a beta-thalassemia carrier or a carrier of another hemoglobin abnormality (such as sickle cell trait)—then there is a 25 percent chance of baby being severely affected.

A CVS or amniocentesis can determine if the baby will be affected, be a carrier, or remain unaffected.

In all hemoglobinopathies, your body breaks down more of your red blood cells than normal. You'll need more folic acid to help make new red blood cells. You should have 4 milligrams a day of folic acid, instead of the 400 micrograms (mcg) a day recommended for other pregnant women.

Reality Check

If your platelet count is too low, you may not be able to have an epidural or spinal **anesthesia**. Why? Because you risk suffering from excessive bleeding in the area where the needle is placed.

18. Deep Venous Thrombosis (DVT)/Pulmonary Embolus (PE)

What is it? A blood clot in the deep veins of the legs or pelvis.

Usual time of onset: Second or third trimester and immediately postpartum.

Symptoms: ***DVT***: Swelling in one leg that is more pronounced than the other one, pain in the same leg, typically in the calf, difficulty walking, and sometimes redness at the site of the clot. ***PE***: Shortness of breath or difficulty breathing, chest pain, severe anxiety, lightheadedness, dizziness, and loss of consciousness.

Cause: You are at risk for blood clots during pregnancy because blood pools in your veins due to your increased weight and big uterus. The uterus is a roadblock that puts pressure on the blood vessels and restricts blood flow from the legs and pelvis back to the heart. Plus, all that progesterone you're making causes the walls of the veins to relax and encourages clotting.

Treatment:

- Blood thinners: heparin, Lovenox (see Appendix A, "Medications," for more details).
- Sometimes a small piece of mesh must be placed in the major vein (vena cava) to catch any potential clots that break free before they make their way to the lungs.

Issues for Mom: DVTs are a concern because they have the potential for a piece of the clot to break off and enter the lung blood vessels, causing a ***pulmonary embolism (PE)***. This is a life-threatening condition, as oxygen flow to other parts of the body can be severely compromised.

Issues for Baby: A DVT itself poses no major risk for the baby. An untreated PE, on the other hand, can lead to very low blood pressure and impaired oxygen delivery, which can compromise the fetus. And since a PE is life-threatening for mom, it is life-threatening for baby, too.

19. Thrombophilia/Clotting Disorder

What is it? Clotting disorders, including Factor V Leiden mutation, prothrombin gene mutation, Protein C or S deficiency, antithrombin III deficiency, and antiphospholipid syndrome, are genetic (hereditary) or acquired defects that affect the blood clotting system, making it easier to form clots in the blood vessels. Five to seven percent of the population have the more common disorders (Factor V Leiden and prothrombin gene mutation). The others are much rarer. Most people who are born with these mutations will never have a blood clot, though their lifetime risk is higher than for other people. So you may not know you even have this disorder, despite being born with it. Among these, only antiphospholipid and other autoimmune antibodies that predispose to blood clots are acquired (meaning you are not born with them).

Usual time of onset: High-estrogen states (like pregnancy or taking birth control pills), extended periods of bed rest or immobilization, and major surgery increase the risk in people already predisposed to clotting.

Symptoms: Usually there are no symptoms until someone develops a blood clot (in the leg or lungs). Only the autoimmune/antiphospholipid antibodies are associated with recurrent first trimester pregnancy losses, and women who have this history can be tested.

Cause: You inherit abnormal genes from one or both parents (depending on the particular disorder you have). Autoimmune antibodies, however, are acquired later in life, and can be recurrent in some families (but they do not occur in a predictable pattern).

Treatment: It depends on the particular disorder and whether you have had affected pregnancies or blood clots in the past.

- Low-dose aspirin and/or heparin or enoxaparin (Lovenox, see Appendix A, "Medications," for more information).
- Stay well hydrated.

Issues for Mom: For people with antiphospholipid antibodies, there are risks for the mother (blood clots) and the pregnancy (miscarriage, growth restriction, preeclampsia). For the other clotting disorders, the risk is only for the mother.

Issues for Baby: See issues for mom.

BOTTOM LINE: Not everyone with a clotting disorder needs to be treated during pregnancy. A high-risk pregnancy doctor (maternal-fetal medicine specialist), along with your doctor, will discuss management options with you.

E. Heart and Blood Vessels

20. Preeclampsia

What is it? Preeclampsia only happens during pregnancy (lucky you!). There are two things required for the diagnosis: 1) You have high blood pressure (greater than or equal to 140 mm Hg systolic OR greater than or equal to 90 mm Hg diastolic on two or more occasions at least four hours apart) beginning after twenty weeks of pregnancy (when you previously had normal blood pressure); and 2) You have protein in your urine. Preeclampsia can be mild or severe. It occurs in 5 to 8 percent of all pregnancies.

Usual time of onset: Almost always in the third trimester, rarely in the second trimester (usually only in women with preexisting medical conditions like lupus or kidney disease), or after recently delivering (postpartum period).

Symptoms: Feeling blah/fatigued, severe headaches that start showing up out of the blue and don't go away with traditional measures, blurred vision, nausea/vomiting, sharp pain under your ribs, on the right side or upper belly area that spreads around the sides or goes deep to the back, and sometimes swelling in the legs/feet/hands/face.

COMPLICATIONS

Cause: We don't know. The result, however, is poor placental function. It is more common in first-time pregnancies, women under eighteen, over forty, having multiples, and those with a pre-pregnancy BMI over 30.

Treatment: Very mild preeclampsia, very early in pregnancy may be observed. Otherwise, delivery is the optimal treatment. If you have severe preeclampsia, you need to deliver regardless of the gestational age of the baby because of the health risk to you and baby.

Observation:

- Non-stress tests (NSTs) twice weekly.
- Periodic ultrasounds.
- Bed rest.
- Check daily fetal kick counts.
- Lab work to look for HELLP Syndrome (see the box on HELLP on page 482).
- Regular blood pressure checks and OB visits.
- Possible blood pressure lowering medication.

Delivery:

- Deliver at hospital that handles high-risk deliveries and newborns, with obstetrician, maternal-fetal medicine specialist, and neonatologist.
- IV of magnesium sulfate to prevent seizures (***eclampsia***) through labor, delivery, and even for a bit afterward (postpartum period).
- Possible blood pressure lowering medication.

Issues for Mom: Without treatment, preeclampsia can progress to full-blown eclampsia (seizures). In rare cases of severe preeclampsia, HELLP syndrome can occur as well as fluid in the lungs (pulmonary edema), a serious problem with blood clotting called disseminated intravascular coagulation (***DIC***), eye problems (retinal detachment), liver rupture, stroke, and kidney damage.

Issues for Baby: Poor placental function can lead to growth restriction, too little amniotic fluid (***oligohydramnios***), ***placental abruption,*** and prematurity.[3]

21. High Blood Pressure (Gestational Hypertension)

What is it? Your blood pressure is higher than it should be, typically higher than 140/90. It occurs in 5 percent of all pregnant women.

Usual time of onset: Either this is a preexisting condition before pregnancy, or it is diagnosed after twenty weeks gestation.

WARNING:

Help, I have HELLP!

H stands for **H**emolysis

EL stands for **E**levated **L**iver enzymes

LP stands for **L**ow **P**latelet count

HELLP syndrome is a serious pregnancy complication that usually occurs with preeclampsia, but occasionally happens on its own. About 0.4 percent of all pregnancies and up to 15 percent of all pregnant women with preeclampsia suffer from HELLP. Why does it happen? We don't know. It usually shows up in the third trimester, but 8 percent of cases occur after delivery.

This is the basic chain of events:

1. Your red blood cells get destroyed, leading to anemia.
2. Your liver malfunctions, leading to poor blood clotting and a buildup of toxins normally processed by the liver.
3. Your platelet count drops, making it harder for your blood to clot.

If you also have preeclampsia, you will have the symptoms discussed in Complication #20 (see earlier). Without preeclampsia, the symptoms can be pretty vague. You may feel crummy, with nausea, vomiting, headaches, all-over itching, and pain or tenderness in the upper right side of the abdomen. Rarely, women who have HELLP syndrome after delivery are only diagnosed when they go into shock. This is really serious. All obstetricians respect the fact that women with preeclampsia can get very sick, very quickly. Don't ignore symptoms, and don't be afraid to ask questions.

About one in four women with HELLP has complications if they are not diagnosed and treated quickly. And even with treatment, there is still a small chance of death (one in 100). Complications include placental abruption, severe blood clotting problems (such as ***DIC***), acute kidney failure, bruising on the liver, and eye problems (retinal detachment).

Women at the greatest risk of having HELLP syndrome have baseline high blood pressure, high blood pressure with pregnancy (***gestational hypertension***), preeclampsia or HELLP in a previous pregnancy, are carrying multiples, have other medical conditions, or are of ***advanced maternal age*** (over thirty-five).

If you have HELLP Syndrome, your baby needs to be delivered immediately. You may also need blood, platelet, and clotting factor transfusions, as well as steroids, if the condition becomes severe.

Symptoms: Usually no symptoms. A person with long-standing, untreated high blood pressure might have headaches, visual changes, or dizziness.

Cause: Several. It can be genetically inherited, or due to other diseases (such as lupus, diabetes, or obesity).

Treatment:

- Close observation by an OB who is comfortable with high-risk pregnancies, along with a maternal-fetal medicine specialist.
- Frequent lab tests (for kidney/liver function, ***HELLP syndrome***).
- Urine samples (looking for protein in the urine, found in ***preeclampsia***).
- Increased fetal surveillance (growth scans every three to four weeks), amniotic fluid level checks weekly or every other week, daily fetal kick counts, sometimes non-stress tests (NSTs) or biophysical profiles beginning at twenty-eight to thirty-two weeks.
- Blood pressure medication, if needed (see Appendix A, "Medications").

Issues for Mom: There is an increased risk of ***preeclampsia, placental abruption***, preterm delivery, delivery by C-section, and stillbirth. Rarely, pregnancy can worsen high blood pressure and lead to having a stroke, kidney or heart failure.

Issues for Baby: ***Fetal growth restriction***, prematurity, increased risk of death as a newborn.[4]

F. Lungs

22. Asthma

What is it? Asthma is fairly common; it's the most common chronic medical condition seen during pregnancy. The tiny airways of the lungs swell up, making it harder to breathe and get enough oxygen into the lungs. People have certain triggers (exercise, allergies to indoor or outdoor pollens, respiratory infections, emotions).

Usual time of onset: Before pregnancy. It can worsen (30 percent), stay the same (47 percent), or improve (23 percent) during pregnancy.

Symptoms: Shortness of breath, difficulty taking a deep breath, chest tightness/pain/pressure, or wheezing and coughing, particularly at night.

Cause: Unknown. Asthma is to the lungs as hay fever is to the nose. It is an allergic response in the lungs. It is unclear why certain triggers cause an attack.

Treatment:

- Avoid potential triggers (if you know what they are).
- Keep your home clean.
- Stay inside on ozone action days (high pollution days).
- Carry an inhaler with you.
- Treat any heartburn or acid reflux since it can trigger asthma flare-ups.

- Review your asthma medications with your doctor (See Appendix A, "Medications," for details about albuterol and steroids).
- Increase fetal surveillance (ultrasounds, non-stress tests).

Issues for Mom: Discomfort, possible worsening of symptoms during pregnancy, possible hospitalization, risk of serious labored breathing. Severe or poorly controlled asthma can lead to ***preeclampsia*** and significant bleeding after delivery.

Issues for Baby: Moms with mild to moderate asthma have healthy babies. Moms with severe, uncontrolled asthma chronically deprive their fetuses of oxygen. That increases the baby's risk of preterm birth and low birth weight.[5]

Reality Check

It's safer for you to take your asthma medication than to have asthma symptoms and flare-ups. Not getting enough oxygen is bad for both you and your baby. Get your asthma under control.

G. Hormonal Issues (Endocrine)

23. Hypothyroidism

What is it? Underactive thyroid makes too little thyroid hormone. FYI: Your thyroid gland sits at the base of your neck and controls many of your body's functions, including metabolism.

Usual time of onset: Before or during pregnancy.

Symptoms: All body systems slow down. Severe fatigue, constipation, hair loss, very dry skin, muscle aches and cramps, cold intolerance, weight gain, intellectual slowness, insomnia (sounds like all pregnant women, right?).

Cause: Hashimoto's disease, subacute thyroiditis, a prior history of complete or partial removal of the thyroid for tumors or cancer, history of Graves' disease that has been treated.

Treatment:

- Thyroid replacement hormone (levothyroxine).
- Increase fetal surveillance (non-stress tests, ultrasounds).
- Consult maternal-fetal medicine specialist and endocrinologist.

Issues for Mom: Untreated hypothyroidism increases the risk of severe preeclampsia.

Issues for Baby: Low birth weight. Moms who are hypothyroid because of iodine deficiency risk having a baby with an intellectual disability. This is, luckily, a rare complication in the United States today.[6]

Reality Check

Women who have one autoimmune disease (such as lupus or diabetes) are at greater risk for developing autoimmune thyroid disease.

24. Hyperthyroidism

What is it? Overactive thyroid makes too much thyroid hormone.

Usual time of onset: Before or during pregnancy.

Symptoms: All body systems speed up. Nervousness, tremors, weight loss, excessive vomiting (***hyperemesis***), intolerance to heat, excessive sweating, rapid heartbeat, palpitations, weight loss, a bulge in the lower portion of your neck (enlarged thyroid gland), frequent loose stools, and insomnia.

Cause: 95 percent of cases are caused by Graves' disease, an autoimmune condition where your body makes antibodies against your own thyroid gland. Other causes: benign tumors of the thyroid, ***molar pregnancies***, ingestion of thyroid hormone (yes, some people take thyroid hormone when they don't need it for a medical reason), toxic multinodular goiter.

Treatment:

- Medications to decrease thyroid hormone production (propylthiouracil or PTU, methimazole).
- Medications to control tremors/palpitations (beta-blockers like propranolol).
- Increase fetal surveillance (non-stress tests, ultrasounds).
- Consult maternal-fetal medicine specialist and endocrinologist.

Issues for Mom: Inadequately treated thyroid disease can lead to preterm labor, increased risk of developing severe ***preeclampsia***, and increased risk of heart failure. Pregnant women with untreated hyperthyroidism may have a medical emergency when excessive amounts of thyroid hormone are released quickly, causing acute heart failure (thyroid storm). Before you go into heart failure reading this book, the risk is quite low—about 1 percent. Just take good care of yourself!

Issues for Baby: If mom is untreated or inadequately treated, there is a greater risk of preterm delivery, low birth weight, and possible stillbirth. There's also a 2 percent chance your newborn will have thyroid dysfunction if you have Graves' disease (because those thyroid antibodies can also affect the baby's thyroid gland). Your baby's pediatrician can check the baby for this by doing a blood test performed at birth and again at two weeks of age.[7]

25. Preexisting Type 1 Diabetes Mellitus (Pregestational Diabetes)

What is it? With pregestational diabetes (not to be confused with gestational diabetes, which starts during pregnancy; see the next complication), the pancreas stops making insulin in normal amounts. Insulin is needed to help glucose (sugar) move into the cells of the body. Lack of insulin makes glucose levels rise, causing complications. (FYI: Type 2 ***diabetes mellitus*** is yet another form of diabetes where someone may make enough insulin but the body becomes relatively resistant to its effects. Type 2 diabetes is due to lack of activity, elevated ***body mass index***, and poor dietary habits.)

Usual time of onset: Before pregnancy.

Symptoms: Excessive thirst, excessive urination, fatigue, dizziness spells, and sweating.

Cause: Diabetes mellitus can be inherited (genetic). It can also be caused by certain viral infections and exposures. They trigger an abnormal immune response, making antibodies that attack and destroy the cells in the pancreas that make insulin.

Treatment:

- Consult a diabetic registered dietitian/nurse, maternal-fetal medicine specialist, obstetrician who cares for high-risk pregnancies.
- Eat a diabetic diet.
- Check your sugars regularly.
- Keep your blood sugar under excellent control to prevent numerous complications.

Issues for Mom: Be diligent about controlling blood sugar or deal with these ugly possibilities: vision problems, kidney disease, high blood pressure, diabetic ketoacidosis, preterm labor, ***polyhydramnios***, ***preeclampsia***, and increased risk of C-section.

Issues for Baby: In poorly controlled mothers: increased risk of intrauterine growth restriction, preterm delivery, stillbirth, ***shoulder dystocia.*** Up to 12 percent of infants born to diabetic moms have a risk of birth defects. These include major heart defects and defects of the brain, spine, and skeleton (***spina bifida***, ***anencephaly***). There are also potential risks for a newborn after delivery: low blood sugar, seizures, respiratory distress syndrome, jaundice.[8]

BOTTOM LINE: Up to 10 percent of pregnant women with preexisting Type 1 diabetes end up in diabetic ketoacidosis (DKA), a life-threatening emergency. Please control your sugars!

---

26. Gestational Diabetes (GDM)

What is it? Problem controlling blood sugars during pregnancy.

Usual time of onset: Typically, late second trimester.

Symptoms: None.

Cause: A hormone made by the placenta (human placental lactogen, hPL) makes it harder for your body to use insulin. Sugar levels rise and your pancreas begins to secrete more insulin. But for some women, the demands on the pancreas are too much, and it can't keep up with the amount of insulin needed by your body. This causes *temporary* diabetes during pregnancy. About 4 percent of women get it, but it's more common in women over the age of thirty-five.

Treatment:

- Check blood sugar levels daily using a home glucose meter or continuous glucose monitor and maintain a diary of all your readings. Do your homework, because your diabetic counselor and OB provider will ask to see it. They need to be sure you are on track to having normal blood sugars.
- Consult a diabetic nurse, dietitian, or counselor to help plan meals/snacks and discuss sugar levels.

COMPLICATIONS

WARNING:

Why You Need to Keep Your Blood Sugar Under Control

Here are the major health concerns for your baby from untreated diabetes. We'd suggest skipping reading this section unless it applies to you. Otherwise, you may not sleep at night.[9]

1. **Big baby** (*macrosomia*). These babies weigh over the ninetieth percentile at birth (which means at least 8½ pounds). Infants of diabetic mothers (IDM) are bigger because of the extra sugar and altered metabolism during development. The bigger the baby, the harder it is for them to pass through the birth canal. So there's a greater risk of having a baby's shoulder get stuck behind mom's pubic bone (***shoulder dystocia***). This can lead to use of forceps or a vacuum during delivery, birth trauma for you (large tears in your genital area or need for an ***episiotomy***), and the baby (nerve injury, broken collar bone or other fractures, insufficient oxygen at birth). And there's a greater risk of needing a C-section.
2. **Delayed lung maturation.** High insulin levels affect the fetus's lung maturation (their ability to utilize the air in the lungs once born). An IDM baby's lungs may be immature prior to thirty-nine weeks.
3. **Low blood sugar (hypoglycemia).** This one may be hard to follow, but stick with us. While an IDM fetus is in the womb, the developing baby has very high blood sugar levels if mom's blood sugar is too high. So their body (the pancreas, specifically) makes extra insulin to deal with the excess sugar. Once the baby is born and the umbilical cord is cut, the baby no longer has excess sugar (since they don't receive mom's blood anymore). But the baby still has excess insulin for the first forty-eight hours until their body's metabolism adjusts. The high insulin levels can lead to a plummeting of baby's blood sugar. Typically, very low blood sugar causes jitteriness, lethargy, and lack of interest in eating (which would fix the problem).
4. **Jaundice (hyperbilirubinemia).** Any newborn can have temporary jaundice (yellowing of the skin). But IDM newborns have a greater risk of having jaundice due to higher levels of ***bilirubin*** (body garbage). IDM babies make more bilirubin than other newborns, so they have more to break down and eliminate. It can be a potential health problem until the body eliminates it properly at around five days of age.
5. **Stillbirth** (fetal death inside the uterus occurring after twenty weeks). The more uncontrolled your sugars are, the higher the likelihood of having a stillborn. If you require medication to control blood sugar, your risk of stillbirth is the same as women who have diabetes prior to pregnancy.

- Don't skip meals. Although it seems counterintuitive, skipping meals will only make things worse. In fact, you'll probably be told to eat a bedtime snack to keep glucose levels constant overnight.
- Moderate exercise (thirty minutes a day) improves glucose control—so do it! But check first with your OB provider before you begin an exercise plan.
- If diet and moderate exercise are not controlling your blood sugars, you will need an oral hypoglycemic (sugar-lowering) pill or insulin.

Issues for Mom: With gestational diabetes, there is an increased risk of ***preeclampsia*** (Complication #20), recurrent urinary tract infections, yeast infections, gestational diabetes in future pregnancies, and diabetes as you get older.

Issues for Baby:

- If mom has excellent blood sugar control: slim to no health risks for baby.
- There are several health concerns if mom has poorly controlled sugars throughout pregnancy. See below.

BOTTOM LINE: Only 15 percent of all women with gestational diabetes require medication to control blood sugars. Don't worry—the medication is safe. The danger to baby if this disease goes untreated is much more serious.

Reality Check

Women with gestational diabetes have a greater risk of developing diabetes later in life. Make healthy lifestyle choices after delivery (diet and exercise) and reach your ideal body weight. Your chance of getting diabetes later drops to less than 25 percent if you take these steps. If not, the risk is 50 percent. Doctors are really aggressive about treating even mild gestational diabetes since this lowers complications at birth.[10]

H. Systemic Autoimmune Diseases

27. Lupus

What is it? Your own immune system attacks you, causing a chronic inflammatory disease.

Usual time of onset: It usually occurs before pregnancy, but a few cases start during pregnancy or right after delivery.

Symptoms: No two cases of lupus are exactly the same. Flares may be mild or severe and may come on slowly or suddenly. It depends which part of your body is currently inflamed. Common symptoms include fever, fatigue, joint pain, stiffness and/or swelling, skin rashes, mouth sores, hair loss, chest pain, dry eyes, shortness of breath, weight gain or weight loss, and easy bruising.

Cause: Autoimmune disease. Instead of your immune system making antibodies that attack foreign threats (like bacteria and viruses), it makes antibodies that fight against your own healthy tissue. Many different body systems can become inflamed (joints, skin, kidneys, blood vessels, heart, lungs, brain) and ultimately damaged.

Treatment:

- Anti-inflammatory medications such as aspirin, ibuprofen, hydroxychloroquine (Plaquenil), steroids (see Appendix A, "Medications," for details on these meds).
- Possibly blood thinners such as heparin, enoxaparin (Lovenox) (see Appendix A, "Medications," for details on these meds).
- If you have antiphospholipid antibodies (lupus anticoagulant or anticardiolipin antibodies) or antiphospholipid syndrome, you'll get daily heparin or enoxaparin (Lovenox) injections.
- Consult with team of specialists regarding management and medication options: high-risk obstetrician, maternal-fetal medicine specialist, rheumatologist.
- Fetal monitoring (non-stress tests, biophysical profiles, periodic ultrasounds—see Chapter 6, "Tests") starting at twenty-six to twenty-eight weeks.
- Special ultrasound of the baby's heart (fetal echocardiogram) to check for heart defects.
- Closely monitor platelet counts, kidney and liver function.

Issues for Mom: Miscarriage, stillbirth, preeclampsia, gestational diabetes, urinary tract infections, and lupus flares during and shortly after pregnancy (first or second trimester or up to four months after delivery). Flares may occur in some pregnancies and not in others. Most flares are mild and can be treated with steroids. But women taking steroids during pregnancy are at higher risk of developing diabetes and high blood pressure. One key point: People with lupus may have antiphospholipid antibodies, which can lead to a miscarriage late in pregnancy. You need to be checked for this prior to or just after you find out you are pregnant.

Issues for Baby: Most babies do fine. Small risk of: miscarriage, stillborn, preterm birth, ***intrauterine growth restriction***, and in 3 percent of babies, *neonatal lupus*. Neonatal lupus causes a rash that resolves within six months of life . . . but more important, half of these babies have a heart defect that requires a permanent pacemaker. Consult your rheumatologist and pediatrician about which medications are safe for you to take while breastfeeding.

Helpful Hint

Yes, you can get pregnant if you have lupus and take medications to control your symptoms. It's a good idea, though, to visit with your obstetrician *before* getting pregnant. And be sure to get checked for antiphospholipid antibodies.

Reality Check

Women with lupus have a higher risk of chronic kidney disease. This should be checked before trying to get pregnant (this can be done with a few simple blood tests), since pregnancy risks are extremely high with both lupus and kidney disease.

I. Brain and Nervous System

28. Epilepsy

What is it? Abnormal pattern of electrical impulses in the neurons (specialized cells) of the brain. Epilepsy is when you have at least two seizures at least twenty-four hours apart that are not caused by fever or substance abuse. There are several types of epilepsy (see below).

Usual time of onset: Before pregnancy.

Symptoms: Depends on the type of seizure. **Generalized seizures:** Total body stiffening with rhythmic movements of arms and legs, open eyes, involuntary urination, temporary lapse of breathing, frothing at the mouth, confusion afterward. **Partial or focal seizures:** Only one area of body may be affected (such as rhythmic jerking of one hand).

Cause: Unknown most of the time.

Treatment:

- Consult with your obstetrician and neurologist, preferably before pregnancy to get seizures under control. This is a condition where pre-pregnancy counseling is critical. Some medications can cause neural tube defects and other deformities in the fetus. Use the lowest possible dose of anti-seizure medication and take only one anti-seizure medication if possible (instead of two or three). You may be able to switch to a newer medication that is less risky for the fetus. If you haven't had a seizure in two to five years, you may be able to discontinue all medication.
- If you didn't know you were pregnant and you take valproate (valproic acid), you need to talk with your doctor prior to stopping your medication. Although valproate is not something doctors want pregnant women taking, it should *never* be stopped cold turkey. Talk to your neurologist.
- Take higher dose folic acid (4 milligrams per day) preferably before pregnancy or starting right now, as it may lower the risk of neural tube defects and other birth defects.
- Get early genetic counseling.
- Get a special ultrasound to look for malformations of the face, brain, spine, or heart.
- Consider doing maternal serum AFP test at sixteen to twenty weeks or an amniocentesis to screen for neural tube defects.
- If you take medication, see your OB and neurologist regularly to check medication levels.
- Vaginal delivery is preferable unless you have repeated seizures in labor.
- Monitor medication levels closely after delivery since they can change quickly.

Issues for Mom: Seizures. Up to one-third of pregnant women with seizure disorders have more seizures during pregnancy. Here are a few reasons: lack of sleep, the liver metabolizes anti-seizure medication differently during pregnancy, and women often stop taking their medications because they worry about adverse effects to the baby. Slightly higher risk of ***preeclampsia***.

Issues for Baby: Most babies do fine. Risk of miscarriage, stillborn, growth restriction. Greater risk (two to five times greater) of birth defects—heart defects, ***cleft lip/palate***. Older children may have abnormal brain wave activity (found on EEG), developmental delays, and lower IQs. The biggest problems are the anti-seizure medications. Carbamazepine and valproic acid increase the risk of neural tube defects. Valproic acid is also associated with an increased risk of autism. Phenytoin can cause a constellation of birth defects in about one-third of fetuses. It's called *fetal hydantoin syndrome* (facial defects, abnormal finger development, and developmental delay).

29. Migraines

What is it? Headaches brought on by certain triggers.

Usual time of onset: Usually before pregnancy, sometimes new onset in first trimester.

Symptoms: Some people know a migraine is coming on about thirty minutes before the pain starts, but many don't. That sixth sense is called an aura (seeing spots, flashing lights, or wavy lines, or numbness/"pins and needles" sensation in the hands, arms, or face). Migraines typically come with throbbing pain usually on one side of the head, worsening with routine activity, nausea and/or vomiting, sensitivity to light/noise/smell.

Cause: Genetics (other family members have them, too), environmental. Some triggers include caffeine, lack of sleep, alcohol, MSG, stress, change in environment (changing elevation or climate), bright lights, loud sounds and intense smells (such as cigarette smoke and perfume), certain medications, extreme physical exertion, and fluctuations in estrogen levels—during the menstrual cycle, menopause, and pregnancy.

Treatment: Lifestyle Measures

- Relaxation exercises (meditation or yoga).
- Get enough sleep.
- Keep a headache diary.
- Avoid known triggers (alcohol, chocolate, caffeine, MSG).
- Exercise.

Complementary Therapies

- Acupuncture.
- Massage.
- Biofeedback.
- A few helpful supplements include riboflavin (vitamin B2), coenzyme Q10, magnesium sulfate supplements. Although there is some evidence that the herbal meds feverfew and butterbur can help prevent or reduce the severity of migraines, do not use these while pregnant.

Medication Options

- Acetaminophen.
- Consider taking medication to prevent migraines (stopping them before they start) with calcium channel blockers or beta-blockers.
- Sumatriptan (Imitrex), rizatriptan (Maxalt), zolmitriptan (Zomig). These medications (called triptans) are possible if absolutely necessary but are not usually recommended due to their ability to increase blood pressure and cause heavy bleeding after delivery.
- Anti-nausea medication.
- Targeted Botox and/or nerve blocks with lidocaine or another local anesthetic.

Issues for Mom: Many women have fewer migraines during pregnancy. Great! Others have more frequent and more intense migraines. Not so great. You're also more likely to have nausea, vomiting, and ***hyperemesis gravidarum*** (Complication #1).

Issues for Baby: None.

Helpful Hint

You should *not* take Migergot, Cafergot, or Migranal (collectively called "ergot" medications) during pregnancy since they can cause uterine bleeding and miscarriage.

J. Mental Health

Welcome! You're in good company. There are about four million pregnancies in the United States annually, and more than 500,000 of pregnant women experience a mental health issue. That may occur before pregnancy, or happen for the first time during pregnancy. It is estimated that up to 33 percent of all fetuses are exposed to some type of psychiatric medication at some point during pregnancy.

For a complete list of medications typically used for mental health conditions, see Appendix A, "Medications."

30. Depression

What is it? This disorder interferes with your ability to carry out activities of daily living. It occurs in 10 to 16 percent of all pregnancies.

Usual time of onset: It usually begins before pregnancy, but some cases arise during pregnancy or in the first four to six weeks after delivery.

Symptoms: Not enjoying life/pleasurable activities, weight loss or weight gain, loss of energy, sleep disturbance, excessive feelings of guilt or worthlessness, depressed mood, and in severe cases, thoughts of committing suicide.

Cause: A chemical imbalance in the brain that may be genetic, environmental (recent loss of a friend, spouse, child, or other family member, loss of a job, loss of finances, divorce), or secondary to substance abuse. The massive hormonal surges that occur during pregnancy and in the postpartum period can trigger an initial episode of depression or can worsen symptoms in someone who was previously doing well.

Treatment: Get treatment, especially during pregnancy, because there are consequences for both mom and baby if you don't get help. Report any of the above symptoms to your OB provider.

- Confirm the diagnosis and receive care from mental health providers (psychologist, psychiatrist, support groups, substance abuse treatment if needed).
- Consult a maternal-fetal medicine specialist.
- Eat well, exercise, get enough sleep.
- Antidepressant medication, if needed.

Issues for Mom: If you aren't treated, you probably won't take good care of yourself. Poor prenatal care, nutrition, and lifestyles can lead to health risks for you and baby and poor maternal-fetal bonding. Depressed pregnant women are also more likely to have substance use disorders.

Issues for Baby: Vicious cycle. Poor prenatal care means pregnancy complications may be missed—which could mean preterm delivery. Growth restriction from poor nutrition. Issues related to substance abuse. Poor maternal-fetal bonding. Possible side effects/withdrawal from psychiatric medications if mom uses them during pregnancy. Newborns of women with untreated depression often cry more and are much more difficult to console.

31. Anxiety Disorders, Obsessive-Compulsive Disorder, or Post-Traumatic Stress Disorder (PTSD)

What is it? An excessive or irrational response to stress, which, if severe, can affect performing activities of daily living. There are eight types: generalized anxiety disorder, specific phobias, social anxiety disorder, panic disorder, agoraphobia, separation anxiety disorder, substance/medication-induced anxiety disorder, and anxiety due to a medical condition. In addition, obsessive compulsive disorder (OCD) and post-traumatic stress disorder (PTSD), although not classified under anxiety disorders, share some similarities.

Usual time of onset: Usually before pregnancy, but some cases first arise during pregnancy or four to six weeks after delivery. PTSD and OCD may worsen after delivery.

Symptoms: It depends on the disorder, but include anxiety, stress, sleep disturbances, feeling of dread, feeling out of control, heart pounding, tingling fingers, avoidance of certain places or activities, ritualistic behaviors, and intrusive thoughts and fears.

Cause: Genetics, brain chemistry, certain life experiences. Massive hormonal surges during pregnancy and in the postpartum period can trigger an initial episode of anxiety or can trigger symptoms in a person whose anxiety was under good control.

Treatment:

- Consult a psychologist, psychiatrist, and support groups.
- Anti-anxiety medication, if necessary (see Appendix A, "Medications," for more information).

Issues for Mom: Excessive worrying, lack of good prenatal care, worsening of symptoms (particularly in women with panic disorder, PTSD, and OCD), postpartum depression. Moms with severe stress and anxiety have a higher risk of miscarriage, preterm labor, and delivery complications (prolonged labor, precipitous labor, fetal distress, use of forceps or vacuum during delivery).

Issues for Baby: Anti-anxiety medications can cause problems for a newborn including low muscle tone (***floppy baby syndrome***), low body temperature, lethargy, and trouble breathing and feeding. Babies can also go through drug withdrawal syndrome and have restlessness, increased muscle tone, diarrhea, vomiting, and tremors. These symptoms may persist up to three months after delivery. They are most common in pregnancies where benzodiazepine medications were used shortly before delivery.

BOTTOM LINE: Anxiety disorders are the most common psychiatric disorders in the United States. About 18 percent of American adults have one these disorders. Some anti-anxiety medications taken during pregnancy can affect your newborn. Talk to your doctor about it.

---

32. Bipolar Disorder

What is it? Involves distinct episodes of highs and lows (abnormal elation and/or irritable mood and separate episodes of depressed mood).

Usual time of onset: Before pregnancy, sometimes new onset during pregnancy, or within six weeks of delivery.

Symptoms: *Depression symptoms*: Lack of pleasure in anything, weight loss or weight gain, loss of energy, sleep disturbance, excessive feelings of guilt or worthlessness, depressed mood, and in severe cases, thoughts of committing suicide. *Mania symptoms*: Sleeplessness, extremely elevated mood, spending sprees, travel, and often substance abuse.

Cause: Genetic, chemical imbalance in the brain. Those hormone surges in pregnancy and after delivery can set off bipolar disorder or trigger symptoms in someone who already carries the diagnosis.

Treatment:

- Be sure your care team includes an obstetrician, maternal-fetal medicine specialist, and psychiatrist.
- Attend support groups.
- Medication, which is usually necessary (mood-stabilizing medication, antidepressants, antipsychotics, antiepileptics). See Appendix A, "Medications," for details on these meds.

Issues for Mom: If you are not appropriately treated, you may not follow up with your prenatal care, may eat poorly, abuse substances, and have poor maternal-fetal bonding. Warning: Many women will have relapses after delivery (30 percent to 70 percent). And up to 45 percent of women develop postpartum psychosis.

Issues for Baby: If you don't take care of yourself, you probably won't follow up with your prenatal care (which detects complications early). So your baby has a higher risk of growth restriction, preterm delivery, substance abuse withdrawal, and psychiatric medication withdrawal. Newborns whose moms had untreated depression often cry more and are more difficult to console.

Partner Tip

If your pregnancy partner has these symptoms, speak up and get her help.

33. Schizophrenia and Schizophrenia-like Disorders

What is it? People with schizophrenia lose touch with reality and have false ideas or see or hear things that are not there.

Usual time of onset: Before pregnancy (late teens to mid-thirties).

Symptoms: Hallucinations (e.g., hearing voices that are not there, seeing things that do not exist), completely unemotional, dysfunctional in social situations.

Cause: Combination of genetics, brain chemistry, and life experiences/situations. It runs in families.

Treatment:

- Be sure your care team includes an obstetrician, maternal-fetal medicine specialist, and psychiatrist.
- Medication, if necessary. Use one medication instead of several, if possible. Older "typical" antipsychotic medications are safe for pregnancy. Newer "atypical" ones lack safety data on use in pregnancy or breastfeeding right now. See Appendix A, "Medications."

Issues for Mom: If you don't take care of yourself, you're likely to have poor nutrition, substance abuse, preterm delivery, increased chance of vaginal delivery with forceps/C-sections, and poor bonding with your baby. If you aren't treated, you may harm yourself or your baby because you are out of touch with reality or hear voices that tell you to do so. Beware: You are at risk of severe postpartum depression and psychosis.

Issues for Baby: Preterm delivery, low birth weight, higher risk of birth defects (especially the heart). If you aren't treated, you might harm your baby. Get treated!

Obstetrical Complications with Mom

K. Uterus/Cervix

34. Cervical Insufficiency

What is it? Cervix begins to open (dilate) very early in pregnancy, often leading to loss of a pregnancy, sometimes as early as thirteen to fifteen weeks.

Usual time of onset: Anytime between thirteen and twenty-four weeks.

Symptoms: You usually don't know your cervix is dilating because it doesn't hurt. One scenario: You have some light spotting and then your membranes rupture abruptly and you deliver.

Cause: Previous surgery on the cervix (LEEP, cold knife conization), overdilation during pregnancy termination, cervical lacerations from previous deliveries, congenital abnormalities of the female genital system, or a deficiency of collagen and elastin in the cervical tissue.

Treatment:

- Placement of a *cerclage* at thirteen to sixteen weeks if you have true cervical insufficiency. What is a cerclage? Your OB sews a large piece of string (suture) around the cervix like a purse string and ties it. The cerclage is removed around thirty-six weeks, just before you would normally break your water or go into labor. A cerclage is 75 to 90 percent effective in preventing preterm delivery.
- Bed rest until you deliver.
- Periodic transvaginal ultrasounds measure the actual length of the cervix to determine whether or not you have cervical insufficiency. This is helpful for women who've had cone biopsies or multiple cervical procedures, as it reduces the need for preventative cerclages and gives time to place one if the cervix starts to shorten too early.

Issues for Mom: Recurrent miscarriage, possible surgical procedure (if you need a cerclage), prolonged bed rest, preterm delivery, risk of cervical insufficiency in subsequent pregnancies.

Issues for Baby: Risk of preterm delivery.[11]

35. Uterine Didelphys or Bicornuate Uterus

What is it? You have an abnormally formed uterus.

Usual time of onset: You're born with it. Many women don't know they have this malformation until they have an ultrasound with a first pregnancy.

Symptoms: Symptoms depend on the actual defect. Some women have no symptoms at all. Possible symptoms: no periods, infertility, recurrent miscarriage, and pain.

Cause: It happened as your female organs developed when you were a fetus. The two Mullerian ducts in the embryo develop into the female organs, the vagina, cervix, uterus, and fallopian tubes. In this complication, your Mullerian ducts formed abnormally.

Treatment: It depends on the abnormality.

- Didelphic uterus: None.
- Uterine septum: Removing the abnormality with a surgical procedure decreases miscarriage rates.

Issues for Mom: It's possible to have a normal pregnancy even if you have a double uterus. But it can increase the risk of miscarriage, premature birth, unusual baby positions (breech, transverse), and delivery by C-section.

Issues for Baby: Possible growth restriction, premature birth.

Reality Check

No surprise, women with a double uterus can have difficulty getting pregnant.

COMPLICATIONS

36. Preterm Contractions/Preterm Labor

What is it? Uterine contractions before thirty-seven weeks gestation.

Usual time of onset: Between twenty-two and thirty-seven weeks.

Symptoms: Painful cramping or tightening in your lower abdomen or back that occur at regular intervals.

Cause: Unknown about half the time. The other half are caused by:

- Stress to mom or baby (severe emotional stress, exhaustion, medical condition, malnutrition in mom and a poor blood supply or birth defect in baby).
- Infections (bladder infections, some vaginal infections, and sexually transmitted infections).
- Bleeding (***placental abruption***, subchorionic clot).
- Overstretching of the uterus (multiple fetuses, too much amniotic fluid, uterus that is abnormally shaped).
- Cervical insufficiency (Complication #34, where the cervix opens too early, often without warning).

Treatment: It depends on the cause of the preterm labor, severity of your contractions, whether your water bag has broken, and whether or not your cervix has dilated.

- Call OB provider if you have more than four to six contractions in an hour and you're less than thirty-five weeks pregnant.
- Possible bed rest.
- Hydration.
- Possible hospitalization (definitely if your water bag has broken).
- Medication to help stop contractions (***tocolytic medication***). See Appendix A, "Medications."
- Antibiotics if an infection is suspected or diagnosed.
- Steroids to mature the baby's lungs if delivery is thought to be imminent.

Issues for Mom: Depends on the cause of the preterm labor.

Issues for Baby: Preterm birth.

See Chapter 20, "Preterm Labor and Babies," for more details.

Helpful Hint

Going on bed rest is not only boring as all heck, it also puts you at risk for having blood clots in your legs (deep venous thrombosis or DVT). Your muscles can get a little weaker as well. Ask your OB provider about getting massages, physical therapy, and doing exercises with light weights in bed to help keep your muscle tone and prevent a DVT. Support stockings are also a good idea.

L. Placenta

37. Placenta Previa

What is it? The placenta implants over part of or all of the cervix. Bleeding when contractions begin and/or the cervix starts to dilate. There are three types:

- *Complete previa*: Placenta completely covers the cervical opening.
- *Partial previa*: Placenta covers a portion of the cervix.
- *Marginal previa:* Placenta extends to the edge of the cervix.

Placenta previa occurs in 1 out of every 200 pregnancies.

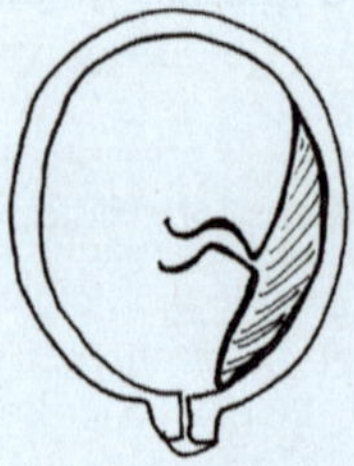

Marginal placenta

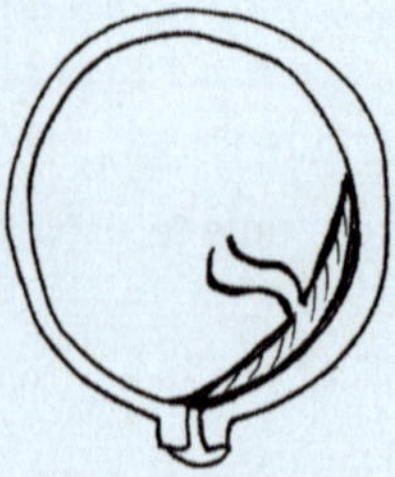

Partial Placenta Previa

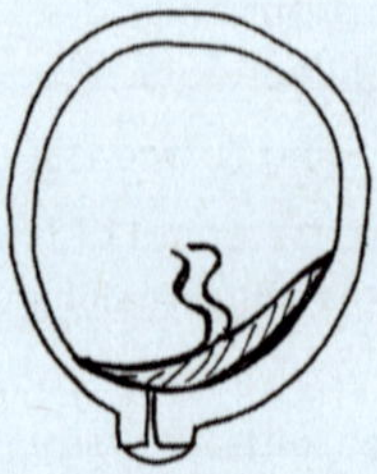

Complete Previa

Usual time of onset: The placenta implants at the beginning of pregnancy, so that's when the problem starts. The good news: Many placenta previas that are diagnosed early in pregnancy move to a safer spot higher up on the uterine wall as the uterus grows.

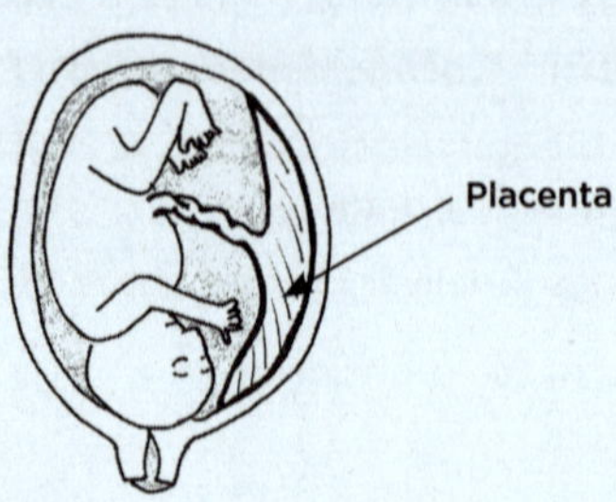

Normal Placenta

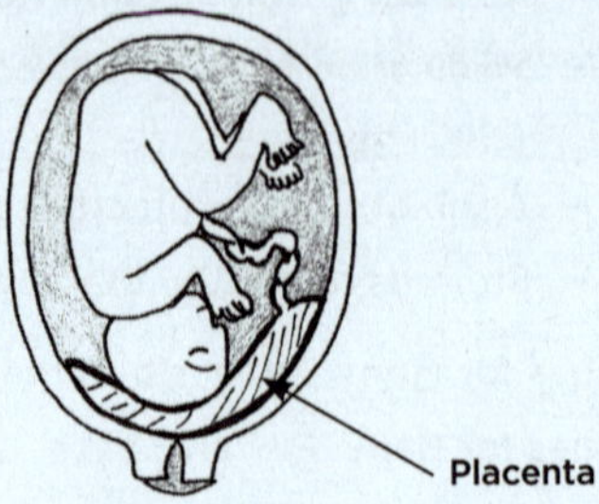

Placenta Previa

Symptoms: Painless bleeding, usually in the third trimester. This ranges from a little bit of spotting to a significant hemorrhage. But you may also be symptom-free during your entire pregnancy.

Cause: Unknown. Several risk factors: mom over thirty-five years old, previous uterine surgery (C-section, myomectomy), carrying multiple fetuses (twins, triplets, etc.), history of more than four pregnancies.

Treatment: Depends on the severity of symptoms.

- Bed rest.
- Pelvic rest (no intercourse or pelvic exams).
- Hospitalization, if there is constant or chronic bleeding.
- Steroid injections to mature your baby's body organs, in case of preterm delivery.
- C-section for complete or partial previas. Some marginal previas can deliver vaginally.

Issues for Mom: Prolonged bed rest, hospitalization, anemia from chronic or severe blood loss (occasionally requires a blood transfusion). ***Placenta previa*** is sometimes associated with ***placenta accreta*** (see Complication #39), which can cause excessive bleeding after delivery and possibly require a hysterectomy.

Issues for Baby: Premature birth. Fetus is also at risk for not getting enough blood or oxygen from the placenta. Occasionally, it can be fatal.

38. Vasa Previa

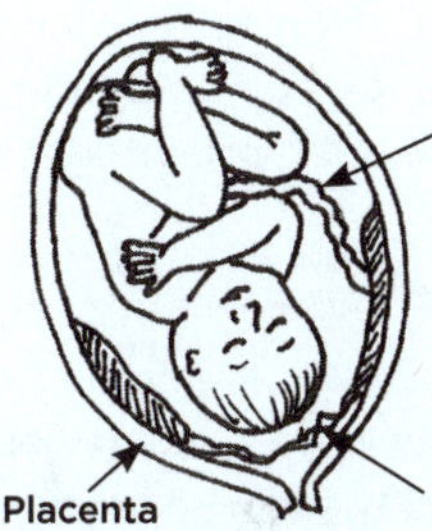

What is it? The blood vessels in the umbilical cord that travel back and forth from the fetus to the placenta are abnormally and dangerously positioned across the cervix. Essentially, the blood vessels are in the way of the baby's exit from the womb. If your water bag breaks, those blood vessels tear and there is excessive bleeding. This can be very serious.

Usual time of onset: The situation occurs when the placenta develops in the first ten weeks of pregnancy. But if there are no symptoms, it may not be diagnosed until you are in labor. It's sometimes possible to discover a vasa previa with a special ultrasound that uses color Doppler (like you see on the Weather Channel) to map blood flow.

Symptoms: There are either no symptoms at all or severe vaginal hemorrhage.

Cause: Cause is unknown, but risk factors include carrying multiple fetuses (twins, triplets, etc.), having two lobes to the placenta, having a low-lying placenta or placenta previa, history of in vitro fertilization (IVF), prior uterine surgery (C-sections, myomectomies, **D&C**), or the umbilical cord inserts into the amniotic sac rather than directly into the placenta (velamentous cord). It is also sure to happen if you are a labor and delivery nurse, doctor, or ER doctor's wife (a little hospital humor, as there is an unwritten rule that really bad things only happen to healthcare personnel).

Treatment: Plan A: If the diagnosis is known prior to delivery:

- Bed rest.
- Hospitalization in the third trimester.
- Early delivery (often at thirty-five weeks) by C-section.

Plan B: If the diagnosis is unknown prior to delivery:

- Emergency C-section is immediately performed. The mother usually has severe vaginal bleeding and the fetus is in distress. (A pathologist confirms the diagnosis after delivery when the placenta and fetal membranes are examined.)

Issues for Mom: Bed rest if diagnosed prior to delivery. Planned C-section at thirty-five weeks.

Issues for Baby: Fetal distress and, unfortunately, often fetal death. Since the blood vessels running over the cervix are those that take blood to and from the fetus, rupture of the amniotic sac leads to rupture of the blood vessels and significant fetal hemorrhage. If hemorrhage occurs, treatment after delivery includes aggressive fetal resuscitation and blood transfusion.

39. Placenta Accreta, Increta, and Percreta

What is it? Placenta attaches too deeply to the wall of the uterus. Typically as the placenta develops, there is a thin layer that forms separating the placenta from the uterine wall. There is no layer with placenta accreta, increta, and percreta. See the following New Parent-to-Be 411 box. Placenta accreta occurs in 1 in every 2,500 pregnancies.

Usual time of onset: It occurs during development of the embryo and placenta. Sometimes it is identified during pregnancy by using ultrasound and Doppler flow technology. But more often it is diagnosed after delivery of the baby and/or the placenta.

Symptoms: None, unless an accreta is present with a placenta previa.

Cause: Unknown. More common with placenta previa (present in 5 to 10 percent), women who have had previous uterine surgery (previous C-sections or fibroid removal), and those who have had multiple previous C-sections (60 percent of women with placenta accreta).

Treatment: There is nothing that can be done to prevent a placenta accreta from happening, and there is very little that can be done once diagnosed. If you are diagnosed prior to delivery:

- Periodic ultrasounds assess the severity/degree of the accreta.
- Scheduled C-section, usually earlier than thirty-nine weeks at a hospital/medical center familiar in dealing with these abnormalities.
- Discuss the game plan with your OB provider regarding possible hysterectomy and blood transfusions (the worst-case scenario).

Issues for Mom: Risk of significant bleeding when an attempt is made to separate the placenta from the uterine wall. If severe, blood loss can be life-threatening and could require further uterine surgery, a hysterectomy, and/or blood transfusions. It's important to diagnose and treat it quickly.

Issues for Baby: Premature delivery if bleeding occurs.

WARNING:
Abnormal Placental Attachments

There are three different types of abnormal placental attachments:

- ***Placenta accreta***: Placenta attaches in an abnormal way to the uterine wall. It does not, however, invade the uterine muscle. This is the most common of the three abnormalities and accounts for 75 percent of all cases.
- ***Placenta increta***: Placenta invades the uterine muscle, but it does not extend through the wall of the uterus. It occurs in 15 percent of all cases.
- ***Placenta percreta***: Placenta penetrates through the entire uterine wall and attaches to another organ, such as the bladder or intestine. This is the least common of the three and accounts for 3 to 5 percent of all cases.

40. Placental Abruption

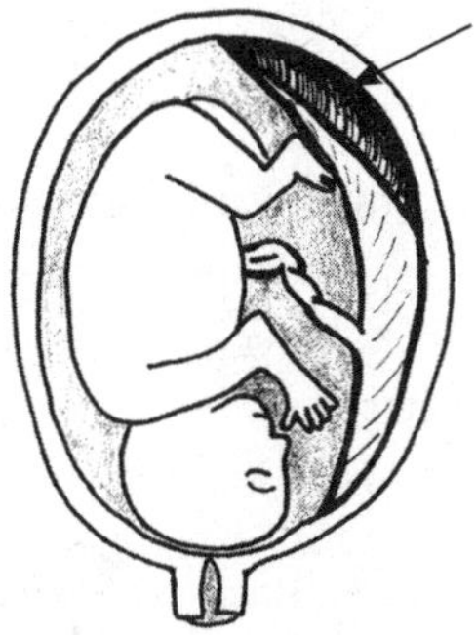

What is it? Placenta separates (partially or completely) from the wall of the uterus prior to delivery of the fetus. It can be serious (depending on the severity of the separation) and occurs in about 1 in 150 deliveries.

Usual time of onset: Mostly third trimester, but any time after twenty weeks.

Symptoms: Usually vaginal bleeding (either slight or heavy) and abdominal pain (with or without contractions), back pain, uterus sometimes tender to touch. If contractions are present, they are usually back-to-back, coming one after another. The amount of blood that is coming from the vagina does not necessarily correlate with how much of the placenta has separated from the wall of the uterus. In one out of five cases, the bleeding is hidden, and a woman can be very ill from losing a large amount of blood before she is diagnosed (symptoms of blood loss are dizziness, low blood pressure, rapid heart rate, and shock).

Cause: Often, there is no specific reason. Direct abdominal injury (such as a car accident or a fall) can cause it. Other risk factors are:

- High blood pressure (chronic or ***preeclampsia***).
- You've had a previous ***placental abruption*** (your risk is about 15 percent in subsequent pregnancies).
- You've been pregnant before.
- Excessive amount of amniotic fluid (***polyhydramnios***).
- Premature rupture of membranes.
- Age (this is more common in women over the age of thirty-five).

- Substance abuse, particularly use of cigarettes, alcohol, cocaine, or methamphetamines during pregnancy.
- Carrying multiples (twins, triplets, or more).

Treatment: Treatment depends on severity of abruption, how far along the pregnancy is, and if the fetus is in any danger. Unfortunately, docs can't reattach the placenta once it has separated from the uterine wall. If you are Rh-negative, you will need RhoGAM.

Scenario #1: Mild abruption, and you are beyond thirty-six to thirty-seven weeks:

- Delivery likely. You will either be induced, if it is safe to do so, or have a C-section.

Scenario #2: Mild abruption, and you are less than thirty-six weeks:

- Check for reassuring fetal heart rate tracing.
- Hospitalization for observation.
- Bed rest at home if bleeding stops and you and baby are stable.
- Frequent follow-up office visits.

Scenario #3: Severe abruption:

- Immediate delivery (usually emergency C-section) no matter how far along you are if you have massive, uncontrollable vaginal bleeding or if you or your baby is unstable.
- Possible blood transfusion, if bleeding is excessive.

Issues for Mom: Bleeding, sometimes excessive. Yes, it's rare, but possible to go into shock or bleed to death without quick medical intervention. Possible C-section, possible hysterectomy after delivery if bleeding cannot be controlled.

Issues for Baby: Premature birth. If too much of the placenta separates from the uterus, the baby can be deprived of oxygen and nutrients. That has the potential to cause neurologic problems or, rarely, stillbirth. The babies at highest risk are those who are unstable before delivery and those delivered by emergency C-section. These babies also have a slightly higher risk of ***sudden infant death syndrome (SIDS)***.[12]

Reality Check

Eighty-five percent of placental abruptions are mild to moderate ones. That's the good news. The bad news: Almost half the women with placental abruptions deliver before thirty-seven weeks.[13]

M. Amniotic Fluid

41. Polyhydramnios

What is it? Too much amniotic fluid. This occurs in 1 to 2 percent of all pregnancies. Most cases are mild and rarely result in any complications. As the level of fluid increases, so does the risk of problems.

Usual time of onset: Usually third trimester, sometimes second trimester.

Symptoms: None, except for a big belly.

Cause: Over half of the time, the cause is unknown. In other cases, the causes could be:

- Birth defects. If a fetus has a malformation (gastrointestinal tract, nervous system) that affects their ability to swallow/digest amniotic fluid, it builds up.
- ***Rh incompatibility.***
- Maternal diabetes, poorly controlled.
- ***Twin-to-twin transfusion syndrome (TTTS)***. One twin gets too much blood flow, and the other too little due to connections between blood vessels in their shared placenta. This leads to too much amniotic fluid for the twin with too much blood flow and too little amniotic fluid for the twin without enough blood flow.

Treatment: Usually none. Increased monitoring by frequent ultrasounds and tests of fetal well-being (non-stress tests, biophysical profiles). Depending on each individual situation, treatments may include:

- Medication that reduces fluid production. It is effective up to 90 percent of the time but is not generally used after about twenty-eight to thirty-two weeks gestation.
- Amnioreduction procedure: A needle drains excess fluid from within the uterine cavity (exactly like an amniocentesis). Risks are premature rupture of membranes, infection, and fluid can build back up again. This procedure is usually only done if the size of the uterus is impairing the ability of mom to breathe.
- Delivery, if baby is at risk (poor growth, lacks signs of well-being).

Issues for Mom: As more fluid accumulates, there is greater risk of premature rupture of the membranes (PROM), increased risk of the umbilical cord protruding through the cervix (***cord prolapse***) with rupture of membranes, preterm labor and delivery, placental abruption, increased risk of needing a C-section, and postpartum hemorrhage.

Issues for Baby: Increased risk of stillborn (although rare, it is twice the risk of a normal pregnancy), possible complications of maternal diabetes (hypoglycemia, seizures, jaundice) if present, possible fetal growth restriction, preterm birth.

WARNING:
What You Need to Know About Blood Transfusions

We know that getting a blood transfusion sounds scary. Rest assured that it is not common to receive blood, either during your pregnancy or afterward. But some people with chronic medical conditions (such as sickle cell anemia) need a blood transfusion during pregnancy.

However, the most common reason for needing a transfusion is excessive bleeding after delivery (***postpartum hemorrhage***). Everyone loses a lot of blood during the delivery of a baby, whether it's a vaginal delivery or a C-section. The average amount of blood lost in a vaginal delivery is about 10 to 13 ounces (300 to 400 ml). In a C-section, the average is about 20 to 27 ounces (600 to 800 ml). Anything greater than 34 ounces (1,000 ml) blood loss in a vaginal delivery or C-section is considered to be a postpartum hemorrhage.

Around the world, a postpartum hemorrhage happens every four minutes. And 140,000 women die each year from this pregnancy complication. Most of those deaths do not occur in the United States because of good medical care and the availability of resources, particularly blood and blood products. But this still happens in the United States, and approximately 700 women a year die from a postpartum hemorrhage in this country. If you have so much blood loss that your blood pressure is dropping, a blood transfusion will save your life. Period. About 0.4 to 0.6 percent of American women need a postpartum blood transfusion.

Obviously, this is not a decision that is taken lightly. If ordered, your OB provider feels the benefits outweigh the potential risks. The risks of transfusion include: a transfusion reaction (an allergic reaction to the blood you receive, even if it is the same blood type), a reaction due to receiving the wrong blood type (pretty rare), or a risk of contracting an infection. Donor blood is screened very thoroughly to prevent infectious disease transmission, so the general risks are about 1 in 1.5 to 2 million to get HIV or hepatitis C from a blood transfusion and 1 in 300,000 for hepatitis B (although most people are vaccinated against hepatitis B so the risk is much lower).[14]

INSIDER SECRET:
Why Is Amniotic Fluid So Important Anyway?

Your baby develops in a fluid-filled bubble. This is why their fingers and toes at birth will look like yours do after a leisurely bath.

Your baby's bubble (the amniotic sac) starts to form just twelve days after conception. Mom makes the initial amniotic fluid (which is mostly water) in the early stages of pregnancy. After about twelve weeks, the placenta and your baby make amniotic fluid. Yes, amniotic fluid is actually your baby's urine—but don't worry, it's all sterile!

The amniotic fluid has several important jobs. Babies not only make the amniotic fluid, they also breathe it into their lungs and swallow it to go through the digestive tract. This helps the lungs and digestive tract develop properly. The fluid cushions and protects your baby, provides them with fluids, allows for fetal movement, allows growth, and helps strengthen the baby's muscles and bones. It also allows the umbilical cord to float around freely. You can see why it's so essential.

Having too much amniotic fluid can be a sign that your baby is not ingesting it as they should or too much is being made. Having too little may mean your baby or the placenta is not producing enough of it, or your membranes have ruptured.

The level of amniotic fluid increases until about twenty-eight to thirty-two weeks of pregnancy, at which time it plateaus and then begins to decrease when your baby reaches thirty-seven to forty weeks.

42. Oligohydramnios

What is it? Too little amniotic fluid. If you are past your due date by at least two weeks, you may be at risk. Oligohydramnios complicates 12 percent of pregnancies that go beyond forty-one weeks.

Usual time of onset: Usually third trimester, but it also happens in the second trimester.

Symptoms: Sometimes none. Or you might feel a decrease in the size of your belly or decreased fetal movement.

Cause: Often unknown. Possible causes include:

- Your membranes have ruptured and you are leaking fluid (preterm or at term).
- You go past your due date, so your placental function declines (see FYI below).
- Birth defects. Your baby's kidneys make urine (amniotic fluid). A problem with the kidneys or urinary tract development can lead to too little amniotic fluid.
- Problems with placenta.
- Maternal complications, such as dehydration, high blood pressure (either chronic/preexisting or preeclampsia), diabetes, lupus, or chronic lack of oxygen that can sometimes occur at higher altitudes or with some diseases.

Certain health conditions will make the placenta "age" prematurely, and as a result, it doesn't function as well (called placental insufficiency). There is less amniotic fluid when there is placental insufficiency since the placenta helps make amniotic fluid. For example, high blood pressure leads to placental insufficiency, which can lead to oligohydramnios.

Treatment: It depends on how far along you are in your pregnancy and the presumed cause. In any scenario, it's possible you will need to get hydrated with either liquids by mouth or an IV.

Scenario #1: You are not full term and not in labor.

- Close monitoring with periodic ultrasounds, non-stress tests, biophysical profiles (see Chapter 6, "Tests").
- Possible hospitalization for observation.
- Possible bed rest.
- Possible infusion of fluid by amniocentesis, if necessary.

Scenario #2: You are full term (or close to it) but not in labor.

- Probable delivery, especially if your water bag has broken.
- Antibiotics, if it is suspected or confirmed that your membranes are ruptured.
- Close monitoring if your membranes are intact and you and baby are stable.
- Delivery if you are at term or there are any signs of fetal distress.

Scenario #3: You are in labor.

- Delivery.
- Amnioinfusion. Obstetrician infuses sterile saline (salt water) through the cervix into the amniotic cavity to help increase buoyancy and prevent compression of the umbilical cord and subsequent fetal distress.

Issues for Mom: Increased risk of C-section if the baby is in distress (***cord compression, meconium-stained fluid***).

Issues for Baby: It depends on when in the pregnancy oligohydramnios occurs. Amniotic fluid is essential for your baby to develop appropriately (see the New Parent-to-Be 411 box on page 504). The baby begins to breathe and swallow the fluid in the second trimester to help their lungs grow and mature. If oligohydramnios occurs earlier in pregnancy (the second trimester), the complications are often more serious: increased risk of miscarriage or stillbirth, birth defects because developing fetal organs are compressed (lung and limb defects). Too little fluid later in pregnancy can lead to growth restriction, preterm birth, passing the first poop (***meconium***) while in the womb (see details below), or cord compression, which stresses the baby.[15]

There are two ways your doc will know if your baby is in distress:

1. **Cord compression:** Umbilical cord (and its blood vessels) is compressed because it can't float around freely. Less oxygen goes to the baby and a non-reassuring fetal heart pattern is seen on the monitor or picked up while listening with a Doppler.
2. **Meconium-stained fluid:** Fetuses do not ordinarily poop while they are in the womb. They poop for the first time once they are born. But they will poop in the womb if they are stressed. So when your water breaks, the fluid looks yellow/green/brown because it is meconium-stained. Unfortunately, this is not only a sign of distress, but it can also become a problem, since this meconium can get into the baby's lungs, causing temporary breathing problems after birth.

BOTTOM LINE: Your baby may be in distress if they don't have enough amniotic fluid.

Red Flags: Amniotic Fluid

Healthy amniotic fluid is clear to straw-colored. If your baby is stressed before delivery, they might poop (pass ***meconium***) for the first time while in the womb (instead of afterward like they are supposed to), making the amniotic fluid stained green/yellow/brown. If you have ***chorioamnionitis*** (an infection), the amniotic fluid can be cloudy and foul-smelling.

Obstetrical Complications with Baby

N. Position

See Chapter 13, "Home Stretch," and 14, "Labor Day," for details on different fetal positions.

43. Breech Position

What is it? It's normal for a baby to come out of the birth canal with their head first. In a breech position (which happens in 3 percent of full-term pregnancies), your baby's head is up near your rib cage with either their feet or bottom down near your cervix. They plan to exit the womb bottom first. There are three types of ***breech presentations***:

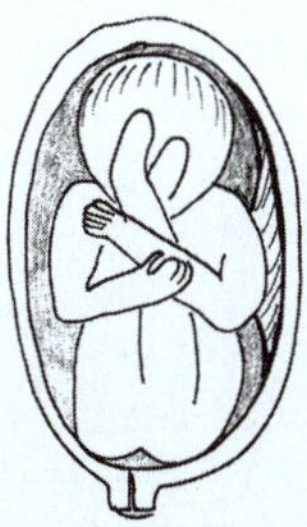

Frank Breech. The baby's butt is over the cervix, with their feet up near their head.

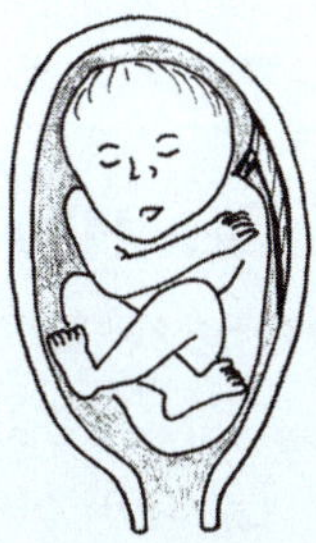

Complete Breech. The baby's butt is over the cervix, but their knees are bent and tucked up against their chest.

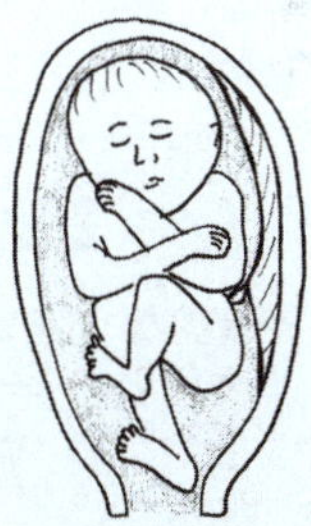

Footling Breech. One or both feet are over the cervix.

Usual time of onset: A baby can be breech at any point during the pregnancy. Many babies start out in the breech position. However, if a baby has not turned by the end of thirty-six weeks, it is unlikely that they will do so in the remaining few weeks of the pregnancy.

Symptoms: Usually none, but some pregnant women can feel their baby's head in their upper abdomen. More kicking may occur lower in the belly, near the cervix and bladder (ouch!).

Cause: Unknown, most of the time. Remember that! Most breech babies are completely healthy and have no medical issues whatsoever. Some situations make a baby feel "more comfortable" with their head up, instead of down. These include maternal uterine abnormalities (see Complication #35), large uterine fibroids or other pelvic tumors, ***polyhydramnios*** (baby has a lot of fluid to move around in), ***oligohydramnios*** (not enough fluid for a baby to move into head down position), ***placenta previa***, birth defects (hydrocephalus, hip dysplasia, for example), multiples.

Treatment: It is much safer to deliver them by C-section. There is substantially less risk of injury to the baby. ACOG recommends delivering all breech babies by C-section (except in the case of twins, when the second twin is breech). But there are some treatments that can move the fetus from a breech position to a head down position before delivery. These include:

- Acupuncture
- Prenatal chiropractor (always check with your OB provider first before seeing one!)
- ***External cephalic version*** (see the Warning box on page 509)

Issues for Mom: Increased chance of more procedures (external cephalic version, possible amniocentesis to assess lung maturity), increased risk of C-section.

Issues for Baby: Growth restriction, possible birth defects, ***cord prolapse*** if rupture of membranes occurs, premature birth (breech position doesn't cause preterm labor . . . many preterm babies just haven't had time to flip around or they are multiples). Check for hip dislocation at six weeks of life (see the Insider Secret box below for more info).

INSIDER SECRET:

The Link Between Hip Dysplasia and Breech Presentation

Breech babies have a slightly higher risk of having a hip deformity called developmental dysplasia of the hips. English translation: It's a hip dislocation similar to what you might see in purebred dogs. The abnormal formation of the hip(s) is what triggers the baby to move into a breech position. Pediatricians screen all breech babies at six weeks of life with a simple hip ultrasound to rule it out. Note: Hip dislocations are uncommon, even for breech babies, but it's something that docs don't want to miss.

COMPLICATIONS

WARNING:

What Is External Cephalic Version Anyway?

This is a procedure that obstetricians use to try to turn a baby who is currently not poised to come out headfirst (vertex presentation). Docs usually attempt this procedure at about thirty-seven weeks of pregnancy in a hospital that is equipped to offer an immediate C-section, should the need arise. Don't worry: The need rarely arises!

Here's how it goes:

- At the hospital, you get hooked up to a fetal heart monitor.
- You have an ultrasound done to be sure there is plenty of amniotic fluid and to reconfirm the position of the baby (because it's really embarrassing to try to turn a baby who is already in the head down position).
- You will have an IV put in, and your blood type should be known (because if you are Rh-negative you will need to receive a shot of RhoGAM).
- You will be offered an epidural. It seems crazy since you aren't in labor, but we have multiple studies showing a much higher success rate if an epidural is placed prior to the version compared to if it isn't.[16] With an epidural, you are more relaxed and so is your uterine muscle, making turning the baby easier. Talk to your doc about this option.
- Someone slathers a bunch of mineral oil or ultrasound gel (hopefully warm) over your belly.
- This is when the fun begins. Have you ever watched WrestleMania? One (or sometimes two) OBs put their hands on your belly, and by applying lots of pressure, attempt to turn the baby, via a forward or backward somersault, into the head down position. It hurts if you don't have an epidural.
- After this attempt, you get another ultrasound to see if your baby moved.

Why bother with all of this? If it turns your baby around, you have the chance to have a vaginal delivery.

Are there risks? Yes, but they are quite rare. It's possible to cause a placental abruption, premature rupture of membranes, labor, and need for emergency C-section. So if your baby is breech, you should talk with your OB provider to see if an external cephalic version is an option for you.

Reality Check

External cephalic version is a procedure that is being done less and less in this country. Most breech babies are born via C-section.

Helpful Hint

Don't worry if your newborn looks frog-legged or their head is flat instead of round. It comes from lying in your womb right-side up instead of down. Your little one's head will round out, and the legs will straighten over the next several weeks. Your pediatrician will monitor your baby's head shape and neck mobility and may give your baby a home exercise routine to help stretch out. Yes, you will be your baby's personal trainer.

44. Transverse Lie

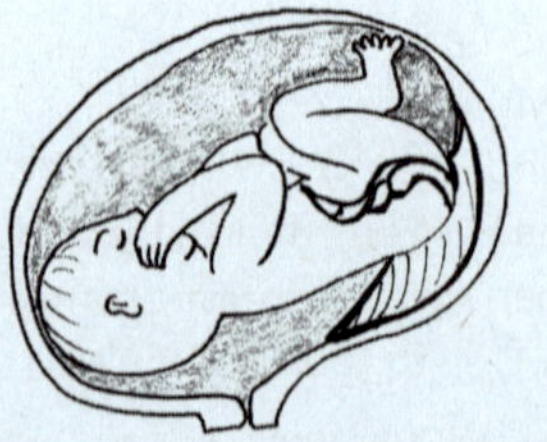

What is it? The baby lies horizontally (sideways) across your belly instead of head down (cephalic/vertex) or bottom/feet down (breech). In 99.5 percent of all term pregnancies, babies are either head down or breech. In 0.5 percent, they are lying in another plane, such as transverse. There are two types of transverse lie:

- *Back up.* The spine of the fetus is oriented upward. Their arms, hands, legs, and feet are the parts intending to exit the birth canal first (the "presenting part" at the cervix).
- *Back down.* The spine of the fetus is oriented downward. Their shoulder intends to exit the birth canal first (the presenting part at the cervix).

Most fetuses that are in the transverse position in early pregnancy turn themselves into a head down (***cephalic/vertex***) or feet/butt down (***breech***) position by the time labor occurs.

Usual time of onset: A baby can be transverse at any point during the pregnancy. It is often seen on an ultrasound early in pregnancy. If your baby has a transverse lie between twenty to twenty-five weeks, there is only a 2.5 percent chance they will be transverse at delivery. After thirty-six weeks, the baby has an 11.5 percent chance of being transverse at the time of labor.

Symptoms: Usually none. A woman might notice a different shape to her belly and feel the fetus's head on one side of her belly.

Cause:

- *Preterm delivery before thirty-two weeks*: Fetuses often don't turn into their final delivery position until after thirty-two weeks.
- *A uterus and abdomen with poor muscle tone*: You've had multiple previous pregnancies.
- *Twins:* The second baby to deliver is more likely to be transverse.
- *Polyhydramnios*: Too much amniotic fluid.
- *Pelvis issue*: Mom's pelvis is too small or abnormally shaped.
- *Extremely large pelvic tumors*: Fibroids or ovarian cysts limit the baby's ability to get into the desired delivery position.
- *Uterus issue:* Mom's abnormal uterus (see Complication #35) also limits the baby's delivery position options.

Treatment: Don't panic. Most babies will turn themselves before labor begins.

- Attempt external cephalic version (see the Warning box on page 509)—there is a 50 to 60 percent success rate.
- Consider acupuncture (unknown success rate).
- C-section, if baby remains in a transverse lie position.

Issues for Mom: Transverse lie is easily treated and unlikely to cause any problems when there is access to excellent medical care. You might have to endure an external cephalic version or C-section. One very rare problem: Rupture of membranes might allow the umbilical cord to come through the cervix into the vagina because there is no head or bottom "blocking" the cervical opening (called a cord prolapse). Even with a cord prolapse, you would probably have enough time to get to the hospital and undergo a cesarean delivery. In underdeveloped countries with inadequate prenatal care, trying to deliver a baby in a transverse lie can be fatal for both mom and baby. That's because these countries may lack adequate medical facilities to perform a C-section.

Issues for Baby: Risks associated with C-section, lack of oxygen or nutrients if cord prolapse occurs (very rare).

O. Size

45. Macrosomia or "Large for Gestational Age" (LGA)

What is it? Big baby. An LGA baby's birth weight is equal to or greater than the ninetieth percentile for a specific gestational age. Macrosomia means the baby weighs over 4 to 4.5 kilograms (8 pounds 13 ounces to 10 pounds), regardless of gestational age. Ten percent of all babies born in the United States weigh more than 8 pounds, 13 ounces, but only 1.5 percent weigh more than ten pounds, thank goodness!

Usual time of onset: Usually diagnosed in the third trimester. Difficult to diagnose. Ultrasounds can be imprecise.

Symptoms: None, other than a really big belly. Your OB provider suspects it when your ***fundal height*** measurements exceed what is expected for your due date. Periodic ultrasound measurements also show a larger weight than expected.

Cause: Here are your risk factors:

- You've already had one or more big babies.
- You were overweight before pregnancy.
- You gain excessive weight during pregnancy.
- You go beyond forty weeks.
- You were a big baby. (You can't control that one!)
- You had diabetes before pregnancy or have gestational diabetes.
- You are younger than seventeen years.
- You are Latina. Unfortunately, you have a better chance of having a big baby than your white, Black, or Asian friends.

Treatment:

- If you have diabetes, control your blood sugars.
- If you have excessive weight gain, meet with a registered dietitian to control further growth.
- Discuss delivery risks with your OB provider, especially if your doc suspects your baby will weigh over 4 kilograms (8 pounds, 13 ounces) and you are diabetic. Or if your baby is over 4.5 kg (10 pounds) and you're not diabetic.
- Discuss a planned C-section for fetuses suspected to be over 4.5 kg (10 pounds) or if you are someone who would appreciate not delivering a baby vaginally who is the size of a two-month-old.

Issues for Mom: Increased risk of a C-section (due to labor abnormalities), genital trauma during delivery (vaginal and perineal lacerations/episiotomies), shoulder dystocia, and excessive bleeding after delivery (postpartum hemorrhage).

Issues for Baby: Rarely, shoulder dystocia can cause nerve injury and occasionally collarbone fractures. Most babies recover without long-lasting problems. Big fetuses also have more trouble with the initial transition to life outside the womb, resulting in lower ***Apgar scores*** at five minutes and a chance of spending some quality time in the newborn intensive care unit. Overweight babies may also remain overweight as they grow up.[17]

46. Fetal Growth Restriction (FGR)

What is it? The short answer: small baby.

The long answer is complicated, so stick with us. Fetal growth restriction (FGR) refers to the limited growth of a *fetus* who is still inside you. If your baby is designated as "small for gestational age" (SGA), your baby is already born; SGA refers to the small *newborn*. A fetus with FGR is estimated to weigh below the tenth percentile for their gestational age. A newborn with SGA has a birth weight below the tenth percentile for gestational age.

SGA babies are either *symmetrically* growth restricted (the entire body is affected) or *asymmetrically* growth restricted (body weight is low, but head and length grow normally). This distinction is important because it helps determine the cause of the problem.

Usual time of onset: FGR is typically diagnosed in the late second or third trimester, sometimes earlier in the second trimester. Diagnosis is difficult and ultrasound can be imprecise.

Symptoms: None. Sometimes a woman notices that her belly has not grown or seems small. Your OB provider discovers that your ***fundal height*** measurements are below what is expected for how far along you are, and periodic ultrasound measurements of your baby will also show a smaller weight than expected.

Cause: FGR risk factors are listed below. It's also possible to have small parents and just be a small baby.

- *Certain maternal medical conditions*: High blood pressure (preexisting and ***preeclampsia***), kidney disease, lupus, blood clotting disorders (***thrombophilias***) like antiphospholipid antibody syndrome, chronic anemia, preexisting diabetes.

- *Abnormal placenta*: Placenta previa, partial placental abruption, placental mosaicism, subchorionic hematoma, placental tumors (very rare).
- *Maternal substance use*: Alcohol use disorder, smoking, use of cocaine or heroin, misuse of methadone.
- *Multiples*: With twins, the placenta is less able to handle nutrition for both (especially when there is only one placenta in monozygotic twins).
- *Certain infections*: Cytomegalovirus (CMV), rubella, chickenpox (varicella), syphilis, toxoplasmosis, trypanosoma (Chagas disease).
- *Genetic disorders*: Chromosome defects cause symmetric growth restriction.
- *Structural defects*: ***anencephaly,*** pyloric stenosis.
- *Teratogen exposure*: Amount and timing of exposure impacts the severity of the growth restriction. Examples: phenytoin (Dilantin), warfarin (Coumadin), methotrexate.

Treatment:

- If possible, figure out the cause. There's usually not much you can do, though, to improve a fetus's growth.
- If you had FGR in a prior pregnancy, talk to your OB provider about possibly adding in baby aspirin, which has been shown in some studies to help.[18]
- Get tested for medical disorders.
- Review any medications you need to take regularly.
- Stop smoking, if you are doing so. Get treatment for substance use or misuse.
- Deliver, if you are at term or anytime after the baby is viable, if the fetus is not growing at all after three to four weeks or if there is immediate concern for fetal well-being.
- Measure your baby by ultrasound every three to four weeks, if you are not at term.
- Periodically assess fetal well-being (non-stress tests, biophysical profiles, Doppler studies on the umbilical arteries).
- Modified bed rest, which means limited activity and no exercise other than short walks.
- Consider zinc supplementation, calcium supplementation, heparin, and maternal oxygen therapy. None of these have been proven to work, however.

Issues for Mom: Possible C-section, and lots of worrying. Sorry, we get it!

Issues for Baby: Although FGR is defined by being less than the tenth percentile, the babies most at risk are less than the third to fifth percentile. One-fourth of all stillbirths are SGA (some of whom also may have too little amniotic fluid).

So when does your doctor decide to proceed with delivery? It depends on your situation and involves your team of specialists. It's time if the fetus has not grown at all between ultrasounds three to four weeks apart or when tests don't confirm fetal well-being.

Your doctors weigh the risks of premature birth against the risk of potential fetal death. C-sections are more common because half of FGR fetuses have abnormal heart rate patterns in labor. Then these babies can have lower Apgar scores initially, and newborn problems that land them in the newborn intensive care unit.[19]

Reality Check

If you smoke, your baby has a three times greater risk of being small for gestational age.

Fact Check

A pregnant woman who eats poorly will have a small baby.

The truth: Studies of women living during famines at the time of World War II showed it takes a diet of less than 1,500 calories per day to affect fetal growth. It is highly unlikely that any poor diet in the United States would be less than that amount.

P. Other

47. Genetic/Chromosomal Defects

Several abnormalities may be detected by CVS or amniocentesis. If your baby is diagnosed with one of these disorders, you should have a consultation with a maternal-fetal medicine specialist or genetic counselor so that you and your partner will have a better idea of what this all means.

48. Post-Term Pregnancy

What is it? You have gone past forty-two weeks. We don't wish this on anyone, but it happens in 7 to 10 percent of all pregnancies.

Symptoms: You feel as big as a house and have irrational thoughts on how to induce labor.

Cause: Usually unknown. First pregnancies, boys more than girls, or your dates may be off. Rarely, things like a placental problem or fetal malformation can prolong a pregnancy.

Treatment:

- Tests of fetal well-being (non-stress test or NST, amniotic fluid index) after forty to forty-one weeks.
- Labor induction if your cervix is favorable (see ***Bishop score*** in Chapter 13, "Home Stretch").
- Deliver by forty-one completed weeks (forty-two weeks) due to risks to baby and mother (although many doctors prefer to deliver babies prior to forty-one weeks or forty completed weeks).

Issues for Mom: Longer and more difficult delivery, genital trauma due to the increased size of the baby, double the chances of needing a C-section, greater risk of stillbirth. Anxiety!

Issues for Baby: Big baby, shoulder dystocia, low blood sugars, seizures, temporary respiratory problems (***meconium aspiration***), infection, too little amniotic fluid, malnourished, increased risk of stillbirth.[20]

INSIDER SECRET:

What Overripe Means

Although we say pregnancy lasts nine months, it's really more like 9 ½ or 9 ⅗ months. A post-term or overripe pregnancy is one that has gone beyond forty-two weeks. About 7 to 10 percent of all pregnancies go post-term.

We know that it is every pregnant woman's nightmare to go a day over your predicted due date. You feel tired and heavy, and you are suffering from leg cramps and heartburn. Every night before you go to bed you pray to the labor gods to please, please, please, at some point before sunrise, make you wake up in a puddle of water or with painful contractions.

From a medical standpoint, doctors also prefer that women don't go too far past their due dates. Why? Why not just let everyone continue until that magical day comes and labor occurs? Well, there are a few risks, both to mom and to baby.

Your baby has an increased risk of stillbirth (the odds are 4 to 7 per 1,000 versus 3 per 1,000 in babies less than forty-two weeks), very large size (***macrosomia***), breathing problems (due to meconium aspiration syndrome) as well as problems related to outgrowing the womb (fetal dysmaturity). The placenta also ages or gets old. Just like our arteries tend to calcify as we age, the placenta does, too. A calcified, or in medical terms ***dysmature***, placenta doesn't work as well and doesn't always provide the right amount of nutrients and/or oxygen to the baby. This can lead to all of the above as well as fetal heart rate abnormalities before and during labor.

Some studies suggest that there is an increased risk of all of the above even after forty-one weeks.[21] Big babies (we are talking about ten-pounders) may have trouble getting through the birth canal, which occasionally leads to broken collar bones and nerve injury. Big babies also have trouble keeping their blood sugars up, which requires close monitoring.

Moms face risks, too. You're more likely to have complications during labor and delivery due to the baby's larger size. These include longer, more difficult labor; increased risk of injury to your vagina, bladder, and rectum; and an increased risk of C-section.

So, for all these reasons, your OB provider will probably suggest an induction if you are post-term.

Bottom line: For pregnancies that go past forty-two weeks, the risk of stillbirth is doubled compared to deliveries at term (37 to 40 weeks). Get the bun out of the oven!

DR. M'S OPINION:

Desperate for Labor?

I know you are desperate enough to do just about anything to go into labor. If you are considering eating hot sauce straight from the bottle . . . drinking gallons of red raspberry leaf tea . . . or walking for hours in the hot sun at an amusement park, without drinking water, while purposefully forgetting the stroller in the car and then having to carry a three-year-old around, we have a word of advice: don't. I tried all these things with my second pregnancy, and none of them worked!

CHAPTER 18

Infections

"I don't think nuclear war will ever get us, but germs will."

—Raymond Martin

What's in This Chapter

- **Group B strep**
- **Chickenpox**
- **Respiratory infections (colds, flu, RSV, COVID-19)**
- **Listeria and toxoplasmosis**
- **Vaginal infections**
- **Vaccines**

Germs don't really care if you are pregnant or not. They follow their mission statement: Infect whoever comes along.

Of course, *you* care about getting sick. First, you will worry that your infection might harm your unborn baby (see—you are already a parent!). Then, you will worry about yourself. It is true that you might become more ill because pregnancy lowers your defenses against infection (remember, this is only temporary).

The good news is that most of the usual players that cause infection—the common cold or stomach virus—are unlikely to have a major impact on your unborn baby.

But there are some infections that can be real problems for both of you, and we'll let you know which ones those are. We'll also cover the routine prenatal infectious disease screening tests and what they mean if they are positive. And since vaccines protect against infections, they are covered here as well.

Let's take a look at some of the common bugs (and vaccinations) during pregnancy:

- **Infections found on routine pregnancy tests.** These include chlamydia and hepatitis B.
- **Other serious infections.** Chickenpox and toxoplasmosis are included in this group.
- **Common infections.** From the common cold to sinus infections, this section also includes the flu, COVID-19, and ***bladder infections***.
- **Vaginal infections.** These include yeast infections, ***bacterial vaginosis***, and genital warts (HPV).
- **Vaccines.** We'll cover all the recommended vaccines in this section.

Helpful Hint: TORCH

TORCH is shorthand for a list of infections that can cause birth defects during pregnancy. If you test positive for one of these infections, you'll be followed more closely for the rest of your pregnancy. We'll discuss these throughout this chapter, but here are the offenders: T for toxoplasmosis, O for Other (syphilis, varicella, parvovirus B19 or fifth disease, HIV), R for rubella, C for cytomegalovirus (CMV), and H for herpes.

Infections Found on Routine Screening

1. Chlamydia/Gonorrhea

Q. I tested positive for chlamydia/gonorrhea. What does that mean?

Chlamydia and gonorrhea are sexually transmitted infections. Both are bacterial infections spread by sexual contact with the penis, vagina, mouth, or anus of an infected partner. They can also spread from mother to baby during delivery.

In gonorrhea, the bacteria grow and multiply easily in the tissues of the female genital tract (cervix, uterus, fallopian tubes).

In chlamydia, the bacteria initially infect the cervix, and the tube leading from the bladder to the outside (urethra). It can also spread into the fallopian tubes.

If untreated, both infections can lead to premature rupture of membranes, preterm labor, and delivery.

During pregnancy, you are screened for both in the first trimester so that if you test positive for one or both, you can be treated early in your pregnancy. People at higher risk may also be screened again in the third trimester.

It's easy to treat both infections with antibiotics. All sexual partners must be treated as well.

After finishing the antibiotics, return to your doctor for re-testing to confirm the infection is completely gone.

Note: It is very important that you not resume sexual relations with anyone who has not been treated. Talk with your provider for exact details.

2. Rubella

Q. My doctor told me that I am not immune to rubella. What is rubella, and what does this mean during my pregnancy?

Rubella (also called German measles or three-day measles) is an infection caused by a virus. Most adults of childbearing age today are immune to rubella because they were vaccinated during childhood with the MMR vaccine.

Ideally, it would be nice to know *before* you got pregnant if you were immune to rubella. You could then be vaccinated before conceiving. (The vaccine for rubella isn't given during pregnancy because there are theoretical health complications for the fetus.)

Women are routinely tested at the beginning of pregnancy to see if they are immune to rubella. If your blood work shows that you are not immune, either you were never vaccinated for rubella, your body never mounted an appropriate response to the vaccine (your body didn't make enough antibodies to protect you), or your immune response has worn off over time (your antibody levels have declined).

Rubella is not an infection you want to get while you are pregnant. Why? If infected with rubella in the first trimester, there is an 85 percent chance your baby will develop congenital rubella syndrome, which can lead to miscarriage, growth restriction, intellectual disability, blindness, deafness, heart defects, and other problems. Exposure to rubella later in pregnancy is also dangerous, but the risk is greatest in the first trimester.

The good news: Most folks are immune. In the United States today, *fewer than ten babies* are born every year with congenital rubella syndrome. Compare that to the 1964 epidemic (prior to the development of rubella vaccine), when 20,000 American babies were born with congenital rubella syndrome.

See information at the end of this chapter regarding the rubella vaccine.

Q. I got vaccinated for rubella and then found out I was pregnant! I'm really worried that I've done some kind of damage to my baby. Have I?

First of all, don't panic.

It is true that the rubella vaccine is not routinely given to pregnant women because it contains a live-attenuated virus. However, there has never been a single documented case of a fetus developing congenital rubella syndrome (severe birth defects) when a mom has accidentally been vaccinated during pregnancy.

It is extremely unlikely your baby has suffered any damage as a result of this vaccine. Of course, doctors err on the side of caution, so you'll probably be monitored more closely and have a few extra ultrasounds.

3. Human Immunodeficiency Virus (HIV)

Q. Why am I being tested for HIV?

HIV is the virus that causes AIDS. It is spread through sexual contact with an infected person or when infected body fluids (like blood and breast milk) come in contact with mucus membranes (inside the eyes, nose, throat, mouth, urethra, rectum, or vagina) or broken skin.

Babies can potentially get infected while developing in the uterus, at the time of delivery, and during breastfeeding. All women are routinely screened for HIV at the beginning of their pregnancies. Yes, it is possible to decline or opt out, but we do not recommend it. People who are at high risk of acquiring HIV can be tested again in the third trimester or at delivery. There are two key reasons:

- If you are HIV positive, you can get treated with antiviral medication. This is important because babies who are born to *untreated* women with HIV have a 25 to 35 percent risk of being infected. If you *do* get treated and don't breastfeed, your baby's risk of getting HIV is less than 2 percent.
- If HIV screening were only offered to women who were thought to be at high risk, OB providers would miss many women who didn't know they were HIV positive. And those women would unwittingly pass along HIV to their babies. Remember, HIV is just a virus—its job is to find another person to infect.

Q. I have had HIV for over five years. What do I need to know now that I am pregnant?

As you probably know, you can have the HIV virus without actually having developed AIDS (acquired immune deficiency syndrome).

Over time, the virus can replicate and may eventually decrease the strength of your immune system. This leaves you susceptible to infections and tumors. Symptoms may include the development of certain cancers (such as cervical cancer, skin cancer, or lymphoma), recurrent infections (such as pneumonia or chronic diarrhea), as well as symptoms including fever, night sweats, chills, weakness, weight loss, and swollen glands.

If you are HIV positive, your healthcare team will include an OB, a maternal-fetal medicine specialist, and an infectious disease specialist. If you are on a regular medication regimen and become pregnant, you should stay on that regimen and talk with your HIV specialist. If you are pregnant and just finding out that you are HIV positive, all of the commonly used multi-drug antiviral medications are safe to use in pregnancy, even in the first trimester. These meds significantly decrease the risk of HIV transmission to your baby, lowering it to 1–2 percent.

While a detailed discussion of HIV and pregnancy is beyond the scope of this book, the goal for any HIV positive woman is to keep her viral load less than 1,000. This reduces the risk of transmission to your baby and means fewer complications for mom-to-be.[1]

4. Hepatitis B and C

Q. I don't have any risk factors, but my doctor wants to test me for hepatitis B and C. Why?

Hepatitis B and C are two of at least six hepatitis viruses that infect the liver. Both viruses spread through sexual contact or contact with infected body fluids (like blood).

As you might know, those at high risk for hepatitis B and C are people who are sexually promiscuous, IV drug users, or who have received multiple blood transfusions throughout their lives (hemophiliacs). However, up to one-third of adults who get a hepatitis B infection are not in those high-risk categories and have no idea where they contracted the illness.

Hepatitis B became part of the routine childhood vaccination series in 1991. While many adults of childbearing age have been vaccinated, doctors still routinely screen all pregnant women to test for immunity or evidence of active or previous infection with hepatitis B. Women with certain risk factors are selectively screened for hepatitis C (for instance, if you have hepatitis B, you also might have hepatitis C).

Pregnant women who are carriers of the hepatitis virus require more specialized prenatal care. Your obstetric provider (OB provider) can discuss medication options as well as questions about delivery and breastfeeding.

If you contract hepatitis B in your first trimester, the fetus has a 10 percent chance of getting infected. If infected during third trimester, there is an 80–90 percent risk of fetal infection. Ninety percent of babies that are born to women with hepatitis B will become lifelong carriers of the disease *unless* they get readily available preventive treatment in the first twelve hours of life.

BOTTOM LINE: Knowing whether you have hepatitis B or C is best for you and your baby. The result is better care for mom and lower risk of spreading the infection to baby.

Q. I tested positive for hepatitis B. What comes next?

The test for hepatitis B gives one of three results:

- You have been vaccinated against hepatitis B.
- You were infected with hepatitis B in the past but no longer have the virus.
- You are a chronic carrier of the infection.

If you are a chronic carrier, your healthcare team should include an OB, a maternal-fetal medicine specialist, and an infectious disease specialist. You should avoid procedures like a ***CVS*** or ***amniocentesis*** (discussed in Chapter 6, "Tests"), if possible, because they risk introducing the infection to the fetus.

You will be able to breastfeed, as long as your baby receives an immune globulin shot and a hepatitis B vaccine after birth.[2]

5. Syphilis

Q. Why am I being screened for syphilis? Does that disease really still exist?

Yes. In fact, syphilis is more popular than ever, unfortunately.

Syphilis is more apparent in men than women—an ugly lesion on the penis is a dead giveaway (yuck, we know). But women with syphilis may not know it, since a lesion may not hurt or be visible.

A test for syphilis is routine at the first prenatal visit (and again in the third trimester for some high-risk populations).

What is the risk for babies? Syphilis infects babies through the placenta or during delivery. If mom is infected and does not receive treatment, there is an increased risk of miscarriage and stillbirth. If the baby survives, they could have congenital syphilis, which can cause blindness, deafness, and bone deformities among other problems. These are preventable with treatment.

Helpful Hint

Looking for more info on sexually transmitted infections? Check out the Centers for Disease Control website at cdc.gov/sti/index.html or call 1-800-CDC-INFO.

6. Group B Strep

See the "Third Trimester Tests" section in Chapter 6, "Tests" (page 146), for information about this infection, screening tests, and treatment.

Other Problem Infections

7. Chickenpox (Varicella)

Q. I've never had chickenpox, so my doctor tested me for it. I was not immune. What does this mean? Can this hurt the baby?

It's easy to do a blood test to see if your immune system has made antibodies to fight off the chickenpox virus (***varicella-zoster virus***). If your test comes back negative, it means one of three things:

- You have never had chickenpox.
- You have never been vaccinated against chickenpox.
- Your body did not mount an appropriate response to the disease or the vaccine.

Why is this important? Because contracting chickenpox for the first time during pregnancy can have a devastating impact on baby (see the discussion on page 524).

If you are not immune to chickenpox, you can get the vaccine after you deliver. Because it is a live-attenuated vaccine, it's not something you can get while you are pregnant. For now, it's best to stay away from young children. We know that is pretty tough if you are, say, a mom already or your job puts you in contact with kids (for example, you are a schoolteacher).

If avoiding little people is impossible, here is the next best advice: Stay home from work if there is a chickenpox outbreak. If your kids were vaccinated against chickenpox (at the twelve- to fifteen-month well-check), they probably won't bring it home.

Helpful Hint

The best time to discuss chickenpox is (ideally) at the pre-conception visit you have with your OB provider. Then you can do the test to see if you have immunity. If you are immune, you won't have to worry if you actually get exposed to someone with chickenpox (varicella) or shingles (zoster). If you are not immune, you can get vaccinated prior to getting pregnant.

Q. How is chickenpox spread?

Chickenpox is spread by coming into contact with an infected person's respiratory droplets (secretions from the nose and mouth in the air) or skin lesions (clear, fluid-filled mini-blisters).

Chickenpox is caused by varicella-zoster virus (VZV), which is a member of the herpes virus family (not the kind that is sexually transmitted, however). Like all herpes viruses, VZV lies dormant forever in previously infected people. So it's possible for the infection to reactivate later in life and cause shingles.

Unlike chickenpox, shingles infects only one group of nerves and causes painful blisters. These blisters contain the virus and are also contagious. But shingles does not spread by a person's respiratory droplets. It is uncommon for someone who isn't immune to get chickenpox by direct contact with the lesions of a person with active shingles. You would have to basically touch or stick your nose right up to the person's active shingles lesions to catch it.

However, with chickenpox, a person is very contagious with chickenpox for twenty-four hours (via those respiratory droplets) *before* the classic chickenpox rash appears. A non-immune person might be exposed to someone who doesn't know they have chickenpox until the next day. That's how these germs used to spread like wildfire through childcare centers and schools before the vaccine came out in 1995. And it's how a non-immune person might get exposed today.

People with chickenpox and shingles are contagious until all the lesions are crusted over.

Helpful Hint

If you are not immune, it takes about ten to twenty-one days to come down with chickenpox after you have been exposed. So breathe a sigh of relief if you are chickenpox free after three weeks.

Q. I have a one-year old, and I am pregnant again. Is it safe for my one-year-old to get the chickenpox vaccine and be around me afterward?

Yes! In fact, you want your child to get this shot and be protected as soon as possible.

The varicella vaccine is a live-attenuated vaccine, which means that your child will mount an immune response to it within one to four weeks of getting the shot.

Occasionally, children will develop a rash that looks like chickenpox when their immune system responds to the vaccine. That rash does *not* mean they have the disease. So you do not have to worry about getting chickenpox from your child.

Q. I found out I was not immune to chickenpox at my preconception visit, so I got the vaccine. I was already pregnant, though, and didn't know it. Will my baby be okay?

The chickenpox vaccine is not routinely given to pregnant women since the vaccine contains live viral particles. However, there has never been a documented case of birth defects or congenital varicella syndrome (see question below) in a fetus born to a pregnant woman who mistakenly received the chickenpox vaccine.

If this happens to you by mistake, yes, your OB provider will watch you more closely. No, you don't need to worry.

Q. I'm in my late second trimester and just got diagnosed with chickenpox. I'm stressed! What do I need to know?

First of all, don't freak out.

Congenital varicella syndrome (fancy words for a baby getting infected with the chickenpox virus while still in the uterus) most often occurs from exposure during the first twenty weeks of pregnancy. It is quite rare, occurring in just 1 to 2 percent of fetuses whose mothers have been infected.

Let's be clear, however: The syndrome is devastating. Babies have skin lesions that scar, abnormal limb formation, eye inflammation, small heads, and varying degrees of intellectual disability.

The other inopportune time for a pregnant woman to get chickenpox is five days before or up to forty-eight hours after delivery. The concern here is the newborn getting chickenpox (neonatal VZV infection). Because newborns have little defense to fend off the infection, death is often the result.

Perhaps the only time your baby would be unaffected by your chickenpox would be during the later part of second trimester. Your doctor will, however, keep a closer eye on the pregnancy.[3]

8. Cytomegalovirus (CMV)

Q. I am pregnant with my first child and work as a kindergarten teacher. My doctor wants to test me for CMV. What is that? Do I have to be worried?

CMV (cytomegalovirus) is another type of herpes virus that spreads through infected blood, saliva, urine, or sexual contact. It is extremely common, and one in three children will have CMV infection by the time they are five years old. By age forty, half of us have had CMV.[4]

Most of the time, people don't even know when they have the infection (which is why it's difficult to diagnose during pregnancy—or any other time, for that matter). Occasionally people feel like they have a flu-like illness with severe fatigue, chills, muscle aches, fever, and abnormal liver function. As a general rule, no one ever gets tested for CMV unless they are donating blood.

It's more likely that a CMV infection is detected after discovering something unusual at the second-trimester ultrasound. The diagnosis is confirmed with amniocentesis.

If a woman gets CMV during pregnancy, her fetus has a 30 to 40 percent chance of becoming infected. In the United States, about 1 in 2,000 babies are born every year with congenital CMV. Of those newborns, 90 percent are healthy and have no signs or symptoms of illness. But one in ten can have significant health issues at birth, some of which are lifelong. This may include hearing loss, a small head, varying degrees of intellectual disability, blindness, and death.

Although CMV is not part of the routine pregnancy screen at the first OB visit, many doctors do check patients who are at higher risk. Those patients include women who have other children at home, those who work with young children (schoolteachers, daycare workers, pediatricians, or pediatric nurses) or work with immune-compromised individuals (such as older adults or AIDS patients).

If blood work shows that you have already been exposed to CMV, you cannot be infected again, and your baby is not at risk. If you are not immune to CMV, you don't have to quit your job and live in a bubble. But you should take preventive measures to help decrease the risk of getting a CMV infection. These include:

- Wear gloves when handling dirty diapers, cleaning small children, or coming in contact with immune-compromised individuals.
- Wash hands vigorously after diaper handling.
- Wash hands vigorously after coming in contact with nasal and respiratory secretions.

Reality Check

CMV is the most common of all congenital infections. It is the leading cause of congenital hearing loss. If your newborn fails their first hearing test at the hospital (and fails again when it is repeated), they will be tested for CMV (via urine, saliva, or a blood test) and treated with an antiviral medication if they have the infection.

9. Parvovirus B19 (aka Fifth Disease or "Slapped Cheek")

Q. I work with kids and was exposed to a child with fifth disease (parvovirus), and I am totally freaked out. Will my baby be okay if I get the infection?

Parvovirus is a very common viral illness that most people get in childhood. It's also called fifth disease because it was the fifth viral illness identified to have a classic rash (called "slapped cheek").

And true to the name, kids get rosy red cheeks about a week or two *after* the time they were contagious with this minor illness. The most annoying part of this infectious disease is that kids have absolutely no symptoms when they are contagious. We only find out two weeks later that the kid had it and exposed their pregnant kindergarten teacher.

Most adults are immune to parvovirus because they had it in childhood. For the rare pregnant woman who actually isn't immune, parvovirus has the potential to cause ***anemia*** in the fetus and, *very rarely,* fetal death.

But you can relax. This is extremely rare. Most fetuses born to women who got parvovirus during pregnancy do just fine. Even if a fetus gets this infection, they tend to clear it all by themselves with no long-term impact. And it doesn't produce birth defects.

The greatest risk to your fetus is if you get parvovirus infection *before* twenty weeks gestation. However, you should talk with your OB provider if you feel you have been exposed at any point during your pregnancy.

If you have been exposed, first get a blood test, no matter how far along in your pregnancy. Odds are, you are immune already, and your blood work will confirm that. Case closed.

If you are one of the few adults who isn't immune, you should get retested three to four weeks later to see if you were, in fact, infected.

If you do contract parvovirus, your OB provider will check your fetus regularly by ultrasound to make sure they aren't becoming anemic, a very rare result of this infection. Doctors can also detect fetal infection by testing the ***amniotic fluid*** via an amniocentesis.

10. Toxoplasmosis

Q. I have three cats at home, and my doctor wants to do a special blood test on me. Should I be worried?

Your doctor wants to test you for toxoplasmosis.

Toxoplasmosis is a parasite that many animals, including cats, can carry. Humans can get the infection by being in direct contact with cat poop (such as when you change the litter box), being scratched or bitten by an infected cat, eating infected meat (particularly pork, lamb, or venison), or coming in contact with soil contaminated with infected cat poop or with unwashed, raw vegetables grown in contaminated soil.

Just a few more drops of blood from you (but, really, who's counting at this point?), and the lab can see if you have two different toxoplasmosis antibodies, IgM and IgG (see the following New Parent-to-Be 411 box to learn more about these antibodies).

Here's what the results mean: If you are negative for both, you have never been exposed to toxoplasmosis. You are *not* immune. Be very careful around your cats or any other cats, particularly strays, outdoor cats, and kittens. Do not change your litter box. Call your OB provider if you are scratched, bitten, or come in direct contact with cat feces, so you can schedule a blood test.

If you are negative for IgM but positive for IgG, you have been exposed to toxoplasmosis in the past. You *are* immune, so neither you nor your baby can become infected even if you are exposed to it again. Whew.

If you are positive for IgM and negative for IgG, it's possible you had a recent infection. But no test is perfect, and neither is this one. Sometimes, a patient's IgM antibody remains high for years after the initial infection. If your OB provider suspects you have a new infection with toxoplasmosis, you will probably need to get your antibody levels retested every three weeks.

NEW PARENT-TO-BE 411:

The Lowdown on Antibodies

If infections are the offense, antibodies are your body's defense—after your body sees a threat (virus, bacteria, parasite, or even a different type of blood), it goes into high gear and cranks out antibodies. These proteins are made by special white blood cells and are sent by your immune system to attack and kill the invaders.

Here's the important part to remember: Tests for infections actually look for antibodies. These antibodies come in several types; two of the most common are IgM and IgG.

When you get sick from ugly virus or bacteria du jour, your body makes IgM antibodies right away. Hence, a test that is positive for IgM means you've had a recent infection.

After the initial antibodies (IgM) do their magic, the body makes a cleanup crew: the IgG antibodies. These protect you in the future should that particular germ make a return visit.

Testing your blood for antibodies tells whether you have:

- Ever come in contact with the germ in question.
- Been exposed recently.
- Been exposed in the past.
- Been vaccinated against a certain bug, in some cases.

Q. My test came back positive for toxoplasmosis. What are the risks to my baby?

It depends. The key issue: When were you infected? That impacts your baby's risk of getting the disease.

In the first trimester, there is a 10 to 15 percent chance that your baby will be infected. The chance is 25 percent in the second trimester. In the third trimester, it is more than 60 percent.

The earlier in pregnancy the fetus is infected, the more severe the consequences. Most infants do not show signs of infection at birth, but between 50 and 80 percent of infected infants later develop problems such as eye damage/blindness, hearing loss, or intellectual disability. Other features of congenital toxoplasmosis infection include a rash, enlargement of the liver and spleen, fever, brain abnormalities, and seizures.

Q. Is there any treatment for toxoplasmosis?

Yes.

There is an antibiotic called spiramycin that may reduce fetal transmission by 60 percent.

However, even if mom is treated, this doesn't *eliminate* the risk of baby contracting the disease.

Doctors can tell if the fetus is infected by ultrasound, amniocentesis, and fetal blood sampling. If so, mom takes three more medications in addition to the spiramycin to attempt to lower the severity of the infection. Unfortunately, these meds rarely cure the infection. A maternal-fetal medicine specialist will do periodic follow-up ultrasounds to make sure the baby is growing appropriately.

11. Genital Herpes (HSV)

Q. I am twenty-two weeks pregnant and have a red bump on the outside of my vagina that is really painful. My doctor told me to come in for a culture. Can this hurt my baby?

Your OB provider probably wants to do a herpes culture or a more specific test (polymerase chain reaction, or PCR) on your lesion.

They will examine you first and decide if this painful red bump (or cluster of fluid-filled bumps) looks enough like herpes to warrant further testing. They will take a bit of fluid from the lesion for the culture and PCR tests. It can be a little painful, especially if you have a fluid-filled blister (vesicle) because your doctor needs to open it up to swab some of the fluid.

Your doctor may also do a blood test to see if this is your first episode of herpes. Antibody tests help determine if you have been exposed to herpes in the past or if the exposure is recent. Unfortunately, herpes tests aren't as helpful or specific as other infectious disease tests. Talk with your OB provider about the pros and cons of herpes testing, given your personal medical history.

People can harbor the virus for years before they have a first outbreak. And a first outbreak during pregnancy doesn't mean you were just infected (so resist making that phone call to the divorce attorney!).

A quick definition: *Primary herpes infection* is the first time you have a herpes infection (painful bumps or vesicles in the genital or rectal area) *and* have evidence that this is a new exposure (through a combination of blood work and a herpes culture).

It is rare to have a primary herpes infection during pregnancy. More common is a first outbreak with a known prior exposure—that is, you knew you had been exposed to herpes in the past.

It's more dangerous to have a primary herpes infection in pregnancy because it poses a greater risk to the fetus than if you have a recurrent herpes outbreak.

If you get a primary infection in the first trimester, the fetus is at risk for eye inflammation, a small head, and, rarely, skin lesions.

If you have a primary outbreak at delivery, the baby has a 30 to 60 percent risk of becoming infected. And once you have herpes, you have it for life. Newborns, in particular, can get very sick with a primary herpes infection. That's why a C-section is recommended if your OB provider detects an active outbreak at the time of delivery.

But don't get too alarmed. You can take prescription antiviral medication (acyclovir) once you recognize you have an outbreak or your OB provider diagnoses it. This helps decrease the duration of the infection and the risk of transmission to baby. Researchers have reviewed acyclovir use during pregnancy extensively over the past fifteen years. It is considered very safe.

Reality Check

Women who have a known history of genital herpes get acyclovir every day, three times a day, starting at thirty-six weeks. The reasons:

- To decrease the amount of virus that is being shed from the cervix and vagina, therefore decreasing the risk to your baby as they make their way down your birth canal.
- To decrease the chance of having an outbreak in labor and needing a C-section.

Q. I have had genital herpes for many years, long before getting pregnant. What precautions do I need to take? Can I still have a vaginal delivery?

You are in good company: More than 45 million adults in the United States have been infected with genital herpes.

Although it's possible recurrent herpes outbreaks can spread the infection to the fetus, the risk is very low (thought to be less than 1 percent). Scientists theorize this is because mom's anti-herpes antibodies pass through the placenta and protect the baby. Even if there is an active herpes lesion at the time of delivery, the risk of transmission to the baby is only about 3 percent.

Despite the low risk, be sure to report all outbreaks to your OB provider so that you can be treated with antiviral medication.

Starting at thirty-six weeks, you should take daily antiviral medication until you deliver your baby (see the Reality Check above for details).

Q. I've heard there are three medications that can treat herpes. Why is acyclovir preferred?

There are three prescription antiviral medications that are used to prevent and treat herpes: acyclovir, famciclovir, and valacyclovir (Valtrex).

We have the most safety information on acyclovir because the Centers for Disease Control and Prevention (CDC) asked drug makers to keep a registry of all pregnant women being treated with this drug over twenty-five years ago.

In this study, more than 700 women took acyclovir, and their babies were all healthy. Unfortunately, there isn't as much data on women taking famciclovir and valacyclovir during pregnancy, which is why they are prescribed less frequently.

All three medications have been proven safe in animal studies, though. (See the explanation of categories of drug safety in Appendix A, "Medications.")

However, valacyclovir is converted to acyclovir in the body, so most doctors are fine with its use.

BOTTOM LINE: It is much safer to take acyclovir than not to take it. The alternative (developing an active herpes infection that in turn infects your baby) is much worse.

Q. Do I need to have a C-section if I have an outbreak at the time I go into labor?

Yes.

A C-section is recommended for all women who either have an active lesion or feel an outbreak is imminent (burning, pain, or itching in the vaginal/vulva area) at the time of delivery. In one study, only 1.2 percent of babies born by C-section to moms with active HSV outbreaks contracted the infection versus 7.7 percent of infants who were born vaginally.

You can still have a vaginal delivery if you don't have an active outbreak or early symptoms that a herpes outbreak is about to happen (itching, tingling, or burning).

Q. Can I still breastfeed my baby if I have active genital herpes?

Yes.

Unless you have a lesion on your breast, you can absolutely breastfeed your baby. You can prevent spreading your infection by washing your hands obsessively. If you have an outbreak, make sure you wash your hands very well before coming in contact with your baby. And yes, acyclovir is safe to take while breastfeeding.

Q. I always get my outbreaks on the back of my thigh and butt. Can I still have a vaginal delivery?

Yes.

Your OB provider can simply cover the lesion with a bandage. But it is very important for your OB provider to closely examine your cervix, vagina, vulva, and rectum to ensure that there are no active lesions elsewhere. The good news: The odds are pretty low of you passing HSV to your baby when you have a recurrent outbreak. In fact, it's less than 1 percent.

12. Oral Herpes

Q. I get cold sores. Are these dangerous during pregnancy?

No.

Cold sores are those painful blisters on the lip that are fluid-filled and then scab over. They are caused by a different form of herpes simplex virus (HSV-1). HSV-1 is a cousin of herpes simplex virus-2 (HSV-2), the most common cause of genital herpes. (Yes, you can get HSV-1 in your genital area and vice versa if your partner has an active cold sore and you receive oral sex.)

Cold sores are not a problem for your fetus, but they can pop up more often during pregnancy while your immune system is suppressed. You can be treated with a topical medication or with antiviral medication taken by mouth, if necessary.

BOTTOM LINE: The biggest issue for the baby is *after* they are born. A person with active cold sores can spread the herpes virus to a newborn, who can in turn get pretty sick. Don't kiss your baby if you have an active cold sore.

INFECTIONS

Reality Check

If you suffer from cold sores or genital herpes, you may have more flare-ups during pregnancy.

NEW PARENT-TO-BE 411:

Neonatal Herpes

So what's the big deal about passing herpes on to your newborn? A herpes infection can go anywhere—including the brain, spinal cord, or eyes. While death rates from neonatal herpes are declining, 20 percent of babies that survive neonatal herpes have long-term neurological issues. There are about 1,500 cases each year in the United States, and one-third of them are due to HSV-1 (oral herpes). About 80 percent of babies who have neonatal herpes are born to moms who have no history of herpes infections.

13. Listeria

Q. I accidentally ate some unpasteurized cheese last night, and this morning I have a high fever with nausea and vomiting. Could this be listeria?

Yes.

Listeria is a bacterial infection most often caused by eating uncooked or undercooked meat (such as hot dogs, deli meat, or lunch meats eaten straight from the package), refrigerated pate or meat spreads, uncooked vegetables, smoked seafood (lox, kipper, jerky), unpasteurized dairy products (soft cheeses like Brie), and random foods like contaminated cantaloupes.

Symptoms include fever, body aches, chills, stomach pain, nausea, and diarrhea. It can feel like the flu or food poisoning. Occasionally, pregnant women infected with listeria can become very ill as the bacteria infects the bloodstream, lungs (pneumonia), or the lining of the spinal cord and brain (meningitis). Some infected pregnant women may only experience mild flu-like symptoms. Pregnant women are twenty times more likely to get listeria infections than other healthy adults.

Your doctor can prescribe antibiotics that can often prevent infection in the fetus . . . but only if symptoms are reported early. It can take several weeks before you feel ill, so report any symptoms to your doctor immediately.

If you have listeria, you will be followed more closely with ultrasounds to ensure the health of your baby. Rarely, the bacteria crosses the placenta and can lead to miscarriage, stillbirth, preterm delivery, or neonatal infection.

Q. How can I protect myself from getting this infection?

The best defense against listeria infection is a good offense. Here's how to avoid it:

- Thoroughly cook all meat such as beef, pork, and poultry.
- Thoroughly wash all raw vegetables before eating them.
- Keep uncooked meat in separate packaging and be sure to keep any liquid from the meat away from other foods.
- Avoid all unpasteurized dairy products.
- Avoid deli meats, cheeses, and hot dogs unless cooked until steaming.
- Wash your hands and all utensils (knives, cutting boards) thoroughly after coming in contact with uncooked meat.

Common Infections

14. Common Cold

Q. I have a cold. Will this harm my baby?

No. Your baby will be fine.

While the common cold is a minor illness, you are more susceptible if you are pregnant. And you'll probably feel more miserable with a cold when pregnant because your immune system isn't firing on all cylinders.

Check with your doctor if you:

- Run a fever over 100.4°F for more than two days straight
- Run any fever over 102°F
- Continue to have a runny nose or cough for more than a couple of weeks.

Check out Appendix A, "Medications," for approved over-the-counter medications to take for a cold while pregnant.

15. Sinus Infection

Q. I have had a cold for the last two weeks, and it is only getting worse. Do I have a sinus infection? Do I need to be treated?

Yes, and you may need an antibiotic to clear it up.

Pregnant or not, a cold that lingers for an extended time or seasonal allergies can be a perfect nesting ground for bacteria to invade your sinuses.

Even during pregnancy, you can use many of the same treatments that you would sans pregnancy. Try taking a hot shower or breathing in warm steam a few times a day. Saline nasal spray, acetaminophen (Tylenol), an expectorant (like Robitussin DM), or decongestant (like Sudafed) are all safe to use.

If you are not getting better after a few days or you have a fever (over 100.4°F), it's time to call your doctor. There are many prescription antibiotics and nasal steroid sprays that are safe during pregnancy. See Appendix A, "Medications," for details.

DR. B'S OPINION:

It's Okay to Have a Cold

I was a senior pediatric resident when I was pregnant with my first child. Needless to say, I suffered my fair share of viral illnesses thanks to my patients. But like you, I worried when I sniffled for the first time during my pregnancy. My OB's comment was, "This is the first of many colds. Relax."

She went on to remind me that it was a good thing because I was giving the antibodies I made to my unborn baby. Not that I felt a whole lot better coughing and sneezing while being pregnant, but at least I was reassured!

16. Influenza (aka The Flu)

Q. I have a fever, body aches, and chills. Do I have the flu? What do I need to do?

Yes, it sounds like you have the flu (technically, an influenza infection).

Although many people refer to the common stomach virus as "stomach flu," this *isn't* the flu. Influenza is a respiratory infection. You start off with fever, chills, body aches, and fatigue. The runny nose, sore throat, and cough come later. Every once in a while, you're unlucky enough to have some vomiting or diarrhea, too.

As a pregnant and thus temporarily immune-compromised person, you are more likely to suffer the complications from the flu: dehydration, pneumonia, meningitis, or bloodstream infection. This infection can also set off preterm labor.

So what should you do? For starters, you can do an at-home flu test (or a combo flu and COVID-19 test). But those tests can produce false negatives early in the course of the illness, and you need to be treated as soon as possible if you do have the flu. So if you feel sick, see your OB provider pronto, even if your home test is negative. You can take antiviral medication like Tamiflu (oseltamivir) to lessen the severity and length of your illness if you start it within forty-eight hours of the first symptoms. You can also take acetaminophen (Tylenol) and cough medication to relieve your symptoms. See Appendix A, "Medications," for details.

And drink lots of fluids to stay hydrated.

Reality Check

Pregnant women are five times more likely to be hospitalized for the flu than non-pregnant women. That's one reason why it is so important for you to get your flu shot!

Q. How do I avoid catching the flu?

Influenza virus spreads by contact with an infected person's cough or sneeze droplets. You can catch it by touching contaminated surfaces like a door handle or an ATM keypad.

Avoid catching the flu by frequently washing your hands and avoiding contact with people who are sick (folks are contagious for one day before symptoms start and until they are fever-free for twenty-four hours). Also limit touching your nose, mouth, and eyes.

Lastly, get a flu shot.

DR. M'S OPINION

When it comes to flu prevention, I no longer think the people who reach for the public bathroom door with a paper towel are nuts!

17. COVID-19

Q. I've had COVID-19 before and, thankfully, was not too sick. Do I need to worry about getting COVID-19 during pregnancy?

It's true, COVID-19 has the potential to be more serious during pregnancy.

This virus really needs no introduction but . . . A novel type of coronavirus called severe acute respiratory syndrome coronavirus 2 (SARS-CoV-2) or its nickname, COVID-19, entered our world for the first time in China in late 2019.

Shortly after the first positive case was identified in the United States, the World Health Organization declared "a public health emergency of international concern" on January 30, 2020. There are many other viruses in the coronavirus family that infect humans as well as other animals. But COVID-19 is unique in how incredibly contagious and easily transmissible it is to others and just how serious the infection can be. The virus is spread via respiratory droplets that stay suspended in the air for a period of time. Infected people begin to be contagious two days prior to symptoms—this then declines over a period of several days.

It is difficult to quantify how many cases have occurred worldwide, as more people now do at-home COVID-19 testing. But there are millions of cases worldwide and over six million deaths in the record books due to this nasty virus. There are likely far more cases than that.

Early in the pandemic, it became clear that the COVID-19 disease was more dangerous for pregnant women and the developing fetus. As we have discussed regarding other infections, pregnant women are uniquely at risk for becoming more seriously ill because they are functionally immunocompromised in order to be able to successfully carry a developing baby inside of them.

Pregnant women are more likely to require hospitalization, require respiratory support with mechanical ventilation, and develop high blood pressure (preeclampsia) or eclampsia if they have a COVID-19 infection. COVID-19 during pregnancy also makes it more likely for a baby to be born prematurely or be stillborn.[5]

ACOG recognizes the risk that COVID-19 infection presents to pregnant women. As a result, it continues to recommend COVID-19 vaccination during pregnancy based on the scientific evidence demonstrating both safety and protection against severe disease for both mother and her newborn.[6] Check out the vaccination content later in this chapter for details about COVID-19 vaccine.

INFECTIONS

Q. If I think I might have COVID-19, what should I do?

You should perform an at-home COVID-19 test (or better yet, a combination home flu and COVID-19 test) or see your primary care doctor or OB doctor to be evaluated. Believe it or not, some people are unlucky enough to have the flu and COVID-19 simultaneously.

Q. If I get COVID-19, can I take an antiviral medication?

Yes, you can safely take nirmatrelvir and ritonavir (Paxlovid) if your doctor prescribes it. You can also take oseltamivir (Tamiflu) simultaneously for the flu, if necessary.

18. Stomach Virus

Q. My toddler came home from daycare with a stomach virus, and now I have it, too. How can I tell if I am getting dehydrated?

People like to call it the "stomach flu," but this illness is not caused by an influenza virus.

If you get a stomach virus (rotavirus, adenovirus, norovirus), you may have one or more of these symptoms: nausea, vomiting, diarrhea (usually watery), abdominal pain/cramps, tiredness, achiness, and maybe a fever.

Less commonly, "the runs" can be caused by bacterial food poisoning (*E. coli*, *Shigella*, or *Salmonella*), or a parasitic infection (Giardia, for example). Any of these can cause wicked diarrhea. Red flags for these illnesses are blood or mucus in your diarrhea or more than a few days of symptoms.

The goal is to stay hydrated since you will lose tons of water in your poop. Dehydration can be pretty serious for pregnant women, sometimes leading to preterm labor.

After your vomiting stops, try to take small sips of a fluid other than water or milk (Gatorade, Vitamin water, 7UP, ginger ale) at five- to ten-minute intervals. If a little sip stays down, wait five to ten minutes and take another little sip.

If you take a big gulp, you will regret it—it will come right back up again.

Take acetaminophen (Tylenol) if you have a fever of 100.4°F or higher.

When to call the doc: if you are unable to keep liquids down for over four to six hours. You might need to be admitted to the hospital for intravenous fluids if you and the toilet bowl are spending too much time together. You can also call your OB provider from the get-go to help determine whether you have a run-of-the-mill stomach bug or something more serious.

19. Bladder Infection

Q. I'm peeing all the time and not that much comes out. It doesn't hurt like it normally does when I've had bladder infections in the past. Should I tell my OB provider?

Yes, you probably have a bladder infection or urinary tract infection (UTI).

UTIs are more common during pregnancy for a number of reasons, and women often have no symptoms. That's one reason docs check your pee at every visit. Typical symptoms include:

- frequent urination.
- urgency (the need to urinate immediately).
- blood in the urine.
- painful urination.

Your doctor will likely prescribe antibiotics to treat it. Drink more cranberry juice and water, and try to urinate often (don't hold it). Untreated UTIs can progress to kidney infections, which are far more serious.

BOTTOM LINE: Bladder infections during pregnancy may not hurt.

Reality Check

Up to 10 percent of pregnant women get bladder infections.

20. Kidney Infection

Q. My doctor is treating me for a bladder infection. I just started taking antibiotics, but now I have back pain, chills, and a fever. Is this a kidney infection?

Yes. Unlike urinary tract infections (which may not have symptoms), this time you'll know you're sick.

Symptoms include back pain on one or both sides, high fever, chills, nausea, vomiting, the need to pee immediately, painful urination, or blood in the urine.

Kidney infections require hospitalization for IV fluids and antibiotics. Your doctor will probably order an ultrasound to look for kidney stones or any obstruction. Once you improve, you can go home and take oral antibiotics for seven to ten days.

OB providers are aggressive about treating kidney infections because they can lead to:

- an infection in the bloodstream that can quickly spread to other organs.
- pneumonia.
- preterm labor and rarely (gulp!) death.

Since women who are susceptible to kidney infections can be repeat offenders, docs usually recommend a daily low-dose antibiotic after the first infection.

BOTTOM LINE: One to two percent of women get a kidney infection during pregnancy.

Vaginal Infections

21. Yeast Infection

Q. I am battling a yeast infection that just won't clear up. Is this a problem for delivery or for the baby?

It's not a problem for your baby, but it's a real pain for you. And it certainly interferes with any desire to have intercourse.

Yeast infections occur more often during pregnancy because of your temporarily depressed immune system. We all have a little yeast growing down there, but pregnancy allows overgrowth and thus you end up with white cottage cheesy vaginal discharge (sometimes it's yellow or green), vaginal irritation, burning, and itching.

The over-the-counter antifungal creams (clotrimazole, miconazole) are safe to use during pregnancy. But if you need a prescription antifungal, you and your OB provider will have to weigh the risks and benefits. See Appendix A, "Medications," for details.

If you are prone to yeast infections, it's wise to take a probiotic (the stuff found in yogurt and kefir) every day for prevention. The more good germs you have living in and on you, the less the yeast is able to grow.

22. Bacterial Vaginosis

Q. I have vaginal discharge, but it doesn't seem like a yeast infection. Is this a problem?

This may be a bacterial infection that causes irritation of the external genital area. Symptoms can mimic a yeast infection because external vaginal itching and burning are common. The increased vaginal discharge is often gray or yellow-white and has a fishy odor, particularly after intercourse. As opposed to a yeast infection that often has "cottage cheesy" discharge, this discharge is often thin and sometimes frothy. Now that we have forever ruined your appetite for cottage cheese, seafood, and beer, be sure to keep reading!

The bacterial culprit here is *Gardnerella vaginalis,* which all women carry around (it's not a sexually transmitted infection). Gardnerella overgrowth is the problem.

Ten to thirty percent of pregnant women will develop bacterial vaginosis (BV) during their pregnancy. In pregnancy, this can be more than just an issue of your bedroom smelling like Eau de Salmon after lovemaking. It has been linked to miscarriage, preterm labor and delivery, breaking your water bag prematurely, and low-birth-weight babies. Obviously, it's very important to tell your OB provider if there is a change in the color, smell, or volume of vaginal discharge!

It is easily treated with oral antibiotics or those inserted directly into the vagina.

DR. M'S OPINION:

More Than You Wanted to Know

Ah, vaginal discharge, the topic of many dinner conversations . . . at least the dinner conversations in my household, as there is an OB-GYN, an obstetric anesthesiologist, and a midwife in my immediate family!

The big question in pregnancy is what is normal and what is not? There is something called ***leukorrhea of pregnancy*** that usually starts to happen in the early first trimester. It's a set of big words that basically mean you will begin to suffer from a lot of vaginal discharge, and I mean a lot.

This is a normal phenomenon that occurs in most pregnant women as a result of the increased blood flow to your cervix and vagina. You will notice large amounts of thin to moderately thick, whitish-yellowish vaginal discharge. It is not clumpy. It is not brown or green. There is no strong odor. You will not have vaginal or external genital pain, burning, or itching. But I can tell you one thing—it is annoying. Any questions? Talk to your OB provider about it. They can decide if this is normal and rule out any infection.

23. Trichomonas

Q. I had a lot of vaginal discharge, so I went in to see my doctor. I have trichomonas. Will this hurt my baby?

This is a sexually transmitted bacterial infection caused by *Trichomonas vaginalis*. It infects the vagina and the cervix. In men, it infects the penis.

It causes yellow-green vaginal discharge, vaginal irritation, and lower abdominal pain. But about 40 percent of women don't have any symptoms at all. It's a problem during pregnancy because it can lead to premature rupture of membranes, preterm labor and delivery, low-birth-weight babies, and possible stillbirth. Very rarely, a baby can get infected while going through the birth canal.

If you test positive for trichomonas, your doctor will prescribe an antibiotic. The cure rate is between 90 and 95 percent, assuming that both you *and* your partner are treated. If you are in a relationship in which one or both of you are sexually active with more than one person, you should always use a condom during intercourse. Refrain from having intercourse with your partner or with anyone new until you and your partner have been fully treated with antibiotics.

24. Genital Warts (HPV)

Q. I have genital warts. Do these need to be treated while I am pregnant?

Yes, genital warts should be treated.

Genital warts are a sexually transmitted infection caused by human papilloma virus (HPV). The warts show up on your external genital area, around your anus, or on your cervix. They look like flesh-colored growths that often occur in clusters. Some clusters are little bumps, and others resemble cauliflower. They do not hurt but often cause itching.

Pregnancy can trigger an outbreak or allow existing lesions to grow more rapidly because of your depressed immune system and hormones gone wild. HPV is one of the most common sexually transmitted infections in the world. There are approximately 5.5 million new cases of sexually transmitted HPV infections annually. At least 20 million Americans are already infected.

Warts should be treated because their increasing size can obstruct the urethra (making it next to impossible to pee), cervix, and vagina (making it difficult to have a vaginal delivery if really large).

Warts are also a possible health risk for your baby. It's rare, but newborns can acquire HPV infection from their moms and get warts on the eyelids or in their throats (laryngeal papillomatosis).

Here are the safe treatment options during pregnancy: trichloroacetic acid (TCA), freezing (cryosurgery), burning (electrocautery), laser treatment, or, rarely, surgical removal.

Vaccines for You

Q. Should I be receiving any vaccines while I'm pregnant?

Here's a quick primer on vaccines and pregnancy. As we have discussed already, pregnant women are essentially immunocompromised to support a growing person inside of them. That puts them at higher risk of serious, significant illness with infectious diseases. That is one reason why certain vaccines are recommended for pregnant women. Additionally, the antibodies that a pregnant woman creates in response to vaccination are passed to the fetus. While these antibodies only last for the first several months after birth, they can provide temporary immunity and protection for a newborn.

The only vaccines given during pregnancy are inactivated ones. In other words, there are no portions of the virus or bacteria contained in the vaccine. Vaccinations for illnesses such as measles, mumps, rubella, or the nasal flu vaccine spray are live-attenuated vaccines, which contain a small fragment of virus that stimulates the immune response. While these are unlikely to be problematic during pregnancy, they are not recommended for this reason.

Q. I got a vaccination before I knew I was pregnant. Is this a problem?

Inactivated vaccinations are not a problem. Live vaccines carry a very small potential risk, which is why they are not recommended during pregnancy.

Typical scenario: A person comes in for a preconception visit and discovers that they are not immune to German measles (rubella) or chickenpox (varicella). They get their shots and are told to wait at least four weeks to conceive. But they end up becoming pregnant before that time. If this happens to you, no worries!

Although we do not give live vaccines during pregnancy because of a potential risk, there has never been a documented case of a fetus coming down with congenital rubella or varicella after a pregnant person was vaccinated either accidentally during the pregnancy or within the one month waiting period. And these are the most common live viral vaccines given to women of childbearing age near the time they conceive.

Reality Check

If a wild animal bites you, get a rabies vaccine whether you are pregnant or not.

Flu Vaccine

All pregnant women should get a flu shot—no matter what stage of pregnancy they are in during flu season.

Numerous studies show that pregnant women who receive the flu shot have a significantly lower risk of complications from the flu—particularly heart and lung problems.[7]

Remember, you are a temporarily immune-compromised sitting duck. You're more likely to get extremely ill or even die (it is rare but possible) from the flu. Studies also show that the flu shot does not harm the fetus at any point during pregnancy. In fact, the flu shot you get during pregnancy has been shown to protect your baby from this respiratory infection for the first six months of life. Newborns and infants whose moms get flu vaccine during pregnancy have a 40 percent lower chance of being hospitalized for flu.[8]

Here are some flu shot dos and don'ts:

- If you are going to be pregnant during flu season (October through April), talk with your OB provider about getting the flu shot.
- The flu vaccine immunizes against the most likely influenza strains expected each annual flu season, typically protecting against two A strains and one or two B strains.
- Yes, you can get a single dose, methylmercury preservative–free flu vaccine.
- No, you cannot get the flu vaccine in the nasal spray form while you are pregnant.
- Yes, you can and should get either the flu shot or the nasal spray while you are breastfeeding.

Fact Check

You can catch the flu from the flu shot.

The truth: The reason you cannot get the flu from the flu shot is because the viruses that are used to create the shot are inactivated or killed. This means they cannot cause the same illness as the live viruses. The shot may have some side effects that can mimic flu-like symptoms, like headache, muscle aches, fatigue, and a low-

NEW PARENT-TO-BE 411:

Mercury Rising

Mercury and vaccines remain in the news, but it is not in your flu shots in the United States. Here's a quick primer. Prior to 2025, the flu shot came in two flavors: 95 percent of the US flu vaccine supply was in individual doses (without preservative) and about 5 percent came in multi-dose vials (with preservative). What's the point of having a preservative, you say? Well, healthcare workers manually take a syringe and draw up vaccine from the multi-dose bottle of liquid several times. The preservative is necessary to prevent contamination of the remaining vaccine in a multi-dose vial (that's bad, trust us). Why not just make individual doses? Because manufacturers must make millions of doses of new flu vaccine every year, the multi-dose vials enabled them to meet the demand. Federal policy changed in 2025, and only preservative-free flu vaccines will be used in the United States. The preservative was never found to cause any health issues, but it's gone now, so it's one less thing you need to ask or worry about!

grade fever, but this is a sign that your body is reacting to the shot and building immunity. Alternatively, some people are exposed to the flu or a flu-like illness prior to getting the flu shot and have symptoms of that disease that they mistakenly attribute to the flu vaccine.

Tdap Vaccine

This is a combination vaccine that protects against tetanus, diphtheria, and pertussis (whooping cough). Whooping cough outbreaks are occurring all over the United States. Because the newborn immune system is weak, many babies have died from this infection. Here's a scary stat: About 70 percent of babies contract whooping cough from a member of their own household, most often their mothers. And newborns can't get the vaccine until two months of age (because the vaccine isn't very effective prior to that).

The vaccine is safe during pregnancy, and if mom gets the shot during the second or third trimester, the antibody protection can be passed from mother to baby, providing temporary immunity for the first several weeks of a newborn's life. As a result, the Centers for Disease Control and Prevention and ACOG recommend that women receive the Tdap vaccine with each pregnancy, preferably between twenty-seven and thirty-six weeks.[9]

Even with a history of vaccination, immunity to whooping cough (pertussis) wanes with time. The best way to protect your newborn is for you and others who will be spending time with your little one (including all family members and caregivers) to get a booster shot and prevent bringing pertussis into your home.

BOTTOM LINE: Anyone who is going to take care of your baby should be vaccinated—dads, grandparents, and so on. Teens and adults can receive a whooping cough booster vaccine that's given in combination with their tetanus shot (called the Tdap vaccine). Moms-to-be should get a Tdap shot with every pregnancy.

COVID-19 Vaccine

COVID-19 infection is something we have all been well educated about over the last few years, but something that most people don't know is that this infection can be more severe in pregnant women. The COVID-19 virus has become less virulent (dangerous) over the last few years compared to the initial few strains in 2020 and 2021. Although most people now get little more than a cold, pregnant moms that contract COVID-19 have an increased risk of being admitted to intensive care and are more likely to need respiratory support with mechanical ventilation. There is also a slightly higher risk of pregnancy complications such as preeclampsia and eclampsia, premature birth, and stillbirth. Because of these risks, albeit small, and because antibody protection produced by the mother is passed to the developing baby (a process called passive immunization), ACOG recommends that all pregnant women receive the COVID-19 vaccine.[10]

It is safe to get the COVID-19 vaccine during any trimester, and it can be given at the same time as other vaccines such as Tdap, the flu, and RSV vaccines. Talk to your obstetric care provider to make the best decision for you.

FEEDBACK FROM THE REAL WORLD:

Dr. B's Patient

A few years back, a mother that I knew well brought her four-week-old son into my office. After having three kids, her mommy instinct told her something was wrong.

The baby was having difficulty breathing. Yes, some newborns have "periodic breathing," where they pant for several breaths, pause, and then breathe again. But this was different. The baby would stop breathing and seemed like he couldn't catch his breath. He was having these episodes a few times a day, and it scared even this seasoned mom.

When I examined him, he appeared perfectly normal until he started choking. I turned to her and asked, "Are you afraid to sleep at night?" Her response: "YES!" That was enough for me: This baby needed to be in the hospital.

The diagnosis: whooping cough. The baby had horrible coughing spells during which he would turn red, choke, and gasp for breath.

It turns out that his mom had a hacking cough toward the end of her pregnancy that she just couldn't shake. It continued in the weeks after she delivered, but she was too busy taking care of her newborn to worry about herself. Mom had whooping cough and gave it to her son.

Fortunately, there was a happy ending. After several scary days in the hospital receiving oxygen and constant monitoring, the boy went home and made a full recovery. Today, he is a healthy, thriving kid.

But not all babies who get whooping cough are so lucky.

That's why it is so important to get vaccinated against this disease. Whooping cough often spreads from adults to those who are the most vulnerable—our babies, who, like my patient, are too young to be vaccinated.

Remember, your baby can only be protected if everyone around them is vaccinated.

RSV Vaccine

RSV, short for respiratory syncytial virus, is a nasty respiratory infection that routinely shows up every fall and winter. It can make babies severely ill, causing difficulty with breathing and dehydration. In fact, it has been the most common cause of hospitalization of infants in the United States in modern times.

There are two different ways to protect your little one from RSV. Both options have significantly reduced severe RSV infections and hospitalization rates in infants since 2023.

Option 1: Get the RSV vaccine during pregnancy. It is an option for pregnant women who are thirty-two to thirty-six weeks pregnant during September through January. It takes two weeks for the antibodies to be passed to the unborn baby, and protection lasts about six months.

Option 2: Give the RSV antibody shot (nirsevimab or clesrovimab-cfor) to your baby after birth. Unlike a vaccine, it provides immediate and long-acting antibody protection without the baby having to work to mount an immune response. All babies under eight months of age whose pregnant mom did not receive the RSV vaccine can get this shot if they are born during RSV season, from October to March. Protection lasts about six months. Children from eight months through nineteen months of age are eligible if they have certain health issues. Newborns can get it at the delivery hospital or at their pediatrician's office.[11]

Hepatitis A Vaccine

The hepatitis A vaccine can be given to pregnant women if they are planning to travel to areas of the world where hepatitis A is more common. It is given in two separate doses, six to twelve months apart.

Rubella Vaccine

The rubella vaccine cannot be given during pregnancy. But if you discover you are not immune, you should absolutely be vaccinated after delivery. Then there are no worries about rubella if you get pregnant again.

Currently, the rubella vaccine is not available in the United States as a single shot. Therefore, you will be vaccinated after delivery with the MMR (measles, mumps, rubella) vaccine. It is safe to get this vaccine even if you are nursing.

Partner Tip

Want to protect your baby? Go get your flu shot, COVID-19 shot, and Tdap booster, too. It's always good to take one for the team.

Infection Prevention

Q. What can I do to boost my immune system while I'm pregnant?

The best thing you can do to support your immune system is to give it the rest and nutrients it needs to function properly. In short, eat right and sleep well. Getting a professional or spouse massage regularly wouldn't hurt, either.

Feel free to take extra vitamin C, zinc, or echinacea—we won't guarantee they will work, but they are safe during pregnancy. We do, however, discourage drinking green tea on a regular basis while you are pregnant. Yes, it is rich in antioxidants. And yes, the active ingredient, epigallocatechin gallate (EGCG), may be beneficial in preventing some types of cancers. But EGCG also interferes with the way the body metabolizes folic acid (folate)—and folic acid is essential to prevent neural tube defects in babies.

CHAPTER 19

Advanced Maternal Age

"Thirty-five is when you finally get your head together and your body starts falling apart."

—Caryn Leschen

What's in This Chapter

- **What it means to be "AMA"**
- **Concerns**
- **Older dads**
- **Delivery issues**

Congratulations! You are among a growing trend of moms-to-be who have a baby later in life. You're ecstatic . . . but concerned about all the risks you keep hearing about—from the media, from your friends, and from your mother (who had three kids by the time she was twenty-six!). We'll go over what you need to know as you dive into pregnancy with more life experience. Find information regarding additional tests you will be offered (including ***amniocentesis*** and ***CVS***) in more detail in Chapter 6, "Tests."

What It Means

Q. I don't feel old. Why am I labeled as "advanced maternal age," or AMA? Isn't forty the new thirty?

The definition of ***advanced maternal age (AMA)*** is any woman who will be thirty-five years of age or older at the time she gives birth to her baby.

Many women today choose to delay childbearing until later in life for a variety of reasons. More women are completing advanced degrees or are busy building careers in their late twenties and early thirties. There is more access to assisted reproductive technology like IVF that help many women conceive later in life. Women are getting married later in life, and some women in their second and third marriages want to have additional children. Whatever the reason, it's trendy to have a baby after age thirty-five. In 1970, 1 in 100 babies were born to moms over age thirty-five. Today, that number is one in five.[1]

Even if forty is the new thirty for many of life's adventures, Mother Nature has not modified her definition when it comes to having babies. You still get the "AMA" rubber stamp on your medical record if you are thirty-five or over.

Q. Are there any advantages to having a baby at this time in my life?

Yes!

Your life experiences may make you more prepared for the rigors of parenthood. Older parents-to-be are usually more educated, and that translates into being more informed.

And, as an added bonus, you are more likely to be financially secure and have better health insurance.

Q. Is it harder for me to become pregnant?

Short answer: yes.

As a woman ages, she has more menstrual cycles where she does not release an egg (***ovulate***). If there is no egg around to fertilize, there's no chance of becoming pregnant! There is a 20 percent chance of a twenty-year-old couple getting pregnant in any one menstrual cycle. That drops to a 3 to 5 percent chance of this happening by the time a woman is forty.

Both egg quality and quantity begin to decline as a woman enters her thirties and forties. And the older a woman gets, the more likely she is to have other issues that may make conception more difficult: ***endometriosis***, ***uterine fibroids, pelvic inflammatory disease***, scarring of the fallopian tubes from previous pelvic surgery, and chronic health conditions like diabetes or thyroid disease.

Although the technical definition of "infertility" is no conception after one year of regular sexual intercourse, the real-life definition of infertility is shorter. The clock is ticking—and there is less time to sit around and see if a thirty-five-year-old woman can become pregnant. Schedule a consultation with your OB provider if you are over the age of thirty-five and have been trying regularly to conceive for six months without success.

BOTTOM LINE: You'll probably still get pregnant, but it just may take more time. It usually takes a woman over age thirty-five about twelve to twenty-four months to conceive.

Concerns During Pregnancy

Q. Are there any more risks during pregnancy because I am a little older?

Yes, but the good news is that most women in their late thirties and early forties end up having perfectly healthy babies. Don't let the list below freak you out.

Here are the risks to keep an eye on:

- **Miscarriage.** The risk is greater because AMA moms are more likely to have a fetus with a major genetic (chromosome) problem.
- **Gestational diabetes.** You are twice as likely to have gestational diabetes as your younger preggo friends.
- **High blood pressure.** There is a greater chance of both ***gestational hypertension*** and ***preeclampsia***.
- **Other medical problems.** You may have some preexisting health problems that can complicate pregnancy (high blood pressure, lupus, diabetes, kidney problems).
- **Placenta problems.** ***Placenta previa*** and placental insufficiency are more common.
- **Preterm delivery.** Women over age thirty-five are 50 percent more likely to deliver before thirty-seven weeks.
- **Low birth weight.** Preterm delivery and having a low-birth-weight baby go together.
- **Stillbirth.** The risk is only *slightly* greater as you age. Women in their twenties have a 4 in 1,000 chance of a stillbirth. Women thirty-five to thirty-nine have a 5 in 1,000 chance. Women forty to forty-four have a 7 in 1,000 chance.[2]

We know all of that can be scary to read. But, like we said in the very first sentence, most women in their late thirties and early forties end up having completely normal pregnancies and, subsequently, normal babies. There is no magic about the day you turn thirty-five where suddenly you are at a much higher risk of pregnancy complications. The risks are small, and we just want you to be aware.

ADVANCED MATERNAL AGE

Reality Check

At thirty-five years of age, the risk of having a fetus with any chromosomal abnormality is 1 in 204. At age forty, that number is 1 in 63. At age forty-five, it is 1 in 19.[3]

Q. Does my risk of miscarriage go up as I get older?

Yes. Miscarriage rates increase with a woman's age.

Studies show that a woman in her twenties has a one in ten chance of losing a recognized pregnancy to miscarriage. A woman who is thirty-five to thirty-nine has a one in five chance. By the time a woman is forty to forty-four years old, she has a 50 percent chance of miscarrying.

The risk goes up primarily because the older you are, the more likely you will conceive a fetus with a major chromosomal defect.

About 85 percent of all miscarriages occur in the first trimester (no matter how old you are).[4]

Q. I'm thirty-six. Is there anything I can do to try to decrease my risk of complications once I get pregnant?

Most of these risks are out of your control. But having a pre-conception visit with your OB provider is helpful if you are not pregnant yet. That gives you a chance to discuss any preexisting health conditions or medications you take regularly with your OB provider. You can start a prenatal vitamin, aim for an ideal body weight, exercise, cut out any bad habits (smoking, alcohol, substance use), get any necessary vaccinations, and take good care of yourself.

But if you are like most of us who do not plan our pregnancies, start those healthy habits now and go to all your prenatal appointments with your OB provider.

Q. Are there any risks to the developing fetus due to my age?

Yes. Genetic defects aside, babies born to moms with advanced maternal age have a slightly greater risk of having some birth defects. Note: We used the word *slightly*, folks. Most babies are healthy and born with ten fingers and ten toes.[5,6]

Q. Should I do additional testing during pregnancy because of my age?

Yes. But the beauty of modern medicine is that every woman who is thirty-five or older does not automatically need to have an amniocentesis. With the advent of noninvasive prenatal screening, fewer women need to get amnios. Take a look at Chapter 6, "Tests," for information on chromosome testing options. The American College of Obstetricians and Gynecologists recommends that women who will be thirty-five or older at the time of delivery be offered diagnostic prenatal testing to diagnose (or, far more likely, rule out) ***Down syndrome*** and other chromosomal problems. Prenatal tests include amniocentesis and chorionic villus sampling (CVS). Most women who have these tests learn that their baby does *not* have a chromosomal problem.

Q. Are older moms and dads a double whammy?

Possibly.

Let's face it—if you are over age thirty-five, it's likely your partner is, too. If both mom and dad are of "advanced" age, there is a greater (although very small) risk of having a baby with a genetic defect. The chances of having a baby with Down syndrome go up significantly if a mother is forty or older *and* the father is thirty-five or older.[7]

It's worth your time to have genetic counseling if you and your partner are AMA and APA.

Reality Check

If you put off childbearing until later in life, you are more likely to need fertility treatments. Over one-third of fertility treatments are performed on women over age forty.

Both advanced maternal age and fertility treatments increase your chances of having multiples. AMA and multiples are a recipe for a high-risk pregnancy.

Partner Tip

Remember your partner may find being stamped as "advanced maternal age" a bit depressing. Treat any discussion of these issues with kid gloves. And do whatever it takes to remind your partner how young she really is!

INSIDER SECRET:

Hey O-Daddy (Older Daddy)!

Okay, guys, while you mostly hear about moms being older during pregnancy and the potential risks, you are not off the hook. Dads who are over the age of forty at conception are considered advanced paternal age (APA). Why is this a potential issue? Well, the reality is that there are more abnormalities with the DNA in older sperm. And with increasing age comes increased exposure to environmental factors that can also negatively impact the health of the sperm (the medical term for this is epigenetics).

APA dads have kids with a greater risk of autism spectrum disorders (almost six times the risk),[8] autosomal dominant chromosome mutations such as achondroplasia and Marfan syndrome, and neurodevelopmental disorders such as schizophrenia.[9]

There may also be a slightly increased risk of certain types of childhood leukemias and brain/spinal cord cancer in kids whose dads are older. There's a reason that the American Society of Reproductive Medicine recommends sperm donors be under age forty (besides the fact that it's easier for younger guys to produce a specimen!). If you compare a thirty-year-old to a fifty-year-old, older guys have fewer sperm, the sperm move around less, and almost one in five sperm are abnormal.

If you are a father-to-be who is fifty or older, there is a greater risk of miscarriage or later fetal loss during pregnancy. While this may all sound like doom and gloom, the good news is that most babies born to more mature daddies are very healthy.

Delivery Considerations

Q. Are there any more risks during labor and delivery because of my age?

Yes. Because as much as you don't want to hear this, your body is older. But overall, you have a very low risk of encountering a problem! The risks include a slightly increased risk of having a preterm delivery (before thirty-seven weeks), having a longer labor, needing a C-section (see more below) and having a postpartum hemorrhage.

Q. Is there any greater risk of having a C-section since I am older than thirty-five?

Yes. Your odds of needing a C-section go up as your age does.

First-time moms over age forty are twice as likely to have a cesarean delivery compared to first-time moms under age thirty. Here are the percentages of first-time moms who have a C-section, based on their age:[10]

- 48 percent of first-time moms over age forty
- 36 percent of first-time moms between thirty and thirty-nine
- 27 percent of first-time moms under age thirty

BOTTOM LINE: Okay, we realize some of this sounds quite depressing. But remember the vast majority of moms over thirty-five give birth to babies who are just fine. And thanks to modern medical science, many of the risks and concerns can be minimized or eliminated. So feel free to have a positive outlook. The odds are in your favor!

CHAPTER 20

Preterm Labor and Babies

"Some babies are born in nine months, by the clock.
Some babies are born, and they sit up and talk.
Some babies are born, and no doctor is there.
But some babies come in on a wing and a prayer."

—Garrison Keillor

What's in This Chapter

- **Signs of preterm labor**
- **Welcome to the NICU**
- **Babies born at less than thirty-four weeks**
- **Late preterm infants**
- **Early term infants**

No one is really prepared to have a baby *before* nine months of pregnancy, but it happens in about one in ten pregnancies. This is reality. Think of this chapter as another one of those "this wasn't in the game plan" discussions.

Thanks to medical advances, OB providers can stall many preterm labors long enough to make delivery safer for the baby. Modern medicine has also come a long way in improving both the short- and long-term outcomes of babies who make a crash-landing arrival.

This chapter will get you through the shock and awe of discovering you are delivering before you've had time to paint the nursery. It will answer the obvious questions swirling around in your head. *Am I actually going to deliver this baby now? How long will my baby stay in the hospital? How sick will my baby be? What lies ahead for our family?* This chapter, above all others, demonstrates why it's nice to have both an OB and a pediatrician here to help you with your pregnancy!

Preterm Labor

Q. How will I know if I am in preterm labor? What are the signs?

The signs of preterm labor often mimic the signs of full-term labor, except they happen before you have reached thirty-seven weeks of pregnancy.

These symptoms include:[1]

- Dull ache in your lower back
- Episodes of hardening or tightening in the lower part of your belly that last thirty to sixty seconds
- Menstrual-like cramping that either comes and goes or is constant
- Increase in vaginal discharge (which may be blood-tinged)
- Feeling of pressure in your pelvis
- Feeling like you need to pee or poop but nothing is coming out

You may have any or all of these symptoms. If something seems awry, get it checked out.

Helpful Hint

Be specific. Tell your OB provider exactly what you are feeling so they have a better idea of what is going on with your body. This is serious—it may save your baby.

Q. What causes preterm labor?

There are many possible causes of preterm labor.

These include bleeding between the uterus and placenta (***subchorionic hemorrhage*** or ***placental abruption***), an overdistended uterus (caused by ***polyhydramnios*** or multiple babies), bacterial infections, and hormonal changes (possibly caused by fetal or maternal stress).

But often, doctors can't find a reason for why a woman goes into preterm labor.

Reality Check

About 10 percent of all births in the United States are babies born before thirty-seven weeks gestation.[2]

Q. My first baby was born prematurely. What are the odds it will happen with this pregnancy?

Your risk is six to eight times greater than a woman who has never had a premature delivery. Your OB provider should keep a close eye on you!

Q. Is there any way to predict if I am at risk for going into preterm labor?

There are a few things that may put you at risk. Your risk is higher if you:

- Are younger than seventeen years of age
- Are older than forty years of age
- Weighed less than 110 pounds before becoming pregnant
- Had a previous preterm birth
- Are pregnant with multiples
- Have a shortened ***cervix*** (your doctor can tell you that) or had a procedure on your cervix that might put it at risk for shortening, such as a loop electrosurgical excision procedure (LEEP) or a conization.
- Had vaginal bleeding at any point during your pregnancy
- Have high blood pressure and protein in urine (***preeclampsia***)
- Are Black American

As you can see by this list, most factors are out of your control.

Q. If I am at risk, is there anything to do to prevent preterm labor?

Short answer: Some things (beyond praying) *may* help prevent labor.

Although we don't usually recommend ***bed rest*** anymore (reclining and relaxing all day), ***pelvic rest*** (no sex, tampons, or douching) and having weekly visits with your doc are very important.

Those extra visits will include frequent ultrasound measurements of your cervix until about thirty-two weeks. The shorter your cervix is before thirty-two weeks, the higher your risk of delivering early. After thirty-two weeks, your OB provider will measure it by doing regular vaginal exams. You may also get screened for specific vaginal infections. In some situations, your OB provider may treat you with progesterone supplementation (see the Insider Secret box on page 554).

Q. What does bed rest really mean?

It means what it says!

If your doctor meant for you to be doing the laundry or shopping for groceries, it would not be called bed rest. Now, your doc may give you some "get out of bed" passes here and there. But in general, you need to hang out in bed or on the couch.

This gives your cervix a break from the weight of your uterus, lowers your blood pressure, and forces you to rest. All these things can help your pregnancy progress a bit further and give your baby more time to mature.

Just to be clear, strict bed rest isn't really a thing anymore because there can be serious downsides to it (mainly an increased risk of a deep vein thrombosis or pulmonary embolism).

Most providers will recommend modified bed rest or pelvic rest, but rarely strict bed rest.

INSIDER SECRET:

Using Progesterone to Prevent Preterm Birth

In 2003, what was initially thought to be an extremely important study conducted by researchers working with the National Institutes of Health reported that progesterone therapy during pregnancy significantly lowered the risk of recurrent preterm delivery for women with a history of unexplained preterm birth. Several smaller subsequent studies confirmed this finding, and, as a result, weekly intramuscular progesterone therapy was recommended by the American College of Obstetricians and Gynecologists and other agencies. However, the company that studied and marketed the progesterone injections delayed conducting and reporting follow-up studies that were required by the FDA when they initially approved the drug for use. When the follow-up study was ultimately completed and reported in 2019, the benefits of progesterone were no longer identified. As a result, in 2020, the FDA withdrew support for progesterone to prevent recurrent preterm birth, followed by reversal of the previous recommendations that were issued by ACOG, the March of Dimes, and the Society for Maternal-Fetal Medicine. Currently, no preventive interventions are approved or recommended for prevention of recurrent preterm delivery. Additionally, current evidence does not support the routine use of progesterone in women with multiple gestations.[3]

Phew! Okay, we know that was a lot of information! For those of you who used progesterone in a prior pregnancy, you should not worry. There was no harm noted to mom or baby—it simply was just not effective in preventing preterm births.

Bottom line: Unfortunately, there are no preventive measures that have been shown to prevent recurrent preterm birth for a pregnant woman with that history. Vaginal progesterone may be suggested, but, like injected progesterone, it hasn't been shown in large studies to be helpful. Vaginal progesterone is recommended for use in women who are incidentally found to have a short cervix in the 2nd trimester, to lower the risk of preterm birth for them, but that is its only current recommended indication in pregnancy.

Q. Is there a way to stop preterm labor once it starts?

Yes, but it depends on the individual situation.

The good news is that 80 percent of women who have signs and symptoms of preterm labor will *not* have a preterm delivery. Part of this depends on whether or not your OB provider identifies a treatable cause of preterm labor. It also depends on if you have any other complications with your pregnancy.

For example, if a woman comes into the hospital at twenty-eight weeks with contractions occurring every five minutes and a cervix that is dilated to two centimeters, there is a good chance her labor may be stopped.

But suppose that same women comes into the hospital at twenty-eight weeks, with contractions every five minutes, her cervix is five centimeters dilated, *and* she has moderate vaginal bleeding due to a placental abruption. In the latter case, it is likely that her labor will not stop. It is also likely that her OB will not try to stop her labor because it is safer for the fetus to deliver a little early than to remain in the uterus with a placenta that is coming off prematurely.

The point is there are many variables that determine whose preterm labor gets treated and whose doesn't.

If your doctor decides to try to stop your preterm labor, they will have a few medication choices at their fingertips. There is no clear first-line drug when it comes to treating preterm labor, and your doctor will take many variables into account before selecting one to use. The following table lists medications that are used to help treat preterm labor and some of their side effects.

Medications That Can Treat Preterm Labor[4]

Generic Name (Drug Class)	Potential Side Effects to Mother
Terbutaline (beta-mimetic)	Fast heart rate, irregular heart rhythm, low blood pressure, an overall "jittery" feeling, fluid in lungs
Nifedipine (calcium channel blocker)	Flushing, headache, dizziness, nausea, low blood pressure
Indomethacin (NSAID)	Nausea, heartburn
Ketorolac (synthetase inhibitor)	Upset stomach, gastritis; no major adverse effects unless given to a patient at increased risk for bleeding (immediately after surgery or in someone with a bleeding disorder)
Sulindac (NSAID)	Upset stomach

Reality Check

A landmark study showed that using intravenous (IV) magnesium sulfate to help stop preterm labor also reduces the chance that a preterm baby will have moderate or severe cerebral palsy. It is now standard treatment at most hospitals, given to pregnant women who are in danger of delivering prematurely.[5]

Q. Do these medications work?

Yes, medication works for a *short* time. But this time is important time.

Most studies show that medication used to stop contractions (***tocolytics***) prolongs pregnancy for up to seven days. Is seven days really worth it? Yes! Although that sounds like no time at all (particularly if you go into preterm labor at twenty-seven weeks), seven days may buy enough time to prepare for a preterm delivery.

The biggest advantage is that you'll be able to take medication to help mature the fetus's lungs, brain, and intestines. The medication is a steroid, usually given in two doses over a forty-eight-hour period. As mentioned above, you will also likely receive IV magnesium sulfate to help mature your baby's brain. This time will also allow you to get a quick course with your OB, a maternal-fetal medicine specialist, and likely a neonatologist, on the consequences of having a premature baby.

Besides medication, you will go on modified bed rest, have your contractions monitored, get tons of fluid either by mouth or IV, and stay in the hospital for close surveillance.

Q. Will I be able to go home, or will I need to stay at the hospital?

If you are in preterm labor (regular uterine contractions with cervical dilation), you will most likely be admitted to the hospital. Your obstetrician and maternal-fetal medicine specialist will work together and develop a plan for the length of your stay, since that depends on many factors.

Premature Rupture of Membranes (PROM)

Before we answer questions, here are a few definitions first:

- **ROM**. Rupture of membranes means your water bag breaks.
- **PROM**. Premature rupture of membranes means rupture of membranes occurs before labor begins.
- **PPROM**. Preterm premature rupture of membranes means rupture of membranes occurs at less than thirty-seven weeks gestation.

Q. I'm thirty weeks. My water broke but I'm not having contractions. What happens now?

In general, here is the step-by-step plan:

1. Your OB provider confirms you have broken your water bag (PPROM).
2. You get admitted to the hospital.
3. You are monitored to check your contraction pattern (or hopefully lack of one) as well as your baby's heart rate pattern.
4. You will get IV fluids for hydration.
5. You will get antibiotics to help prevent infection.
6. You will most likely get medication to stop contractions (if present).
7. You will get steroids and magnesium sulfate (if indicated).
8. Then we watch and wait.

If it looks like your baby is in trouble, your OB provider will recommend that you proceed to delivery. It's more likely you will have a C-section because fetuses born prematurely are often not in the head down position yet and there is also a higher risk of fetal distress, which will make your OB want your baby out sooner rather than later.

Q. Why does my doctor want to give me steroids? Will they help my baby?

Yes, if you are delivering between twenty-four and thirty-four weeks.

Steroids, formally known as corticosteroids, are a family of drugs that have a variety of therapeutic uses. (These steroids are very different than what some professional athletes use, by the way.)

If a preterm delivery is imminent, steroids are *the* single most beneficial thing your doctor can do for your baby.

Steroids cross the placenta and enter into the baby's system. They trigger the cells in the fetus's lungs, brain, and intestines to mature. And when a baby is born prematurely, we worry most about these organs. The concerns:

- Immature lungs cannot expand properly to hold air (***respiratory distress syndrome***).
- Immature brain has fragile blood vessels that bleed easily (***intraventricular hemorrhage***).
- Immature intestines have poor blood supply that can lead to injury and death of the tissues (necrotizing enterocolitis).

Giving mom a dose of steroids (preferably within seven days of delivery) may help these organs mature and prevent these major complications in preterm babies. In short, steroids lower the risk of your preterm baby dying. The goal here is to get two doses of betamethasone in before delivery.

Reality Check

More is not better. Women in preterm labor need just two doses before delivery. Giving multiple doses does not improve a baby's health outcome and can even lead to an increased risk of a newborn infection as well as low sugar levels in the baby.

However, a "booster" dose of steroids may be given four to six weeks after the first course if you're still pregnant, still under thirty-four weeks, and still at increased risk of early delivery. The two-dose regimen has not been shown to increase any risk of fetal or newborn infection.

Q. My friend broke her bag at thirty-two weeks, and her doctor gave her steroids. I am thirty-five weeks and just broke my bag. Why won't my doctor give them to me?

Steroids are most useful between twenty-four and thirty-four weeks.

If you are past thirty-four weeks, research shows there is no significant benefit. In most cases of PPROM, there is a "stressful event" like placental bleeding or infection that triggers the water bag to break.[6] When there is stress, your fetus releases their own stress hormones (adrenaline), which accelerate lung, brain, and intestine maturation . . . just like the steroids.

And FYI, there is a gray zone (medicine is rarely black or white) between thirty-two and thirty-four weeks. Some experts recommend giving steroids to women with PPROM who fall in this category, and others do not.

Reality Check

If you rupture your membranes prematurely (PPROM), you have a 60 to 70 percent chance of going into labor on your own and delivering within a week. It is rare for the fluid to stop leaking and for the pregnancy to continue. That's because up to 60 percent of women with PPROM develop an infection of the amniotic sac (***chorioamnionitis***).

When the bag breaks, there is no longer a sterile protective barrier that keeps vaginal bacteria out of the uterus. This makes it easy for bacteria to enter the amniotic sac and uterus.

In fact, OB providers recommend immediate delivery if there is an obvious infection in the uterus (such as maternal fever, elevated maternal white blood cell count, foul-smelling ***amniotic fluid***, rapid maternal heart rate, rapid fetal heart rate, or nonreassuring fetal heart rate).

Q. I'm thirty weeks. My water broke, and I am having contractions. What happens now?

It really depends on your particular situation.

Your doctor will look at your medical history, current vital signs and lab work, physical exam, and the health of the fetus (by fetal monitoring).

If you are in active labor and your cervix is five to six centimeters dilated, medications will probably not help, and you will be delivering a baby today. You will get IV antibiotics to protect the baby from infection.

But if you are in early labor and you have no other complications besides a broken water bag, your doctor may give you medication to stop labor.

Q. What caused my water bag to break so early?

There are many possible causes.

They include premature contractions, infection, second and third trimester bleeding, severe nutritional deficiencies, smoking, an overdistended uterus (***polyhydramnios***, multiple fetuses), having prior cervical surgery (LEEPs, cervical conization, ***cerclage***), severe lung disease, or a history of ***amniocentesis***. If your water bag broke before thirty-seven weeks with your first pregnancy, the risk of having it happen in any subsequent pregnancy is between 16 percent and 32 percent.

In many cases, however, docs never identify a clear risk factor.

Q. What is the youngest age that a fetus can survive outside the womb?

- Wow. This is a tough question. The official term for surviving outside the womb is "viability," and it is based on both the baby's gestational age and their birthweight. ACOG and the Society for Maternal-Fetal Medicine carefully and thoughtfully review the data. Here are their most recent findings:[7]
- Babies at twenty-three weeks gestation have a 23 to 27 percent survival rate.

- Babies at twenty-four weeks have a 42 to 59 percent survival rate.
- Babies at twenty-five weeks have a 67 to 76 percent survival rate.

The National Institute of Child Health and Human Development has a useful tool to calculate survival rates based on several factors. Find it here: nichd.nih.gov/research/supported/EPBO/use.

Of note, babies who are born extremely early and survive may face significant neurodevelopmental impairment. So it's not just about survival—it's about quality of life as well.

We'll talk about life in the neonatal intensive care unit (NICU) later in this chapter. But the reality is that very premature newborns have the most serious health complications to overcome even if they survive delivery.

Any time a woman will potentially deliver a very premature baby (twenty-one to twenty-five weeks gestation), parents-to-be should have an in-depth discussion with all healthcare team members (OB, maternal-fetal medicine specialist, neonatologist, and pediatrician). The team can go over the baby's potential health outcome based on the age, estimated weight, and gender of the fetus.

When it comes to extremely preterm and low-birth-weight babies, there will be a discussion on whether or not to perform rescue procedures on the baby (neonatal resuscitation). Example: A 0.8 lb. (400 gram) fetus at twenty-two weeks gestation has an extremely poor chance of survival. Many parents choose to avoid intervention. Other parents want providers to take all measures to aid survival. Additionally, if you

NEW PARENT-TO-BE 411:

Preemie Lingo

Your baby's category based on their gestational age:

Early term:	37 through 38 weeks gestation
Late preterm:	34 to under $36\frac{6}{7}$ weeks gestation
Very preterm:	Under 32 weeks gestation
Extremely preterm:	At or below 25 weeks gestation

Your baby's category based on their birth weight:

Low birth weight (LBW):	Birth weight less than 2,500 g (less than 5.5 pounds)
Very low birth weight (VLBW):	Birth weight less than 1,500 g (less than 3.3 pounds)
Extremely low birth weight (ELBW):	Birth weight less than 1,000 g (less than 2.2 pounds)
"Micropreemies":	Birth weight less than 800 g (less than 1.8 pounds)

are delivering at a hospital that does not have a neonatal ICU (NICU), you or your baby may be transferred to one that does.

If you are faced with this scenario, gather all the facts and ask questions to feel satisfied that you are making an informed decision.[8]

Reality Check

Premature baby girls are stronger than baby boys. They have lower mortality rates as well as a lower risk of cerebral palsy.

Q. My doctor cannot stop my labor. Once the baby is born, will my baby be able to room in with me?

It depends on the maturity of the baby.

Usually babies beyond thirty-five weeks can stay with mom if they know how to breathe, eat, maintain their body temperature, and do not have any risk of infection.

Some babies born between thirty-four through thirty-five weeks are typically observed in the NICU for twenty-four to forty-eight hours and then return to their mother's hospital room for the remainder of the stay.

Babies born earlier than thirty-four weeks will stay in the NICU long after you have been discharged.

Q. What happens during/after delivery?

When delivery is imminent, the neonatal care team (neonatologist/neonatal nurse practitioner, OB provider, and neonatal nurse) arrives in your delivery suite or operating room. Your OB will hand your baby immediately over to them for care.

The first priorities for the team are to make sure your baby is breathing and their heart is beating. The team will perform CPR (cardiopulmonary resuscitation) if needed and give medications, if necessary.

If your baby is very preterm, the team will place a tube into their throat to breathe for them, give them oxygen, and administer a medication (***surfactant***) that helps keep the tiny air sacs in the lungs open.

The team will also dry your baby off and warm them up on a radiant warming exam table.

Once your baby is stabilized, you will be able to take a quick peek at your little one. But if your baby is ill, they will need to head to the NICU fairly quickly. You will get to visit your baby (assuming the NICU is at your hospital) a few hours after a vaginal delivery.

If you've had a C-section, though, you'll need to wait until at least the next day to visit in person. Your partner will be able to visit and snap some pictures for you. Some NICUs also have iPads set up to FaceTime with parents who can't make it up to the NICU, so that's an option, too.

Neonatal Intensive Care Unit 411

Having your baby whisked away to the neonatal intensive care unit (NICU) is a scary, surreal experience that often follows a whirlwind, unexpected delivery. But once you get used to the place and your baby's amazing healthcare team, it becomes more familiar and less terrifying.

DR. M'S OPINION

I always tell my patients that in a matter of days, they will be more proficient with the medical lingo used in the NICU than I am!

Q. My baby was born before thirty-four weeks. What should I be prepared for?

This is a topic that is a book in and of itself, but the basic concept is this: Your baby needs to mature outside the womb and will not go home until they are ready to face the world. Discharge Day usually equates to near or at their actual due date. Hopefully, that path to maturity goes smoothly, but there can be some unpredictable bumps along the road.

Q. What are all these machines doing for my baby?

The first time you enter a NICU, it feels a bit overwhelming. It may also feel like you walked into a sci-fi movie. There will be rows of tiny babies, each in their own little incubator or open warmer table, attached to numerous machines with tubes and wires. Premature babies have weak and immature lungs, so they frequently need oxygen and mechanical support to help them breathe. They may need one or more tubes attached to veins (IV lines) for fluid and for medication, if needed. They also may need nutrition via intravenous fluid or a tube going from the nose into the stomach (NG tube) until they are able to eat by mouth. Then, there are tons of devices constantly monitoring a baby's heart rate, blood pressure, and oxygen saturation. In short, these are all necessary items to support your baby and detect any changes quickly.

Q. How often can I visit my baby at the NICU?

While every NICU has its own protocol, parents can typically visit anytime they desire. Once a mom is discharged home after recovering from delivery, some neonatal units also offer a limited number of family suites so that a parent can stay overnight and be near their baby.

Q. Can I hold my baby?

Yes! Your baby may be medically fragile initially and may not be able to safely move from the open warmer. But once they are stabilized, the medical staff will assist you in holding your baby.

Q. When can my baby be discharged?

There are some general requirements for your baby to head home from the NICU.

Premature babies have very little body fat, and their nervous systems are immature. They have to prove that they can maintain their core body temperature and not get cold.

Premature babies get tired quickly and have immature oral motor skills. They need to prove they can eat and grow. You'll get used to their daily weigh-ins.

Premature babies have immature lungs and nervous systems. They need to breathe effectively to maintain their oxygen without needing support. And they need to remember to breathe. Many premature babies have spells where they briefly pause and stop breathing (called ***apnea of prematurity***). They need to prove they don't have any significant and prolonged apnea spells, where their heart rate also drops, for several days before they are allowed to go home.

Q. How long is the typical stay in the NICU?

Premature babies may need medical support in the hospital until they grow, mature, and get closer to their actual due date. But it really depends on each baby's medical situation.

While we don't have enough room in this book to go over all the medical issues you could face with a premature baby, there are two books we recommend for further reading: *Preemies: The Essential Guide for Parents of Premature Babies* by Dana Wechsler Linden, Emma Trenti Paroli, and Mia Wechsler Doron and *The Preemie Primer* by Dr. Jennifer Gunter.

Late Preterm Infants

(Babies Born Thirty-Four Through Thirty-Six Weeks)

Q. What is a late preterm infant?

Babies born between thirty-four weeks through thirty-six weeks are considered premature, and get the designation "late preterm infant." Late preterm infants account for 70 percent of all preemies.

The good news is that late preterm infants usually do not encounter the major health complications that younger preemies do. But they still deserve special treatment. They are different from their full-term friends.

Q. Will my baby need to stay in the NICU?

Your baby will likely be cared for in the NICU if you deliver at thirty-four to thirty-five weeks. If you deliver in the thirty-sixth week, your baby might be able to room in with you and be cared for by your pediatrician and the nursery staff. It really depends on the factors that led to the preterm delivery. But rest assured, whether in the NICU or

FEEDBACK FROM THE REAL WORLD:

Find a Support Network

Here are some specific tips to get through your NICU experience (and beyond) from seasoned parents of preemies:

- Become your child's advocate.
- Take breaks from the unit when you can.
- Rest when you can.
- Read to your child in a soft voice.
- Make relationships with other parents with children in the NICU.
- Learn the medications and orders written for your child.
- Trust the advice of your doctors, but don't be afraid to ask questions.
- Listen to advice from nurses. Nurses have lots of interaction with your baby and can be a huge asset during extended stays in the hospital.
- Ask for help when you get home.
- Avoid public places during winter infection season (October to April), especially the child's first winter.
- Make sure to ask lots of questions and get well educated on your own.
- Be prepared to feel helpless and wonder if the staff is giving your baby the best care possible.
- Be with your baby as much as possible (both parents).
- Partners need to support each other. This is a critical time in your lives.
- Keep in mind how resilient babies are.
- Be clean, clean, clean—infections and the NICU don't mix.
- Be involved as much as possible—help the nurses with daily tasks.
- If your baby is born under two pounds, you can sign them up for Supplemental Security Income (SSI). This is a federal income support program. Go to ssa.gov/ssi/ for details.
- Keep your own medical records. You may need them for future reference.
- Keep an open dialogue with case managers and doctors and take notes to help you remember. The intensity of the situation makes it difficult to remember details of conversations.
- Don't ever give up.

Special thanks for these tips to Kelli Kelley, mom of two preemies and founder of the organization A Hand to Hold.

in the regular nursery, the medical staff will watch your baby to be sure they remember to breathe, know how to eat well enough to maintain a normal blood sugar, and can maintain their body temperature.

Q. My baby is a late preterm infant. Is there anything special I need to look out for?

Yes. Here is a list of their unique issues:

- **Neurologic:** About one-third of a baby's brain volume grows in the last eight weeks of gestation, so it's no surprise that your newborn is not as prepared as a full-term baby to face the world. Your little peanut will probably be very sleepy, and you'll need to awaken them for feedings. They may suck ineffectively, which can make feedings (especially breastfeeding) a real challenge. Your baby may be kind of cranky, startle, and have difficulty being soothed (don't get too discouraged). All of these things resolve; they just take a little time until your baby's brain and body matures.
- **Temperature regulation:** Your baby may have trouble regulating their body temperature (besides having very little body fat to retain heat). Swaddle your baby with two or three receiving blankets and have them wear a hat for those first days after birth. Once you are home, you no longer need to continue this practice.
- **Respiratory:** Your baby is being born just about the time their lungs are fully mature. If your baby is on the younger end of the spectrum of late preterm infants (thirty-four to thirty-five weeks), it's still possible that they will have respiratory distress and need temporary breathing support because of immature lungs. Due to neurologic immaturity, your baby is also at risk for forgetting to breathe (also known as ***apnea of prematurity*** or AOP). Your baby won't be allowed to go home from the hospital until they prove that they do remember to breathe! You also need to take extra care when holding your newborn upright, as they have very poor head control and being upright can collapse their airway.
- **Infectious diseases:** Being born early is considered a risk factor for newborn bloodstream infection (***sepsis***). Although the chance of this is very small, your baby may have lab work and tests done to rule it out.
- **Gastrointestinal:** Your baby will be a pickey eater in the beginning and so won't poop very much. This, and an immature liver, make your baby more at risk of developing ***jaundice.*** Some babies either have a delay in eliminating ***bilirubin*** (a body byproduct) or produce higher levels than their bodies can eliminate effectively. Late preterm infants may have jaundice issues for the first five to seven days.
- **Growth/nutrition:** This is a major issue with late preterm infants. They are notoriously difficult feeders. As we discussed above, they are sleepy. They don't wake up on their own for feedings. They tire easily and fall asleep feeding. And their sucking ability, to put it bluntly, sucks. This means your baby is at risk for excessive weight loss or poor weight gain—both of which can lead to dehydration. To complicate matters even further, your baby is also at risk for low blood

sugar in the first twenty-four hours of life—which would prevent just about anyone from having the energy to eat.

Reality Check

Many late preterm infants need to bottle feed with expressed breast milk, donor milk, or infant formula while they mature and learn to breastfeed. Supplements help reduce weight loss and give babies energy to learn to nurse. If you are breastfeeding, you'll probably find that your little one gets tired out long before they fill their tummy. And since your baby is small or weak, they may not be able to rev up your breast milk supply with their demand. Therefore, it's a good idea to pump after nursing sessions to improve your milk production. Check out our companion book, *Baby 411*, for many tips on feeding a late preterm infant. See the back of this book for more info.

Q. Will I be able to take my late preterm baby home when I am discharged from the hospital?

Maybe. It really depends on your baby's age and maturity.

Here is what the American Academy of Pediatrics says your baby needs to do to get their walking papers:

- Stable vital signs (body temperature, blood pressure, heart rate, and respiratory rate) for at least twelve hours before discharge
- Proof they have the skill to eat by mouth (twenty-four hours of successful feedings with coordinated sucking/swallowing/breathing)
- Formal breastfeeding assessment with a trained caregiver
- At least one spontaneous poop
- No significant dehydration
- No significant jaundice
- Follow-up planned with pediatrician in twenty-four to forty-eight hours

The AAP developed these guidelines to decrease hospital readmissions in the first two weeks of life for dehydration, severe jaundice, lack of breathing (apnea), and infections.[9] Even with late preterm infants, watch for developmental delays and subtle learning problems later in life.

Early Term Infants

(Babies Born Thirty-Seven through Thirty-Eight Weeks)

Q. What is an early term infant?

This term applies to babies who are born between thirty-seven weeks and thirty-eight weeks. While they are not premature, they may or may not act like a full-term baby. Giving them this special label is a reminder that these babies may need special care and grace.

Q. My baby is an early term infant. Is there anything special I need to look out for?

Yes. We don't trust them to be strong, efficient, or effective feeders, and we need to watch them more closely to ensure they are not losing too much weight or not getting too jaundiced.

Early term infants may get tired out from a feeding before they fill up. They may also not have mature sucking and swallowing skills to effectively latch to the breast and transfer milk at the breast.

If you plan to breastfeed, it's helpful to have a certified lactation consultant (IBCLC) support you and your baby in the early days or weeks. Your pediatrician will monitor your baby's weight closely. Your pediatrician and lactation consultant may advise something called "triple feeding," which involves nursing, then pumping, and then offering expressed breast milk in a bottle. This short term, labor-intensive protocol gives your baby a safety net. It ensures your baby is getting enough to eat and you are getting enough stimulation to develop and protect your milk supply.

Because early term infants have a tendency to be poor feeders, they could also be more at risk for getting jaundiced because they are not effectively eliminating a body byproduct called bilirubin. Your pediatrician will also follow your newborn closely for jaundice in the first several days.

DR. B'S OPINION:

Every Day Is a New Day!

Every day, your baby is a day older and wiser. Once these babies approach their due date, they act more like full-term babies, and we trust them a little more to do what they need to do—that is, eat and poop!

CHAPTER 21

Multiples

"When I have a kid, I want to put him in one of those strollers for twins, then run around the mall looking frantic."

—Steven Wright

What's in This Chapter

- **All about twins**
- **Extra weight gain**
- **Health risks**
- **Delivery issues**
- **Breastfeeding multiples**

Most pregnant couples reading this book are nervous about the prospect of caring for one newborn. Those parents have no idea how easy they have it.

You, however, have hit the daily double (or triple or more). Your pregnancy will be different than your friends who are only carrying one fetus. There's more to it than getting bigger sooner or eating more than most teenage boys do.

INSIDER SECRET:

Fun Facts about Multiples

- **Twins are the most common type of multiple birth.** In 2023, 3 percent of all births were twins. Rates of triplets and higher-order births have been declining since 1998 and now make up only 0.07 percent of all births.
- **More twins are left-handed.** 18 to 22 percent of twins are left-handed compared with under 10 percent for non-twins.
- **The world record for giving birth to multiples is held by Leontina Albina.** From Chile, Albina gave birth to fifty-eight children, including three sets of triplets.
- **Cryptophasia.** This is the term for when twins develop their own "language" that only they understand.

Multiples, Facts and Figures[1]

Statistic	Twins	Triplets
Average birth weight	5 pounds, 3 ounces	3 pounds, 12 ounces
Average gestational age at delivery	35.3 weeks	32.2 weeks
Percent with growth restriction	14–25 percent	50–60 percent
Percent requiring admission to neonatal intensive care unit	25 percent	75 percent
Average length of stay in NICU	18 days	30 days
Risk of **cerebral palsy** (compared to singletons)	4 times	17 times
Risk of death by age one year (compared to singletons)	7 times	20 times

How Did This Happen?

Q. What's the difference between fraternal and identical twins? Does it matter?

The short answer: Most twins are fraternal, which means they do not share all of their genetic material. They are siblings with the same birthdays. Identical twins have exactly the same genetic material.

The long answer: Bear with us, this gets technical.

Fraternal Twins (Dizygotic or DZ):

- Mom has two separate eggs (instead of just one) in her cycle, and each egg gets fertilized by an individual sperm. In short: two eggs, two sperm.
- Two-thirds of all twins are fraternal.
- The babies do not share all of their genetic material. They are siblings with the same birthdays.
- The babies can be the same or different sex.
- They are dizygotic, which means they are from two ("di") separate fertilized eggs ("zygotes"). With two fertilized eggs, there are always two placentas, two inner fetal membranes (**amnion**), and two outer fetal membranes (chorion). Technically, that's called ***diamniotic/dichorionic*** placentas.
- Women who used fertility medications to stimulate ovulation, as well as in vitro fertilization and **embryo** transfer, are more prone to having fraternal twins.
- Women over thirty-five also have more fraternal twins.

Reality Check

Male and female twins are always fraternal. They cannot be identical because, clearly, they have different genetic material when it comes to their plumbing!

Identical Twins (Monozygotic or MZ):

- Mom has one egg that gets fertilized by one sperm, but the fertilized egg spontaneously divides into two separate embryos. In short: one egg, one sperm, plus one extra split.
- Only one-third of all twins are identical.
- The babies have the same exact genetic material.
- The babies must be the same sex.
- The placenta and fetal membranes of identical twins vary, depending on when that extra split occurs after fertilization. So identical twins can be:
    1. **Diamniotic/dichorionic** = 2 placentas, 2 amnions, 2 chorions
    2. **Diamniotic/monochorionic** = 1 placenta, 1 chorion, 2 amnions (2 sacs)
    3. **Monoamniotic/monochorionic** = 1 placenta, 1 chorion, 1 amnion (both babies are in the same sac—the rarest and most dangerous type of pregnancy involving twins)
- Why do docs care about identical twins' fetal membranes? Identical twins with just one chorion and amnion have more health risks and need to be followed more closely.
- Identical twins have more birth defects (neural tube defects, abdominal wall defects, urinary tract abnormalities).
- Identical monoamniotic/monochorionic twins may be mirror images. One could be right-handed, and the other left-handed. Or hair whorls may go in opposite directions. They also have nearly identical brain wave patterns on EEG.

Reality Check

Your OB provider can usually figure out what type of twins you are having by ultrasound or at delivery. But if your same-sex twins have two placentas, two amnions, and two chorions (***diamniotic/dichorionic***), they can be either fraternal or identical. You can have the babies' DNA tested after birth to figure it out.

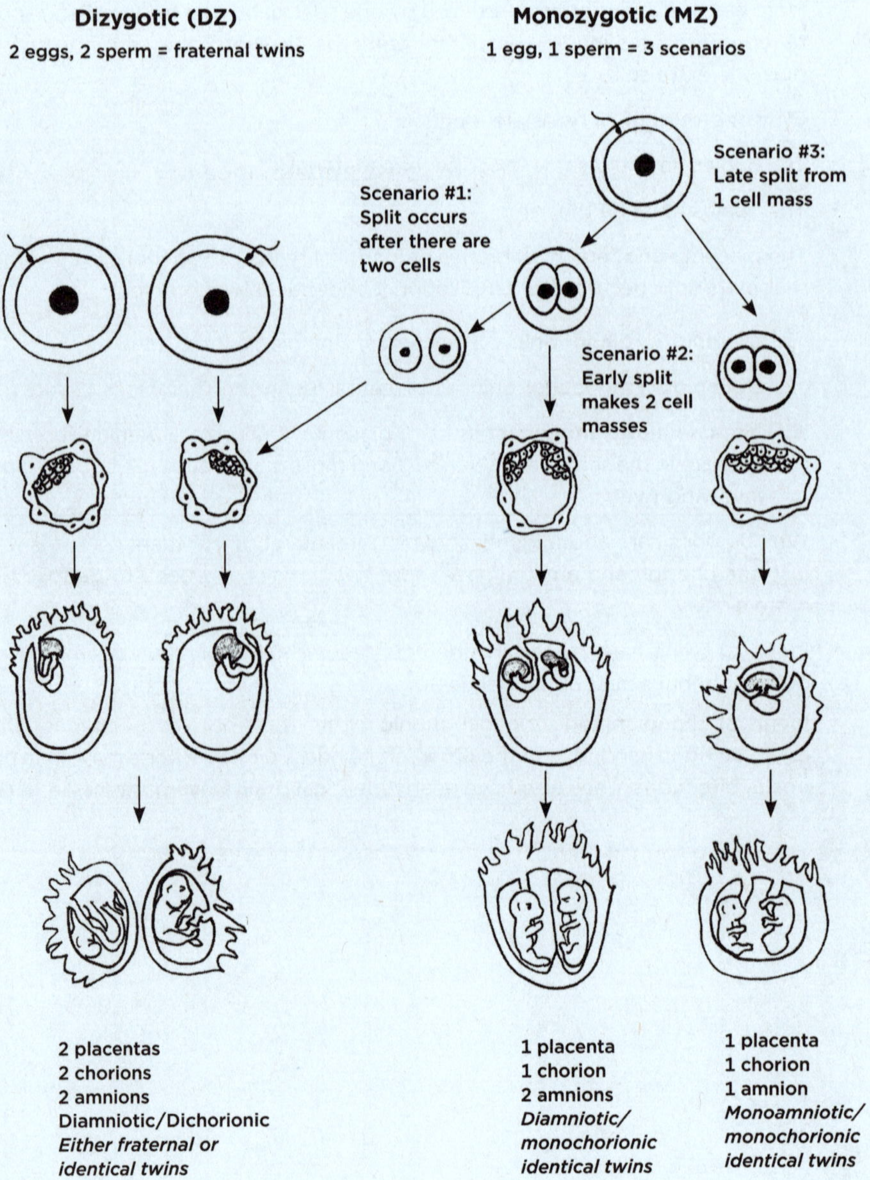

Q. Twins run in my family. What are the odds that I will have twins?

Identical twins happen randomly and do not run in families. *Fraternal* twins can be hereditary—but only if they run in the mother-to-be's family.

In the general population, the chance of having twins is between 1 in 80 to 1 in 250. Triplets occur by chance in 1 out of every 8,000 pregnancies. But if you yourself are a fraternal twin, your chance of having twins goes up to 1 in 60. If fraternal twins run in your family, your chances increase as well. But the hereditary factor only pertains to a *woman's* family history. It doesn't matter if your husband has two sets of aunts who are twins and four sets of twin cousins once removed!

Q. Is there anything else that increases my chance of having multiples?

Other than assisted reproductive technology, here are the other factors that come into play:

- **Advanced maternal age.** Yes, older woman do have one advantage here—more hormones (specifically, follicle stimulating hormone, or FSH)! FSH makes our eggs ripen and motivates the ovaries to work. As we age and our ovarian function declines, FSH levels rise to stimulate the ovaries. Extra FSH may cause more than one egg to be released per menstrual cycle, resulting in twins if both eggs are fertilized. Although women over the age of thirty-five are less likely to get pregnant in a menstrual cycle, they are more likely to have twins.
- **Race.** Your chances are greater if you are of African descent (1 in 70). Your chances are lower if you are Japanese (1 in 150) or Chinese (1 in 300).
- **Previous pregnancies.** Your chances are greater if this is not your first pregnancy.
- **Previous pregnancy with twins.** Chances increase if you have already been pregnant with fraternal twins.
- **Taller women.** Women who are taller with a larger body frame have more twins.

Q. What are the odds of having multiples if I have been treated by a fertility specialist?

It really depends on what kind of treatment you have. Here is a general breakdown for having *fraternal* twins:

- Clomiphene citrate (Clomid) alone: 3 to 8 percent chance of multiples.
- Injectable ovulation induction medications (gonadotropins): 20 percent.
- In vitro fertilization (IVF): 20 to 40 percent—depending on how many embryos are transferred into your uterus.

But guess what? You also have better odds of *identical* (monochorionic) twins, too. The rate is about 3 to 5 percent, compared to a rate of 0.4 percent in the general population.

How does this happen? Example: You have two embryos placed into the uterus via

IVF—but one decides to split—now you have three fetuses (one fraternal sibling, and two identical twins!). This little phenomenon is how some fertility patients end up with multiples beyond twins (higher-order multiples). It also increases the complications. This is why most fertility offices now only transfer *one* embryo into a patient.

Q. How early in my pregnancy will I know if I am carrying twins?

Doctors can diagnose twins between six and ten weeks by ultrasound. If your OB provider doesn't do an ultrasound, they may still pick it up in the first trimester when the size of your uterus is larger than your dates indicate. Then they will refer you to have an ultrasound to confirm their suspicions. It's almost unheard of in today's world for women to be surprised at birth with a second baby!

What You Need to Know

Q. Why is carrying multiple babies considered a high-risk pregnancy?

Short answer: more babies = more pregnancy complications = more preterm deliveries.

Just about every pregnancy complication you hear about happens more often in women who are carrying multiples. That includes ***preeclampsia***, **anemia**, gestational diabetes, **acute fatty liver**, gallstones, blood clots, kidney infections, skin problems, premature rupture of membranes, preterm labor, and excessive bleeding after delivery. Whew! Yes, that is a long list. See Chapter 17, "The Complicated Pregnancy," for details.

And babies who are born prematurely also have their unique set of issues (detailed in Chapter 20, "Preterm Labor and Babies").

Fun, eh? Believe it or not, most women carrying multiples have healthy pregnancies and healthy babies. But we point these facts out to you to make you realize you have a special pregnancy that requires closer observation on your part and your doctor's. Be sure to ask your OB provider if they are comfortable caring for a twin pregnancy and delivery, as many may not be and will refer you to another OB.

Q. Are there any special tests or additional prenatal visits because I am carrying twins?

Yes. You visit your doctor more often, you get more tests, and you meet more doctors. Enter the maternal-fetal medicine specialist—a doctor who is a high-risk obstetric specialist.

Your doctor will watch for pregnancy complications and signs of preterm labor. It's also wise to have a maternal-fetal medicine specialist who will work with your obstetrician to ensure that any medical issues are identified early.

For the first twenty-four weeks, you will likely have the same number of office visits as your friends who are only carrying one baby. But from twenty-two to twenty-eight weeks, you get to visit your OB or maternal-fetal medicine specialist every other week (as opposed to once a month).

Starting at thirty-two weeks, you will see your OB or maternal-fetal medicine specialist every week. If any complications arise, you may have even more appointments!

And yes, you get to do more tests. Here is what lies ahead:

1. **More ultrasound exams.** Starting at eighteen to twenty weeks, you will likely get an ultrasound (sorry, but many are with a vaginal probe) every few weeks. Your doctor measures the length of your **cervix** to ensure that it is not shortening prematurely (a risk factor for preterm labor).
2. **Non-stress tests.** You will probably have these on a weekly basis starting at some point in your third trimester. Identical twins with one placenta and one sac are tested the earliest and the most often.

For a full discussion of these tests, see Chapter 6, "Tests."

Q. Do pregnant moms of multiples have more morning sickness? I feel awful!

Yes! The more babies you carry, the more morning sickness you will have.

Morning sickness seems to be linked to elevated amounts of two hormones: ***beta-hCG*** and progesterone. When you are carrying multiple babies, your body makes more of these hormones. So it's no surprise that you may have more "all-day" sickness. You are also at greater risk of having ***hyperemesis gravidarum.***

Q. Will I need to go on bed rest, stop working, exercising, or having sex any earlier in my pregnancy because I'm carrying multiples?

While most obstetricians and perinatologists will restrict certain activities for a multiples mom-to-be, there is very little scientific data to prove that these restrictions work.

Based on the precautionary principle alone, your doctor may recommend that you go on modified bed rest, restrict your activity, and go on pelvic rest. Yes, it may be horrible for your mental state. But think of it this way: It just might help your babies stay in your incubator for as long as possible.

> DR. B'S OPINION
>
> *With multiples, the bigger your babies are at birth, the healthier they will be. Do what you need to do to give your babies the best shot!*

The Institute of Medicine's (now part of the National Academies of Sciences, Engineering, and Medicine) guidelines (based on pre-pregnancy weights) have special recommendations for moms-to-be of twins:[2]

- A woman with a normal ***body mass index (BMI)*** before pregnancy should gain thirty-seven to fifty-four pounds with a twin pregnancy.
- A woman who is overweight before pregnancy should gain thirty-one to fifty pounds.
- A woman who is obese before pregnancy should gain twenty-five to forty-two pounds.

If you are carrying triplets, expect to gain fifty to sixty pounds. And you wild and crazy moms carrying quadruplets should gain up to sixty-five pounds.

Here is a key point: It's not only how much you gain, but when you gain it. You want to gain most of your weight in the first twenty-eight weeks of your pregnancy. This is particularly important for women who were underweight before their pregnancy began.

Q. Am I going to gain more weight since I am carrying more than one baby?

Definitely.

We suggest you discuss your own personal goals with your obstetrician and maternal-fetal medicine specialist. One of the challenges: You may have already gained five to twelve pounds from fertility medications if you conceived using one of many assisted reproductive technologies (such as IUI or IVF).

Your OB provider will keep an eye on everything and let you know if you are too far ahead or too far behind on the weight curve.

Q. I have twins and have been having a few contractions. My doctor wants to give me steroids. Why?

We go over this in detail in Chapter 20, "Preterm Labor and Babies." But the short answer is this: Steroids help mature your babies' lungs, brains, and intestines if they are born prematurely. They are the most beneficial if you get treated within seven days of delivery.

Q. Is it more likely that I will have premature babies?

Yes. Seventeen percent of all preterm births (occurring before thirty-seven weeks) are multiples. They account for 23 percent of all early preterm births (those that occur before thirty-two weeks). It's wise to be prepared for an earlier delivery and for the significance of delivering preterm babies. For more information, see Chapter 20, "Preterm Labor and Babies."

Helpful Hint

Since you may deliver early, take your childbirth classes, have your baby shower, and do the hospital tour in your second trimester.

Reality Check

The guidelines for treating preterm labor in single fetus pregnancies (modified bed rest, progesterone injections, ***cerclage*** placement) may not be as helpful for women carrying multiples.[3]

Complications When Carrying Multiples

Although most women carrying multiples have uncomplicated pregnancies and deliveries, you are at higher risk for certain issues. We mention a few below for those of you who have been given a specific diagnosis or who are interested in seeing what could lie ahead. But this can be scary info, so proceed with caution.

Q. Will my babies have any more health risks?

If you have identical twins with one placenta, they are at risk for something called ***twin-twin transfusion syndrome (TTTS)*** (see the next question).

All types of identical twins are at slightly greater risk of birth defects including club foot, nervous system abnormalities, and urinary tract abnormalities.

Even if the babies do not have major complications, many have a low birth weight or have been growth restricted in the womb.

Reality Check

Any set of multiples is at risk for having *discordant growth*. That means there is a greater than 20 percent difference in the size of the fetuses. Growth restriction happens in 14 to 25 percent of twins, while 50 to 60 percent of triplets and quads experience growth restriction. And sometimes when one baby isn't growing well, the only treatment is delivery of both of them.

Q. What exactly is twin-twin transfusion syndrome?

First of all, this only happens with identical twins that share a placenta (***monochorionic***). The blood vessel connections within the placenta allow one twin to get more blood than the other one. The "recipient" twin gets more blood from the "donor" twin. It usually occurs and is diagnosed in the second trimester. And this is one of the things that your doc is looking for with all of those ultrasounds you are getting every few weeks!

The donor twin is significantly smaller. They may be anemic, with too little ***amniotic fluid*** and poor growth. At birth, this twin looks kind of pale and scrawny.

The recipient twin can be really big and have too much amniotic fluid and too many red blood cells. At birth, this twin looks really pink and healthy. (However, the recipient twin is more likely to run into problems with jaundice.)

Twin-twin transfusion can lead to premature rupture of membranes and preterm labor. In rare, severe cases, one or both fetuses can die.

There are a few treatments that can be undertaken during pregnancy if either of the fetuses is at risk. These are among the highest-risk pregnancies doctors deal with. If this happens, your OB and maternal-fetal medicine specialist will discuss this in detail with you.

DR. B'S OPINION:

Pick Your Hospital Carefully!

If you are having multiples, assume your babies will be coming earlier than planned. That means there is a decent chance your babies will need a special care nursery or NICU.

Think about that when you decide where to deliver. If you deliver in a ***community hospital*** and then your babies need to be transferred to a regional care center with a NICU across town or fifteen miles away, you will not get to see your babies until you are discharged from the hospital. That may be a very long two to four days.

Q. I had ART (assisted reproductive technology) and had three embryos transferred. All three took, and now I am carrying triplets. What are the pros and cons of "selectively reducing" the number of babies I carry?

The official term is "multifetal pregnancy reduction (MPR)." This is obviously a touchy subject for anyone. It's a medical, ethical, and emotional dilemma for all parents-to-be and their OB provider.

Here is the health concern: When you start multiplying the number of fetuses in a pregnancy, you also multiply their health risks. Higher order multiples are smaller and are born earlier. They have a lower chance of survival and potentially face lifelong impairment. And the mom-to-be has greater risks as well when she is carrying more babies. Reducing the number of fetuses may improve the health of both the mother and her surviving babies.

Multifetal pregnancy reduction can be done with twin pregnancies but is really only a consideration with higher-order pregnancies (triplets or more). It's a bit riskier when fetal reduction is done with a twin or triplet pregnancy. In fact, there is a 4 to 6 percent chance of losing all the fetuses with a triplet to twin reduction. Pregnancy reduction may also be discussed when one of the fetuses is chromosomally or structurally abnormal.

If you choose reduction, the procedure is usually done at ten to thirteen weeks. The fetus selected for termination may have a genetic or structural abnormality, or it may be in a safer location to reach in the womb. The doctor injects a medication into the fetus's heart to make it stop beating. The remnants of that fetal tissue do not interfere with the surviving fetus(es).[4]

Reality Check

The United Kingdom only allows two embryos to be transferred in a woman under forty years of age. It's called restricted embryo transfer. The United States currently has no federal laws on the books. Individual states have different laws and approaches to IVF and embryo transfer. And despite guidelines from the

American Society for Reproductive Medicine (ASRM) that strongly recommend a single-embryo transfer to decrease the risk of multiple pregnancies, none are legally enforceable.

Q. I've just learned that one of the fetuses has a very serious problem. Is there a way to terminate this pregnancy without risking the health of the other twin?

This is yet another difficult decision. This process is called ***selective fetal termination***.

The procedure is similar to a multifetal pregnancy reduction. However, the risks of this procedure are greater because most selective fetal terminations are done later in pregnancy (between sixteen and twenty-two weeks).

The decision to proceed with selective fetal termination is made based on risks. It's possible to lose the entire pregnancy if the abnormal fetus is situated in a difficult place (like lying over the cervix). But an abnormal twin with major malformations can put the healthy twin at risk. This is a very difficult decision to make. Ask for a referral to a support group or counselor who can be a resource for you.

Q. What if one of the twins dies in the womb? Will the other baby be okay?

It depends on when the loss occurs and whether the babies share one placenta (***monochorionic***).

The average rate of loss of a twin or triplet fetus is about 6 percent. The loss rate in higher-order multiples is probably much higher. If you lose a twin or triplet in the first trimester (***vanishing twin***), the other fetus/fetuses usually do just fine.

It gets riskier for the surviving fetus/fetuses if the loss occurs *after* the first trimester. If the fetal death occurs after the first trimester and you are nowhere near delivery (at twenty weeks, for example), your OB will probably watch you closely and let the pregnancy continue. This is particularly true if the fetal death has nothing to do with the uterus, placenta, or medical issues with mom.

If the fetal death occurs close to term, most experts recommend immediate delivery of the remaining fetus(es) because their survival is at risk.

The highest risk is for twins that share one placenta. That's because there are almost always connections between the blood vessels in the placenta. If one twin dies, the surviving twin experiences an immediate drop in blood pressure. And blood clots can form later on that may travel from the deceased twin to the live twin. This can cause major health problems for the surviving fetus.

Delivery Considerations

Q. Will I be able to deliver twins vaginally?

Yes, it is possible if a few criteria are met. If you have had a vaginal delivery before with a previous pregnancy, you have even better odds of avoiding a C-section.

Here's how the stars have to line up to make it work:

- The first twin to come out (also known as the *presenting twin* or "Twin A") must be facing head down (***vertex***).
- The second twin ("Twin B") is also facing head down (vertex).
- Or, if the second twin ("Twin B") is *not* facing head down, the first twin must be the same size or bigger than the second twin for a safe vaginal delivery.

It's possible to deliver the second twin, even if they are ***breech*** (head comes out last) as long as the first, larger, twin has paved the way. The last thing we want to do is to end up with a second twin whose head gets stuck in the birth canal. Forty-two percent of twins are both head down (vertex/vertex) at delivery.

Rarely, if you attempt a vaginal delivery with twins, you may deliver the first twin vaginally and need a C-section for the second. That's why docs deliver all twins in an operating room, not a regular delivery room.

If your twins are breech/vertex, breech/breech, or breech/transverse, your safest option is to have a C-section from the get-go.

Reality Check

If you are having twins or higher-order multiples, you need to deliver at a hospital with an obstetrician for the safety of you and your babies. It is not safe to have a home birth for this delivery.

Q. Is there any advantage to being the first born?

Other than bragging rights when they get older, there are a few medical reasons why the first twin often does better than the second.

The second twin (Twin B) is often in an abnormal position in the uterus (***breech*** or ***transverse***), making delivery more difficult. Delivery of the second twin, particularly if the delivery is vaginal, can be risky because there are more cases of umbilical ***cord prolapse***, placental abruption, and breech head entrapment with the second born.

Any of these situations can cause a temporary lack of oxygen to the baby's brain. And yes, that means there is a slightly greater risk of brain injury and cerebral palsy.

Q. How long is it between the first and second (and third . . .) deliveries?

If you are having a C-section, the deliveries of all babies occur within seconds or minutes of each other. Your doctor delivers one baby, cuts the cord, and hands the baby to the neonatal nurse. Then the doctor ruptures the second amniotic sac, delivers that baby, and cuts its cord (and so on . . .).

But if you are delivering your twins vaginally, there can be a significant delay between the first and second baby. The average time between delivery of the first twin and second twin is seventeen minutes. However, the time between delivery of the first and second twin can range from just a minute or two . . . to many hours. Occasionally, twins have different birth dates. Sometimes one twin is born before midnight and the second twin takes their time and is born after midnight!

Q. If I go into preterm labor, is it possible to deliver one twin and keep the other one from delivering until later?

Yes, but it is rare. If one twin delivers prematurely, the second twin usually delivers within hours.

Postpartum Considerations

While it's true that having two or three babies at home after delivery is certainly challenging, your body will recover very similarly to women who delivered only one (except you get to brag about the fact that you delivered more!). See, things are already getting easier!

Q. Am I going to have more trouble losing my pregnancy pounds?

That depends on how much weight you have gained. Most women carrying multiples gain more weight (ten pounds on average) than women carrying only one fetus. This means that there is more weight to lose.

Here's another good reason to breastfeed: You burn even more calories when you nurse or pump for two or more babies.

Start exercising as soon as you have your doctor's blessing. Walk or hike regularly with your kids. Put one in an infant carrier and one in a stroller, or both in a double stroller. It's a great way to get outside, and you'll get to spend time together. As they get a little older, you will also get to spend time picking leaves and goldfish crackers out of your hair afterward. An added bonus.

Q. Will I be able to breastfeed multiples?

Yes. And every ounce counts.

Breast milk is the ideal nourishment for newborns, especially for those who may be born prematurely. Don't worry if you do not have enough breast milk to feed all your babies exclusively.

Q. Am I less likely to produce enough breast milk if I'm feeding multiples?

One of the many remarkable things about breastfeeding is that the body makes the volume of milk that is needed to feed a baby or multiple babies. Breastfeeding follows the principles of supply and demand. If the demand is there, your body should produce more milk. Now, the reality of this is it's exhausting! Many moms will try tandem feeding, with one baby at each breast simultaneously, to reduce the time it takes to nurse more than one baby.

But every nursing mom's experience is unique, influenced by medical issues prior to and during pregnancy, and if the babies are born prematurely. Be prepared to do what needs to happen to feed your babies. It may involve pumping to stimulate your milk supply, feeding your babies expressed breast milk in a bottle, or feeding them a combination of breast milk and infant formula if necessary. The goal is to feed your babies to help them gain weight and grow.

Reality Check

Multiple needy newborns multiply the stress in the household, so it shouldn't surprise you that moms of multiples are even more likely to suffer from postpartum depression. See Chapter 15, "Postpartum: What's Next?" to learn about signs of postpartum depression. Get professional help if you need it!

CHAPTER 22

When It Doesn't Work

"Perhaps, they are not stars in the sky, but rather openings where our loved ones shine down to let us know they are happy."

—Inuit proverb

What's in This Chapter

- → Miscarriage
- → Stillbirth
- → D&C procedure

This is the chapter no one really wants to read. If your pregnancy is progressing smoothly, you can just skip right past it.

But if your pregnancy ends abruptly, we will walk you down this road and help you to understand what happened, what comes next, and what you need to know to make key decisions.

Miscarriage

Q. What is a miscarriage?

A miscarriage (***spontaneous abortion***) is the loss of a pregnancy occurring before twenty weeks. More than 80 percent occur within the first twelve weeks, with most of those occurring before the eighth week.

Your risk of having a miscarriage drops significantly if you make it past fifteen weeks. Only 6 in every 1,000 pregnancies miscarry after fifteen weeks.

Q. How many pregnancies end up miscarrying?

This will shock you. *Up to 30 percent of all known pregnancies end in miscarriages.*

This rate may be even higher than what's reported because many women miscarry without even knowing they were pregnant. For example, you might be a few days late for your period and then have a heavier than normal period, with or without more cramping. This may have been a very early miscarriage.

Q. Why do miscarriages happen?

There are many reasons.

By far the most common reason is that the embryo or fetus is chromosomally abnormal. Remember we talked about mom and dad's chromosomes lining up (twenty-three from the egg and twenty-three from the sperm) back in Chapter 2. Well, sometimes an embryo gets too many or too few chromosomes during this lineup. Some embryos with chromosomal abnormalities can survive life outside the womb (such as ***Down syndrome***). Others cannot. When survival is impossible, the body often spontaneously aborts that embryo.

The older the mother, the higher the risk of having a fetus with abnormal chromosomes. Thus, your risk of having a miscarriage also goes up as your age goes up. The general risk of having a fetus with any chromosomal abnormality at age thirty-three is 1 in 208, but at age forty, the risk increases to one in forty.

Other reasons for miscarriages include:

- A medical condition that interferes with successful pregnancy (severe lupus, uncontrolled diabetes, or uncontrolled thyroid disease)
- Infection
- Substance use (including smoking, alcohol, marijuana, cocaine, and opioids)
- Exposure to large doses of ionizing radiation
- Physical trauma

As you can see by the list, there are a few factors that you can control to ensure a successful pregnancy. There are also quite a few that are out of your control.

Q. Why do miscarriages happen more as women get older?

Older eggs mean more risk of damage to them.

Remember that we women are born with all of our eggs. They are buried deep within the ovaries until puberty and then each month when we ovulate, one of those eggs (and occasionally two) is released.

Women never make more eggs after we are born with them, and all the eggs we do have are subject to all the exposures we have had during our lifetime (such as CT scans and X-rays, pesticides, and drugs).

As we get older, our eggs are more likely to have been damaged from some exposure that has occurred in the past. This can lead to embryos with abnormal chromosomes.

Q. What are some of the warning signs that a miscarriage may occur?

- Lower abdominal pain and vaginal bleeding
- Painful cramping occurring every five to fifteen minutes

- Brown or bright red bleeding with or without abdominal pain
- Increased mucusy discharge with pink or red streaks
- Passing tissue from the vagina
- Sudden decrease in the signs of "feeling pregnant"

If you are having any of these symptoms, discuss them with your doctor.

Q. I am six weeks pregnant and have been having a small amount of vaginal bleeding. What is the chance I will have a miscarriage?

Twenty to thirty percent of pregnancies have some bleeding in the early part of pregnancy (first trimester). Of the early pregnancies (less than seven weeks) that have bleeding, 50 percent of those will go on to have a normal pregnancy and will ultimately deliver a baby. The other 50 percent will end in miscarriage. As you get further along and approach the second trimester, you are less likely to miscarry, even if bleeding occurs.

Q. Is there anything I can do to prevent a miscarriage from progressing?

Unfortunately, in most cases, the answer is no. Your OB provider will likely recommend modified bed rest as well as pelvic rest. This means that they are recommending that you remain fairly sedentary (reclined on your bed, a couch, or a big comfy chair) until your bleeding stops. It also means that you should refrain from intercourse, using tampons, douching, or putting anything in the vagina until the bleeding stops.

Q. I am eight weeks along, and I just passed a few large clots of blood. What do I do?

If you are having heavy vaginal bleeding at any point in your pregnancy, you should call your OB provider (day or night).

Although there is nothing docs can do to save a pregnancy before ***viability*** (twenty-three to twenty-four weeks), there are a few things that your OB provider will evaluate.

First, they will decide if you need to be seen right away or if the amount of bleeding you are having can wait to be evaluated. If this occurs during daylight hours, you will probably be asked to come into the office to have a pelvic exam and an ultrasound.

While waiting to see your OB provider, make sure you rest and drink a lot of water. Being active will only increase your bleeding. If you passed tissue (and you can stomach it), bring it in for your OB provider to examine. They may decide to send it out to a lab for further testing. This is especially important if you have a loss after the first trimester or if you have a history of recurrent miscarriages.

If this occurs in the middle of the night or on a weekend, you will likely be advised to go to the emergency room or an urgent care facility if your bleeding is severe.

WARNING:
What Happens After a Miscarriage?

If you miscarry before six weeks, you will most likely need some rest at home and a few ibuprofen tablets.

But other types of miscarriages, particularly those that happen when someone is further along in their pregnancy, may require medication or a surgical procedure to clear out any remaining products of conception. Here are those scenarios:

- **Complete abortion.** A miscarriage where the entire pregnancy (all the products of conception) come out and there is no tissue left behind. No further treatment is needed other than making sure the ***beta-hCG*** (a pregnancy hormone) is followed by your OB provider until it is zero.
- **Incomplete abortion**. Some of the pregnancy has miscarried or come out, and some is still in the uterus. A surgical procedure called a dilation and curettage (D&C) can help remove all remaining tissue (products of conception or POC) and decrease bleeding and pain. In some cases, when the miscarriage happens before seven weeks, medication can be used to manage this complication.
- **Missed abortion.** There is no longer growth of the pregnancy and/or no heartbeat, but a woman hasn't had any pain or bleeding. All of the tissue is still in the uterus. Again, a D&C or medication (if less than seven weeks) can be used to remove all of the products of conception. Observation is also an option if you are less than six weeks.

Q. I'm six weeks pregnant, and I've been having some bleeding. My doctor just confirmed that I miscarried and had a "complete abortion." How long will the bleeding last?

Your bleeding will probably continue for seven to ten days, although occasionally it can last for up to fourteen days. It will be heaviest at the beginning and should become lighter and less red in color near the end.

If your bleeding lasts for more than fourteen days, is associated with a fever, or is heavier than a heavy period, you should contact your OB provider.

Q. I just miscarried. When will I get my period again?

Your next period should come four to six weeks after your miscarriage or ***dilation and curettage (D&C)*** procedure. If you had irregular periods in the past, it may take longer. If you had normal periods in the past (every twenty-eight to thirty days) and you haven't gotten your period within six weeks, call your OB provider.

Q. I was just told my fetus doesn't have a heartbeat, and I'm seven weeks. What are my options?

There are three.

1. **Allow nature to take its course**. Most women who miscarry before seven to eight weeks have the option of miscarrying on their own. As long as you are not bleeding heavily, you can choose to wait to see if your body is able to pass all the tissue on its own. It involves some pretty intense cramping and heavy bleeding for a day or two, followed by lighter amounts of bleeding for up to seven to ten days afterward. There is always a small risk that not all of the tissue will be passed and you will need a D&C. This is possible up to about eight weeks. After that time, there is often too much tissue to pass and women lose too much blood, so other methods are recommended.
2. **Take medication to make the tissue come out.** Mifeprex and misoprostol are medications used to help expel a miscarriage that hasn't come out. Typically, these medications are only used up to seven weeks, but occasionally can be used past this point. Mifeprex is given orally, and misoprostol is given either orally or vaginally. Depending on your individual situation, how far along you are when you miscarry, the state you live in, and your conversation with the person caring for you, one or both of these medications can be given in lieu of having a surgical procedure.
3. **Have a D&C procedure.** A D&C is a surgical procedure used to remove pregnancy tissue from the uterus. See the question below for more details about the procedure. If you miscarry later in pregnancy, often after eight to ten weeks, there is a lot of tissue that needs to be passed, and the risk of having some of the tissue remain inside the uterus increases. The possibility of heavy bleeding and even hemorrhage rises as well. This is why most OB providers recommend a D&C for missed abortions that are more than eight weeks along.

The ultimate decision is yours. Some women do not want to undergo a surgical procedure and prefer to wait. If you decide to wait, you have two weeks for your body to take care of business. If nothing has happened after two weeks or so, your doctor may suggest a D&C to prevent infection or excessive bleeding leading to the inability to clot blood (a rare complication). Other women find it easier, both physically and emotionally, to get everything taken care of quickly.

Q. What is the name of the procedure to clear out any remaining tissues?

If you need a procedure to remove tissue after a miscarriage, you will either have a ***dilation and curettage (D&C)***, which is done before twelve weeks, or a ***dilation and evacuation (D&E)***, which is done after twelve weeks. Which one depends on how far along you were when you miscarried. Both are surgical procedures that remove the contents of the uterus.

Q. Where is the procedure done?

Some docs will do a D&C in their office if it is in the first trimester. Others prefer surgery centers. High-risk patients may have the procedure done at a hospital.

Q. Do I need to have any tests done first?

Before you have any procedure, your doctor needs to know a few things.

They will want to do an ultrasound (if you haven't already had one) to document that your pregnancy is in fact in the uterus and not in the fallopian tube or another abnormal location (***ectopic pregnancy***). Also, there needs to be confirmation that the pregnancy has, in fact, ended (for example, there is no fetal heart rate).

Your OB provider also needs to know your blood type and Rh. If you are Rh-negative (see Chapter 17, "The Complicated Pregnancy," Complication #14), you will need an injection called ***RhoGAM*** at the time of your procedure.

RhoGAM can be given up to seventy-two hours after the procedure, but it is best to give it at the same time. This protects you from making antibodies that could potentially cross the placenta and harm a fetus in any future pregnancy.

Helpful Hint: RhoGAM

If your blood type is Rh-negative, you will need RhoGAM if you miscarry, regardless of whether you pass everything on your own or need a D&C.

Q. What do these procedures involve?

The D&C procedure itself is relatively simple. You are often given oral or IV pain medication. You will lie down on your back with your feet or knees placed in stirrups. Your doctor places a speculum in your vagina (just like when you get a Pap smear). Then they clean the cervix with a special type of soap to make things sterile.

If your OB provider is using local anesthesia to block the nerves in your cervix, they will administer it now. It pinches and burns for a few seconds, very similar to getting a shot of Novocaine at your dentist's office.

They will then dilate your cervix using a series of small, thin instruments. Once the cervix has been dilated, in most cases, they will insert a suction device into the uterus and turn on the machine.

I warn my patients in advance that this part is pretty loud. If you have the procedure done in your doctor's office, bring some headphones and listen to music so you don't hear the noise. After most of the contents of the uterus have been removed, your doc inserts another instrument to check the walls of the uterus to make sure all products of conception have been removed.

That's it. The whole thing takes about ten minutes.

If you are having a D&E, you may be asked to come into your OB provider's office the day before the procedure to have something called laminaria placed into the cervical canal. Laminaria are thin dilators made out of seaweed. They absorb moisture from the cervix and vagina, and slowly expand over the next twelve hours so that the cervix begins to dilate. It makes further dilatation easier during the procedure the next day.

A D&E procedure usually takes longer than ten minutes, and it is performed at an outpatient surgery center or hospital while you are under general anesthesia (asleep).

Q. Will I be uncomfortable?

Most OB providers performing D&Cs will give some kind of pain medication. If you have it done at your doctor's office, you will likely get oral pain medication (such as ibuprofen, Vicodin, Percocet, Valium, Ativan, in different combinations, not all at once!). There is also an injection of a local anesthetic to numb the area, just like when the dentist numbs a tooth. You should be comfortable, but you won't be put to sleep. At most, you will feel a bit of cramping like a period.

If you have the D&C done at a surgery center or hospital with an anesthesiologist present, you will have IV pain medication and possibly IV sedation.

If you have a D&E procedure, you are given IV sedation (usually propofol) because this procedure is very painful.

Q. How long will I bleed after receiving a D&C or D&E?

This depends on how far along you are when you miscarry. Early miscarriages (under eight weeks) usually have a few days of bleeding after the procedure. The bleeding trails off and usually stops completely by seven to ten days. If you are further along when you have your D&C or D&E, you may bleed for up to two weeks.

Q. I'm worried that the D&C my doctor is recommending will make it harder for me to get pregnant again. Are there any risks to this procedure?

A D&C (dilatation and curettage) is the standard of care for incomplete abortions, missed abortions, miscarriages after about eight weeks, or when there is a need for specialized testing on the fetal tissue.

Your risk of having a complication is very low (about 1 percent) if a trained OB provider performs a D&C using sterile technique. The risks include infection (because no matter how sterile we are, bacteria are everywhere), bleeding (occasionally requiring medication and very rarely requiring a blood transfusion), and uterine perforation, which can occur when one of the surgical instruments makes a small hole through the wall of the uterus.

It is extremely rare to become infertile after having a D&C. You have an increased risk of infertility if you develop an infection of the uterine lining or if you undergo vigorous scraping of the uterine walls that leads to scarring. This scarring, called Asherman's syndrome, is more likely if you have multiple D&Cs, a postoperative infection, or a D&C after the first trimester.

Q. I went into my doctor's office for a routine visit at eighteen weeks, and she told me there wasn't a heartbeat. I'm devastated and now need to have a D&E procedure. What can I expect physically afterward?

Physically, it takes three to four weeks to recover from a D&E.

You will probably have moderate vaginal bleeding for up to seven days after your procedure. Following the heavier bleeding, expect some lighter bleeding or spotting for another few days to a week.

If you had normal monthly periods before the miscarriage, your period should resume four to six weeks after the procedure. If you haven't had a period by the sixth week, call your doctor.

Other symptoms include lower abdominal pain or cramping, similar to what you get with your period. These usually go away two to three days after the procedure. You may also have breast pain, ***engorgement***, or leaking. Try using ice packs and wrapping your breasts with a tight bandage or tight sports bra. This may last for about a week.

Your pregnancy hormones may continue to circulate for about a month after your miscarriage. It all depends on how advanced your pregnancy was when the miscarriage occurred.

Q. Is there anything I can do to decrease my risk of infection after the procedure?

Yes.

First, some OB providers give an antibiotic at the time of surgery. You can ask your OB provider if you will be receiving one.

After the procedure, you need ***pelvic rest*** for two to four weeks (or until the bleeding stops). Pelvic rest means no tampons, douching, or intercourse. It is also recommended that you avoid swimming pools, hot tubs, and bathtubs.

Helpful Hint

You can shower after a D&C. It's the bathtub that is off-limits.

Q. When will I be able to exercise again and return to all of my normal daily activities after a D&E?

Your doc will tell you to take it easy and avoid exercise for a few days afterward. Ease back into your activities. Remember you had surgery, even though you don't have a scar or stitches. Speak with your doctor for specific instructions on strenuous exercise and other activities.

Q. I am really sad about losing my pregnancy. Everyone keeps telling me that I will feel better, but I don't. Is this normal?

It is normal. Many women go through it. You are grieving, and there are several phases of emotions during this process.

You may feel shock, denial, guilt, depression, sadness, disbelief, and anger. Sometimes, the extreme emotional pain causes physical symptoms, such as difficulty sleeping, loss of appetite, anxiety, fatigue, and chest tightness. Don't ignore all of your emotions, because they will only build up inside. Get through them and you will reach a phase of acceptance. It is okay to need help, counseling, and in some cases, even medication.

During your healing process, situations will likely make you relive the pain and sadness you felt at the beginning. You may find it hard to go to a friend's baby shower, see a mother nursing her child, or have a checkup in your doctor's office in the same room where you were given the news that you miscarried. Allow yourself to go through these setbacks and give yourself the space and time to heal.

Q. My husband doesn't seem to be sad about the fact that I just miscarried. Is that possible?

Men and women grieve differently.

While this isn't true in all cases, women typically are more expressive about their loss, feel the need to talk about it, and are ten times more likely to ask for help or seek out counseling.

Men tend to use distraction as a technique to deal with grief and are more likely to investigate and problem solve than join a support group, go to therapy, or talk to their friends. A grieving man might bury himself in work or other projects and keep quiet, avoiding conversations with friends or family.

You also must realize that you were the one carrying the baby in your body. This allowed you, and not your partner, to form a unique bond. You saw and felt your body changing. Some women even report feeling a bond the second they get a positive pregnancy test. Partners may not experience real bonding until after the baby is born.

Recognize the differences in how you are each coping and grieving. Keep the lines of communication open. You need to let your partner know how you feel and vice versa. This way, you can both begin to heal in your own way.

Partner Tip

Admit to your partner that you, too, are also grieving. You might not be in the mood to share your feelings, and that's okay. Just telling your partner that you are grieving privately will help.

Q. None of my friends have miscarried, and I just don't know where to turn. Are there any resources for me?

It's so important to talk about what has happened and to voice your feelings and concerns. Sadness and anger are normal parts of healing, and you have to let yourself go through these steps.

Talk with your OB provider to get all of your questions answered. Talk with your partner so you understand how the other is feeling. Talk with anyone you feel close with—a mother, sister, friends. Chances are that many of them will have been through the same thing. Two helpful websites for women who have miscarried are miscarriagesupport.org.nz and mend.org

DR. M'S OPINION

Know that you are not alone. So many women have gone through one or more miscarriages. It's something that we don't talk about enough. We don't have villages like we used to, and women often hide their feelings of shame, embarrassment, sadness, anger, and despair. Know that there is help and there is hope.

DR. M'S OPINION:

The Truth About Miscarriage

It may be stating the obvious, but having a miscarriage is tough on anyone. This is especially true for women who don't have any children yet. I can tell you from personal experience that the miscarriage I had prior to my first child being born was far more difficult emotionally than the one I had between my two children.

Q. I've had a miscarriage in the past, and I just had another one at eight weeks. I am going in for a D&C tomorrow, and my doctor wants to send the tissue to a lab to test the fetus's chromosomes. Is this a good idea?

Many things can cause a miscarriage, but abnormal chromosomes in the fetus are the most common explanation, by far.

Doctors don't typically send the fetal tissue for testing for just one miscarriage because it is not likely to happen again and the testing can be expensive. If, however, a woman has had two or more miscarriages, many physicians recommend checking the fetus's chromosomes (karyotyping) to see if there is a chromosomal issue. If the chromosomes are normal, your OB provider knows to search for another cause.

Q. My doctor just did an ultrasound and told me I had a blighted ovum. What does that mean?

A ***blighted ovum*** means that there is an amniotic sac present, but no embryo. It is the cause of about 40 to 50 percent of all miscarriages occurring before twelve weeks. It is usually the result of a chromosomal abnormality. The pregnancy doesn't continue to grow, since there is some signal that tells the fertilized egg it would never develop into a healthy fetus.

Fact Check

A miscarriage can be caused by exercise or carrying around a toddler.

The truth: It is normal to feel some guilt after losing a pregnancy. Women rack their brains trying to pinpoint what past event led to the loss of their fetus. Was it bending over to pick up the plate that fell on the ground? Was it getting your hair colored? Was it the five-hour plane ride you took last week?

The truth is none of these things cause a miscarriage. Miscarriages happen commonly and are often due to genetic reasons where the chromosomes are abnormal. It's very normal to feel guilty, but having a miscarriage is not your fault.

Q. Is there a way to prevent a miscarriage from happening?

Since most miscarriages result from chromosomal abnormalities, there is not much that can be done to prevent them.

Once you find out you are pregnant, do what you can to make your uterus the best possible home for your baby.

Helpful Hint: Five Potentially Treatable Medical Reasons for Miscarriage

While many times there may not be an identifiable reason, it's worth doing a medical workup just in case. Here are five treatable medical disorders that increase the risk of miscarriage:

1. Celiac disease
2. Lupus (systemic lupus erythematosus, SLE)
3. Uncontrolled/undiagnosed thyroid disease
4. Uncontrolled/undiagnosed diabetes
5. Cigarette, alcohol, or substance use

If you have a chronic medical condition, try to plan your pregnancy when your disease is under control (as best as possible). A pre-pregnancy consultation with your internist, obstetrician, and a high-risk pregnancy specialist can be very important for planning a healthy pregnancy.

Q. Can stress can cause a miscarriage?

Some people think this is a myth, but there may be a wee bit of truth to it.

Recent studies show a relationship between significant chronic psychological and severe acute stress and miscarriage as well as stress and preterm labor.[1] It's hard to prove stress causes miscarriage because we all have some level of stress in our daily lives. And most women give birth to healthy babies.

Here's what we know: Stress increases the release of a hormone called cortisol. This hormone is being actively investigated as a link to miscarriage, preterm labor, and other unfortunate pregnancy outcomes.

It's unlikely that the day-to-day stress that we all encounter will have any negative effect on your pregnancy. However, it is possible that major levels of stress that occur with the loss of a spouse or child, a divorce, or major financial disaster could cause miscarriage or other pregnancy complications.

Helpful Hint: Will I Miscarry Again?

Here are the stats. But keep in mind that whatever your risk, there is a much greater chance that you will have a successful pregnancy rather than another miscarriage, no matter what your history is:

- One prior miscarriage: 20 percent chance of another miscarriage.
- Two prior miscarriages: 28 percent chance of another miscarriage.
- Three or more miscarriages: 43 percent chance of miscarriage.

The flip side is that a history of even one successful pregnancy improves your chances of being successful again.

- One live birth: 5 percent chance of miscarriage.
- More than one live birth: 4 percent chance of miscarriage.
- One live birth and then one miscarriage: 6 percent chance of miscarriage.

Considering the frequency of miscarriage, about one in thirty-six women will have two miscarriages due to nothing more than chance. This is why many doctors will wait until a woman has had three or more consecutive miscarriages to begin a full investigation into the problem.

It's possible to improve your odds of success if you figure out why you have miscarried in the past. For example, if you had two miscarriages and then discovered that you had Hashimoto's thyroiditis (a form of thyroid disease), getting treated with thyroid replacement medication will lower your chance of having another miscarriage.

Q. I had a miscarriage. How long do I need to wait before trying to conceive again?

There is no amount of time that is perfect for everyone. And it depends on how your miscarriage ended. Passing everything on your own only truly requires one menstrual cycle to go by prior to trying again. But having a D&C, where more of the uterine lining is removed, is different, and most OB providers usually advise a woman to wait for two or three menstrual cycles before conceiving again. This is because it takes time for the lining of the uterus to fully regenerate and be healthy enough to carry another pregnancy.

It is also important to take time to grieve your loss and be emotionally ready to go through another pregnancy.

But it really depends on your own situation. A very early pregnancy loss may differ from a loss in the second trimester. Check with your OB provider to see what they recommend.

Stillbirths

Q. What is the difference between a miscarriage and stillbirth? What are the odds of a stillbirth happening?

A stillbirth is when the fetus dies after twenty weeks gestation. These occur in about 1 in 200 pregnancies. Term stillbirths (a stillbirth that occurs after thirty-seven weeks) are much less common and occur in 1 out of every 1,200 deliveries. The majority of stillbirths happen before labor begins. A very small percentage occur during labor and delivery.

Q. My doctor just told me that my baby is a stillborn. I'm in shock. What should I do?

This is one of the most difficult things for a person/couple to ever go through. About 28,000 families in the United States suffer the loss of a viable baby prior to birth each year. There were no obvious problems in about half of those pregnancies.

Most couples are initially in shock. Everyone grieves differently, but it is very important to let yourself grieve. Let yourself cry. Let yourself feel numb. Let yourself get angry. And then let yourself heal.

And in the face of all this pain, you still have to deliver the baby. If you are not already in labor, you usually have to be induced to deliver vaginally or have a D&E (see info earlier in this chapter about this procedure). In some circumstances, it's also possible to wait until you go into labor on your own.

It's rare to have a cesarean section for a stillbirth unless an unforeseen complication occurs during labor or delivery, or your previous deliveries were C-sections.

Doctors prefer to induce labor or perform the D&E as soon as possible after the diagnosis, although it is probably safe from a medical standpoint to wait up to two weeks. Waiting more than two weeks is dangerous because it increases your risk of developing a blood clotting problem or an infection in the uterus.

One important note: If you wait until you go into labor on your own or wait a week or two to be induced, it will affect how a baby looks at the time of delivery. This can be extremely distressing for parents, so talk to your OB provider about this in advance.

Q. My best friend just had a stillbirth at thirty-eight weeks. I am currently pregnant in my second trimester and am absolutely terrified that this will happen to me, too. Is there anything I can do to prevent a stillbirth?

Many stillbirths are not preventable. And having a stillbirth at term is rare.

But there are some things that can be done to decrease your risk. All women should do daily ***fetal kick counts*** after about twenty-six weeks. Set aside some time each day to be aware of and/or record your baby's movements. You will begin to know when your baby is most active at about this time.

If you notice that your baby hasn't been as active (their pattern of movement changes) or isn't moving at all after a twelve-hour period, contact your OB provider.

Avoid smoking, alcohol, and drug use during pregnancy. If you have been classified as "high risk," talk to your OB provider about whether you will need increased monitoring with ultrasounds and/or fetal heart rate monitoring (non-stress tests or NSTs).

If you have had a previous stillbirth, your OB provider will monitor you very closely with any subsequent pregnancy.

Q. I'm devasted. I'm thirty-seven weeks and just found out at my doctor's office that my baby doesn't have a heartbeat. My doctor said I need to go to the hospital to deliver the baby. What does that process look like? Do I have to see the baby after I deliver?

This is an incredibly difficult time, and we are so very sorry. Let us walk you through the options.

Option 1 is to be induced and have a vaginal delivery (this is normally recommended). Option 2 is to have a cesarean section (only usually recommended if you have had one or more C-sections in the past).

The induction process is identical to the process for any other woman in labor. Your OB provider will discuss the possible induction methods with you depending on what number pregnancy this is for you and what your cervical exam is on admission. You can choose to have an epidural or not. You can also choose to have a sheet up between your torso and the lower half of your body so that you don't have to watch your delivery.

Once you've delivered, some people want to see the baby and some don't. As difficult as it is, it is highly recommended to see the baby afterward and say goodbye. We know this seems impossible, but it helps exponentially with the grieving process. Women have less postpartum depression when they are able to hold their baby after delivery. Additionally, most hospitals have special personnel (or it may be your labor and delivery nurse) who can discuss options for tissue and anatomic evaluation if the reason for the stillbirth is unknown (pathology), burial, or cremation.

Choosing Termination

Q. We just found out that our fetus has a serious genetic defect. We are interested in terminating the pregnancy. What are the next steps?

The first step once you have learned that something may be wrong with your fetus is to speak with as many people as you can.

Schedule a consultation visit with your OB provider as well as a maternal-fetal medicine specialist (high-risk obstetric doctor) or genetic counselor if possible to make sure that you are fully educated before making a final decision. Do some research on the particular problem and bring questions. Getting a second opinion won't hurt, either. Although questions will differ based on the individual condition, here are a few that may be helpful:

- What does this diagnosis/problem/condition mean?
- What organ systems are affected?
- Is there a chance that I will have a stillborn?
- Is there a chance the baby will die after birth?
- Will the baby need to have surgery? More than one?
- Is there any chance of intellectual disability?
- Is this condition something that we can accept/live with/embrace?
- Is this condition something that we are not prepared to accept/live with/embrace?

Once all of your questions have been answered, you will be able to make an informed decision. Mind you, it's never an *easy* decision. Even if you are quite sure that you would never want to deliver a baby with trisomy 13, for example, your emotions may influence your decision.

Have a long talk with your partner. Sometimes, it is also helpful to talk with friends and family. For others, it is easier to talk with a therapist or religious advisor. If you have decided that termination is the right choice for you, the details of the procedure (D&C or D&E) itself are described earlier in this chapter.

DR. M'S OPINION:

Don't Forget to Grieve

Even if you never got to know your baby, you formed a bond as a parent to your unborn child, and you will have feelings of loss, guilt, and yes, even anger. Going through the grieving process is normal and a natural human emotion.

Everyone goes through it at their own pace and in their own way. And it doesn't matter if you lost your baby at eight weeks, twenty-two weeks, or thirty-four weeks. It is a loss any way you look at it. Women who have miscarried often have many unanswered questions, and it is extremely important to be in open communication with your OB provider, family, and friends.

APPENDIX A

Medications[1]

This chapter focuses on detailed info on medication use during pregnancy and breastfeeding. There are several medications that are off-limits or to be used with caution during these times. See Appendix B, "Complementary Medicines and Therapies," for complementary/alternative therapies (such as herbs, homeopathic remedies, and acupuncture). If you have questions, always ask your OB provider.

First up, the most common over-the-counter medications you may be wondering about.

What Can I Take, Doc?

Here's a summary of over-the-counter medications you can take for symptoms you might encounter:

SYMPTOM	OTC MEDICATION
Constipation	Docusate (Colace), calcium polycarbophil (FiberCon), polyethylene glycol 3350 (MiraLAX), psyllium fiber (Metamucil)
Cough	Dextromethorphan (Robitussin DM)
Diarrhea	Loperamide (Imodium A-D)
Flu symptoms	Acetaminophen and pseudoephedrine (Tylenol Cold & Sinus)*, acetaminophen and diphenhydramine (Tylenol PM)
Headache, fever	Regular strength acetaminophen (Tylenol)
Heartburn	Calcium carbonate (TUMS), calcium carbonate and magnesium hydroxide (Mylanta, Maalox, Rolaids), cimetidine (Tagamet)
Hemorrhoids	Hydrocortisone cream (Anusol HC), witch hazel pads (Tucks)
Nasal congestion	Nasal saline spray (Ocean Spray), diphenhydramine (Benadryl), loratadine (Claritin only, not Claritin-D)**
Nausea	Vitamin B6 (100 mg/day) and doxylamine succinate (Unisom), glucose (Emetrol), acupressure (Sea-Band), ginger root capsules, sour candy
Sore throat	Throat lozenges, salt water rinses, benzocaine and menthol (Cepacol)

*Pseudoephedrine-containing products should be used for forty-eight hours or less.

**While pseudoephedrine (Tylenol Cold) is safe to take during pregnancy for short periods of time (less than forty-eight hours), Claritin-D is not. The D stands for decongestant in the form of pseudoephedrine, and it's a higher dose than what is found in Tylenol Cold.

Notes:

- If your symptoms don't improve in three days, call your OB provider!
- Regarding pain and fever-reducing medication: Avoid ibuprofen (Advil, Motrin) and naproxen (Aleve) throughout pregnancy. And painkillers, like Vicodin and Tylenol 3, taken just prior to or just after conception may be linked to certain birth defects. Take acetaminophen (Tylenol)—and even then, only when you really need it.

Helpful Hint

Some people use a combination of traditional care and complementary/alternative medicine, or CAM (herbs, homeopathy, acupuncture, etc.). Some CAM therapies are effective and safe. Others may be ineffective or downright dangerous. Our mantra is: Show us the scientific evidence that a therapy is both safe and effective and we are happy to recommend it. Unfortunately, much of that data is lacking when it comes to CAM. Inform your OB provider of *any* therapies you are using that your OB provider has not prescribed.

Q. How do I know which medications require a prescription?

We've included some handy tables later in this chapter with information on common medicines. In the tables, you'll note the following symbols.

- **Rx**: Denotes that a product is available with a doctor's prescription only.
- **OTC**: Denotes that a product is available over the counter (that is, without a prescription).

Q. How can I find out if a generic equivalent is available for the medicine my doctor has prescribed?

Ask your doctor or pharmacist. For the medication tables below, the generic name is the first name listed. The brand name is listed in parentheses. Note: While all medications have a generic name, not all of them are available to be purchased in generic form.

Q. How do I know if a medication is safe for me to take while I am pregnant or breastfeeding?

Some information is listed in the medication tables later in this appendix. Unfortunately, pregnancy and lactating people are not uniformly included in pre-licensure medication trials. Think about it—who wants to volunteer for that study while a person is carrying such precious cargo?! The FDA used to label medications into five categories based on risk versus benefit during pregnancy. They discontinued that categorization about a decade ago. Now OB providers are left to counsel their patients on the relative risk of a particular treatment during pregnancy.

While the FDA no longer has easy-to-use categories for medications and pregnancy, many OB providers rely on the Infant Risk Scale (infantrisk.com) for medication safety while breastfeeding. The safety categories were developed by lactational pharmacologist Thomas Hale, PhD, RPh, one of the top authorities in breastfeeding medicine and perinatal medication safety. We have included that information to give our readers some basic guidance.

Your obstetrician, pediatrician, pharmacist, and lactation consultant can all help provide safety and risk information. If you have doubts, contact them.

Breastfeeding Categories

- **L1**: Okay to use while nursing. Studies have been done on nursing parents to prove safety.
- **L2**: Okay, but use with caution. Safety research is limited.
- **L3**: Unknown whether there is a risk, because there are no studies in humans. Consult your OB provider.
- **L4**: Possible health hazards, so the benefit to the nursing parent must outweigh the risk to the baby.
- **L5**: Definitely harmful to baby. Do not use while nursing.

Q. How do I know if there is a problem taking more than one medicine at a time?

The official term is drug interaction.

Your doctor or pharmacist can answer this question. However, don't assume that your doctor knows all the medications you are taking. If you received a prescription from another doctor/specialist, it might not be recorded in your chart. Remind your doctor about *all* the drugs you are taking.

Reality Check

Tell your doctor if you are taking any herbal remedies. Just because they are natural doesn't mean they aren't drugs. Case in point: Cannabis, cocaine, and alcohol are natural, and they certainly have an effect on your body and your fetus.

Q. Is it safe to take acetaminophen (Tylenol) during pregnancy?

Yes. Of all of the pain and fever reducer medications, acetaminophen (Tylenol) is considered the safest to take when it is necessary. As with any non-routine medication use during pregnancy, it is best to limit use to the lowest dose and shortest duration as much as possible. But if you need it, you need it! Some observational studies have reported an association between acetaminophen use in pregnancy and autism.[2] But a recent, well-designed, large-scale study shows no associated risk.[3] And one key point that ACOG (the American College of Obstetricians and Gynecologists) makes very clear: No studies have proven that acetaminophen use *causes* autism.[4]

Pregnant people often take acetaminophen when they are running a fever, because of an infection, for example. And we know that certain infections (and fevers) during particularly sensitive periods of embryonic and fetal development in pregnancy can, in fact, lead to neurodevelopmental issues in the child. The fever or the infection may be the link here, not the medication.

There are additional studies looking at acetaminophen use in the third trimester and a weak association to wheezing in childhood.[5] We share this with you so you can weigh the potential risks and benefits of using this medication.

We concur with ACOG's recommendations: If you need to take a pain reliever or fever reducer during pregnancy, acetaminophen is your safest choice, and it is fine to use if it is needed. Do not feel guilty about using it.

Q. Can you use Tylenol and an antibiotic at the same time?

It is okay to use acetaminophen (Tylenol), cough medicine (like Robitussin DM), and an antibiotic simultaneously.

Q. I took some medications before I knew I was pregnant. What effect will it have on the baby?

The answer depends on the specific medications you took. Most medications will not cause a serious problem for your fetus, especially if you stop using them once you know you are pregnant. Talk to your OB provider about any medications (over the counter, herbal, or prescription) you have been taking.

Q. I was taking birth control pills before I realized I was pregnant. Is this a problem?

Oops! So you were still using some form of birth control and you were already pregnant? Worried it might have caused a problem for the baby? Well, you are not alone! Here is a list of common contraceptives and what (if any) potential issues could arise:

- **Depo-Provera.** This is a progesterone-only (no estrogen) injectable form of birth control. It is 97 to 99.2 percent effective in preventing pregnancy. If you become pregnant while using Depo-Provera, there may be a small risk of going into preterm labor.
- **Spermicides.** No need to worry. Spermicides do not cause birth defects or any other harm to a developing fetus if a woman becomes pregnant while using them. It's also not a problem if a pregnant woman accidentally uses a spermicide.
- **Intrauterine device (IUD).** This is the most effective form of birth control (99.9 percent effective in preventing pregnancy), but it is possible to become pregnant despite having an IUD in place—your odds are about 2 in 1,000 (rare but not impossible). This form of birth control can cause problems for a developing fetus. There is a risk of having your pregnancy located outside the uterus (see ***ectopic pregnancy***). Call your OB provider right away if you have an IUD and think you are pregnant. There is also a risk of infection, miscarriage, premature delivery, and—in extremely rare cases—death when an IUD is kept in place after an intrauterine pregnancy is diagnosed. That said, your OB provider may suggest removing your IUD, even though that procedure could cause a miscar-

riage. If your IUD cannot be removed, talk with your OB provider about the risks and benefits of continuing the pregnancy.

- **Combination oral contraceptives** (run-of-the-mill birth control pills containing both estrogen and progesterone). Besides condoms, this is the most common method of birth control. They are 99.2 percent effective at preventing a pregnancy when used correctly. Don't get too alarmed if you become pregnant while taking the pill, do not recognize that you are pregnant, and continue taking the pill. This little accident has been happening for decades and thus we know there's very little risk of birth defects from the hormones found in birth control pills. But once you find out you are pregnant, you should immediately stop using your pills. Why? You don't need them anymore! Plus, the pill contains synthetic estrogen. You want to limit your exposure to this hormone as soon as possible and let the hormones of pregnancy do their job.

Medications: The Details

Use this appendix to check on medications you may need to take during pregnancy or while you are breastfeeding. If you have questions, always ask your OB provider.

Anti-Infective Medications

Antivirals

Generic Name	Brand Name	Safety in Pregnancy	Safety in Breastfeeding
Acyclovir	Zovirax	Compatible	L2
Amantadine	Symmetrel	Avoid in first trimester	L3
Baloxavir	Xofluza	Consult your OB provider (no studies in humans)	Consult your OB provider
Bictegravir, emtricitabine, and tenofovir	Biktarvy	Human studies show no risk to mother or fetus	N/A*
Famciclovir	Famvir	Animal data suggests low risk	L2
Oseltamivir	Tamiflu	Consult your OB provider (no studies in humans)	L2
Rimantadine	Flumadine	Consult your OB provider (no studies in humans)	L3
Valacyclovir	Valtrex	Consult your OB provider (no studies in humans)	L2
Zanamivir	Relenza	Consult your OB provider (no studies in humans)	L3

*Breastfeeding is not recommended for a person who is HIV positive.

Note: No studies have been conducted to assess the safety of giving antivirals to treat the flu (influenza virus) for pregnant people. But these medications are used during pregnancy when needed, and there have never been any adverse effects on the fetus. ACOG recommends that pregnant people who become ill with the virus take oseltamivir (Tamiflu) to help prevent serious complications.[6] However, just like with most other medication, consult your OB provider before taking one of these antiviral medications.

Antibiotics

Generic Name	Brand Name	Rx or OTC?	Safety in Pregnancy	Safety in Breast-feeding
Amoxicillin	No brand names	Rx	Compatible	L1
Amox-Clavulanate	Augmentin	Rx	Compatible	L1
Azithromycin	Zithromax	Rx	Animal data shows low risk	L2
Cefaclor	Ceclor	Rx	Compatible	L1
Cefadroxil	Duricef	Rx	Compatible	L1
Cefdinir	Omnicef	Rx	Compatible	L2
Cefepime	Maxipime	Rx	Compatible	L2
Cefixime	Suprax	Rx	Compatible	L2
Cefpodoxime	Vantin	Rx	Consult your OB provider (no studies in humans)	L2
Cefprozil	Cefzil	Rx	Compatible	L1
Cefuroxime	Ceftin	Rx	Compatible	L2
Cephalexin	Keflex	Rx	Compatible	L1
Ciprofloxacin	Cipro	Rx	Not recommended if alternatives available	L3
Clarithromycin	Biaxin	Rx	Not recommended if alternatives available	L1
Clindamycin	Cleocin	Rx	Compatible	L2
Co-trimoxazole	Bactrim	Rx	No in first and third trimesters	L3
Doxycycline	Vibramycin	Rx	No, stains baby's teeth	L3
Erythromycin	E-mycin	Rx	Compatible	L2
Levofloxacin	Levaquin	Rx	Not recommended if alternatives available	L3
Metronidazole	Flagyl	Rx	Compatible	L2
Minocycline	Minocin	Rx	No, stains baby's teeth	L2
Moxifloxacin	Avelox	Rx	Not recommended if alternatives available	L2
Nitrofurantoin	Macrobid	Rx	No in first and third trimesters.	L2
Tetracycline	Achromycin V	Rx	No, stains baby's teeth	L2

Helpful Hint

Antibiotics kill both bad and certain "good" bacteria that live in our mouths and on our skin. If you lack the normal bacteria, you may be at risk for getting a yeast infection in the genital area. Consider taking a probiotic (or start downing yogurt) if you are taking antibiotics.

Antifungals

Generic Name	Brand Name	Rx or OTC?	Safety in Pregnancy	Safety in Breast-feeding
Amphotericin B	No brand name	Rx	Compatible	L3
Ciclopirox	Loprox	Rx	Topical application okay	L3
Clotrimazole*	Lotrimin*	OTC	Topical application okay	L1
Fluconazole	Diflucan	Rx	Human data suggests risk	L2
Miconazole*	Monistat*	OTC	Animal data suggests risk	L2
Nystatin*	Mycostatin*	Rx	Topical application okay	L1
Terconazole	Terazol 3 or 7	Rx	Limited data	L3

*Typically, clotrimazole and miconazole are thought to be safe during pregnancy. Nystatin cream or ointment can also help with the itching and burning in your outer genital area. Other commonly used yeast medications such as terconazole have limited safety data, and fluconazole (Diflucan) has human safety data that suggest risk. Although these two medications are commonly used during pregnancy, they should be used only after first consulting your OB provider.

Helpful Hint

Do you have toenail fungus? Nails infected with this fungus turn white or yellow, and appear thick and hard, with white debris. Whether you are pregnant or not, it can be a real challenge to treat. But during pregnancy, many of the medications docs typically use are off-limits due to potential side effects, so your only treatment option for now (and through breastfeeding) is to use a topical prescription lotion called terbinafine (Lamisil). Alternatively, you can just wait until pregnancy and breastfeeding are over with to treat your toenails. Trust us, the fungus will still be there waiting for you. And so will your dermatologist, who can then treat it with an oral medication.

Other Vaginal Medications

Generic Name	Brand Name	Rx or OTC?	Safety in Pregnancy	Safety in Breast-feeding
Clindamycin cream	Cleocin	Rx	Compatible	L2
Metronidazole cream	Metrogel	Rx	Human data suggests low risk	L2

Note: If you are diagnosed with ***bacterial vaginosis*** during pregnancy, we recommend using metronidazole (Metrogel) vaginal cream to treat it. While clindamycin (Cleocin) vaginal cream is safe to use, there is no evidence that it helps reduce the risk of preterm labor or delivery associated with this type of vaginal infection.

Allergy and Asthma Medications

Antihistamines/Allergy Medications

Generic Name	Brand Name	Rx or OTC?	Safety in Pregnancy	Safety in Breast-feeding
Azelastine	Astelin nasal spray	Rx	Consult your OB provider (no studies in humans)	L3
Brompheniramine/Phenylephrine	Dimetapp	Rx	Limited human data	L3
Budesonide	Rhinocort nasal spray	Rx	Animal data shows no risk	L1
Cetirizine	Zyrtec	Rx	Low risk	L2
Chlorpheniramine	Chlor-Trimeton	Rx	Compatible	L3
Clemastine	Tavist	Rx	Consult your OB provider (no studies in humans)	L4—passes through breast milk
Desloratadine	Clarinex	Rx	No human data	L2
Dimenhydrinate	Dramamine	Rx	Animal data shows no risk	L2
Diphenhydramine	Benadryl	Rx	Compatible	L2
Fexofenadine	Allegra	Rx	Animal data suggests moderate risk	L2
Fluticasone	Flonase nasal spray	Rx	Animal data suggests low risk	L3
Loratadine	Claritin	Rx	Compatible	L1

Asthma Medications

Generic Name	Brand Name	Rx or OTC?	Safety in Pregnancy	Safety in Breast-feeding
Albuterol inhaler	Ventolin HFA	Rx	Compatible	L1
Budesonide inhaler	Pulmicort Flexhaler	Rx	Compatible	L1
Fluticasone inhaler	Arnuity HFA	Rx	No human data	L3
Fluticasone/Salmeterol	Advair HFA	Rx	No human data	L3
Ipratropium Bromide	Atrovent HFA	Rx	Human data suggests low risk	L2
Ipratropium/Albuterol	Combivent Respimat	Rx	Human data suggests low risk	L2

Helpful Hint

Always rinse your mouth after taking an inhaled steroid. It will help prevent you from getting a yeast infection in your mouth (aka thrush).

Heart/Blood Pressure Medications

Certain heart and blood pressure medications (such as methyldopa and some drugs classified as calcium channel blockers and beta blockers) are okay to take during pregnancy. Drugs classified as angiotensin-converting enzyme inhibitors ACE inhibitors and angiotensin II receptor blockers (ARBs) are not safe to take during pregnancy.

Blood Pressure Medications

Generic Name	Brand Name	Rx or OTC?	Safety in Pregnancy	Safety in Breast-feeding
Acebutolol	Sectral	Rx	Animal data shows low risk	L3
Amlodipine	Norvasc	Rx	No human data	L3
Atenolol	Tenormin	Rx	Human data suggests risk	L3
Clonidine	Catapres	Rx	Animal data suggests risk	L3
Furosemide	Lasix	Rx	Human data shows low risk	L3
Hydralazine	Apresoline	Rx	Potential risk in third trimester	L2
Hydro-chlorothiazide	Oretic	Rx	Compatible	L2
Irbesartan	Avalide	Rx	Risk in second and third trimesters	L3
Labetalol	Trandate	Rx	Human data shows low risk	L2
Methyldopa	Aldomet	Rx	Use for gestational hyper-tension	L2
Nifedipine	Adalat	Rx	Human data shows low risk	L2
Spironolactone	Aldactone	Rx	Animal data suggests risk	L2

MEDICATIONS

Cholesterol-Lowering Medications

Generic Name	Brand Name	Rx or OTC?	Safety in Pregnancy	Safety in Breast-feeding
Atorvastatin	Lipitor	Rx	No in all trimesters	L3
Cholestyramine	Questran	Rx	Lacks human data	L1
Lovastatin	Mevacor	Rx	No in all trimesters	L3
Simvastatin	Zocor	Rx	No in all trimesters	L3

Pain and Fever Reducers

Generic Name	Brand Name	Rx or OTC?	Safety in Pregnancy	Safety in Breast-feeding
Acetaminophen	Tylenol	OTC	Compatible	L1
Acetaminophen with codeine	Tylenol 3	Rx	Human data suggests risk	L3
Acetaminophen with hydro-codone	Vicodin	Rx	Animal data suggests risk	L3
Aspirin (baby)	Bayer Low Dose	OTC	Compatible	L3
Celecoxib	Celebrex	OTC	Animal data suggests risk	L2
Codeine	Tylenol 3	OTC	Human data suggests risk	L3
Ibuprofen	Motrin, Advil	OTC	Avoid in all trimesters. Okay only after delivery.	L1
Naproxen	Aleve	OTC	Avoid in all trimesters. Human data suggests risk.	L3

The risk of using ibuprofen (Motrin/Advil) is highest in the first and third trimesters. We suggest using acetaminophen (Tylenol) during pregnancy instead. However, use acetaminophen *only as needed* in the third trimester as there is an increased risk of wheezing in kids at five years of age whose pregnant parents used acetaminophen regularly.

Skin and Acne Medications

Generic Name	Brand Name	Rx or OTC?	Safety in Pregnancy	Safety in Breast-feeding
Acitretin	Soriatane	Rx	Avoid in all trimesters	L5
Adapalene	Differin	OTC	Not recommended	L3
Azelaic acid	Azelex, Finacea	Rx	Okay for spot treatment*	L3
Benzoyl peroxide	Oxy10, Proactiv	OTC	Okay for spot treatment*	L2
Botulinum toxin A	Botox	N/A	Animal data shows risk	L3
Calamine lotion	Several brands	OTC	Compatible	L2
Clindamycin	Cleocin-T	Rx	Compatible	L2
Hyaluronic acid dermal filler	Restylane	Rx	Not recommended	L3
1 percent hydrocortisone cream	Cortaid	OTC	OTC is compatible; higher potency (Rx) is of more concern	L2
Salicylic acid	Several brands	OTC	Okay for spot treatment*	L3

*It's okay to use acne preparations that contain benzoyl peroxide and/or salicylic acid for a blemish here or there. Doctors don't recommend using them in large quantities over your entire face.

Mental Health

Anxiety Medications

Generic Name	Brand Name	Rx or OTC?	Safety in Pregnancy	Safety in Breast-feeding
Alprazolam	Xanax	Rx	Animal data suggests risk	L3
Buspirone	BuSpar	Rx	Animal data suggests low risk	L3
Clonazepam	Klonopin	Rx	Animal data suggests risk	L3
Diazepam	Valium	Rx	Risk in first and third trimesters	L3
Eszopiclone	Lunesta	Rx	Not recommended unless benefit to mother exceeds risk to fetus. No human studies.	L3
Lorazepam	Ativan	Rx	Animal data suggests risk	L3
Zaleplon	Sonata	Rx	Not recommended unless benefit to mother exceeds risk to fetus. No human studies.	L2
Zolpidem	Ambien	Rx	Not recommended unless benefit to mother exceeds risk to fetus. No human studies.	L3

Note: The medications most often used to treat anxiety disorders are the benzodiazepines (clonazepam, lorazepam, alprazolam). Older research suggested that these medications could cause an increased risk of cleft lip and cleft palate. A few recent studies have not found this association.

Antidepressants

Generic Name	Brand Name	Rx or OTC?	Safety in Pregnancy	Safety in Breast-feeding
Amitriptyline	Elavil	Rx	Human data suggests low risk	L2
Amoxapine	Asendin	Rx	Animal data suggests risk	L2
Bupropion	Wellbutrin	Rx	Human data suggests low risk	L3
Citalopram*	Celexa*	Rx	Animal data shows risk	L2
Clomipramine	Anafranil	Rx	Possible risk if taken in first and third trimesters	L2
Desipramine	Pertofrane	Rx	Human data suggests low risk	L2
Doxepin	Sinequan	Rx	Human data suggests low risk	L5
Duloxetine	Cymbalta	Rx	Risk in third trimester	L3

MEDICATIONS

Generic Name	Brand Name	Rx or OTC?	Safety in Pregnancy	Safety in Breast-feeding
Escitalopram*	Lexapro*	Rx	Discuss potential risks/ benefits in third trimester with healthcare provider	L2
Fluoxetine	Prozac*	Rx	Animal data shows risk	L2
Mirtazapine	Remeron	Rx	Animal data suggests risk	L3
Paroxetine*	Paxil*	Rx	Human data suggests risk	L2
Sertraline*	Zoloft*	Rx	Potential risk in third trimester	L2
Trazodone	Desyrel	Rx	Human data, low risk	L2
Venlafaxine	Effexor	Rx	Potential risk in third trimester	L3

*Denotes antidepressants that are in the selective serotonin reuptake inhibitor (SSRI) category.

Note: Recent studies show concern for selective serotonin reuptake inhibitor (SSRI) use in the first trimester. These drugs may cause birth defects, especially heart defects. The most recent research suggests that patients at highest risk for having fetuses with cardiac malformations are those who change their SSRI medications during their pregnancy. Use in third trimester may have temporary effects on baby's behavior after birth. Talk to both your OB provider as well as your newborn's healthcare providers.

Antipsychotics

Generic Name	Brand Name	Rx or OTC?	Safety in Pregnancy	Safety in Breast-feeding
Aripiprazole	Abilify	Rx	Animal data suggests risk	L3
Olanzapine	Zyprexa	Rx	Human data, low risk	L2
Quetiapine	Seroquel	Rx	Animal data suggests risk	L2

Sleep Aids

Generic Name	Brand Name	Rx or OTC?	Safety in Pregnancy	Safety in Breast-feeding
Doxylamine	Unisom	OTC	Compatible	L4
Estazolam	Prosom	Rx	Avoid in all trimesters	L3
Eszopiclone	Lunesta	Rx	No human data	L3
Zolpidem	Ambien	Rx	Data shows low risk but is limited	L3

Smoking Cessation

Generic Name	Brand Name	Rx or OTC?	Safety in Pregnancy	Safety in Breast-feeding
Bupropion	Zyban	Rx	Low risk	L3
Varenicline	Chantix	Rx	No human data	L4

Blood-Related Issues

Platelet/Clotting Agents

Generic Name	Brand Name	Rx or OTC?	Safety in Pregnancy	Safety in Breast-feeding
Anagrelide	Agrylin	Rx	Limited human data	L4
Apixaban	Eliquis	Rx	No human studies, could increase risk of hemorrhage at delivery	L4
Enoxaparin	Lovenox	Rx	Animal data shows no risk	L3
Heparin	No brand name	Rx	Animal data shows no risk	L1
IVIG	No brand name	Rx	Animal data shows risk	L2
Magnesium sulfate	No brand name	Rx	Animal data shows no risk	L1
Rivaroxaban	Xarelto	Rx	No, animal studies show risk of birth defects in fetus	L3
Warfarin	Coumadin		No, animal studies show risk of birth defects.	L2

Anemia

Generic Name	Brand Name	Rx or OTC?	Safety in Pregnancy	Safety in Breast-feeding
Iron	Slow FE	OTC	Compatible	L1
Folic Acid	No brand name	OTC	Compatible	L1

Gut Issues

Anti-Nausea/Vomiting Medications

Generic Name	Brand Name	Rx or OTC?	Safety in Pregnancy	Safety in Breast-feeding
Cyclizine	Marezine	OTC	Compatible	L3
Dextrose/Glucose	Emetrol	OTC	Compatible	L3
Doxylamine	Unisom	OTC	Compatible	L4
Doxylamine+B6	Diclegis, Bonjesta	Rx	Compatible	L3
Metoclopramide	Reglan	Rx	Animal data shows no risk	L2
Ondansetron	Zofran	Rx	Animal data shows no risk	L2
Promethazine	Phenergan	Rx	Compatible	L2

Note: Diclegis (doxylamine and pyridoxine) is a popular, safe prescription product for morning sickness. It's really a combination of Unisom, an over-the-counter sleep aid, and pyridoxine (vitamin B6). As you might guess, it should only be used at night, as it will cause drowsiness. You don't want to drift off to la-la land in the middle of your day just before carpool.

Helpful Hint

Don't want to take Emetrol? A home remedy is to take one to two teaspoons of heavy fruit syrup (fruit cocktail juice) every twenty to thirty minutes. This occasionally works to relieve nausea, even though the thought of it could potentially induce nausea.

Constipation

Generic Name	Brand Name	Rx or OTC?	Safety in Pregnancy	Safety in Breast-feeding
Bisacodyl	Dulcolax	OTC	Risk in second and third trimesters	L3
Castor Oil	No brand name	OTC	Limited data suggests risk	L3
Docusate sodium	Colace	OTC	Compatible	L2
Docusate calcium	Surfak	OTC	Compatible	L2
Lactulose	Kristalose	Rx	Compatible	L3
Magnesium hydroxide	Milk of Magnesia	OTC	Compatible	L2
Polyethylene Glycol PEG 3350	MiraLAX	OTC	Lacks human data	L3
Psyllium	Metamucil	OTC	Compatible	L2
Wheat dextrin	Benefiber	OTC	Compatible	L3

Hemorrhoids

Generic Name	Brand Name	Rx or OTC?	Safety in Pregnancy	Safety in Breast-feeding
Hydrocortisone/ Lidocaine	AnaMantle	Rx	Compatible	L1
Hydrocortisone/ Pramoxine	Analpram	Rx	Compatible	L1
Hydrocortisone 2.5 percent	Anusol HC	Rx	Compatible	L1
Pramoxine/ Phenylephrine	Preparation H	Rx	Compatible	L1

Digestive Agents (Probiotics)

Generic Name	Brand Name	Rx or OTC?	Safety in Pregnancy	Safety in Breast-feeding
Lactobacillus species	Several brands	Rx	Compatible	L3

Diarrhea

Generic Name	Brand Name	Rx or OTC?	Safety in Pregnancy	Safety in Breast-feeding
Bismuth Subsalicylate	Pepto Bismol	OTC	Human data shows low risk	L3
Diphenoxylate	Lomotil	Rx	Animal data shows risk	L3
Loperamide	Imodium A-D	OTC	Animal data shows low risk	L2

Acid Reflux/Heartburn

Generic Name	Brand Name	Rx or OTC?	Safety in Pregnancy	Safety in Breast-feeding
Aluminum/ Magnesium	Maalox	OTC	Compatible	L2
Calcium carbonate	TUMS	OTC	Compatible	L3
Cimetidine	Tagamet	OTC	Compatible	L2
Esomeprazole	Nexium	OTC	No human data	L2
Famotidine	Pepcid	OTC	Animal data shows low risk	L1
Lansoprazole	Prevacid	OTC	Animal data shows no risk	L3
Magnesium Hydroxide	Mylanta	OTC	Compatible	L1
Metoclopramide	Reglan	OTC	Animal data shows no risk	L2

Generic Name	Brand Name	Rx or OTC?	Safety in Pregnancy	Safety in Breast-feeding
Omeprazole	Prilosec	OTC	Animal data shows risk	L2
Rabeprazole	Aciphex	Rx	Lacks human data	L3

Cholestasis of Pregnancy

Generic Name	Brand Name	Rx or OTC?	Safety in Pregnancy	Safety in Breast-feeding
Cholestyramine	Questran	Rx	Compatible	L1
Ursodeoxycholic acid	Actigall	Rx	Animal data shows no risk	L3

Nervous System/Brain

Seizure Medications

Generic Name	Brand Name	Rx or OTC?	Safety in Pregnancy	Safety in Breast-feeding
Carbamazepine	Tegretol	Rx	Only if benefit to mother outweighs risk	L2
Clonazepam	Klonopin	Rx	Human data shows low risk	L3
Ethosuximide	Zarontin	Rx	Human data shows low risk	L4
Felbamate	Felbatol	Rx	Animal data shows modest risk	L4
Levetiracetam	Keppra	Rx	Animal data shows risk	L3
Phenytoin	Dilantin	Rx	Risk of birth defects	L2
Valproic acid	Depakote	Rx	Risk of birth defects, lower IQ	L2

Migraines

Generic Name	Brand Name	Rx or OTC?	Safety in Pregnancy	Safety in Breast-feeding
Almotriptan	Axert	Rx	Animal data, low risk	L3
Butalbital	Fioricet	Rx	Animal data shows risk	L3
Eletriptan	Relpax	Rx	Animal data shows modest risk	L2
Ergotamine	Cafergot, Migranal	Rx	Avoid in all trimesters	L4
Rimegepant	Nurtec ODT	Rx	Animal studies suggest benefits exceed risk	L2

Generic Name	Brand Name	Rx or OTC?	Safety in Pregnancy	Safety in Breast-feeding
Rizatriptan	Maxalt	Rx	Animal data shows risk	L3
Sumatriptan	Imitrex	Rx	Animal data shows risk	L3
Topiramate	Topamax	Rx	Risk of birth defects	L3
Ubrogepant	Ubrelvy	Rx	No data, cannot rule out risk to fetus	L3
Zolmitriptan	Zomig	Rx	No human data	L3

In general, the popular "triptan" class of medications (Imitrex, Maxalt, Zomig) are not considered the best options to use while pregnant, although a recent study suggested they are safe to use. And medications that are in the opiates class are only used as a last resort since they can be addictive. Other migraine meds like ergotamine (Cafergot) and dihydroergotamine (Migranal) are complete no-nos because they are extremely unsafe, and any benefit is outweighed by the potential risk to the fetus.

So what's a pregnant woman with migraines to do? Medications that prevent the onset of the migraine may be an option for you. These are meds in the "calcium channel blocker" and "beta-blocker" groups. They are safe during pregnancy and can be very effective.

Autoimmune Disorders

Lupus

Generic Name	Brand Name	Rx or OTC?	Safety in Pregnancy	Safety in Breast-feeding
Aspirin (baby)	Bayer Low Dose	Rx	Compatible	L3
Enoxaparin	Lovenox	Rx	Animal data suggests no risk	L3
Folic acid*	No brand name	Rx	Compatible in first and second trimester	L1
Heparin	No brand name	Rx	Animal data suggests no risk	L1
Hydroxychloro-quine	Plaquenil	Rx	Lacks data	L2
Prednisone	No brand name	Rx	Human data suggests risk	L2

*Folic acid, used in very high doses for autoimmune disorders, is compatible for use only in the first and second trimester. It should only be used if the benefit to the mother outweighs the risk in the third trimester. The dose of folic acid found in prenatal vitamins is just fine throughout pregnancy.

Note: There are some medications used to treat lupus that are not safe during pregnancy. For example, Coumadin (a blood thinner) and ACE inhibitors (a class of high blood pressure medication) should not be used during pregnancy. We suggest you consult with both a perinatologist and rheumatologist for advice during pregnancy and with breastfeeding.

Multiple Sclerosis

Generic Name	Brand Name	Rx or OTC?	Safety in Pregnancy	Safety in Breast-feeding
Adalimumab	Humira	Rx	Animal data shows low risk	L3
Azathioprine	Imuran	Rx	Human data shows risk	L3
Baclofen	Lioresal	Rx	Animal data shows risk	L2
Carbamazepine	Tegretol	Rx	Known human risk	L2
Corticotropin	ACTH	Rx	Known human risk	L3
Cyclophospha-mide	Cytoxan	Rx	Known human risk	L5
Dantrolene	Dantrium	Rx	Limited human data	L4
Diazepam	Valium	Rx	Known human risk	L3
Etanercept	Enbrel	Rx	Animal data shows no risk	L3
Glatiramer	Copaxone	Rx	Animal data shows no risk	L3
Interferon Beta-1A	Avonex, Rebif	Rx	Risk of miscarriage	L2
Interferon Beta-1B	Betaseron	Rx	Animal data shows low risk	L2
Natalizumab	Tysabri	Rx	Animal data shows risk	L3
Phenytoin	Dilantin	Rx	Known human risk	L2
Prednisone	No brand name	Rx	Human data suggests risk	L2

Hormonal/Endocrine Disorders

Diabetes

Generic Name	Brand Name	Rx or OTC?	Safety in Pregnancy	Safety in Breast-feeding
Acarbose	Precose, Prandase	Rx	Animal data, low risk	L3
Glipizide	Glucotrol	Rx	Animal data shows risk	L3
Glyburide	Diabeta	Rx	Human data, low risk	L2
Insulin	No brand name	Rx	Compatible	L1
Metformin	Glucophage	Rx	Animal data, no risk	L1
Pioglitazone	Actos	Rx	Animal data shows risk	L3
Sitagliptin	Januvia	Rx	Animal data, no risk	L3

Note: GLP-1 (glucagon-like peptide-1) agonists including semaglutide (such as Wegovy and Ozempic) and tirzepatide (Zepbound) are not recommended for use during pregnancy or breastfeeding. Ideally, they should be stopped at least one month before conceiving.

Thyroid Disease

Generic Name	Brand Name	Rx or OTC?	Safety in Pregnancy	Safety in Breast-feeding
Carbimazole	Neo-Mercazole	Rx	Known human risk	L3
Levothyroxine	Synthroid	Rx	No risk	L1
Methimazole	Tapazole	Rx	Potential risk	L3
Propylthiouracil	PTU	Rx	Can cause goiter in baby	L2

Note: Although propylthiouracil (PTU) and methimazole are known to have risk to the fetus, both are considered acceptable to use during pregnancy and safe for breast-feeding if needed. The benefit to the mother may outweigh the risk to the fetus.

Fibroids

Generic Name	Brand Name	Rx or OTC?	Safety in Pregnancy	Safety in Breast-feeding
Indomethacin	Indocin	Rx	Avoid in third trimester	L3

Note: Indomethacin as well as ibuprofen (brand names: Motrin, Advil) and aspirin can cause reduced amounts of amniotic fluid (***oligohydramnios***) and premature closure of an important fetal blood vessel that should remain open until after birth (***ductus arteriosus***). This problem typically happens with prolonged use (short courses are advised) or if these medications are used after twenty-eight to thirty-two weeks gestation.

Cough and Cold Remedies

Generic name	Brand Name	Rx or OTC?	Safety in Pregnancy	Safety in Breast-feeding
Dextromethorphan	Robitussin DM, Delsym	OTC	Compatible	L1
Guaifenesin	Mucinex, Robitussin	OTC	Compatible	L2
Phenylephrine	Contact-D	OTC	Human data suggests risk	L3
Pseudoephedrine	Sudafed	OTC	Animal data suggests risk	L3

Note: Decongestant nose sprays (like Afrin, see below) are usually okay as are antihistamines. Some cough medicines are *not* okay. Pseudoephedrine, a popular decongestant, may reduce milk supply by 25 percent.

MEDICATIONS

INSIDER SECRET:

A Round-up of Cough and Cold Remedies

- **Decongestants:** Intended to reduce or relieve nasal congestion. They can be taken by mouth (absorbed into bloodstream) or sprayed into the nose.
- **Oral decongestants:** Pseudoephedrine, phenylephrine, ephedrine. Avoid oral decongestants during pregnancy or use them for short periods (typically forty-eight to seventy-two hours) after you get permission from your OB provider. They all cause temporary narrowing of the blood vessels in your nose and sinus passages, which relieves congestion. But this also means that they can temporarily narrow other blood vessels (including placental vessels) if used for longer periods of time.
- **Nasal spray:** Oxymetazoline (Afrin), phenylephrine (Neosynephrine). It's safe during pregnancy. But avoid getting addicted to this stuff! You can get rebound nasal congestion if you use it more than four days in a row.
- **Saline:** Saline is just salt water. It is effective in loosening mucus and can be used as often as needed.
- **Antihistamines:** The purpose of antihistamines is to combat the effect of histamine in the body. Histamine is released as an allergy response and causes nasal congestion, among other things. Antihistamines are frequently found in cough and cold medicines because they are sedating, improve the cough suppressant effect, and dry up a runny nose. Common ingredients: brompheniramine, chlorpheniramine, diphenhydramine.
- **Expectorants:** These medications make thick mucus looser. By loosening mucus in the in the bronchial tubes (lungs) it can be coughed up more easily. These medications do not suppress the cough. Common ingredients: guaifenesin.
- **Cough suppressants:** Used to reduce the brain's "cough center" activity. For common cold and flu viruses, this is the type of cough medicine you want to use to stop coughing at night. Common ingredients: dextromethorphan.

Vitamin/Nutritional Supplements to Treat or Help You Avoid Colds

Generic Name	Rx or OTC?	Safety in Pregnancy	Safety in Breastfeeding
Co-enzyme Q10 (CoQ10)	OTC	No human data	L3
Riboflavin (B2)	OTC	Compatible	L1
Vitamin C	OTC	Avoid excessive intake	L1
Zinc	OTC	Compatible	L2

APPENDIX B

Complementary Medicines and Therapies

Complementary and integrative health blends conventional medicine and less mainstream approaches to a person's health.

Some people like to use a combination of conventional medicine and complementary approaches. Please inform your OB provider of *any* therapies you are using that your OB provider has not prescribed. There can be significant drug interactions.

Some complementary therapies may be effective and safe. Others may be ineffective or downright dangerous. Our mantra is: Show us the scientific evidence that a therapy is both safe and effective and we are happy to recommend it. Unfortunately, much of that data is lacking when it comes to complementary medicine and therapies.

Herbal Remedies

As a consumer, you need to ask a few questions about herbal remedies before you start using them:

1. **Are they effective?** There are very few scientific studies that prove with statistical significance that herbal remedies work. The National Center for Complementary and Integrative Health, part of the National Institutes of Health, is investigating many of these products.
2. **Are they safe?** There are no required clinical research trials that test herbal products on humans to prove that they are safe before they are sold to the public. Herbal remedies are categorized as "foods" by the Food and Drug Administration (FDA). This is a convenient loophole for herbal product manufacturers. This means that they do not need to do any of the scientific research that a pharmaceutical company does to market their medications. This is based on federal legislation from 1994. Attempts to revise this act have failed in the past due to political pressure (and money) from the dietary supplements lobbying group.[1]

3. **Are production standards uniform?** Production is not standardized. The potency and purity of the product may vary tremendously. This is especially true for products that contain expensive herbs (e.g., ginseng). In fact, herbs produced in China are often laced with unlabeled products such as steroids and antibiotics to make them more potent. Also know that developing countries may sell products that are contaminated with mercury, arsenic, and lead.[2] In the United States, researchers found that only 7 percent of the studied echinacea supplements complied with FDA labeling standards, and some of the supplements contained no measurable amounts of echinacea![3] A recent study showed that melatonin gummies contained varying amounts of melatonin ranging from 74 percent to 347 percent of the amount listed on the label. And some melatonin supplements contained no melatonin but instead prohibited cannabidiol (CBD), that was not listed on the label.[4]
4. **Can I trust the label?** The claims on the label for marketing purposes do not require scientific evidence that the information is accurate. Bottom line: Consumers don't have any protection against misleading information.

Compare herbs to conventional medicine. Many conventional medications are based on naturally occurring products. Penicillin is derived from a mold. Digoxin, a popular heart drug, is based on the digitalis plant. It is true that certain naturally occurring products have medical value. The difference between herbs and medications is how they are tested and regulated. Some herbs have absolutely no therapeutic value. And some herbs are so potent, they can be harmful.

We suggest you look at reliable resources to examine the evidence before you try these alternative meds. Here are a couple of free online sources:

- National Center for Complementary and Integrative Health (nccih.nih.gov/)
- Cochrane Reviews (cam.cochrane.org/cochrane-reviews-related-complementary-medicine)

BOTTOM LINE: Just because it's natural doesn't mean it is safe.

Herbs and Pregnancy

Q. What is safe to use during pregnancy?

In pregnancy, you'll want to be even more cautious about herbal therapies.

There are three herbs that are generally considered safe to use in moderation during pregnancy:

1. **Ginger root:** Ginger root is popular and seems to help relieve morning sickness. But use it with caution because there may be an increased risk of bleeding and unknown effects on the fetus.
2. **Red raspberry leaf tea** ("pregnancy tea"): Midwives commonly prescribe it to help reduce nausea and labor pains. It is probably safe for use after first trimester.
3. **Peppermint leaf:** This may be used for morning sickness and gas.

Reality Check

Yes, it is safe to cook with rosemary, garlic, sage, or ginger. The dangers we are talking about may occur when these products are used in concentrated doses for medicinal purposes.

Q. What herbs are not safe to use during pregnancy?

Other than the ones mentioned above, the rest of them should be avoided. They may increase the risk of uterine contractions or adversely affect the fetus.[5]

Herbs and Breastfeeding

Here's a summary of herbs that you can take while breastfeeding. The herbs are categorized using the same categories from Appendix A, "Medications."

Breastfeeding Categories[6]

- **L1**: Okay to use while nursing. Studies have been done on breastfeeding moms to prove safety.
- **L2**: Okay, but use with caution. Safety research is limited.
- **L3**: Unknown whether there is a risk, because there are no studies in humans.
- **L4**: Possible health hazards, so the benefit to the mother must outweigh the risk to the baby.
- **L5**: Definitely harmful to baby. Do not use while nursing.

Herb	Safety in breastfeeding
Black cohosh	L4
Blessed thistle	L3
Blue cohosh	L5
Buckthorn bark and berry	L5
Calendula	L3
Chamomile	L3
Comfrey	L5
Echinacea	L3
Evening primrose oil	L3
Fennel	L4
Fenugreek	L3
Gingko biloba	L3
Ginseng	L3
Gordolobo yerba tea	L5
Kava kava	L5
St. John's wort	L2
Tea tree oil	L3
Valerian root	L3

Homeopathy

According to the National Center for Complementary and Integrative Health (NCCIH), a branch of the National Institutes of Health, "Homeopathy is a controversial topic. A number of the key concepts underlying the theory of homeopathy are not consistent with fundamental scientific concepts as we understand them. For example, homeopathic preparations can be so dilute that a substance considered to be the 'active ingredient' becomes unmeasurable, which creates major challenges to the rigorous investigation of such products. However, recent research has begun to examine physical attributes of these preparations to determine if it will be possible to characterize them in the future."[7]

DR. B'S OPINION

The NCCIH sums it up nicely. If there is no science to back it up, don't use these therapies.

Acupuncture

Q. Is acupuncture safe during pregnancy?

Yes, it is safe. And it may be an effective way to reduce some of the aches and pains of pregnancy. However, your acupuncturist needs to avoid areas that could potentially trigger uterine contractions. Steer clear of inner or outer ankle bones and the webbing between the thumb and index finger (stimulating these areas can cause uterine contractions).

Massage Therapy

Q. Is massage therapy safe during pregnancy?

Yes. Just be sure the massage therapist has experience with prenatal massage. After eighteen to twenty weeks, you cannot lie on your back. The therapist should either have a cut-out table for your belly, or they will have you lie on your side. There are few other restrictions: no essential oils, no warming blankets, and no massages of the inner or outer ankle bones/webbing between the thumb and fingers (which, like acupuncture, can stimulate uterine contractions).

APPENDIX C

Glossary

Abdominoplasty. Aka "a tummy-tuck." A surgical procedure that helps tighten up loose fascia and the muscles of the belly, while also removing excess skin and fat in the area.

ABO incompatibility. Occurs when mom and baby's blood types are different (mom is O and baby is A or B). Mom's blood can potentially mount a response that destroys some of baby's red blood cells and increases their risk of developing jaundice as a newborn. See **jaundice**.

Acute fatty liver. A rare but serious and potentially life-threatening condition where the liver is unable to break down fatty acids and they begin to accumulate in the pregnant woman's liver. This can lead to liver insufficiency or liver failure.

Adnexae. A term that refers to the female reproductive organs, including the fallopian tubes and ovaries.

Adnexal torsion. The ovary and, sometimes, the fallopian tube twists. Twisting cuts off the blood flow to these structures. This most often happens when an ovarian or tubal cyst is present. It's possible for everything to untwist on its own, but if the twisted ovary or fallopian tube gets stuck, surgery is required to untwist the ovary/fallopian tube, and removal of the affected body part is occasionally required.

Advanced maternal age (AMA). A woman who will be thirty-five years of age or older when she gives birth.

Alpha-fetoprotein (AFP) test. This is a screening blood test done that measures a hormone that helps potentially identify neural tube defects (such as spina bifida) and some chromosomal defects (such as Down syndrome and trisomy 18) in the developing fetus. Also known as maternal serum AFP test.

Amniocentesis. A diagnostic test that can determine if a fetus has chromosomal defects. A thin needle goes through the skin into the uterus, and a little bit of amniotic fluid is taken for analysis. The test is done between fifteen and twenty weeks of pregnancy. This test is also done at times to determine whether a baby's lungs are mature enough to induce labor or perform a C-section at a time in pregnancy that is earlier than one week prior to the due date.

Amnioinfusion. Sterile water is injected into the uterus to help the umbilical cord float or to dilute thick meconium (if the fetus poops while still in the womb).

Amnion. Inner fetal membranes. The membranes that expand and enclose the embryo in a big, fluid-filled space (the amniotic cavity).

Amniotic fluid. Fluid that surrounds the fetus. It cushions the fetus and allows vital organs to grow and develop appropriately. The placenta makes some of it, and some of it is made from your unborn baby's urine.

Amniotic fluid embolism. A rare, serious condition where amniotic fluid (or other debris from the amniotic sac) ends up in the mother's blood. It can be fatal.

Amniotomy. Also known as artificial rupture of membranes (AROM). This is an obstetric procedure that involves intentionally breaking the amniotic sac or water bag during labor.

Analgesia. A term to describe pain relief without sedation or immobilization.

Anemia. Decreased ability of the red blood cells to carry an adequate amount of oxygen to body tissues. Examples of different forms of anemia include iron-deficiency anemia and sickle cell disease.

Anencephaly. A neural tube defect where there is partial or complete absence of the brain/skull.

Anesthesia. Medication that provides pain relief, immobilization, and/or sedation.

Anesthesiologist. A medical doctor specializing in the administration of anesthesia and management of patients' pain and critical care. In obstetrics, this is the doctor who performs that epidural or spinal.

Apgar score. An assessment done at one and five minutes (and occasionally at ten minutes) after delivery of your baby to see how they are transitioning to life outside the womb.

Apnea of prematurity. Babies who are born early may have temporary, prolonged pauses in their breathing. Preemies eventually outgrow this problem. Until they do, they are placed on a monitor with an alarm to warn parents if breathing stops.

Adult respiratory distress syndrome (ARDS). A life-threatening emergency where there is fluid buildup in the lungs.

Areola (plural: areolae). The colored tissue surrounding the nipples.

Arrest of descent. A condition that can occur in labor where the baby's head stops moving down the birth canal despite adequate contractions.

Arrest of dilation. A condition where the cervix stops dilating during labor despite adequate contractions.

Atelectasis. A temporary situation where part of the lung tissue does not fully expand. Symptoms include shortness of breath or difficulty breathing.

Baby blues. Moodiness and irritability occurring from a few days after delivery to two weeks afterward. You don't have trouble sleeping when you get the chance to.

Bacterial vaginosis. An overgrowth of the bacteria *Gardnerella vaginalis* that causes irritation (often itching and burning) of your external genital area and a fishy smelling discharge.

Bed rest. Exactly what it says. Resting and reclining 24/7.

Beta-hCG. See **human chorionic gonadotropin.**

Bicornuate uterus. Some women are born with a malformed uterus. This particular abnormality describes a heart-shaped womb with two "horns."

Bilirubin. A waste product of the body. It is broken down by the liver and intestines, and then excreted in our poop. When bilirubin levels get too high, the body can't get rid of all of it via poop, and it collects in the skin—this condition is called **jaundice.**

Bishop score. A calculation that helps predict whether inducing labor will be successful.

Bladder infection. See **urinary tract infection.**

Blighted ovum. Fertilized egg attaches to the uterine wall, but an embryo never develops.

Bloody show. Blood-tinged vaginal discharge seen during labor.

Body mass index (BMI). This is a calculation that measures your weight relative to your height.

Brachial plexus injury. Injury to the nerves supplying the shoulder, arm, and hand. Can occur in the fetus during a difficult delivery (for example, if there is **shoulder dystocia**).

Braxton-Hicks contractions. Your uterus is made out of muscle. Braxton-Hicks contractions occur when your uterus flexes its muscles before you need to use them in labor. You will feel your uterus harden up and then relax. Some women, especially those who have had babies before, will feel these practice contractions in their second trimester, but you are more likely to feel them in the third trimester.

Breast shield. A soft plastic artificial nipple that is placed over mom's nipple. It is used for two reasons: 1) a baby has a larger target to latch onto; and 2) a mother gains protection from baby's mouth to allow existing nursing-related injuries to heal.

Breech presentation. The baby's buttocks or foot/feet is the first body part preparing to exit the uterus. A procedure may be attempted to move the fetus (see **external cephalic version**). Or a C-section is recommended.

C-section (cesarean section): This is a surgical procedure used to deliver a baby. The obstetrician makes a small cut or incision in a woman's lower belly and uterus to remove the baby.

Carcinogen. A toxin that is known to cause cancer. Examples: arsenic, tobacco.

Cephalhematoma. Literally, a head bruise. This happens to newborns due to birth trauma. Some bruises are quite large and take one to two months to go away. Since the bruise is a collection of blood, it sometimes creates an additional bilirubin load (the breakdown product of red blood cells). This, in turn, can lead to newborn jaundice.

Cephalic. Refers to the head.

Cephalopelvic disproportion. Baby's head is too big to get through the mother's pelvic bones and thus the birth canal.

Cerclage. Stitches temporarily placed around the edge of the cervix to keep it closed.

Cerebral palsy. Muscle and posture dysfunction that varies in severity but does not get progressively worse.

Cervical insufficiency. Cervix begins to open (dilate) very early in pregnancy, often leading to loss of pregnancy. It happens between thirteen and twenty-four weeks of pregnancy.

Cervix. The opening to your uterus (womb).

Chemical pregnancy. Your body makes enough pregnancy hormone to produce a positive pregnancy test, but the pregnancy doesn't progress. You were pregnant, but a very early miscarriage occurred before anything could be detected by ultrasound.

Cholecystitis. Inflammation of the gallbladder.

Cholestasis of pregnancy. The normal flow of bile in the gallbladder and liver is decreased or stops altogether. The bile eventually enters the bloodstream and makes your skin turn yellow (see **jaundice**).

Cholasma. See **melasma.**

Chorioamnionitis. An infection of the amniotic sac.

Chorion. Fetal membranes that surround the embryo. Part of the chorion (the chorionic villi) invade the wall of the uterus and eventually form the placenta.

Chorionic villus sampling (CVS). A diagnostic test that determines whether a fetus has chromosomal defects. A thin catheter is placed into the uterus (either through the cervix or through the abdominal wall), and a small bit of tissue from the placenta is analyzed. The test is done between ten to thirteen weeks of pregnancy.

Chromosomes. Thin strands of DNA that are found in most cells in our body and serve as our genetic building blocks. We get half of our chromosomes from our mom and half from our dad.

Clavicular fracture. Broken collarbone. It can happen to newborns during a difficult delivery. It happens more commonly if mom is small and baby is big or the baby's shoulder gets stuck during delivery. The bone heals nicely within six to eight weeks without a cast.

Cleft lip. A defect occurring during fetal development that causes a gap in the middle of the upper lip. It may or may not be associated with a cleft palate. See **cleft palate**.

Cleft palate. A defect occurring during fetal development involving the roof of the mouth, leaving an opening in the middle. It may be a partial defect, or a complete one that involves the lip as well. See **cleft lip**.

Clitoral hood. The tissue lying directly above the clitoris that is a popular place for body piercings. Ouch!

Colostrum. Early breast milk. Some women begin producing and releasing it in their late second or third trimesters. This early milk is rich with the antibodies you have made over your lifetime. It is lower in calories than the mature milk produced three to five days after delivery. It looks clearer and waterier than mature milk.

Community hospital. A hospital designed to handle routine medical and surgical issues.

Complete abortion. When a miscarriage happens and all of the products of conception are expelled from the uterus.

Conception. This is the moment when the egg and sperm meet. It is also called fertilization.

Congenital heart defect. This can be a defect in the formation of the muscle wall, valve, or a chamber of the heart. Many congenital heart defects are treatable with surgery.

Cord compression. The umbilical cord and its blood vessels get compressed because they cannot float around freely (sometimes from too little amniotic fluid). Less oxygen goes to the baby, and the fetal heart rate may show a non-reassuring pattern (fetal distress).

Cord prolapse. The woman's cervix is open (dilated), and the baby's umbilical cord drops through it prior to delivery. This is serious stuff because it can reduce blood flow and oxygen to the baby. It's most commonly seen in non-vertex presentations (when something other than baby's head is first—butt, knee, foot).

Corpus luteum. A cyst that forms on the ovary during pregnancy and secretes a hormone called progesterone.

CRNA: an advanced practice registered nurse specializing in administering anesthesia and providing care before, during, and after surgical procedures. In obstetrics, this is the practitioner that may give you an epidural or in the case of a cesarean section, a spinal.

Deep venous thrombosis (DVT). A blood clot in the deep veins of the legs or pelvis.

Degenerating fibroid. Benign tumors that commonly grow in the uterus. They can enlarge during pregnancy and not get enough blood flow to sustain them, so they begin to break down and become painful.

DHA. Stands for docosahexaenoic acid. It is an omega-3 fatty acid that is needed for brain, eye, and nervous system functioning.

Diabetes mellitus. A disease where the body either does not make enough insulin or does not utilize it to properly metabolize sugar.

Diamniotic/dichorionic. Twins who have two amniotic sacs, two chorions (fetal membranes), and two placentas. These twins can be identical or fraternal.

Diamniotic/monochorionic. Twins who have two amniotic sacs, one shared chorion (fetal membrane), and one placenta. These twins can only be identical.

Diastasis recti. Also called rectus diastasis. A pregnant woman's expanding belly allows the area between the abdominal wall muscles to get bigger (creating a gap between the right and left sides). It is worse with multiples or repeated pregnancies. Consider doing Pilates after you deliver to help get those core muscles back in shape!

Dilation. The process of the cervix opening to let the baby out. This ranges from closed (not dilated at all) to ten centimeters (maximum dilation, occurring just before delivery occurs).

Dilation and curettage (D&C). Procedure where the cervix is opened (dilated) and the contents within the uterus are removed (curettage).

Dilation and evacuation (D&E). Procedure where the cervix is opened (dilated) and the contents within the uterus are removed (evacuation). This term applies to removal of a pregnancy within the uterus after the first trimester.

Disseminated intravascular coagulation (DIC). A serious blood clotting problem where tiny blood clots form throughout the body and block the blood flow to vital organs. The clots use up the blood proteins needed for your body to properly stop bleeding and excessive bleeding occurs.

Down syndrome. Also known as trisomy 21. Chromosomal defect where there are three copies of the twenty-first chromosome instead of two. It comes with characteristic facial features and causes intellectual disability as well as other abnormalities.

Ductus arteriosus. This is a connection in the fetus between the major blood vessels connected to the heart (main pulmonary artery and the aorta). At birth, this connection usually closes off on its own.

Early term. Babies who are born between thirty-seven and thirty-eight weeks gestation.

Eclampsia. Seizures that occur in severe cases of **preeclampsia**.

Ectopic pregnancy. A fertilized egg implants in an incorrect location, outside of the uterus. It can implant in the fallopian tube, ovary, cervix, or even in a woman's abdominal cavity. Since none of these places are fit for the embryo to grow, it usually dies within the first eight weeks. This is a medical emergency for a woman as it can cause severe bleeding (and, yes, pain).

Edema. Fluid accumulates in a body part, resulting in swelling of the area. The lay term for this is fluid retention.

Effacement. The cervix starts to thin out in preparation for birth. A normal cervical length is about 3 to 4 centimeters. When fully effaced (fully thinned out), the cervix can be as thin as a piece of paper.

Egg. A woman's contribution to the baby-making process. This is what is released from the ovary each month. Each egg contains half of the genetic material required to make a baby.

Elective C-section. A cesarean delivery that is desired by a woman without a medical or obstetric reason and planned before labor begins.

Embryo. This is what your unborn baby is called from the time of conception through the first eight weeks of development.

Emergency C-section. A cesarean delivery that is determined to be the best/safest mode of delivery. It can occur after labor is already in progress or may be the only mode of delivery in cases when labor has not yet begun (such as severe hemorrhage from a placenta previa at thirty-four weeks or non-reassuring fetal heart pattern found during an office visit).

Endometritis. Infection of the lining of the uterus. Symptoms include fever, chills, lower abdominal pain, bleeding, uterine tenderness, and foul-smelling discharge.

Endometriosis. Tissue from the lining of the uterus that inappropriately grows outside of the uterus. Patients can be symptom-free or suffer from severe pelvic pain.

Endometrium. Inner lining of your womb (uterus).

Engaged. When your baby's presenting body part moves down and settles into the pelvic cavity. The lay term is lightening.

Engorgement. The milkman cometh. Period of excessive breast milk production around three to five days after childbirth. Women's breasts feel full and often uncomfortable until milk demand and milk supply even out.

Epidural anesthesia. Pain relief medication that numbs the nerves from the waist down. A thin catheter tube remains in place for the duration of labor and delivery, providing a continuous flow of medication.

Episiotomy. A surgical cut in the tissue of the vagina and perineum (the tissue between the vagina and rectum) to widen the opening. Performed just before delivery of the fetal head.

Estimated date of confinement (EDC). How long you will be having company in your womb. Synonymous with estimated date of delivery (EDD).

Estimated date of delivery (EDD). How long you will be having company in your womb. Synonymous with estimated date of confinement (EDC)

External cephalic version. A procedure attempting to change a fetus's position before delivery by using ultrasound jelly and brute strength.

Fallopian tube. These muscular tubes are an extension of the uterus. We have one tube for each ovary, and each tube sits right next to its respective ovary. A mature egg leaves the ovary and travels through the fallopian tube, where it is either fertilized (and a pregnancy occurs) or not (and a menstrual period occurs).

Fecal incontinence. Lack of control over defecation leading involuntary loss of stool, gas, liquid stool, and mucus.

Fetal alcohol syndrome disorders (FASD). A range of health issues that babies experience due to alcohol exposure in the womb.

Fetal growth restriction. A fetus that does not grow as much as expected. It can be due to a problem with the fetus, the mother, or the placenta.

Fetal hypoxia. Lack of oxygen to the fetus leading to brain cell death.

Fetal ketoacidosis. A serious condition in the fetus that occurs when a diabetic pregnant woman's blood sugar is out of control. When her body is unable to process glucose properly, it breaks down fat for energy, producing ketones and acidic blood. The sugar, ketones, and acidic blood crosses the placenta, putting the fetus at risk for lack of oxygen and potential fetal demise.

Fetal kick counts. A method of monitoring how your baby is doing in the womb. The official method asks you to relax for an hour and see if you can feel your baby kicking and moving around at least ten times. It is a sign that your baby is healthy and doing well. The more realistic goal? Be sure you feel movement within every twelve-hour period. Do this every day around starting at about twenty-six weeks of pregnancy.

Fetus. This is what your unborn baby is called from nine weeks of development until they are born.

Floppy baby syndrome. Abnormally low muscle tone due to a variety of medical or genetic conditions.

Full term. A baby who is born between thirty-nine and forty weeks gestation.

Fundal height. The measurement from your pubic bone to the top of your uterus. Your fundal height in centimeters should approximately equal your gestational week (for example: a baby who is thirty-two weeks should have a fundal height of approximately 30–34 centimeters).

Gastroenteritis. An inflammation of the stomach and intestines caused by either a virus or bacteria. The inflammation can cause both vomiting and diarrhea. Viral gastroenteritis is commonly known as the stomach flu and tends to cause watery diarrhea. Bacterial gastroenteritis is commonly known as food poisoning and tends to cause diarrhea mixed with blood or mucus.

Gastroesophageal reflux disease (GERD). Lay terms: acid reflux or heartburn. A chronic condition where stomach acid comes up into the esophagus, causing burning discomfort/nauseated feeling/pain.

Gestation. The period of time that the embryo/fetus develops in the womb.

Gestational age. The number of weeks or days that the embryo/fetus has been in the womb. The countdown starts on the first day of your last menstrual period.

Gestational diabetes. Diabetes that occurs during pregnancy.

Gestational hypertension. High blood pressure that occurs during pregnancy.

Gingivitis. Bleeding, swollen gums.

Glucola test. This is a one-hour test that all pregnant women receive to screen for gestational diabetes. It is done at twenty-four and twenty-eight weeks of pregnancy, in most cases. It involves consuming a sugary drink containing 50 grams of glucose and getting your blood drawn one hour later. If your value on this test is too high, you get to take the three-hour glucose tolerance test. See **three-hour glucose tolerance test**.

Group B streptococcus (GBS). A bacteria that most often lives in harmony with a woman in her gut/bowels and vagina. It occasionally causes a vaginal or urinary tract infection in mom. It can lead to serious infection for a newborn, though, if not properly treated.

HELLP syndrome. A severe form of preeclampsia. H stands for hemolysis (red blood cells are broken down), EL stands for elevated liver enzymes, and LP stands for low platelets. Immediate delivery is necessary.

Hemoglobin electrophoresis. Special blood test that detects some of the inherited red blood cell abnormalities. See **hemoglobinopathy**.

Hemoglobinopathy. Inherited (genetic) red blood cell abnormality. Examples: sickle cell disease, thalassemia.

Hemorrhoids. Swollen veins (varicose veins) around your anus. They are itchy, and occasionally they bleed. Aren't you glad you looked this one up?

High-risk pregnancy. A pregnancy that is monitored more closely and more often, and one that is more likely to require specialized tests. Reasons for a high-risk pregnancy include having multiples, a history of repeated miscarriages or an ectopic pregnancy, conception with the help of a fertility specialist, having a chronic medical condition, being thirty-five years of age or older, or having a complication arise during pregnancy (gestational diabetes, gestational hypertension, etc.).

Human chorionic gonadotropin (beta-hCG). Hormone produced by the placenta that turns a pregnancy test positive. It tells the body to build a nest for a growing baby, and it tells the ovaries to stop producing mature eggs every month.

Humerus fracture. A break in the humerus bone in the upper arm.

Hyperbilirubinemia. See **jaundice**.

Hyperemesis gravidarum. Constant nausea and vomiting that causes dehydration and weight loss. It's thought to be due to elevated hormone levels (particularly beta-hCG) during pregnancy.

Hyperpigmentation. Area of the skin that has a darker color than normal. It occurs more commonly in darker-skinned people.

Hypertension. High blood pressure.

Hyperthyroidism. Thyroid gland produces excess amount of thyroid hormone.

Hypoglycemia. Low blood sugar.

Hypopigmentation. Area of the skin that lacks color.

Hypothyroidism. Thyroid gland does not produce adequate amounts of thyroid hormone.

Implantation. When your little peanut (embryo) attaches to the lining of the womb (uterus) and settles in.

Implantation bleeding. When the fertilized egg attaches to your womb (uterus), you may have some light spotting (mild vaginal bleeding). You may not even realize you are pregnant when this occurs because you have not missed your period yet.

Incomplete abortion. Some but not all of the tissues of pregnancy pass. The tissue that remains can cause heavy bleeding. A D&C is often needed to remove the remaining tissue.

Intertrigo. Skin chafing.

Intracranial hemorrhage. Bleeding within the skull or brain.

Intravenous fluid. A mixture of fluid and electrolytes (sodium, chloride, etc.) that goes directly into a person's vein.

Intraventricular hemorrhage. A particular type of brain bleed (intracranial hemorrhage). Bleeding occurs within the brain's spinal fluid highway (ventricles). It occurs most commonly in babies born at or before thirty-two weeks gestation, babies delivered vaginally, and those that have had asphyxia or occasionally severe birth trauma.

Jaundice. A yellowing of the skin and the whites of the eyes due to excess amounts of body waste (bilirubin) in the blood. It can be due to a liver problem or to increased breakdown of red blood cells.

Kegel exercises. Exercises to help get your pelvic floor muscles back into shape.

Ketones. The breakdown products of fat.

Large for gestational age (LGA). Over ninetieth percentile birth weight compared to other babies born at the same age.

Last menstrual period (LMP). The first day you began bleeding in your monthly cycle before becoming pregnant.

Late preterm infant. A baby born between thirty-four and thirty-six weeks of pregnancy.

Leukorrhea of pregnancy. Also known as vaginal discharge. Yellowish-white, thick, and mucousy on the underwear. We know . . . yuck.

Lightening. As in "lightening your load." The lay term is dropping. Your baby starts to head downward into your pelvis in preparation for being born. Some babies drop several weeks before delivery; others drop when labor begins. See **engaged**.

Linea alba. Translation: white line. Everyone has a line from the belly button to the top of the pubic hair. But it's invisible when you aren't pregnant.

Linea nigra. Translation: black line. A dark line from your belly button to your pubic hair that appears due to increased melanin production.

Lochia. Bloody discharge you will pass after delivery for about six weeks.

Macrosomia. The term used to refer to a big baby, at least 8.5 pounds.

Mastitis. Breast infection usually caused by cracks in the nipples, blocked milk ducts, and germs that enter through the broken skin.

Maternal-fetal medicine specialist. A physician who cares for women with high-risk pregnancies.

Meconium. Your baby's first poop. It's black, tarry, and a real mess to clean up. Ideally, it is supposed to come out after your baby is born. Unborn babies who are under stress may pass their first meconium poop in the uterus prior to delivery. This can cause a temporary breathing problem at birth if the baby breathes it into their lungs (see **meconium aspiration syndrome**).

Meconium aspiration syndrome. The baby's first poop ends up in their lungs. It can cause difficulty breathing and pneumonia. More commonly seen in babies that go past their due date.

Meconium-stained fluid. Amniotic fluid that is stained with baby poop (meconium). Seen after the amniotic sac is ruptured (you break your water bag) and the fluid begins to leak out.

Melasma. A common skin condition characterized by brownish patches on the face, also known as the mask of pregnancy. Melasma often develops during pregnancy due to rising estrogen levels.

Menstrual period. Also known as your period. If an egg does not get fertilized by a sperm in a monthly cycle, the egg dies and the lining of the uterus that has been preparing to nurture a growing baby will slough off. The result is bleeding for three to seven days.

Miscarriage. The loss of a pregnancy occurring before twenty weeks of pregnancy. There are specific types of miscarriage: complete abortion, incomplete abortion, inevitable abortion, missed abortion, recurrent abortion, and threatened abortion.

Missed abortion. The fetus dies, but there is no pain or bleeding.

Modified bed rest. Limitations on certain activities in an effort to improve pregnancy outcomes.

Molar pregnancy. A pregnancy that does not develop normally. Sometimes it is just pregnancy tissue (products of conception). Sometimes there is also an abnormal embryo growing, but it cannot survive. It can occasionally lead to a malignancy, but women are followed closely during and after molar pregnancies because of that potential.

Monochorionic. Twins who share one set of fetal membranes.

Monochorionic/monoamniotic. Twins who share one set of fetal membranes, one placenta, and one amniotic sac. They can only be identical. This type of twin pregnancy is extremely high risk.

Monounsaturated fats. Good fats, found in nuts, olives, avocados, olive and canola oil.

Mucus plug. The tissue that protects the cervix (opening to the uterus) during pregnancy. It may fall out several weeks before you go into labor—so don't get too excited if you see it in your undies or in the toilet. It looks like a glob of snot. Double yuck! Some women never see it when it falls out. And sometimes it comes out at delivery.

Neonatologist. A doctor who cares for ill and premature newborn babies.

Neural tube. The name for the beginnings of the brain, spinal cord, and nerves in an embryo or fetus.

Neural tube defect. Abnormality in the developing brain, spinal cord, and nervous system (the neural tube). Examples: spina bifida, anencephaly.

Nipple shells. Plastic devices placed over mom's nipple to help relieve soreness or help draw out flat or inverted nipples.

Non-elective C-section. See **emergency C-section**.

Non-vertex presentation. A fetus who does not plan to come out headfirst. Stubborn little thing!

Nuchal cord. Umbilical cord is wrapped around the baby's neck. It's very common and rarely a problem.

Nuchal lucency. The thickness of the fetus's neck, measured on a first trimester ultrasound. It is a helpful screening tool as a thicker size can be associated with certain chromosomal abnormalities.

Oblique lie. Baby lies diagonally when preparing to exit the womb.

Occiput anterior (OA). The typical position a baby is in at the time of delivery. The back part of the baby's head is closer to mom's pubic bone, and the baby is looking down.

Occiput posterior (OP). Baby is facing "sunny-sice up" at birth. The back of the baby's head is closer to mom's spine, and the baby is looking up toward the sky. This position can cause additional pain for the laboring mom (called back labor).

Occiput transverse. The baby plans to come out head down, but their head is turned horizontally in relationship to the mother's pelvic bones. If they face mom's left thigh, they are "right occiput transverse" or ROT. If they face mom's right thigh, they are "left occiput transverse" or LOT.

Oligohydramnios. Too little amniotic fluid.

Ovary. Women are born with two of these small, oval-shaped body organs. It's their job to store a woman's eggs. Each month, female hormones stimulate the ovary to mature one of the eggs (occasionally two) and ready it for fertilization.

Ovulation. When an egg leaves the ovary (home base) and makes the trek through the fallopian tube with the intention of meeting a nice sperm and uniting to become a baby.

Palpitations. When you sense your heart beating, like you had a double shot espresso.

Pancreatitis. Inflammation of the pancreas (an abdominal organ that releases enzymes that help in digesting food).

Pelvic inflammatory disease (PID). An infection of the uterus and fallopian tubes that can damage the female organs. Chlamydia and gonorrhea (sexually transmitted infections) are notorious for causing this problem. PID can lead to abscess formation, infertility, ectopic pregnancy, and chronic pain.

Pelvic rest. No sexual intercourse, no tampons, no douching.

Pfannenstiel incision. The name for the most common surgical cut made on the skin for a C-section. It is horizontal and made just low enough that you could still wear a bikini afterward (if you so desire!).

Placenta. Organ that interfaces between your body and your fetus while in your womb. It brings nourishment to and removes waste from the unborn baby (fetus). The umbilical cord, which contains blood vessels, is what serves as the conduit between the placenta and the fetus.

Placental abruption. Placenta pulls off the wall of the uterus prematurely. This compromises the fetus's blood flow and oxygen supply.

Placenta accreta. The placenta attaches too deeply to the inner layer of the uterus.

Placenta increta. The placenta invades too deeply and attaches to the muscle layer of the uterus.

Placenta percreta. The placenta attaches and invades through the muscle layer of the uterus, often growing into the bladder or other surrounding organs.

Placenta previa. If a fertilized egg implants in the uterus in an incorrect position (near the opening of the womb over the cervix), the placenta will then lie right over the cervix, which can lead to significant bleeding in the later part of pregnancy.

Pneumonia. Lung infection.

Polyhydramnios. Too much amniotic fluid.

Polyunsaturated fats. Fats that include omega-3 and omega-6 fatty acids.

Postdates. A pregnancy that goes beyond forty-two weeks or more than 294 days after the first day of your last menstrual period.

Postdural puncture headache. Also known as a spinal headache. A complication of having epidural anesthesia that results in a pretty severe headache.

Postpartum. "Post" means after. Postpartum refers to the six-week window after a woman gives birth.

Postpartum D&C. Procedure where the cervix is opened (dilated) and the contents of the uterus (such as leftover placenta) are removed (curettage). Occurs after delivery to stop heavy bleeding. See **retained products of conception**.

Postpartum depression. Severe fatigue, overwhelming feelings of sadness, trouble eating and sleeping after delivery.

Postpartum hemorrhage. Excessive bleeding after delivery. That means more than 500 ml of blood loss in a vaginal delivery and more than 1 liter of blood loss after a C-section.

Postterm pregnancy. A pregnancy that goes beyond forty-two weeks or more than 294 days after the first day of your last menstrual period.

Precipitous labor. A rapid labor resulting in the birth of a baby in under three hours from start to finish.

Preconception. Before you are pregnant.

Preconception visit. This is a consultation appointment with your obstetrician/OB provider before you decide to become pregnant.

Preeclampsia. You develop high blood pressure after twenty weeks of pregnancy (you previously had normal blood pressure) and you have protein in your urine.

Premature rupture of membranes (PROM). You break your water bag before labor starts.

Prenatal. "Pre" means before and "natus" means birth—so prenatal refers to the time after conception until birth. Some countries use the words "antenatal" and "prenatal" interchangeably. Confusing, we know.

Preterm premature rupture of membranes (PPROM). You break your water bag before thirty-seven weeks of pregnancy.

Public hospital. A hospital that provides services to all, regardless of ability to pay.

Pulmonary embolism (PE). A blood clot, usually from the legs (see **deep venous thrombosis**), obstructs the blood vessel to the lungs (the pulmonary artery). This can be life-threatening.

Pruritic urticarial papules and plaques (PUPPS). Really itchy red patches on the belly, thighs, legs, and arms.

Pyelonephritis. Kidney infection.

Quickening. Technical term for you feeling your baby kick or move around in the womb. It usually happens between eighteen and twenty-two weeks gestation. Women who have been pregnant before may feel it as soon as fifteen or sixteen weeks.

Respiratory distress syndrome (RDS). A premature baby whose lungs are not yet mature who has difficulty breathing on their own.

Retained products of conception (retained POC). Remnants of the placenta or amniotic membranes that are not expelled during delivery (or after a miscarriage). Their presence can interfere with the uterus contracting properly, and thus lead to excessive bleeding (postpartum hemorrhage). A D&C is sometimes necessary to remove the remaining tissue.

Retinal hemorrhage. Bleeding in the inner lining of the eye (retina).

Rh disease/isoimmunization/incompatibility. There is a blood type incompatibility between a mom who is Rh-negative and her fetus, who is Rh-positive. This can have serious effects on the fetus.

RhoGAM. A medication given to a pregnant woman who has a Rh-negative blood type to prevent her body from making antibodies to a Rh-positive fetus in a future pregnancy.

Ripe cervix. Your cervix is thinning or softening in preparation of labor.

Round ligament pain. Sharp pain in your abdomen or hip area, on one or both sides. Due to a rapidly growing uterus stretching some connections between the uterus and the abdominal wall.

Rupture of the amniotic sac. Lay term for your water breaking. Clear, watery fluid. It does not smell like urine.

Rupture of membranes. See **rupture of amniotic sac**.

Ruptured ovarian cyst. The bursting of a fluid-filled sac on the surface of or in the ovary. It hurts.

Selective fetal termination. The decision to end a pregnancy with an abnormal fetus in a multiple gestation pregnancy (twins, triplets, or more).

Sepsis. A serious bacterial infection in the bloodstream.

Shoulder dystocia. The baby's shoulder gets stuck behind mom's pubic bone during delivery. This is an emergency in which multiple maneuvers are used to deliver the baby safely.

Sickle cell disease. Blood disorder in which the red blood cells have an abnormal crescent shape. These cells get stuck in blood vessels and interfere with oxygen transport to the body tissues and organs.

Singleton. Carrying one baby during pregnancy.

Small for gestational age (SGA). A baby's birth weight is less than the tenth percentile compared to other babies born at the same number of weeks of pregnancy.

Spina bifida. A neural tube defect in which part of the spinal cord tissue (rarely brain tissue) sits in an exposed sac. It is associated with hydrocephalus. See **hydrocephalus**.

Spinal anesthesia. Pain relief via a single injection of medication into a specific area in the back, causing numbing from the waist down.

Spinal headache. See **postdural puncture headache**.

Spontaneous abortion. See **miscarriage**.

Station. The measurement that compares where your baby's head is in relation to specific bones in your pelvis. It is a way that your OB provider can track your baby's descent into the birth canal.

Stillbirth. A fetal death inside the uterus occurring after twenty-two weeks.

Stretch marks. Areas of the skin that begin as dark, purple/red streaks and eventually fade to pink/white/silver. The rapid growth of certain body parts (your breasts, your belly) causes a layer of skin to tear, resulting in these beautiful badges of courage.

Subchorionic hematoma. A collection of blood between the uterine wall and the fetal membranes. It can be a cause of vaginal bleeding.

Subgaleal hemorrhage. Bleeding between the skull bone and the layer of tissue overlying it. It happens to newborns at delivery and can be quite serious. It's rare, but it happens more often in vacuum-assisted deliveries than in standard vaginal deliveries.

Sudden infant death syndrome (SIDS). Infants who die in their sleep for no obvious reason. Risk factors include moms who smoke, warm room temperature, fluffy bedding and pillow, and babies sleeping on their tummies.

Sulcal tears. Deep tears along the sides of the vagina after a vaginal childbirth.

Surfactant. A soapy substance produced by the lungs that keeps the tiniest airways (alveoli) open. Fetuses begin making surfactant around twenty-six weeks gestation. Because lung function is critical for survival, it is difficult for a fetus to survive before they begin making surfactant.

Teaching hospital. A hospital that participates in the training of physicians and other health personnel.

Teratogens. Any environmental exposure that causes a negative effect on the development of an embryo or fetus.

Thalassemias. A group of inherited blood disorders that affect the production of hemoglobin, a protein in red blood cells that carries oxygen. Examples are alpha-thalassemia and beta-thalassemia.

Three-hour glucose tolerance test. If you don't pass your one-hour glucola test, you get further testing to see if you really have gestational diabetes. In a nutshell, it involves getting four separate blood draws, drinking a really sugary drink (yes, again), and sitting in your OB provider's office or at a lab for three to four hours.

Thrombophilias. An inherited predisposition to making blood clots.

Tocolytic medication or **tocolytics.** Medication used to stop preterm labor.

Transient tachypnea of the newborn (TTN). A newborn has some residual amniotic fluid in their lungs and thus breathes faster than normal to help clear it out. It is more common in C-sections. But, true to the name, it is temporary (transient).

Transvaginal ultrasound. Placing a probe into the vaginal canal to see an image of the womb, developing embryo/fetus and other female organs (ovaries/fallopian tubes). It is useful early in pregnancy.

Transverse lie. Fetus lying sideways when preparing to leave the womb. Not a good exit strategy. It is unsafe for both mother and baby, and a C-section is recommended.

Trimester. Your pregnancy lasts about forty weeks. That time is divided into three stages or trimesters, and each is about thirteen weeks. The first trimester is zero to thirteen weeks. The second trimester is fourteen to twenty-seven weeks. The third trimester is twenty-eight to forty weeks.

Twin-twin transfusion syndrome. Twins who share one placenta (monochorionic) may have blood vessel connections that allow one twin to get a larger share of blood flow and nutrients ("recipient twin") and one twin to get less ("donor twin").

Type 1 diabetes. Type 1 diabetes is caused by an insulin deficiency. There are not enough insulin-making cells in the pancreas because they have been destroyed. Type 1 diabetes usually begins in childhood.

Type 2 diabetes. See **diabetes mellitus** for details. Type 2 diabetes is primarily caused by the body's diminished response to insulin (resistance) as well as decreased insulin secretion. Type 2 diabetes is more common in overweight and obese people.

Umbilical cord. The tissue that connects the placenta to the baby. It contains three blood vessels: one blood vessel brings nutrients, oxygen, and antibodies to the unborn baby and the other two send back the baby's waste products to its mom.

Umbilical cord prolapse. See **cord prolapse**.

Unfavorable cervix. Your cervix is not ready to deliver yet.

Urethral sphincter. The muscle between the bladder and the urethra that prevents leakage of your urine.

GLOSSARY

Urinary incontinence. Inability to hold urine. Laughing and coughing make it worse in certain cases.

Urinary tract infection (UTI). Lay term: bladder infection. Bacterial infection starting in the urine and leading to infection of the bladder walls.

Uterine atony. The uterine muscles are soft after delivery and do not contract. This can lead to excessive bleeding.

Uterine didelphys. A double uterus. There is a double uterus and cervix. It is also possible to have additional duplications (example: vagina).

Uterine fibroid. Benign smooth muscle tumor in the womb (uterus).

Uterine rupture. The wall of the uterus opens, usually at the site of a uterine scar from a previous C-section.

Uterus. This is the female organ commonly known as the womb. It is where the developing baby grows until they are ready to be born.

Vagina. This is the muscular passageway between the opening of the womb (cervix) and the outside world. It is there for sexual intercourse and for menstrual bleeding. And it is the birth canal that your baby will travel through if you deliver without needing a C-section.

Vaginal delivery. A baby is delivered after traveling through the birth canal (the vagina). The vagina is basically a muscular tube that goes from the uterus and cervix to the outside.

Vaginal discharge. See **leukorrhea of pregnancy**.

Vaginitis. Inflammation and irritation of the vagina. Itchy and red.

Vanishing twin. Death of one fetus early on in a twin pregnancy.

Varicella-zoster virus. The virus that causes both chickenpox and shingles.

Vasa previa. The blood vessels of the placenta are abnormally found coursing through the amniotic sac and lie directly over the cervix. This can occur when there are two lobes (pieces) of the placenta instead of one, or when there is an abnormal insertion of the umbilical cord into the placenta. Rupture of membranes may be life-threatening for the fetus.

Vasovagal event. Blood flow shifts away from the brain, causing someone to faint.

VBAC. Abbreviation for vaginal birth after cesarean.

Vernix. Cheesy substance that covers your unborn baby's skin to protect them from their watery environment. You'll see it on them once they are born.

Vertex. When your baby plans to be born with their head coming out first. This is the most common, and preferred, position.

Viability. The age that a fetus is capable of surviving outside the womb. Ballpark is around twenty-three to twenty-four weeks of pregnancy.

Vulva. The external female genitals. It includes both sets of "lips" or folds of tissue (called the labia majora and labia minora), the clitoris, and the outer part of the vagina.

Yeast infection. Infection caused by yeast (candida). Yeast likes warm, moist places where there is little competition from bacteria. It will often infect the vagina, nipples, and a baby's mouth. If inadequately treated, it can be passed back and forth between a nursing mother/baby pair.

ACKNOWLEDGMENTS

Michele: I am profoundly grateful for those who stood by me through the late nights and weekends filled with reading and typing, the frequent deadlines and all of my doubts.

Neil, you have been and continue to be my guru for all things obstetrics! Thank you for your expertise and time on yet another edition.

Michael, your repeated encouragement helped me to do this again. Thank you and I love you.

Leila and Ava, thank you for choosing me to be your Mama. I love you both so much.

Ari: To Elysia Liang, Marnie Cochran, and the rest of the team at Rodale Books, and Kristin von Ogtrop at InkWell Management—thank you for believing in this project and helping the next generation of parents on their journey.

NOTES

Chapter 1. It's Positive. . . . Now What Do I Do?

1. American College of Obstetricians and Gynecologists, *Your Pregnancy and Childbirth: Month to Month* (American College of Obstetricians and Gynecologists Women's Health Care Physicians, 2021).
2. Neville F. Hacker, Joseph C. Gambone, and Calvin J. Hobel, *Hacker & Moore's Essentials of Obstetrics and Gynecology* (Elsevier Health Sciences, 2015).
3. Thomas W. Sadler, *Langman's Medical Embryology*, 14th edition (LWW, 2018).

Chapter 2: The First Trimester

1. Thomas W. Sadler, *Langman's Medical Embryology*, 14th edition (LWW, 2018).
2. Jason C. Birnholz, "The Development of Human Fetal Eye Movement Patterns," *Science* 213, no. 4508 (August 7, 1981): 679–81, https://doi.org/10.1126/science.7256272.

Chapter 3: The Second Trimester

1. "Periviable Birth," ACOG, n.d., https://www.acog.org/clinical/clinical-guidance/obstetric-care-consensus/articles/2017/10/periviable-birth.

Chapter 4: The Third Trimester

1. "Prevention of Group B Streptococcal Early-Onset Disease in Newborns," *Obstetrics and Gynecology* 135, no. 2 (January 24, 2020): e51–72, https://doi.org/10.1097/aog.0000000000003668.

Chapter 5: Is This Normal?

1. "Breast Cancer During Pregnancy," Cancer.gov, December 14, 2022, https://www.cancer.gov/types/breast/patient/pregnancy-breast-treatment-pdq.
2. Nicola R. Young et al., "Does Greater Morning Sickness Predict Carrying a Girl? Analysis of Nausea and Vomiting During Pregnancy from Retrospective Report," *Archives of Gynecology and Obstetrics* 303, no. 5 (October 24, 2020): 1161–66, https://doi.org/10.1007/s00404-020-05839-1.
3. Hilary Baldwin and Jerry Tan, "Effects of Diet on Acne and Its Response to Treatment," *American Journal of Clinical Dermatology* 22, no. 1 (August 3, 2020): 55–65, https://doi.org/10.1007/s40257-020-00542-y.

Chapter 6: Tests

1. "Hemoglobinopathies in Pregnancy," ACOG, n.d., https://www.acog.org/clinical/clinical-guidance/practice-advisory/articles/2022/08/hemoglobinopathies-in-pregnancy.
2. Mark B. Landon et al., *Gabbe's Obstetrics: Normal and Problem Pregnancies* (Saunders, 2020).

3. Toni Medina, "Testing & Diagnosis," NFXF, May 22, 2025, https://fragilex.org/fx/testing-diagnosis/#:~:text=Specific%20indications%20for%20testing%20include,learning%20disabilities%20of%20unknown%20cause.
4. "Current ACOG Guidance," ACOG, n.d., https://www.acog.org/advocacy/policy-priorities/non-invasive-prenatal-testing/current-acog-guidance.
5. Jessica M. Turner et al., "Evaluation of Pregnancy Outcomes Among Women with Decreased Fetal Movements," *JAMA Network Open* 4, no. 4 (April 8, 2021): e215071, https://doi.org/10.1001/jamanetworkopen.2021.5071.
6. "Prevention of Group B Streptococcal Early-Onset Disease in Newborns," ACOG, n.d., https://www.acog.org/clinical/clinical-guidance/committee-opinion/articles/2020/02/prevention-of-group-b-streptococcal-early-onset-disease-in-newborns#:~:text=Introduction-,Group%20B%20streptococcus%20(GBS)%20is%20the%20leading%20cause%20of%20newborn,the%20genitourinary%20and%20gastrointestinal%20tracts.

Chapter 7: Nutrition

1. "Obesity and Pregnancy," ACOG, n.d., https://www.acog.org/womens-health/faqs/obesity-and-pregnancy.
2. "Obesity and Pregnancy," ACOG, n.d., https://www.acog.org/womens-health/faqs/obesity-and-pregnancy.
3. U.S. Department of Agriculture and U.S. Department of Health and Human Services, *Dietary Guidelines for Americans, 2020–2025*, report, 2020, https://DietaryGuidelines.gov.
4. U.S. Department of Agriculture and U.S. Department of Health and Human Services, *Dietary Guidelines for Americans, 2020–2025*, report, 2020, https://DietaryGuidelines.gov.
5. U.S. Department of Agriculture and U.S. Department of Health and Human Services, *Dietary Guidelines for Americans, 2020–2025*, report, 2020, https://DietaryGuidelines.gov.
6. Bianka Hoxha et al., "Folic Acid and Autism: A Systematic Review of the Current State of Knowledge," *Cells* 10, no. 8 (August 3, 2021): 1976, https://doi.org/10.3390/cells10081976.
7. "MTHFR Gene Variant and Folic Acid Facts," Folic Acid, May 27, 2025, https://www.cdc.gov/folic-acid/data-research/mthfr/index.html.
8. "Neural Tube Defects," ACOG, n.d., https://www.acog.org/clinical/clinical-guidance/practice-bulletin/articles/2017/12/neural-tube-defects.
9. Julie E.H. Nevins et al., "Omega-3 Fatty Acid Dietary Supplements Consumed During Pregnancy and Lactation and Child Neurodevelopment: A Systematic Review," *Journal of Nutrition* 151, no. 11 (June 28, 2021): 3483–94, https://doi.org/10.1093/jn/nxab238.
10. Irene Cetin et al., "Omega-3 Fatty Acid Supply in Pregnancy for Risk Reduction of Preterm and Early Preterm Birth," *American Journal of Obstetrics & Gynecology MFM* 6, no. 2 (December 7, 2023): 101251, https://doi.org/10.1016/j.ajogmf.2023.101251.
11. Irene Cetin et al., "Omega-3 Fatty Acid Supply in Pregnancy for Risk Reduction of Preterm and Early Preterm Birth," *American Journal of Obstetrics & Gynecology MFM* 6, no. 2 (December 7, 2023): 101251, https://doi.org/10.1016/j.ajogmf.2023.101251.
12. Kat Gál, "The Complete Guide to Omega-3-Rich Foods," Medical News Today, November 15, 2023, https://www.medicalnewstoday.com/articles/323144#vegetarian-and-vegan.
13. Chrysoula Giourga et al., "Vitamin D Deficiency as a Risk Factor of Preeclampsia During Pregnancy," *Diseases* 11, no. 4 (November 2, 2023): 158, https://doi.org/10.3390/diseases11040158.
14. H.P.M. Smedts et al., "High Maternal Vitamin E Intake by Diet or Supplements Is Associated with Congenital Heart Defects in the Offspring," *BJOG an International Journal of*

Obstetrics & Gynaecology 116, no. 3 (January 21, 2009): 416–23, https://doi.org/10.1111/j.1471-0528.2008.01957.x.

15. *Weight Gain During Pregnancy*, *National Academies Press eBooks*, 2009, https://doi.org/10.17226/12584.
16. "Weight Gain During Pregnancy," ACOG, n.d., https://www.acog.org/clinical/clinical-guidance/committee-opinion/articles/2013/01/weight-gain-during-pregnancy.
17. Mark B. Landon et al., *Gabbe's Obstetrics: Normal and Problem Pregnancies* (Elsevier, 2024).
18. Katherine J. Stothard et al., "Maternal Overweight and Obesity and the Risk of Congenital Anomalies," *JAMA* 301, no. 6 (February 10, 2009): 636, https://doi.org/10.1001/jama.2009.113.
19. U.S. Department of Agriculture and U.S. Department of Health and Human Services, *Dietary Guidelines for Americans, 2020–2025*, report, 2020, https://DietaryGuidelines.gov.
20. Adi Y. Weintraub et al., "Effect of Bariatric Surgery on Pregnancy Outcome," *International Journal of Gynecology & Obstetrics* 103, no. 3 (September 2, 2008): 246–51, https://doi.org/10.1016/j.ijgo.2008.07.008.
21. Anatte Karmon and Eyal Sheiner, "Pregnancy After Bariatric Surgery: A Comprehensive Review," *Archives of Gynecology and Obstetrics* 277, no. 5 (February 25, 2008): 381–88, https://doi.org/10.1007/s00404-008-0608-5.

Chapter 8: Environmental Health

1. Line Mathiesen et al., "Fetal Exposure to Environmental Chemicals: Insights from Placental Perfusion Studies," *Placenta* 106 (February 15, 2021): 58–66, https://doi.org/10.1016/j.placenta.2021.01.025.
2. Jessica L. Gleason et al., "Association Between Maternal Caffeine Consumption and Metabolism and Neonatal Anthropometry," *JAMA Network Open* 4, no. 3 (March 25, 2021): e213238, https://doi.org/10.1001/jamanetworkopen.2021.3238.
3. "Moderate Caffeine Consumption During Pregnancy," ACOG, n.d., https://www.acog.org/clinical/clinical-guidance/committee-opinion/articles/2010/08/moderate-caffeine-consumption-during-pregnancy.
4. Human Foods Program, "Aspartame and Other Sweeteners in Food," U.S. Food and Drug Administration, February 27, 2025, https://www.fda.gov/food/food-additives-petitions/aspartame-and-other-sweeteners-food.
5. Carla R. Toop et al., "Impact of Perinatal Exposure to Sucrose or High Fructose Corn Syrup (HFCS-55) on Adiposity and Hepatic Lipid Composition in Rat Offspring," *The Journal of Physiology* 595, no. 13 (April 27, 2017): 4379–98, https://doi.org/10.1113/jp274066.
6. "Nutrition During Pregnancy," ACOG, n.d., https://www.acog.org/womens-health/faqs/nutrition-during-pregnancy.
7. Human Foods Program, "Questions & Answers From the FDA/EPA Advice About Eating Fish for Those Who Might Become or Are Pregnant or Breastfeeding and Children Ages 1 to 11 Years," U.S. Food And Drug Administration, February 17, 2022, https://www.fda.gov/food/consumers/questions-answers-fdaepa-advice-about-eating-fish-those-who-might-become-or-are-pregnant-or.
8. Angela Zacharasiewicz, "Maternal Smoking in Pregnancy and Its Influence on Childhood Asthma," *ERJ Open Research* 2, no. 3 (July 1, 2016): 00042–02016, https://doi.org/10.1183/23120541.00042-2016.
9. "Smoking, Pregnancy, and Babies," Centers for Disease Control and Prevention, March 15, 2023, https://www.cdc.gov/tobacco/campaign/tips/diseases/pregnancy.html.
10. Johanna M. Jaakkola et al., "Childhood Exposure to Parental Smoking and Life-course

Overweight and Central Obesity," *Annals of Medicine* 53, no. 1 (December 11, 2020): 208–16, https://doi.org/10.1080/07853890.2020.1853215.

11. Maria Vlachou et al., "Perinatal Smoking and Sleep Disorders in Neonatal Age: A Systematic Review," *Tobacco Prevention & Cessation* 10, no. Supplement 1 (October 17, 2024), https://doi.org/10.18332/tpc/194364.
12. "Marijuana Use During Pregnancy and Lactation," ACOG, n.d., https://www.acog.org/clinical/clinical-guidance/committee-opinion/articles/2017/10/marijuana-use-during-pregnancy-and-lactation#:~:text=Because%20of%20concerns%20regarding%20impaired,encouraged%20to%20discontinue%20marijuana%20use.
13. Abay Woday Tadesse et al., "Prenatal Cannabis Use and the Risk of Attention Deficit Hyperactivity Disorder and Autism Spectrum Disorder in Offspring: A Systematic Review and Meta-analysis," *Journal of Psychiatric Research* 171 (January 23, 2024): 142–51, https://doi.org/10.1016/j.jpsychires.2024.01.045.
14. Gale A. Richardson et al., "Pathways from Prenatal Cocaine Exposure to Adult Substance Use and Behavior," *Neurotoxicology and Teratology* 102 (February 17, 2024): 107335, https://doi.org/10.1016/j.ntt.2024.107335.
15. "Child Welfare Information Gateway," childwelfare.gov, accessed July 4, 2025, https://Childwelfare.gov.
16. "About Zika," Zika Virus, January 30, 2025, https://www.cdc.gov/zika/about/index.html.
17. "Dengue During Pregnancy," Dengue, January 30, 2025, https://www.cdc.gov/dengue/hcp/clinical-signs/pregnancy.html#:~:text=Pregnant%20women%20can%20transmit%20dengue,birth%20weight%2C%20and%20premature%20birth.
18. Linda M. Frazier, "Reproductive Disorders Associated with Pesticide Exposure," *Journal of Agromedicine* 12, no. 1 (July 31, 2007): 27–37, https://doi.org/10.1300/j096v12n01_04.
19. American Academy of Pediatrics. Council on Environmental Health, *Pediatric Environmental Health*, 2018.
20. Geneviève Van Maele-Fabry, Laurence Gamet-Payrastre, and Dominique Lison, "Household Exposure to Pesticides and Risk of Leukemia in Children and Adolescents: Updated Systematic Review and Meta-analysis," *International Journal of Hygiene and Environmental Health* 222, no. 1 (September 26, 2018): 49–67, https://doi.org/10.1016/j.ijheh.2018.08.004.
21. Michelle C. Turner, Donald T. Wigle, and Daniel Krewski, "Residential Pesticides and Childhood Leukemia: A Systematic Review and Meta-analysis," *Ciência & Saúde Coletiva* 16, no. 3 (March 1, 2011): 1915–31, https://doi.org/10.1590/s1413-81232011000300026.
22. American Academy of Pediatrics Committee on Nutrition, *Pediatric Nutrition Handbook.*, ed. Frank R. Greer and Steven A. Abrams, 9th ed. (American Academy of Pediatrics, 2025).
23. World Health Organization: WHO, "Pesticide Residues in Food," September 15, 2022, https://www.who.int/news-room/fact-sheets/detail/pesticide-residues-in-food.
24. Sharon K. Sagiv et al., "Prenatal and Childhood Exposure to Organophosphate Pesticides and Behavior Problems in Adolescents and Young Adults in the CHAMACOS Study," *Environmental Health Perspectives* 131, no. 6 (June 1, 2023), https://doi.org/10.1289/ehp11380.
25. "Protecting Children from Pesticides: Information for Parents," HealthyChildren.org, n.d., https://www.healthychildren.org/English/safety-prevention/all-around/Pages/Protecting-Children-from-Pesticides-Information-for-Parents.aspx.
26. "Known and Probable Human Carcinogens," American Cancer Society, n.d., https://www.cancer.org/cancer/risk-prevention/understanding-cancer-risk/known-and-probable-human-carcinogens.html.
27. "Are GMO Foods Safe for My Child? AAP Policy Explained," HealthyChildren.org, n.d., https://www.healthychildren.org/English/healthy-living/nutrition/Pages/are-GMO-foods-safe-for-my-child-AAP-policy-explained.aspx.

28. "Our Current Understanding of the Human Health and Environmental Risks of PFAS | US EPA," US EPA, November 26, 2024, https://www.epa.gov/pfas/our-current-understanding-human-health-and-environmental-risks-pfas.
29. "Fish, Mercury, and the Developing Brain," *URMC Newsroom*, February 5, 2025, https://www.urmc.rochester.edu/news/publications/neuroscience/fish-mercury-and-the-developing-brain.
30. Richard L. Canfield et al., "Intellectual Impairment in Children with Blood Lead Concentrations Below 10 Mg per Deciliter," *New England Journal of Medicine* 348, no. 16 (April 16, 2003): 1517–26, https://doi.org/10.1056/nejmoa022848.
31. Dunzhu Li et al., "Microplastic Release from the Degradation of Polypropylene Feeding Bottles During Infant Formula Preparation," *Nature Food* 1, no. 11 (October 19, 2020): 746–54, https://doi.org/10.1038/s43016-020-00171-y.
32. Yufei Wang and Haifeng Qian, "Phthalates and Their Impacts on Human Health," *Healthcare* 9, no. 5 (May 18, 2021): 603, https://doi.org/10.3390/healthcare9050603.
33. Dennis R. Ownby, Christine Cole Johnson, and Edward L. Peterson, "Exposure to Dogs and Cats in the First Year of Life and Risk of Allergic Sensitization at 6 to 7 Years of Age," *JAMA* 288, no. 8 (August 28, 2002): 963, https://doi.org/10.1001/jama.288.8.963.
34. "Electric and Magnetic Fields," National Institute of Environmental Health Sciences, n.d., https://www.niehs.nih.gov/health/topics/agents/emf.
35. "Do Cell Phones Cause Cancer? | Cellphones and Cancer," American Cancer Society, n.d., https://www.cancer.org/cancer/risk-prevention/radiation-exposure/cellular-phones.html.
36. "Travel Tips: Pregnant Travelers," Transportation Security Association, accessed July 4, 2025, https://TSA.gov.
37. "Risk Factors for Childhood Leukemia," American Cancer Society, n.d., https://www.cancer.org/cancer/types/leukemia-in-children/causes-risks-prevention/risk-factors.html.
38. "Guidelines for Diagnostic Imaging During Pregnancy and Lactation," ACOG, n.d., https://www.acog.org/clinical/clinical-guidance/committee-opinion/articles/2017/10/guidelines-for-diagnostic-imaging-during-pregnancy-and-lactation.
39. "Guidelines for Diagnostic Imaging During Pregnancy and Lactation," ACOG, n.d., https://www.acog.org/clinical/clinical-guidance/committee-opinion/articles/2017/10/guidelines-for-diagnostic-imaging-during-pregnancy-and-lactation.

Chapter 9: Lifestyles

1. "Physical Activity and Exercise During Pregnancy and the Postpartum Period," ACOG, n.d., https://www.acog.org/clinical/clinical-guidance/committee-opinion/articles/2020/04/physical-activity-and-exercise-during-pregnancy-and-the-postpartum-period.
2. Enrico M. Camporesi, "Diving and Pregnancy," *Seminars in Perinatology* 20, no. 4 (August 1, 1996): 292–302, https://doi.org/10.1016/s0146-0005(96)80022-x.
3. ME Aronson and Nelson, "Fatal Air Embolism in Pregnancy Resulting from an Unusual Sex Act," *Obstetrics and Gynecology* 30, no. 1 (1967): 127–30.
4. S Ashai et al., "Assessment of Medical Care," *New England Journal of Medicine* 295, no. 2 (July 8, 1976): 117–18, https://doi.org/10.1056/nejm197607082950235.
5. "Air Travel During Pregnancy," ACOG, n.d., https://www.acog.org/clinical/clinical-guidance/committee-opinion/articles/2018/08/air-travel-during-pregnancy.
6. A. J. Greenwald, T. H. Allen, and R. W. Bancroft, "Abdominal Gas Volume at Altitude and at Ground Level," *Journal of Applied Physiology* 26, no. 2 (February 1, 1969): 177–81, https://doi.org/10.1152/jappl.1969.26.2.177.
7. "Home | U.S. Equal Employment Opportunity Commission," US Equal Employment Opportunity Commission, accessed July 5, 2025, https://www.eeoc.gov/.

8. "Fact Sheet #28A: Employee Protections Under the Family and Medical Leave Act," DOL, n.d., https://www.dol.gov/agencies/whd/fact-sheets/28a-fmla-employee-protections.

Chapter 10: Self-Care

1. Jasmin Eatman et al., "Personal Care Product Use Is Associated With Elevated Phthalate Levels During Pregnancy in the Atlanta African American Maternal Child Cohort [ID 1393]," *Obstetrics and Gynecology* 145, no. 6S (May 15, 2025): 78S-79S, https://doi.org/10.1097/aog.0000000000005918.074.
2. Office of the Commissioner, "Hair Smoothing Products That Release Formaldehyde When Heated," U.S. Food And Drug Administration, October 15, 2024, https://www.fda.gov/cosmetics/cosmetic-products/hair-smoothing-products-release-formaldehyde-when-heated#:~:text=What%20Should%20Consumers%20Know?,Methylene%20glycol.
3. Che-Jung Chang et al., "Use of Straighteners and Other Hair Products and Incident Uterine Cancer," *JNCI Journal of the National Cancer Institute* 114, no. 12 (October 17, 2022): 1636–45, https://doi.org/10.1093/jnci/djac165.
4. "BOTOX® (onabotulinumtoxinA) - Official BOTOX® Cosmetic Site," BOTOX®, n.d., https://www.botoxcosmetic.com/.
5. Megha Trivedi, Takeshi Inouye, and Jenny Murase, "Safety of Cosmetic Procedures During Pregnancy and Lactation: A Review [24E]," *Obstetrics and Gynecology* 129, no. 1 (May 1, 2017): 58S, https://doi.org/10.1097/01.aog.0000514815.26206.d6.
6. *HIGHLIGHTS OF PRESCRIBING INFORMATION*, prescribing information, 2023, https://www.rxabbvie.com/pdf/botox_pi.pdf.
7. Meaghan E. Coyle, Caroline Smith, and Brian Peat, "Cephalic Version by Moxibustion for Breech Presentation," *Cochrane Library* 2023, no. 5 (May 9, 2023), https://doi.org/10.1002/14651858.cd003928.pub4.
8. Elma D Baron, "Selection of Sunscreen and Sun Protective Measures," ed. Rosamarie Corona, *UpToDate*, March 2025, https://www.uptodate.com/contents/selection-of-sunscreen-and-sun-protective-measures.
9. American Academy of Dermatology, "10 Surprising Facts About Indoor Tanning," accessed July 6, 2025, https://www.aad.org/public/diseases/skin-cancer/surprising-facts-about-indoor-tanning.
10. Office of the Commissioner, "Nail Care Products," U.S. Food And Drug Administration, October 15, 2024, https://www.fda.gov/cosmetics/cosmetic-products/nail-care-products#:~:text=Toluene%20is%20used%20as%20a,containing%20toluene%20had%20dropped%20sharply.

Chapter 11: Parenthood Prep

1. "About Vitamin K Deficiency Bleeding," Vitamin K Deficiency Bleeding, January 17, 2025, https://www.cdc.gov/vitamin-k-deficiency/about/index.html.
2. Rachael Schulte et al., "Rise in Late Onset Vitamin K Deficiency Bleeding in Young Infants Because of Omission or Refusal of Prophylaxis at Birth," *Pediatric Neurology* 50, no. 6 (February 28, 2014): 564–68, https://doi.org/10.1016/j.pediatrneurol.2014.02.013.
3. J. J. Nietfeld et al., "Lifetime Probabilities of Hematopoietic Stem Cell Transplantation in the U.S.," *Biology of Blood and Marrow Transplantation* 14, no. 3 (February 15, 2008): 316–22, https://doi.org/10.1016/j.bbmt.2007.12.493.
4. William T. Shearer et al., "Cord Blood Banking for Potential Future Transplantation," *PEDIATRICS* 140, no. 5 (October 30, 2017): e20172695, https://doi.org/10.1542/peds.2017-2695.
5. "Umbilical Cord Blood Banking," ACOG, n.d., https://www.acog.org/clinical/clinical-guidance/committee-opinion/articles/2019/03/umbilical-cord-blood-banking.

6. "Circumcision | Boston Children's Hospital," n.d., https://www.childrenshospital.org/treatments/circumcision.
7. Thomas C. Quinn, "Circumcision and HIV Transmission," *Current Opinion in Infectious Diseases* 20, no. 1 (December 20, 2006): 33–38, https://doi.org/10.1097/qco.0b013e328012c5bc.
8. "Herpes - STI Treatment Guidelines," n.d., https://www.cdc.gov/std/treatment-guidelines/herpes.htm.
9. Nader Shaikh et al., "Prevalence of Urinary Tract Infection in Childhood," *The Pediatric Infectious Disease Journal* 27, no. 4 (March 31, 2008): 302–8, https://doi.org/10.1097/inf.0b013e31815e4122.
10. S. Collins, "Effects of Circumcision on Male Sexual Function: Debunking a Myth?," *Journal of Urology* 167, no. 5 (May 2002): 2111–12.
11. S. Masood et al., "Penile Sensitivity and Sexual Satisfaction After Circumcision: Are We Informing Men Correctly?," *Urologia Internationalis* 75, no. 1 (January 1, 2005): 62–66, https://doi.org/10.1159/000085930.
12. DaiSik Kim and Myung-Geol Pang, "The Effect of Male Circumcision on Sexuality," *BJU International* 99, no. 3 (November 28, 2006): 619–22, https://doi.org/10.1111/j.1464-410x.2006.06646.x.
13. Susan Blank et al., "Circumcision Policy Statement," *PEDIATRICS* 130, no. 3 (August 28, 2012): 585–86, https://doi.org/10.1542/peds.2012-1989.
14. "Circumcision - American Urological Association," n.d., https://www.auanet.org/about-us/aua-statements/circumcision.
15. Aletha C. Huston and Stacey Rosenkrantz Aronson, "Mothers' Time with Infant and Time in Employment as Predictors of Mother–Child Relationships and Children's Early Development," *Child Development* 76, no. 2 (March 1, 2005): 467–82, https://doi.org/10.1111/j.1467-8624.2005.00857.
16. "Immunization Schedules," June 4, 2025. Accessed June 17, 2025. https://publications.aap.org/redbook/resources/15585/Immunization-Schedules.
17. Ranee Seither et al., "Coverage with Selected Vaccines and Exemption Rates Among Children in Kindergarten — United States, 2023–24 School Year," *MMWR Morbidity and Mortality Weekly Report* 73, no. 41 (October 17, 2024): 925–32, https://doi.org/10.15585/mmwr.mm7341a3.
18. Michael J. Smith and Charles R. Woods, "On-time Vaccine Receipt in the First Year Does Not Adversely Affect Neuropsychological Outcomes," *PEDIATRICS* 125, no. 6 (May 25, 2010): 1134–41, https://doi.org/10.1542/peds.2009-2489.
19. Frank DeStefano, Cristofer S. Price, and Eric S. Weintraub, "Increasing Exposure to Antibody-Stimulating Proteins and Polysaccharides in Vaccines Is Not Associated With Risk of Autism," *The Journal of Pediatrics* 163, no. 2 (March 30, 2013): 561–67, https://doi.org/10.1016/j.jpeds.2013.02.001.
20. "Immunization Schedules," June 4, 2025. Accessed June 17, 2025. https://publications.aap.org/redbook/resources/15585/Immunization-Schedules.

Chapter 12: Feeding Your Newborn

1. Noel T. Mueller et al., "The Infant Microbiome Development: Mom Matters," *Trends in Molecular Medicine* 21, no. 2 (December 11, 2014): 109–17, https://doi.org/10.1016/j.molmed.2014.12.002.
2. M. M. Vennemann et al., "Does Breastfeeding Reduce the Risk of Sudden Infant Death Syndrome?," *PEDIATRICS* 123, no. 3 (March 1, 2009): e406–10, https://doi.org/10.1542/peds.2008-2145.
3. Alison M. Stuebe et al., "Lactation and Incidence of Premenopausal Breast Cancer," *Archives of Internal Medicine* 169, no. 15 (August 10, 2009): 1364, https://doi.org/10.1001/archinternmed.2009.231.

4. "Breastfeeding Report Card," Breastfeeding Data, February 24, 2025, https://www.cdc.gov/breastfeeding-data/breastfeeding-report-card/index.html.
5. Nina R. O'Connor et al., "Pacifiers and Breastfeeding," *Archives of Pediatrics and Adolescent Medicine* 163, no. 4 (April 6, 2009): 378, https://doi.org/10.1001/archpediatrics.2008.578.
6. Nina R. O'Connor et al., "Pacifiers and Breastfeeding," *Archives of Pediatrics and Adolescent Medicine* 163, no. 4 (April 6, 2009): 378, https://doi.org/10.1001/archpediatrics.2008.578.
7. Ruth A. Lawrence and Robert M. Lawrence, *Breastfeeding: A Guide for the Medical Profession* (Elsevier, 2021).

Chapter 13. Home Stretch

1. Marian F. MacDorman and Eugene Declercq, "Trends and State Variations in Out-of-Hospital Births in the United States, 2004–2017," *Birth* 46, no. 2 (December 10, 2018): 279–88, https://doi.org/10.1111/birt.12411.
2. Edward H. Bishop, "Pelvic Scoring for Elective Induction," *Obstetrics and Gynecology* 24 (August 1964): 266–68.
3. "Total Cesarean Deliveries: United States, 2023," March of Dimes | PeriStats, n.d., https://www.marchofdimes.org/peristats/data?reg=99&top=8&stop=86&lev=1&slev=1&obj=9&dv=ms.
4. "ACOG Committee Opinion No. 761: Cesarean Delivery on Maternal Request," *Obstetrics and Gynecology* 133, no. 1 (January 1, 2019): e73–77, https://doi.org/10.1097/aog.0000000000003006.
5. Antonio Braga et al., "Increase in Cesarean Sections in Brazil – a Call to Reflection," *Revista Brasileira Ginecologia E Obstetrícia* 45, no. 03 (March 1, 2023): 109–12, https://doi.org/10.1055/s-0043-1768454.
6. "ACOG Committee Opinion No. 761: Cesarean Delivery on Maternal Request," Obstetrics and Gynecology 133, no. 1 (January 1, 2019): e73–77, https://doi.org/10.1097/aog.0000000000003006.
7. "NIH State-of-the-Science Conference Statement on Cesarean Delivery on Maternal Request," *NIH Consens State Sci Statements* 23, no. 1 (March 2006): 1–29.
8. S. Liu et al., "Maternal Mortality and Severe Morbidity Associated With Low-risk Planned Cesarean Delivery Versus Planned Vaginal Delivery at Term," *Canadian Medical Association Journal* 176, no. 4 (February 12, 2007): 455–60, https://doi.org/10.1503/cmaj.060870.
9. Ahmad F Bakr and Mohammad M Abbas, "Severe Respiratory Distress in Term Infants Born Electively at High Altitude," *BMC Pregnancy and Childbirth* 6, no. 1 (February 16, 2006), https://doi.org/10.1186/1471-2393-6-4.
10. ACOG Practice Advisory, Counseling Regarding Approach to Delivery After Cesarean and the Use of a Vaginal Birth After Cesarean Calculator, December 2021.
11. "Vaginal Birth After Cesarean Delivery," ACOG, n.d., https://www.acog.org/clinical/clinical-guidance/practice-bulletin/articles/2019/02/vaginal-birth-after-cesarean-delivery.
12. "Counseling Regarding Approach to Delivery After Cesarean and the Use of a Vaginal Birth After Cesarean Calculator," ACOG, n.d., https://www.acog.org/clinical/clinical-guidance/practice-advisory/articles/2021/12/counseling-regarding-approach-to-delivery-after-cesarean-and-the-use-of-a-vaginal-birth-after-cesarean-calculator.
13. "Macrosomia," ACOG, n.d., https://www.acog.org/clinical/clinical-guidance/practice-bulletin/articles/2020/01/macrosomia.
14. B. J. McGuinness and A. N. Trivedi, "Maternal Height as a Risk Factor for Caesarean Section Due to Failure to Progress in Labour," *Australian and New Zealand Journal of Obstetrics and Gynaecology* 39, no. 2 (May 1, 1999): 152–54, https://doi.org/10.1111/j.1479-828x.1999.tb03360.x.

Chapter 14. Labor Day

1. Grazia Rutigliano et al., "Peripheral Oxytocin and Vasopressin: Biomarkers of Psychiatric Disorders? A Comprehensive Systematic Review and Preliminary Meta-analysis," *Psychiatry Research* 241 (May 5, 2016): 207–20, https://doi.org/10.1016/j.psychres.2016.04.117.
2. Linmarie Sikich et al., "Intranasal Oxytocin in Children and Adolescents with Autism Spectrum Disorder," *New England Journal of Medicine* 385, no. 16 (October 13, 2021): 1462–73, https://doi.org/10.1056/nejmoa2103583.
3. Simon G. Gregory et al., "Association of Autism with Induced or Augmented Childbirth in North Carolina Birth Record (1990–1998) and Education Research (1997–2007) Databases," *JAMA Pediatrics* 167, no. 10 (August 13, 2013): 959, https://doi.org/10.1001/jamapediatrics.2013.2904.
4. Anna Sara Oberg et al., "Association of Labor Induction with Offspring Risk of Autism Spectrum Disorders," *JAMA Pediatrics* 170, no. 9 (July 25, 2016): e160965, https://doi.org/10.1001/jamapediatrics.2016.0965.
5. The Leapfrog Group, "The Leapfrog Group 2025 Report on Trends: State of Maternity Care in U.S. Hospitals," report, *The Leapfrog Group 2025 Report on Trends*, 2025, https://www.leapfroggroup.org/sites/default/files/Files/MaternityCare-report-2025-FINAL_0.pdf.
6. "Delayed Umbilical Cord Clamping After Birth," ACOG, n.d., https://www.acog.org/clinical/clinical-guidance/committee-opinion/articles/2020/12/delayed-umbilical-cord-clamping-after-birth.
7. Nicole K. Yamada et al., "2023 American Heart Association and American Academy of Pediatrics Focused Update on Neonatal Resuscitation: An Update to the American Heart Association Guidelines for Cardiopulmonary Resuscitation and Emergency Cardiovascular Care," *PEDIATRICS*, November 16, 2023, https://doi.org/10.1542/peds.2023-065030.
8. Dana Figueroa et al., "Surgical Staples Compared with Subcuticular Suture for Skin Closure After Cesarean Delivery," *Obstetrics and Gynecology* 121, no. 1 (January 1, 2013): 33–38, https://doi.org/10.1097/aog.0b013e31827a072c.
9. "ACOG Practice Bulletin No. 209: Obstetric Analgesia and Anesthesia," *Obstetrics and Gynecology* 133, no. 3 (February 28, 2019): e208–25, https://doi.org/10.1097/aog.0000000000003132.
10. R. Russell, R. Dundas, and F. Reynolds, "Long Term Backache After Childbirth: Prospective Search for Causative Factors," *BMJ* 312, no. 7043 (June 1, 1996): 1384–88, https://doi.org/10.1136/bmj.312.7043.1384a.
11. Cynthia A. Wong et al., "The Risk of Cesarean Delivery with Neuraxial Analgesia Given Early Versus Late in Labor," *New England Journal of Medicine* 352, no. 7 (February 16, 2005): 655–65, https://doi.org/10.1056/nejmoa042573.
12. Gonen Ohel et al., "Early Versus Late Initiation of Epidural Analgesia in Labor: Does It Increase the Risk of Cesarean Section? A Randomized Trial," *American Journal of Obstetrics and Gynecology* 194, no. 3 (March 1, 2006): 600–605, https://doi.org/10.1016/j.ajog.2005.10.821.
13. Kristi Watterberg et al., "Providing Care for Infants Born at Home," *PEDIATRICS* 145, no. 5 (April 20, 2020), https://doi.org/10.1542/peds.2020-0626.

Chapter 15. Postpartum: What's Next?

1. "Risks and Complications," n.d., https://www.redcrossblood.org/donate-blood/blood-donation-process/what-happens-to-donated-blood/blood-transfusions/risks-complications.html.
2. Roger Y. Dodd, "Current Risk for Transfusion Transmitted Infections," *Current Opinion in Internal Medicine* 7, no. 1 (September 26, 2007): 45–50, https://doi.org/10.1097/moh.0b013e3282e38e8a.

3. Gladys M. Martinez and Kimberly Daniels, "Fertility of Men and Women Aged 15–49 in the United States: National Survey of Family Growth, 2015–2019," *Natl Health Stat Report.* 179 (2023): 1–22.
4. Lucy J. Puryear, *Understanding Your Moods When You're Expecting: Emotions, Mental Health, and Happiness—Before, During, and After Pregnancy* (Houghton Mifflin Harcourt, 2008).

Chapter 16. Pregnancy 911

1. Haywood L. Brown, "Trauma in Pregnancy," *Obstetrics and Gynecology* 114, no. 1 (July 1, 2009): 147–60, https://doi.org/10.1097/aog.0b013e3181ab6014.

Chapter 17. The Complicated Pregnancy

1. Eero Kajantie, "Fetal Origins of Stress-Related Adult Disease," *Annals of the New York Academy of Sciences* 1083, no. 1 (November 1, 2006): 11–27, https://doi.org/10.1196/annals.1367.026.
2. Shoboo Rahmati et al., "The Relationship Between Maternal Anemia During Pregnancy with Preterm Birth: A Systematic Review and Meta-analysis," *The Journal of Maternal-Fetal & Neonatal Medicine* 33, no. 15 (December 7, 2018): 2679–89, https://doi.org/10.1080/14767058.2018.1555811.
3. "Gestational Hypertension and Preeclampsia," ACOG, n.d., https://www.acog.org/clinical/clinical-guidance/practice-bulletin/articles/2020/06/gestational-hypertension-and-preeclampsia.
4. "Gestational Hypertension and Preeclampsia," ACOG, n.d., https://www.acog.org/clinical/clinical-guidance/practice-bulletin/articles/2020/06/gestational-hypertension-and-preeclampsia.
5. Mitchell P. Dombrowski and Michael Schatz, "ACOG Practice Bulletin No. 90: Asthma in Pregnancy," *Obstetrics and Gynecology* 111, no. 2 (February 1, 2008): 457–64, https://doi.org/10.1097/aog.0b013e3181665ff4.
6. "Thyroid Disease in Pregnancy," ACOG, n.d., https://www.acog.org/clinical/clinical-guidance/practice-bulletin/articles/2020/06/thyroid-disease-in-pregnancy.
7. "Thyroid Disease in Pregnancy," ACOG, n.d., https://www.acog.org/clinical/clinical-guidance/practice-bulletin/articles/2020/06/thyroid-disease-in-pregnancy.
8. "Pregnancy With Type 1 or Type 2 Diabetes," ACOG, n.d., https://www.acog.org/womens-health/faqs/pregnancy-with-type-1-or-type-2-diabetes.
9. Wing Hung Tam et al., "Glucose Intolerance and Cardiometabolic Risk in Children Exposed to Maternal Gestational Diabetes Mellitus in Utero," *PEDIATRICS* 122, no. 6 (December 1, 2008): 1229–34, https://doi.org/10.1542/peds.2008-0158.
10. Diaz-Santana, Mary V et al. "Persistence of Risk for Type 2 Diabetes After Gestational Diabetes Mellitus." *Diabetes Care* vol. 45,4 (2022): 864–870. doi:10.2337/dc21-1430.
11. "Cerclage for the Management of Cervical Insufficiency," ACOG, n.d., https://www.acog.org/clinical/clinical-guidance/practice-bulletin/articles/2014/02/cerclage-for-the-management-of-cervical-insufficiency.
12. Mark B. Landon et al., *Gabbe's Obstetrics: Normal and Problem Pregnancies* (Saunders, 2020).
13. Mark B. Landon et al., *Gabbe's Obstetrics: Normal and Problem Pregnancies* (Saunders, 2020).
14. "Risks and Complications," n.d., https://www.redcrossblood.org/donate-blood/blood-donation-process/what-happens-to-donated-blood/blood-transfusions/risks-complications.html.
15. "Oligohydramnios," March of Dimes, n.d., https://www.marchofdimes.org/find-support/topics/planning-baby/oligohydramnios#:~:text=Oligohydramnios%20is%20when%20you%20have,the%20amniotic%20sac%20(membrane).

16. Liming Lei et al., "Effect of Anesthesia on the Success Rate of External Cephalic Version: GRADE-Assessed Systematic Review and Meta-analysis of Randomized Controlled Trials," *Systematic Reviews* 13, no. 1 (July 30, 2024), https://doi.org/10.1186/s13643-024-02616-y.
17. "Macrosomia," ACOG, n.d., https://www.acog.org/clinical/clinical-guidance/practice-bulletin/articles/2020/01/macrosomia.
18. ACOG Committee Opinion No. 743 Summary: Low-Dose Aspirin Use During Pregnancy, *Obstetrics and Gynecology* 132, no. 1 (June 26, 2018): 254–56, https://doi.org/10.1097/aog.0000000000002709.
19. "ACOG Practice Bulletin No. 204: Fetal Growth Restriction," *Obstetrics and Gynecology* 133, no. 2 (January 25, 2019): e97–109, https://doi.org/10.1097/aog.0000000000003070.
20. "Management of Late-Term and Postterm Pregnancies," ACOG, n.d., https://www.acog.org/clinical/clinical-guidance/practice-bulletin/articles/2014/08/management-of-late-term-and-postterm-pregnancies.
21. Tim A. Bruckner, Yvonne W. Cheng, and Aaron B. Caughey, "Increased Neonatal Mortality Among Normal-weight Births Beyond 41 Weeks of Gestation in California," *American Journal of Obstetrics and Gynecology* 199, no. 4 (July 18, 2008): 421.e1-421.e7, https://doi.org/10.1016/j.ajog.2008.05.015.

Chapter 18. Infections

1. "Prenatal and Perinatal Human Immunodeficiency Virus Testing," ACOG, n.d., https://www.acog.org/clinical/clinical-guidance/committee-opinion/articles/2018/09/prenatal-and-perinatal-human-immunodeficiency-virus-testing.
2. "Viral Hepatitis in Pregnancy," ACOG, n.d., https://www.acog.org/clinical/clinical-guidance/clinical-practice-guideline/articles/2023/09/viral-hepatitis-in-pregnancy.
3. "Cytomegalovirus, Parvovirus B19, Varicella Zoster, and Toxoplasmosis in Pregnancy," ACOG, n.d., https://www.acog.org/clinical/clinical-guidance/practice-bulletin/articles/2015/06/cytomegalovirus-parvovirus-b19-varicella-zoster-and-toxoplasmosis-in-pregnancy.
4. "Clinical Overview of CMV and Congenital CMV," Cytomegalovirus (CMV) and Congenital CMV Infection, November 6, 2024, https://www.cdc.gov/cytomegalovirus/hcp/clinical-overview/?CDC_AAref_Val=https://www.cdc.gov/cmv/clinical/congenital-cmv.html.
5. "COVID-19, Pregnancy, Childbirth, and Breastfeeding: Answers from Ob-Gyns," ACOG, n.d., https://www.acog.org/womens-health/faqs/coronavirus-covid-19-pregnancy-and-breastfeeding.
6. "ACOG Statement on HHS Recommendations Regarding the COVID Vaccine During Pregnancy," ACOG, May 27, 2025, https://www.acog.org/news/news-releases/2025/05/acog-statement-on-hhs-recommendations-regarding-the-covid-vaccine-during-pregnancy.
7. "Influenza in Pregnancy: Prevention and Treatment," ACOG, n.d., https://www.acog.org/clinical/clinical-guidance/committee-statement/articles/2024/02/influenza-in-pregnancy-prevention-and-treatment.
8. A. A. Eick, "Maternal Influenza Vaccination and Effect on Influenza Virus in Young Infants," *Archives of Pediatric and Adolescent Medicine* 165, no. 2 (Feb 2011): 104–11.
9. "Update on Immunization and Pregnancy: Tetanus, Diphtheria, and Pertussis Vaccination," ACOG, n.d., https://www.acog.org/clinical/clinical-guidance/committee-opinion/articles/2017/09/update-on-immunization-and-pregnancy-tetanus-diphtheria-and-pertussis-vaccination#:~:text=The%20American%20College%20of%20Obstetricians%20and%20Gynecologists%20encourages%20obstetrician%E2%80%93gynecologists,of%20gestation%20in%20each%20pregnancy.
10. "COVID-19 Vaccines and Pregnancy: Conversation Guide for Clinicians," ACOG, n.d.,

https://www.acog.org/covid-19/covid-19-vaccines-and-pregnancy-conversation-guide-for-clinicians.

11. "RSV Immunization Guidance for Infants and Young Children," Respiratory Syncytial Virus Infection (RSV), August 30, 2024, https://www.cdc.gov/rsv/hcp/vaccine-clinical-guidance/infants-young-children.html.

Chapter 19. Advanced Maternal Age

1. Andrea Brown et al., "Trends in Mean Age of Mothers in the United States, 2016 to 2023," *National Vital Statistics Reports*, n.d., https://doi.org/10.15620/cdc/174598.
2. Ralitza H. Peneva and Matthew M. Finneran, "278 Is Age Just a Number? Advanced Maternal Age and Stillbirth Risk," *American Journal of Obstetrics and Gynecology* 230, no. 1 (January 1, 2024): S160–61, https://doi.org/10.1016/j.ajog.2023.11.300.
3. "Screening for Fetal Chromosomal Abnormalities," ACOG, n.d., https://www.acog.org/clinical/clinical-guidance/practice-bulletin/articles/2020/10/screening-for-fetal-chromosomal-abnormalities.
4. Linda J. Heffner, "Advanced Maternal Age—How Old Is Too Old?," *New England Journal of Medicine* 351, no. 19 (November 3, 2004): 1927–29, https://doi.org/10.1056/nejmp048087.
5. Damin Ahn et al., "Congenital Anomalies and Maternal Age: A Systematic Review and Meta-analysis of Observational Studies," *Acta Obstetricia Et Gynecologica Scandinavica* 101, no. 5 (March 14, 2022): 484–98, https://doi.org/10.1111/aogs.14339.
6. Jennita Reefhuis and Margaret A. Honein, "Maternal Age and Non-chromosomal Birth Defects, Atlanta—1968–2000: Teenager or Thirty-something, Who Is at Risk?," *Birth Defects Research* 70, no. 9 (September 1, 2004): 572–79, https://doi.org/10.1002/bdra.20065.
7. Harry Fisch et al., "The Influence of Paternal Age on Down Syndrome," *The Journal of Urology* 169, no. 6 (June 1, 2003): 2275–78, https://doi.org/10.1097/01.ju.0000067958.36077.d8.
8. Abraham Reichenberg et al., "Advancing Paternal Age and Autism," *Archives of General Psychiatry* 63, no. 9 (September 1, 2006): 1026, https://doi.org/10.1001/archpsyc.63.9.1026.
9. Rakesh Sharma et al., "Effects of Increased Paternal Age on Sperm Quality, Reproductive Outcome and Associated Epigenetic Risks to Offspring," *Reproductive Biology and Endocrinology* 13, no. 1 (April 17, 2015), https://doi.org/10.1186/s12958-015-0028-x.
10. Fay Menacker and Division of Vital Statistics, "Trends in Cesarean Rates for First Births and Repeat Cesarean Rates for Low-Risk Women: United States, 1990–2003," *National Vital Statistics Reports* (2005) 54, no. 4.

Chapter 20. Preterm Labor and Babies

1. "Management of Preterm Labor," ACOG, n.d., https://www.acog.org/clinical/clinical-guidance/practice-bulletin/articles/2016/10/management-of-preterm-labor.
2. Brady E. Hamilton, Joyce A. Martin, and Michelle J.K. Osterman, "Vital Statistics Rapid Release Report No. 38 April 2025 Births: Provisional Data for 2024," April 2025, https://www.cdc.gov/nchs/data/vsrr/vsrr038.pdf.
3. Updated Clinical Guidance for the Use of Progestogen Supplementation for the Prevention of Recurrent Preterm Birth," n.d., https://www.acog.org/clinical/clinical-guidance/practice-advisory/articles/2023/04/updated-guidance-use-of-progestogen-supplementation-for-prevention-of-recurrent-preterm-birth.
4. Amy E. Hearne and David A. Nagey, "Therapeutic Agents in Preterm Labor: Tocolytic Agents," *Clinical Obstetrics & Gynecology* 43, no. 4 (December 1, 2000): 787–801, https://doi.org/10.1097/00003081-200012000-00009.

5. Dwight J. Rouse et al., "A Randomized, Controlled Trial of Magnesium Sulfate for the Prevention of Cerebral Palsy," *New England Journal of Medicine* 359, no. 9 (August 27, 2008): 895–905, https://doi.org/10.1056/nejmoa0801187.
6. "Antenatal Corticosteroid Therapy for Fetal Maturation," ACOG, n.d., https://www.acog.org/clinical/clinical-guidance/committee-opinion/articles/2017/08/antenatal-corticosteroid-therapy-for-fetal-maturation.
7. "Periviable Birth," ACOG, n.d., https://www.acog.org/clinical/clinical-guidance/obstetric-care-consensus/articles/2017/10/periviable-birth.
8. "Periviable Birth," ACOG, n.d., https://www.acog.org/clinical/clinical-guidance/obstetric-care-consensus/articles/2017/10/periviable-birth.
9. Dan L. Stewart et al., "Updates on an At-Risk Population: Late-Preterm and Early-Term Infants," *PEDIATRICS* 144, no. 5 (October 21, 2019), https://doi.org/10.1542/peds.2019-2760.

Chapter 21. Multiples

1. "Multifetal Gestations Twin Triplet and Higher-Order Multifetal Pregnancies," ACOG, n.d., https://www.acog.org/clinical/clinical-guidance/practice-bulletin/articles/2021/06/multifetal-gestations-twin-triplet-and-higher-order-multifetal-pregnancies.
2. "Weight Gain During Pregnancy Reexamining the Guidelines," n.d., https://doi.org/10.17226/12584.
3. "Management of Preterm Labor," ACOG, n.d., https://www.acog.org/clinical/clinical-guidance/practice-bulletin/articles/2016/10/management-of-preterm-labor.
4. M. Evans et al., "International, Collaborative Experience of 1789 Patients Having Multifetal Pregnancy Reduction: A Plateauing of Risks and Outcomes," *Journal of the Society for Gynecologic Investigation* 3, no. 1 (January 1, 1996): 23–26, https://doi.org/10.1016/1071-5576(95)00037-2.

Chapter 22. When It Doesn't Work

1. Fan Qu et al., "The Association Between Psychological Stress and Miscarriage: A Systematic Review and Meta-analysis," *Scientific Reports* 7, no. 1 (May 4, 2017), https://doi.org/10.1038/s41598-017-01792-3.

Appendix A: Medications

1. Lexi-Drugs. Wolters Kluwer Health, Inc; May 17, 2025. UpToDate, n.d. https://www.uptodate.com
2. Diddier Prada et al., "Evaluation of the Evidence on Acetaminophen Use and Neurodevelopmental Disorders Using the Navigation Guide Methodology," *Environmental Health* 24, no. 1 (August 13, 2025), https://doi.org/10.1186/s12940-025-01208-0.
3. Viktor H. Ahlqvist et al., "Acetaminophen Use During Pregnancy and Children's Risk of Autism, ADHD, and Intellectual Disability," *JAMA* 331, no. 14 (April 9, 2024): 1205, https://doi.org/10.1001/jama.2024.3172.
4. "ACOG Affirms Safety and Benefits of Acetaminophen During Pregnancy," September 22, 2025, https://www.acog.org/news/news-releases/2025/09/acog-affirms-safety-benefits-acetaminophen-pregnancy.
5. Elizabeth M. Kang et al., "Prenatal Exposure to Acetaminophen and Asthma in Children," *Obstetrics and Gynecology* 114, no. 6 (November 21, 2009): 1295–1306, https://doi.org/10.1097/aog.0b013e3181c225c0.
6. "Physician FAQ: Influenza," ACOG, n.d., https://www.acog.org/programs/immunization-for-women/physician-tools/influenza-faqs-for-providers.

Appendix B: Complementary Medicines and Therapies

1. United States Congress, "Dietary Supplement Health and Education Act of 1994," *Public Law*, 1994, https://www.congress.gov/103/statute/STATUTE-108/STATUTE-108-Pg4325.pdf.
2. Kathi J. Kemper, *The Holistic Pediatrician, Twentieth Anniversary Revised Edition: A Pediatrician's Comprehensive Guide to Safe and Effective Therapies for the 25 Most Common Ailments of Infants, Children, and Adolescents* (Harper Paperbacks, 2016).
3. Christine M Gilroy et al., "Echinacea and Truth in Labeling," *Archives of Internal Medicine* 163, no. 6 (March 24, 2003): 699, https://doi.org/10.1001/archinte.163.6.699.
4. Pieter A. Cohen et al., "Quantity of Melatonin and CBD in Melatonin Gummies Sold in the US," *JAMA* 329, no. 16 (April 25, 2023): 1401, https://doi.org/10.1001/jama.2023.2296.
5. "Dietary and Herbal Supplements," NCCIH, n.d., https://www.nccih.nih.gov/health/dietary-and-herbal-supplements.
6. InfantRisk.com. Accessed July 26, 2025.
7. "Homeopathy," NCCIH, n.d., https://www.nccih.nih.gov/health/homeopathy.

EXPECTING 411 MEDICAL ADVISORY BOARD

Michael J. Hakakha, MD
Diplomate, American Board of Obstetrics and Gynecology
Assistant Clinical Professor, Obstetrics and Gynecology
David Geffen School of Medicine at UCLA
Southern California Kaiser Permanente
Los Angeles, CA

Linda Hill, RN, IBCLC
Lactation Consultant
The Breast Connection
Midland, TX

Andy Hooper, MD
Anesthesiologist
Austin, TX

Elieke Kearns, PhD, RD
Nutrition scientist and registered dietitian
Chicago, IL

Susan Landers, MD, FAAP, FABM
Neonatologist
Austin, TX

Heather Milovina
Certified Nurse Midwife
Maui, HI

Steve Rutman, MD
Anesthesiologist
Austin, TX

Michael R Sanchez, MD
Obstetric Anesthesiologist
Attending Physician, Cedars-Sinai Medical Center

Neil S. Silverman, MD, FACOG
Professor of Clinical Obstetrics and Gynecology
Director, Maternal-Fetal Medicine Fellowship Program
Director, Infections in Pregnancy Program
David Geffen School of Medicine at UCLA

Mark Zamutt, RPh
Pharmacist
Austin, TX

CREDITS

Photo of teddy bear: Kunut/Adobe Stock

Icons:

Reality Check (checkmark): owngraphic1/Adobe Stock

Helpful Hints (pencil): TVHAPPYLINE/Adobe Stock

Red Flags (flag): ssstocker/Adobe Stock skull: YSStock/Adobe Stock

Fact Check (conversation bubbles): lanastace/Adobe Stock

New Parent-to-Be 411 (clipboard): Belashova/Adobe Stock

Insider Secrets (magnifying glass): YSStock/Adobe Stock

Feedback from the Real World (radio tower): YSStock/Adobe Stock

Dr. B's Opinion (stethoscope): YSStock/Adobe Stock

Dr. M's Opinion (medical bag): Craft Studio/Adobe Stock

Warning sign: Graphic asset/Adobe Stock

Partner Tip (couple): Yusuf/Adobe Stock

INDEX

ABOUT THE AUTHORS

MICHELE MILOVINA, MD, FACOG, is an obstetrician/gynecologist with twenty-seven years of experience in caring for pregnant women and delivering their babies. She is in private practice in Beverly Hills, California.

Dr. Milovina graduated with honors from the University of California, Santa Barbara, with a Bachelor of Science degree in biopsychology. She then returned to her home state of Hawai'i to complete her medical school training at the John A. Burns School of Medicine at the University of Hawai'i, where she was inducted into the Alpha Omega Alpha Medical Honor Society. After deciding to pursue a career in women's health, Dr. Milovina began a rigorous four-year residency program at Cedars-Sinai Medical Center in Los Angeles, California, under the chairmanship of world-famous perinatologist, Dr. Lawrence Platt.

Dr. Milovina has contributed to numerous articles, educational videos and podcasts on pregnancy, and appeared in *Little Man*, a 2005 award-winning documentary on preterm birth. She has received many awards during her career including the Janet M. Glasgow award for academic excellence in women's health and the Prematurity Champion Award given by the March of Dimes. Dr. Milovina is board-certified, a process she maintains annually and is a fellow of The American College of Obstetricians and Gynecologists.

Dr. Milovina's interest in caring for women extend internationally as well, and since 2018, she has been the head of the OB-GYN portion of the Los Angeles Medical Mission. This group travels annually to remote villages in Guatemala to provide poverty-stricken populations with life-saving medical care and surgery. She also initiated the first midwife training course in rural Guatemala which she continues to teach annually. She and other OB-GYNs help educate and train rural lay midwives about postpartum hemorrhage, preeclampsia, neonatal resuscitation, and other pregnancy and labor complications.

Dr. Milovina is married to Dr. Michael Sanchez, an obstetric anesthesiologist, and is the mother of two delightful daughters, Leila and Ava.

For more information about Dr. Milovina, visit her website: www.michelemilovinamd.com.

ARI BROWN, MD, FAAP, is a pediatrician with thirty years of experience in primary care, working with children and families. She is the founder of 411 Pediatrics in Austin, Texas.

Dr. Brown graduated magna cum laude from the University of Texas at Austin with a bachelor's degree in child development. She received her medical degree from Baylor College of Medicine and completed her pediatric residency and fellowship training in developmental/behavioral pediatrics at Harvard Medical School, Boston Children's Hospital.

Her passion to advocate for children and educate families extends beyond the office setting. Her superpower is her unique ability to translate science-based child health information and keep it real!

She is a trusted voice for children's health, serving as a spokeswoman for the American Academy of Pediatrics (AAP) for more than twenty years. Over the span of her career, she has appeared in countless national news outlets, including NBC's *Today* show and the *New York Times*, and has authored articles published in the *Wall Street Journal*, *Newsweek*, and *Parents* magazine.

Dr. Brown has received the American Academy of Pediatrics Lifetime Achievement Award for child health advocacy and was voted Austin's favorite pediatrician several times by *Austin Family Magazine*.

She is the author of the bestselling parent education books *Baby 411*, *Expecting 411*, and *Toddler 411.* She also teaches online classes on newborn care and infant sleep. Since the first edition of *Baby 411* was published twenty years ago, more than a million families have relied on these books for a trusted reassuring voice in the middle of the night, straight talk, and facts to guide them. After freshly updating all three titles, Dr. Brown is ready to take a much-needed vacation!

Of all her accomplishments, the greatest one is being a mom. She has proudly raised two children who are now very grown-up.

Instagram and TikTok: @aribrownmd

www.draribrown.com
Check Dr. Brown's website to make sure you
have the most current version.

Dr. Brown is available for select speaking engagements.
To inquire about a possible appearance, please contact
Penguin Random House Speakers Bureau at
speakers@penguinrandomhouse.com
or visit www.prhspeakers.com.